Exercise Physiology

Exercise Physiology

Theory and Application to
Fitness and Performance

third edition

Scott K. Powers
University of Florida

Edward T. Howley
University of Tennessee-Knoxville

McGraw WCB
Hill McGraw-Hill

Boston, Massachusetts   Burr Ridge, Illinios   Dubuque, Iowa
Madison, Wisconsin   New York, New York   San Francisco, California   St. Louis, Missouri

Book Team

Executive Managing Editor *Ed Bartell*
Developmental Editor *Theresa Grutz*
Production Editor *Marilyn Rothenberger*
Proofreading Coordinator *Carrie Barker*
Designer *Christopher E. Reese*
Art Editor *Miriam Hoffman*
Production Manager *Beth Kundert*
Production/Costing Manager *Sherry Padden*
Marketing Manager *Pam Cooper*
Copywriter *Sandy Hyde*
Proofreader *Mary Svetlik Anderson*

Basal Text *10/12 Novarese*
Display Type *Rotis*
Typesetting System *Macintosh™ QuarkXPress™*
Paper Stock *50# Restorecote*

WCB/McGraw-Hill

A Division of The McGraw·Hill Companies

President and Chief Executive Officer *Bob McLaughlin*
Vice President, Business Development *Russ Domeyer*
Vice President of Production and New Media Development *Victoria Putman*
National Sales Manager *Phil Rudder*
National Telesales Director *John Finn*

Cover photographs © Chuck Pefley/Tony Stone Images

Proofread by Denise A. Kieler

The credits section for this book begins on page 503 and is considered an extension of the copyright page.

Copyedited by Rose Kramer

Library of Congress Catalog Card Number: 96–83127

ISBN 0–697–25798–3

Printed in the United States of America

10 9 8 7 6 5 4 3

dedicated to Lou and Ann

for their love, patience,

and support

Brief Contents

SECTION I
Physiology of Exercise

1 Physiology of Exercise in the United States—Its Past, Its Future   3

2 Control of the Internal Environment   13

3 Bioenergetics   21

4 Exercise Metabolism   45

5 Hormonal Responses to Exercise   63

6 Measurement of Work, Power, and Energy Expenditure   95

7 The Nervous System: Structure and Control of Movement   107

8 Skeletal Muscle: Structure and Function   125

9 Circulatory Adaptations to Exercise   151

10 Respiration During Exercise   177

11 Acid–Base Balance During Exercise   205

12 Temperature Regulation   215

13 The Physiology of Training
       Effect on $\dot{V}O_2$ Max, Performance, Homeostasis, and Strength   229

SECTION II
Physiology of Health and Fitness

14 Patterns in Health and Disease
       Epidemiology and Physiology   255

15 Work Tests to Evaluate Cardiorespiratory Fitness   265

16 Exercise Prescriptions for Health and Fitness   285

17 Exercise for Special Populations   299

18 Body Composition and Nutrition for Health   317

SECTION III
Physiology of Performance

19 Factors Affecting Performance   361

20 Work Tests to Evaluate Performance   371

21 Training for Performance   391

22 Training for the Female Athlete, Children, and Special Populations   409

23 Nutrition, Body Composition, and Performance   419

24 Exercise and the Environment   439

25 Erogenic Aids   459

Contents

Preface   xiii

SECTION 1

Physiology of Exercise

CHAPTER 1

Physiology of Exercise in the United States–Its Past, Its Future   3

European Heritage   3
Harvard Fatigue Laboratory   4
Physical Fitness   5
Physical Education to Exercise Science   7
Graduate Study and Research in the Physiology of Exercise   8
Professional Societies and Research Journals   9
Translation of Exercise Physiology to the Consumer   10

CHAPTER 2

Control of the Internal Environment   13

Homeostasis: Dynamic Constancy   14
Control Systems of the Body   15
Nature of the Control Systems   15
    Negative Feedback   16
    Gain of a Control System   16
Examples of Homeostatic Control   17
    Regulation of Arterial Blood Pressure   17
    Regulation of Blood Glucose   17
Exercise: A Test of Homeostatic Control   18

CHAPTER 3

Bioenergetics   21

Cell Structure   22
Biological Energy Transformation   24
    Cellular Chemical Reactions   24

Fuels for Exercise   27
    Carbohydrates   27
    Fats   27
    Proteins   28
High-Energy Phosphates   28
Bioenergetics   29
    Anaerobic ATP Production   29
    Aerobic ATP Production   33
Aerobic ATP Tally   39
Efficiency of Oxidative Phosphorylation   39
Control of Bioenergetics   39
    Control of ATP-PC System   40
    Control of Glycolysis   40
    Control of Krebs Cycle and Electron Transport Chain   40
Interaction Between Aerobic/Anaerobic ATP Production   41

CHAPTER 4

Exercise Metabolism   45

Rest-to-Exercise Transitions   46
Recovery from Exercise: Metabolic Responses   47
Metabolic Responses to Exercise: Influence of Duration and Intensity   49
    Short-Term Intense Exercise   49
    Prolonged Exercise   50
    Incremental Exercise   50
Estimation of Fuel Utilization During Exercise   53
Factors Governing Fuel Selection   53
    Exercise Intensity and Fuel Selection   54
    Exercise Duration and Fuel Selection   55
    Interaction of Fat/Carbohydrate Metabolism   55
    Body Fuel Sources   56

CHAPTER 5

Hormonal Responses to Exercise   63

Neuroendocrinology   64
   Blood Hormone Concentration   65
   Hormone-Receptor Interaction   66
Hormones: Regulation and Action   68
   Hypothalamus and the Pituitary Gland   68
   Thyroid Gland   71
   Parathyroid Gland   72
   Adrenal Gland   72
   Pancreas   75
   Testes and Ovaries   76
Hormonal Control of Substrate Mobilization During Exercise   80
   Muscle-Glycogen Utilization   81
   Blood Glucose Homeostasis During Exercise   82
   Hormone-Substrate Interaction   89

CHAPTER 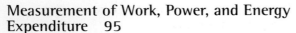 6

Measurement of Work, Power, and Energy Expenditure   95

Units of Measure   96
   Metric System   96
   SI Units   96
Work and Power Defined   96
   Work   96
   Power   97
Measurement of Work and Power   97
   Bench Step   97
   Cycle Ergometer   98
   Treadmill   98
Measurement of Energy Expenditure   99
   Direct Calorimetry   99
   Indirect Calorimetry   100
Estimation of Energy Expenditure   101
Calculation of Exercise Efficiency   102
   Factors That Influence Exercise Efficiency   103
Running Economy   104

CHAPTER 7

The Nervous System: Structure and Control of Movement   107

General Nervous System Functions   108
Organization of the Nervous System   108
   Structure of the Neuron   109
   Electrical Activity in Neurons   111
Sensory Information and Reflexes   115
   Proprioceptors   115
   Muscle Chemoreceptors   115
   Reflexes   116
Somatic Motor Function   117
Vestibular Apparatus and Equilibrium   117

Motor Control Functions of the Brain   118
   Brain Stem   118
   Cerebrum   119
   Cerebellum   119
Motor Functions of the Spinal Cord   119
Control of Motor Functions   120
Autonomic Nervous System   121

CHAPTER 8

Skeletal Muscle: Structure and Function   125

Structure of Skeletal Muscle   126
Neuromuscular Junction   128
Muscular Contraction   129
   Overview of the Sliding Filament Model   129
   Energy for Contraction   131
   Regulation of Excitation-Contraction Coupling   131
Fiber Types   135
   Biochemical and Contractile Characteristics of Skeletal Muscle   135
   Characteristics of Individual Fiber Types   136
   Fiber Types and Performance   139
Alteration of Muscle Fiber Types by Exercise Training   139
Age-Related Changes in Skeletal Muscle   140
Isometric and Isotonic Contractions   141
Speed of Muscle Contraction and Relaxation   142
Force Regulation in Muscle   142
Force-Velocity/Power-Velocity Relationships   144
Receptors in Muscle   145
   Muscle Spindle   146
   Golgi Tendon Organs 146

CHAPTER 9

Circulatory Adaptations to Exercise   151

Organization of the Circulatory System   152
   Structure of the Heart   152
   Pulmonary and Systemic Circuits   153
Heart: Myocardium and Cardiac Cycle   153
   Myocardium   153
   Cardiac Cycle   154
   Arterial Blood Pressure   155
   Electrical Activity of the Heart   157
Cardiac Output   160
   Regulation of Heart Rate   160
   Regulation of Stroke Volume   161
Hemodynamics   163
   Physical Characteristics of Blood   163
   Relationships Between Pressure, Resistance, and Flow   163
   Sources of Vascular Resistance   164

Changes in Oxygen Delivery to Muscle During Exercise 165
  Changes in Cardiac Output During Exercise 165
  Changes in Arterial-Mixed Venous O_2 Content During Exercise 166
  Redistribution of Blood Flow During Exercise 167
  Regulation of Local Blood Flow During Exercise 167
Circulatory Responses to Exercise 169
  Emotional Influence 169
  Transition from Rest to Exercise 169
  Recovery from Exercise 169
  Incremental Exercise 170
  Arm versus Leg Exercise 170
  Intermittent Exercise 171
  Prolonged Exercise 171
Regulation of Cardiovascular Adjustments to Exercise 172

CHAPTER 10

Respiration During Exercise 177

Function of the Lung 178
Structure of the Respiratory System 178
  Conducting Zone 179
  Respiratory Zone 180
Mechanics of Breathing 181
  Inspiration 182
  Expiration 182
  Airway Resistance 182
Pulmonary Ventilation 184
Pulmonary Volumes and Capacities 184
Diffusion of Gases 185
Blood Flow to the Lung 187
Ventilation-Perfusion Relationships 188
O_2 and CO_2 Transport in Blood 188
  Hemoglobin and O_2 Transport 188
  Oxyhemoglobin Dissociation Curve 189
  O_2 Transport in Muscle 191
  CO_2 Transport in Blood 191
Ventilation and Acid-Base Balance 192
Ventilatory and Blood-Gas Responses to Exercise 193
  Rest-to-Work Transitions 193
  Prolonged Exercise in a Hot Environment 194
  Incremental Exercise 194
Control of Ventilation 195
  Ventilatory Regulation at Rest 195
  Ventilatory Control During Submaximal Exercise 198
  Ventilatory Control During Heavy Exercise 198
  Do the Lungs Limit Maximal Exercise Performance? 200

CHAPTER 11

Acid-Base Balance During Exercise 205

Acids, Bases, and pH 206
Hydrogen Ion Production During Exercise 207
Importance of Acid-Base Regulation During Exercise 207
Acid-Base Buffer Systems 208
  Intracellular Buffers 208
  Extracellular Buffers 208
Respiratory Influence on Acid-Base Balance 209
Regulation of Acid-Base Balance via the Kidneys 210
Regulation of Acid-Base Balance During Exercise 210

CHAPTER 12

Temperature Regulation 215

Overview of Heat Balance During Exercise 216
Temperature Measurement During Exercise 217
Overview of Heat Production/Heat Loss 217
  Heat Production 217
  Heat Loss 218
Body's Thermostat-Hypothalamus 220
  Shift in the Hypothalamic Thermostat Set Point Due to Fever 221
Thermal Events During Exercise 221
Exercise in the Heat 224
  Gender and Age Differences in Thermoregulation 224
  Heat Acclimatization 225
Exercise in a Cold Environment 226
  Cold Acclimatization 226

CHAPTER 13

The Physiology of Training: Effect on $\dot{V}O_2$ Max, Performance, Homeostasis, and Strength 229

Principles of Training 230
  Overload 230
  Specificity 231
Research Designs to Study Training 231
Endurance Training and $\dot{V}O_2$ Max 231
  Training Programs and Changes in $\dot{V}O_2$ Max 232
$\dot{V}O_2$ Max: Cardiac Output and the Arteriovenous O_2 Difference 232
  Stroke Volume 234
  Arteriovenous O_2 Difference 235
Detraining and $\dot{V}O_2$ Max 236
Endurance Training: Effects on Performance and Homeostasis 236
  Biochemical Adaptations and the Oxygen Deficit 237
  Biochemical Adaptations and the Plasma Glucose Concentration 239
  Biochemical Adaptations and Blood pH 240
  Biochemical Adaptations and Lactate Removal 241
Endurance Training: Links Between Muscle and Systemic Physiology 243
  Peripheral Feedback 243
  Central Command 244
Physiological Effects of Strength Training 245
Physiological Mechanisms Causing Increased Strength 246
  Neural Factors 246
  Muscular Enlargement 247
  Simultaneous Strength and Endurance Training 247

CHAPTER 14

Patterns in Health and Disease: Epidemiology and Physiology   255

Epidemiology   255
Coronary Heart Disease   258
    Physical Inactivity as a Risk Factor   259
Physiology   261
Synthesis   262

CHAPTER 15

Work Tests to Evaluate Cardiorespiratory Fitness   265

Testing Procedures   266
    Screening   266
    Resting and Exercise Measures   268
Field Tests for Estimating CRF   268
    Maximal Run Tests   268
    Walk Tests   270
    Canadian Home Fitness Test   270
Graded Exercise Tests: Measurements   271
    Heart Rate   271
    Blood Pressure   272
    ECG   272
    Rating of Perceived Exertion   272
    Termination Criteria   273
$\dot{V}O_2$ Max   273
    Estimation of $\dot{V}O_2$ Max from Last Work Rate   274
    Estimation of $\dot{V}O_2$ Max from Submaximal HR Response   274
Graded Exercise Test: Protocols   275
    Treadmill   277
    Cycle Ergometer   278
    Step Test   281

CHAPTER 16

Exercise Prescriptions for Health and Fitness   285

Prescription of Exercise   286
    Dose-Response   287
    Physical Activity and Health   287
General Guidelines for Improving Fitness   289
    Screening   289
    Progression   289
    Warm-Up, Stretch, and Cool-Down, Stretch   290
Exercise Prescription for CRF   290
    Frequency   290
    Duration   290
    Intensity   291

Sequence of Physical Activity   292
    Walking   292
    Jogging   293
    Games and Sports   294
Strength Training   294
Environmental Concerns   295

CHAPTER 17

Exercise for Special Populations   299

Diabetes   300
    Exercise and the Diabetic   301
Asthma   304
    Causes   304
    Prevention/Relief of Asthma   304
    Exercise-Induced Asthma   305
Chronic Obstructive Pulmonary Disease   307
    Testing and Training   307
Hypertension   308
Cardiac Rehabilitation   309
    Population   309
    Testing   309
    Exercise Programs   309
Elderly   310
Pregnancy   312

CHAPTER 18

Body Composition and Nutrition for Health   317

Nutritional Goals   318
Standards of Nutrition   319
Classes of Nutrients   320
    Water   320
    Vitamins   321
    Minerals   323
    Carbohydrates   327
    Fats   328
    Protein   328
Meeting the Guidelines and Achieving the Goals   329
    Food Group Plans   329
    Evaluating the Diet   329
Body Composition   331
    Methods of Measuring Body Composition   331
    Two-Component System of Body Composition   335
    Body Fatness for Health and Fitness   338
Obesity and Weight Control   339
    Obesity   339
Diet, Exercise, and Weight Control   342
    Energy and Nutrient Balance   342
    Diet and Weight Control   343
    Energy Expenditure and Weight Control   344

CHAPTER 19

Factors Affecting Performance   361

Sites of Fatigue   362
  Central Fatigue   362
  Peripheral Fatigue   363
Factors Limiting All-Out Anaerobic Performances   365
  Ultra Short-Term Performances (Less than Ten Seconds)   366
  Short-Term Performances (10 to 180 seconds)   366
Factors Limiting All-Out Aerobic Performances   367
  Moderate-Length Performances (Three to Twenty Minutes)   367
  Intermediate-Length Performances (Twenty-One to Sixty Minutes)   367
  Long-Term Performances (One to Four Hours)   368
Athlete as Machine   369

CHAPTER 20

Work Tests to Evaluate Performance   371

Laboratory Assessment of Physical Performance   372
  Physiological Testing: Theory and Ethics   372
What the Athlete Gains by Physiological testing   372
What Physiological Testing Will Not Do   373
Components of Effective Physiological Testing   373
Direct Testing of Maximal Aerobic Power   374
  Specificity of Testing   374
  Exercise Test Protocol   374
  Determination of Peak $\dot{V}O_2$ in Paraplegic Athletes   375
Laboratory Tests to Predict Endurance Performance   375
  Use of the Lactate Threshold to Evaluate Performance   375
  Measurement of Critical Power   377
Tests to Determine Exercise Economy   378
Estimating Success in Distance Running Using the Lactate Threshold and Running Economy   379
Determination of Anaerobic Power   380
  Tests of Ultra Short-Term Maximal Anaerobic Power   380
  Tests of Short-Term Anaerobic Power   382
Evaluation of Muscular Strength   383
  Criteria for Selection of a Strength-Testing Method   384
  Isometric Measurement of Strength   384
  Isotonic Measurement of Strength   385
  Isokinetic Assessment of Strength   386
  Variable Resistance Measurement of Strength   386

CHAPTER 21

Training for Performance   391

Training Principles   392
  Overload, Specificity, and Reversibility   392
  Influence of Gender, Initial Fitness Level, and Genetics   393
Components of a Training Session: Warm-Up, Workout, and Cool Down   394

Training to Improve Aerobic Power   394
  Interval Training   395
  Long, Slow Distance   396
  High-Intensity, Continuous Exercise   396
Injuries and Endurance Training   397
Training for Improved Anaerobic Power   397
  Training to Improve the ATP-PC System   397
  Training to Improve the Glycolytic System   398
Training to Improve Muscular Strength   398
  Progressive Resistance Exercise   398
  General Strength-Training Principles   398
  Free Weights versus Machines   399
  Combined Strength and Endurance Training Programs   399
  Gender Differences in Response to Strength Training   400
  Muscle Soreness   401
Training for Improved Flexibility   402
Year-Round Conditioning for Athletes   402
  Off-Season Conditioning   403
  Preseason Conditioning   403
  In-Season Conditioning   403
Common Training Mistakes   403

CHAPTER 22

Training for the Female Athlete, Children, and Special Populations   409

Factors Important to Women Involved in Vigorous Training   410
  Exercise and Menstrual Disorders   410
  Training and Menstruation   411
  The Female Athlete and Eating Disorders   411
  Bone Mineral Disorders and the Female Athlete   412
  Training During Pregnancy   412
Sports Conditioning for Children   413
  Training and the Cardiopulmonary System   413
  Training and the Musculoskeletal System   414
Competitive Training for Diabetics   415
Training for Asthmatics   415
Epilepsy and Physical Training   416
  Does Exercise Promote Seizures?   416
  Risk of Injury Due to Seizures   416

CHAPTER 23

Nutrition, Body Composition, and Performance   419

Nutrition and Performance   420
  Carbohydrate   420
  Protein   423
  Water and Electrolytes   426
  Minerals   429
  Vitamins   430
  Pregame Meal   431

Body Composition and Performance   432
    Somatotype   432
    Body Fatness and Performance   434

CHAPTER

24

Exercise and the Environment   439

Altitude   440
    Atmospheric Pressure   440
    Short-Term Anaerobic Performance   440
    Long-Term Aerobic Performance   441
    Maximal Aerobic Power and Altitude   442
    Adaptation to High Altitude   443
    Training for Competition at Altitude   444
    The Quest for Everest   445
Heat   448
    Hyperthermia   448
Cold   451
    Environmental Factors   451
    Insulating Factors   452
    Energy Production   453
    Dealing with Hypothermia   454
Air Pollution   454
    Ozone   454
    Sulfur Dioxide   455
    Carbon Monoxide   455

CHAPTER

25

Erogenic Aids   459

Research Design Concerns   460
Nutritional Supplements   461
Aerobic Performance   462
    Oxygen   463
    Blood Doping   464

Anaerobic Performance   465
    Blood Buffers   465
Drugs   466
    Amphetamines   466
    Caffeine   467
    Cocaine   470
    Nicotine   470
Physical Warm-Up   471

APPENDICES

Appendix A
Calculation of Oxygen Uptake and Carbon Dioxide Production   477

Appendix B
Estimated Energy Expenditure During Selected Activities   481

Appendix C
Physical Activity Prescriptions   485

Appendix D
1989 Recommended Dietary Allowances   486

Appendix E
1989 RDAs—Estimated Safe and Adequate Daily Dietary Intakes of Selected Vitamins and Minerals   488

Appendix F
1989 RDSs—Median Heights and Weights and Recommended Energy Intake   489

Appendix G
Percent Fat Estimate for Men: Sum of Triceps, Chest, and Subscapula Skinfolds   490

Appendix H
Percent Fat Estimate for Women: Sum of Triceps, Abdomen, and Suprailium Skinfolds   491

GLOSSARY   493

INDEX   503

Preface

S imilar to previous editions, the third edition of *Exercise Physiology: Theory and Application to Fitness and Performance* is intended for students of exercise science; clinical physiologists; physical educators; coaches; and physical therapists interested in exercise physiology, sports performance, adult fitness, or cardiopulmonary rehabilitation. The goal of this text is to provide the student with an up-to-date understanding of the physiology of exercise. In addition, the book contains extensive practical applications, including work tests to evaluate cardiorespiratory fitness, and information on training for improvements in health-related fitness and sports performance.

This volume is intended for use in a one-semester, upper-level undergraduate or beginning graduate exercise physiology course. Clearly, the text contains more material than can be covered during a typical fifteen-week semester. This is by design. The book was written to be comprehensive in order to afford instructors a large degree of freedom to select the material that they consider most important for the makeup of their class.

New to This Edition

The third edition of this book has undergone extensive revision. The major changes include:

- New **4-color** format enhances and enlivens the presentation
- **New color illustrations** to improve student understanding of complex concepts
- **New references** related to the **latest research** have been added to all chapters
- Addition of **"Research Focus"** boxes in several chapters. This feature is designed to highlight exciting and new research in exercise physiology.
- **Section summaries** now follow major topical sections of each chapter. This feature provides a brief summary of the major points presented to immediately help the student internalize key concepts and reinforce their mastery of the material.

- **Chapter 8, Skeletal Muscle: Structure and Function** has undergone extensive revision to include the latest research on muscle fiber types and the details of how muscles contract.
- **Chapter 14.** The introductory chapter to the section on health and fitness has been modified to examine patterns in health and disease from an epidemiological as well as a physiological perspective.
- **Chapter 18** has been revised to provide new information on the 3- and 4-component models of body composition, and presents information contrasting energy balance with fat balance in weight control.
- **Chapter 22** has been revised to include new information on special concerns for the female athlete.

Contents and Organization

All topics in exercise physiology addressed within this text are presented in a contemporary fashion supported by up-to-date references. The text is divided into three sections: (I) Physiology of Exercise, (II) Physiology of Health and Fitness, and (III) Physiology of Performance. Section I (Physiology of Exercise) contains thirteen chapters that provide the necessary background for the beginning student of exercise physiology to understand the role of the major organ systems of the body in maintaining homeostasis during exercise. Indeed, a major theme in Section I of the book is that almost all organ systems of the body work to help maintain a relatively stable internal environment during exercise. Included in Section I are chapters covering an overview of biological control systems, bioenergetics, exercise metabolism, endocrine function during exercise, techniques for measurement of work, power, and energy expenditure, neuromuscular function during exercise, cardiopulmonary responses to exercise, acid-base regulation during exercise, temperature regulation, and the effects of endurance training on various organ systems.

The chapters in the first section provide an up-to-date presentation of exercise physiology without consideration as to how that information is applied to fitness or performance. The purpose of the second and third sections of the text is to address these concerns. These last two sections distinguish between exercise programs that are appropriate for attainment of health-related fitness goals versus those needed to realize world-class or individual maximal performance goals. Section II of the text (Physiology of Health and Fitness) contains five chapters dealing with health-related fitness: (1) patterns in health and disease: epidemiology and physiology, (2) work tests used to evaluate cardiorespiratory fitness, (3) training methods for fitness, (4) exercise concerns for special populations and (5) body composition and nutritional concerns for health.

Section III includes seven chapters dealing with the physiology of performance: (1) factors affecting performance, (2) work tests to evaluate performance, (3) training techniques for improvement of performance, (4) training concerns for special populations,

(5) nutrition, body composition, and performance, (6) environmental influences on performance, and (7) ergogenic aids. A unique aspect of Sections II and III of the book is the inclusion of two chapters on exercise training for special populations. These chapters include discussions of exercise for women, asthmatics, diabetics, and the elderly.

Writing Style

The concepts in this text are presented in a simple and straightforward style. Illustrations and examples are commonly used to clarify or further explain a concept. Technical terms are defined as they are presented and are also organized in a glossary at the end of the book.

Pedagogical Aids

As an aid to help students study and learn the material within *Exercise Physiology*, the following pedagogical devices are included in the text:

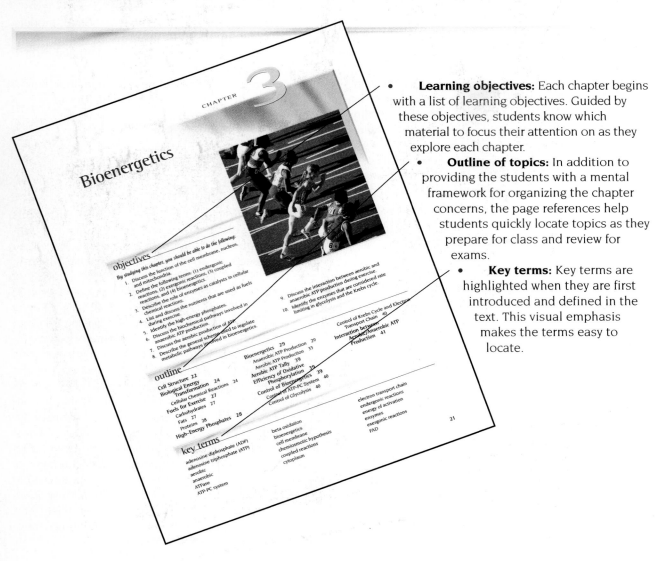

- **Learning objectives:** Each chapter begins with a list of learning objectives. Guided by these objectives, students know which material to focus their attention on as they explore each chapter.
- **Outline of topics:** In addition to providing the students with a mental framework for organizing the chapter concerns, the page references help students quickly locate topics as they prepare for class and review for exams.
- **Key terms:** Key terms are highlighted when they are first introduced and defined in the text. This visual emphasis makes the terms easy to locate.

- **In Summary:** At the end of major sections throughout the text, students are given a summary of the important ideas presented in the section. These summaries ensure that students grasp the key concepts and immediately reinforce the main ideas.

Figure 8.14
(a) Isotonic contractions occur when a muscle contracts and shortens. (b) Isometric contractions occur when a muscle exerts force but does not shorten.

of fast fibers (particularly Type slow fibers (65a). See refer-

and strength observed in related to aging popula- use muscle atrophy in in muscle size ob- period of immobi- (3). This simple tal muscle is a both use and

in summary
- Aging is associated with a loss of muscle mass. This age-related loss of muscle mass is slow from age 25 to 50 years but increases rapidly after 50 years of age.
- Regular exercise training can improve skeletal muscular strength and endurance in the elderly but cannot completely eliminate the age-related loss in muscle mass.

Isometric and Isotonic Contractions

It is possible for skeletal muscle to exert force without a large amount of muscle shortening. This might occur when an individual pulls against a wire attached to the wall of a building (see figure 8.14b). What happens here is that muscle tension increases but the body does not move and therefore neither does the wall does not arm) that applies the force. Contractions of this type are called **isometric**, or **static**. Isometric contractions are

---

A Closer Look 13.1
Role of Exercise Intensity and Duration on Mitochondrial Adaptations

A muscle fiber's oxidative capacity can improve only if the muscle fiber is recruited during the exercise session. Figures 13.6a and 13.6b show changes in citrate synthase (CS) activity, a marker of mitochondrial oxidative capacity, due to exercise programs differing in duration (30, 60, and 90 minutes) and intensity (~55%, ~65%, and ~75% VO₂ max). Figure 13.6a shows that CS activity increased in the red gastrocnemius (primarily Type IIa fibers) for all treatments, but the magnitude of the change was independent of the intensity and duration of the activity. In contrast, figure 13.6b shows that for the white gastrocnemius (primarily Type IIb fibers) CS activity increased due to both intensity and duration of activity. Why the difference? The Type IIa fibers were easily recruited by the lowest exercise intensity while very strenuous exercise was required to recruit the Type IIb fibers (44a). These observations support our understanding of the specificity of exercise—light to moderate exercise will improve or maintain the oxidative capacity of high oxidative fibers (Type I and Type IIa), while strenuous exercise is

needed to change low oxidative (Type IIb) fibers (16a, 56d). Given the rapid loss of a muscle's oxidative capacity with cessation of training, it is

Figure 13.6
Changes in citrate synthase act of exercise

no surprise that high-level endurance performances, which require the recruitment of Type IIb fibers, fall off quickly when training ceases.

training, when the number of mitochondria has doubled, the ADP concentration increases only half as much, since each mitochondrion needs only half the stimulation to take up 1.0 liter of O₂ per minute. The increase in the capillary density in the muscle cell after endurance training is a parallel change that support this process. In essence, after an endurance training program, it takes less change in the ADP concentration to stimulate the mitochondria to take up (28). Since less of a change in the ADP concentration causing ATP → ADP + Pᵢ will cat needed to stimulate the mitochondria, the phosphorylation to be activated earlier into a faster rise in the oxygen upta onset of work, resulting in the stea achieved earlier (see figure 4.2) (25 in oxygen uptake at the onset of

238

Research Focus 9.2
Discovery of a New Vasodilator Substance: Nitric Oxide

Recent research has lead to the discovery of a new and important vasodilator called nitric oxide (see reference 39a for a review). Nitric oxide is produced in the endothelium of arterioles. After production, nitric oxide promotes smooth muscle relaxation in the arteriole which results in vasodilation and therefore causes an increase in blood flow. Current evidence suggests that ni-

tric oxide works in conjunction with other local factors in autoregulation of blood flow.

How important is nitric oxide in the autoregulation of muscle blood flow during exercise? At present, a definitive answer to this question is not available. Nonetheless, it seems likely that nitric oxide is one of several factors involved in regulation of muscle blood flow

during exercise. Current speculation is that muscular contraction results in increased production of nitric oxide which promotes vasodilation in those arterioles leading to the working muscle. Improving our understanding of the role of nitric oxide in the regulation of muscle blood flow is an exciting area for future research.

Figure 9.19
Distribution of cardiac output during rest and maximal exercise. At rest, the cardiac output is 5 l/min (bottom of figure); during maximum exercise, the cardiac output increased five-fold to 25 l/min. Note the large increases in blood flow to the skeletal muscle and the reduction in flow to the liver/GI tract.
From P. Åstrand and K. Rodahl, *Textbook of Work Physiology*, 3d ed. Copyright © 1986 McGraw-Hill, Inc. New York. Reprinted by permission of the authors.

168

Section One Physiology of Exercise

- **Informational boxes:** Most chapters include special or practical applications that are contained within a "box" format called "A Closer Look" or "Research Focus."

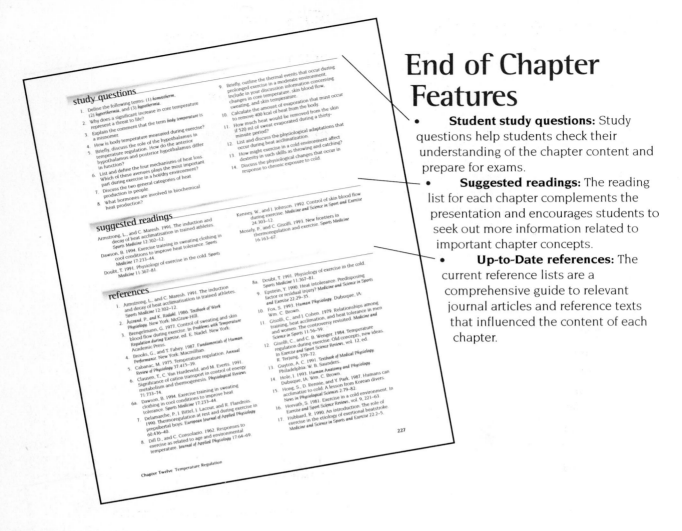

End of Chapter Features

- **Student study questions:** Study questions help students check their understanding of the chapter content and prepare for exams.
- **Suggested readings:** The reading list for each chapter complements the presentation and encourages students to seek out more information related to important chapter concepts.
- **Up-to-Date references:** The current reference lists are a comprehensive guide to relevant journal articles and reference texts that influenced the content of each chapter.

End of Book Features

- **Appendices:** Supplementary appendices include: (1) Calculations of oxygen uptake and carbon dioxide production; (2) Estimated energy expenditure during selected activities; (3) Physical activity prescriptions; (4) Recommended dietary allowances for vitamins and minerals; (5) Recommended energy intake; (6) Estimate of percent body fat from skinfold measurements.
- **Glossary:** The end-of-book glossary of terms is a helpful study aid, providing quick access to the definitions of all key terms.

Ancillary Material

The following materials are available from Brown & Benchmark Publishers to qualified adopters of *Exercise Physiology: Theory and Application to Fitness and Performance*:

- **Instructor's Manual** by Scott K. Powers and Edward T. Howley. The Instructor's Manual provides a chapter-by-chapter overview of key concepts to be stressed by the instructor as well as a multiple-choice test bank. The

Instructor's Manual also provides suggestions for laboratory exercises.

- **Exercise Physiology Transparency Set.** Color transparency acetates complement the textbook.
- **Computerized testing software** eases the task of preparing tests. The test items can be edited, and test items can be added to customize the testing program.
- **Exercise Physiology Videolabs** show clear and complete demonstrations of common lab experiments to support students with limited access to labs. Also included is an Instructor's Guide which provides guidance on using the videolabs.
- **Student Video manual** actively involves students in the videolab presentations and reinforces concepts through worksheets and activities. This manual is available for student purchase.

Also available:

- **Student study guide:** The student study guide includes a chapter on study skills, summaries of all chapters, and an ample supply of study questions for each chapter. The guide is available for student purchase.

Acknowledgments

A text like *Exercise Physiology* is not the effort of two authors, but represents the contributions of hundreds of scientists throughout the world. While it is not possible to acknowledge every contributor to this work, we would like to recognize the following scientists who have greatly influenced our thinking, careers, and lives in general: Drs. Bruno Balke, Ralph Beadle, Ronald Byrd, Jerome Dempsey, Stephen Dodd, H. V. Forster, B. D. Franks, Steven Horvath, Henry Montoye, Francis Nagle, Robert N. Singer, and Hugh G. Welch. Additional thanks are due to the following scholars who reviewed this and earlier editions of this book and offered comments for improvement that we trust they will recognize:

Dr. Phillip A. Bishop
University of Alabama

Dr. Marilyn Cairns
Northeastern University

Dr. Greg Cartee
University of Wisconsin

Dr. Cheryl Cohen
Western Illinois University

Dr. Mitchell Collins
Kennesaw State College

Dr. William Floyd
University of Wisconsin–LaCrosse

Dr. Laura Gerace
Penn State University

Dr. Robert Grueninger
Eastern Montana College

Dr. Roger Hammer
Central Michigan University

Dr. Craig G. Johnson
St. Mary's College

Dr. James H. Johnson
Smith College

Dr. Martin W. Johnson
Mayville State University

Dr. John Kelly
St. Cloud State University

Dr. Francis J. Nagle
University of Wisconsin–Madison

Dr. Roberta L. Pohlman
Wright State University

Dr. Robert Staron
Ohio University

Dr. Anthony A. Sucec
San Diego State University

Dr. Phil Watts
Northern Michigan University

Dr. Hugh Welch
Texas A & M University

Finally, we wish to offer thanks to our editors, Theresa Grutz and Marilyn Rothenberger of Brown & Benchmark, for their excellent support and cooperation during the completion of this work.

Scott K. Powers, Gainesville, Florida

Edward T. Howley, Knoxville, Tennessee

Physiology of Exercise

Physiology of Exercise in the United States— Its Past, Its Future

objectives

By studying this chapter, you should be able to do the following:

1. Name the three Nobel Prize winners whose research work involved muscle or muscular exercise.
2. Describe the role of the Harvard Fatigue Laboratory in the history of exercise physiology in the United States.
3. Describe factors influencing physical fitness in the United States over the past century.

outline

European Heritage   3
Harvard Fatigue Laboratory   4
Physical Fitness   5
Physical Education to Exercise
   Science   7

Graduate Study and Research in the
   Physiology of Exercise   8
Professional Societies and Research
   Journals   9

Translation of Exercise Physiology
   to the Consumer   10

---

oes one have to have a "genetic gift" of speed to be a world-class runner, or is it all due to training? What happens to your heart rate when you take a fitness test that increases in intensity each minute? What changes occur in your muscles as a result of an endurance training program that allows you to run at faster speeds over longer distances? The answers to these and other questions are provided throughout this text. However, we go beyond simple statements of fact to show how information about physiology of exercise is applied to the prevention of and rehabilitation from coronary heart disease, the performances of elite athletes, and the ability of a person to work in adverse environments such as high altitudes. The recent acceptance of terms such as *sports physiology*, *sports nutrition*, and *sports medicine* is evidence of the growth of interest in the application of physiology of exercise to real-world problems. Before we take you on this journey, a brief look at the history of exercise physiology is needed to understand where we are and where we are going.

European Heritage

A good starting place to discuss the history of exercise physiology in the United States is in Europe. Three scientists, A. V. Hill of Britain, August Krogh of Denmark, and Otto Meyerhof of Germany, received Nobel Prizes for research on muscle or muscular exercise (5). Hill, who is well known for his work on O_2 debt, introduced the term "maximal oxygen intake" in 1924 as a description of the upper limit of performance. We will discuss both of these topics in detail in later chapters. Meyerhof is recognized for his work on the metabolism of glucose, which can lead to the production of lactic acid, a factor long implicated in fatigue. Although

Krogh received his Nobel Prize for his research on the function of the capillary circulation, he is also known for designing a considerable amount of instrumentation used in exercise physiology research. A precise gas analyzer to measure CO_2 within 0.001%, and a precision balance to weigh human subjects within a few grams (9) are but two examples of Krogh's resourcefulness. The August Krogh Institute in Denmark contains some of the most prominent exercise physiology laboratories in the world.

There are several other European scientists who must be mentioned, not only because of their contributions to the physiology of exercise, but because their names are commonly used in a discussion of exercise physiology. J. S. Haldane did some of the original work on the role of CO_2 in the control of breathing. Haldane also developed the respiratory gas analyzer that bears his name (9). C. G. Douglas did pioneering work with Haldane in the role of O_2 and lactic acid in the control of breathing during exercise, including some work conducted at various altitudes. The canvas-and-rubber gas collection bag used for many years in exercise physiology laboratories around the world carries Douglas's name. A contemporary of Douglas, who did the classic work on how O_2 binds to hemoglobin, was Christian Bohr of Denmark. The "shift" in the oxygen-hemoglobin dissociation curve due to the addition of CO_2 bears his name. It was in Bohr's lab that Krogh got his start on a career studying respiration and exercise in humans (9).

in summary

- Three physiologists, A. V. Hill, August Krogh, and Otto Meyerhof received the Nobel Prize for work related to muscle or to muscular exercise.

Harvard Fatigue Laboratory

A focal point in the history of exercise physiology in the United States is the Harvard Fatigue Laboratory. Professor L. J. Henderson organized the laboratory within the Business School to conduct physiological research on industrial hazards. Dr. David Bruce Dill was the research director from the time the laboratory opened in 1927 until it closed in 1947 (12). Table 1.1 shows that the laboratory conducted research in numerous areas, in the laboratory and in the field, and the results of those early studies have been supported by recent investigations. Dill's classic text, *Life, Heat, and Altitude* (8), is recommended reading for any student of exercise and environmental physiology. Much of the careful and precise work of the laboratory was conducted using the now-classic Haldane analyzer for respiratory gas analysis

Table 1.1	Active Research Areas in the Harvard Fatigue Laboratory

Metabolism
    Maximal oxygen uptake
    Oxygen debt
    Carbohydrate and fat metabolism during long-term work
Environmental physiology
    Altitude
    Dry and moist heat
    Cold
Clinical physiology
    Gout
    Schizophrenia
    Diabetes
Aging
    Basal metabolic rate
    Maximal oxygen uptake
    Maximal heart rate
Blood
    Acid-base balance
    O_2 saturation: role of PO_2, PCO_2, and carbon monoxide
Nutrition
    Nutritional assessment techniques
    Vitamins
    Foods
Physical fitness
    Harvard Step Test

and the van Slyke apparatus for blood-gas analysis. The advent of computer-controlled equipment in the 1980s has made data collection easier, but has not improved on the accuracy of measurement (see figure 1.1).

The Harvard Fatigue Laboratory attracted doctoral students as well as scientists from other countries. Many of the alumni from the laboratory are recognized in their own right for excellence in research in the physiology of exercise. Two doctoral students, Steven Horvath and Sid Robinson, went on to distinguished careers at the Institute of Environmental Stress in Santa Barbara and Indiana University, respectively. Foreign "Fellows" included E. Asmussen, E. H. Christensen, M. Nielsen, and the Nobel Prize winner August Krogh from Denmark. These scientists brought new ideas and technology to the lab, participated in laboratory and field studies with other staff members, and published some of the most important work in the physiology of exercise between 1930–1980. Rudolpho Margaria, from Italy, went on to extend his classic work on oxygen debt, and describe the energetics of locomotion. Peter F. Scholander, from Norway, gave us his chemical gas

Figure 1.1

Comparison of old and new technology used to measure oxygen consumption and carbon dioxide production during exercise. (*Left*: The Carnegie Institute of Washington, D.C.; *Right*: Quinton Instrument Co.)

analyzer that is now the primary method of calibrating tank gas used to standardize electronic gas analyzers (12).

In summary, under the leadership of Dr. D. B. Dill, The Harvard Fatigue Laboratory became a model for research investigations into exercise and environmental physiology, especially as it relates to humans. When the laboratory closed and the staff dispersed, the ideas, techniques, and approaches to scientific inquiry were distributed throughout the world, and with them, Dill's influence in the area of environmental and exercise physiology. Dr. Dill continued his research outside Boulder City, Nevada, into the 1980s. He died at the age of 93 in 1986.

in summary

- The Harvard Fatigue Laboratory was a focal point in the development of exercise physiology in the United States. Dr. D. B. Dill directed the laboratory from its opening in 1927 until its closing in 1947. The body of research in exercise and environmental physiology produced by that laboratory forms the basis of much of what we know today.

Physical Fitness

Physical fitness is a popular topic today and its popularity has been a major factor in motivating college students to pursue careers in physical education, physiology of exercise, health education, nutrition, physical therapy, and medicine. In 1980 the Public Health Service listed "physical fitness and exercise" as one of fifteen areas of concern related to improving the country's overall health (23). While this might

appear to be an unprecedented event, similar interests and concerns about physical fitness existed in this country over one hundred years ago. Between the Civil War and the First World War (WW I) physical education was primarily concerned with the development and maintenance of fitness, and many of the leaders in physical education were trained in medicine (6, p. 5). For example, Dr. Dudley Sargent, hired by Harvard University in 1879, set up a physical training program with individual exercise prescriptions to improve a person's structure and function to achieve "that prime physical condition called fitness—fitness for work, fitness for play, fitness for anything a man may be called upon to do" (26, p. 297).

Sargent was clearly ahead of his time in promoting health-related fitness. Later, a primary force driving this country's interest in physical fitness was war. Concerns about health and fitness were raised during WW I and WW II when large numbers of draftees failed the induction exams due to mental and physical defects (11, p. 407). These concerns influenced the type of physical education programs in the schools during these years, making them resemble pre-military training programs (28, p. 484).

The present interest in physical activity and health was stimulated in the early 1950s by two major findings: (1) autopsies of young soldiers killed during the Korean War showed that significant coronary artery disease had already developed, and (2) Hans Kraus showed that American children performed poorly on a minimal muscular fitness test compared to European children (28, p. 516). Due to the latter finding, President Eisenhower initiated a conference in 1955 that resulted in the formation of the President's Council on Youth Fitness. The American Association for Health, Physical Education, and Recreation (AAHPER) supported these activities and

Figure 1.2
A group of businessmen in a dancing class under the direction of Oliver E. Hebbert.

Figure 1.3
Roof of the John Wanamaker store, Philadelphia, showing running track, basketball, and tennis courts.

in 1957 developed the AAHPER Youth Fitness Test with national norms to be used in physical education programs throughout the country. Before he was inaugurated, President Kennedy expressed his concerns about the nation's fitness in an article published in *Sports Illustrated*, called "The Soft American" (16).

> For the physical vigor of our citizens is one of America's most precious resources. If we waste and neglect this resource, if we allow it to dwindle and grow soft, then we will destroy much of our ability to meet the great and vital challenges which confront our people. We will be unable to realize our full potential as a nation.

During Kennedy's term the council's name was changed to the "President's Council on Physical Fitness" to highlight the concern for fitness. The name was changed again in the Nixon administration to the current "President's Council on Physical Fitness and Sports," which supports fitness not only in schools but in business and industry. Items in the Youth Fitness Test were changed over the years and in 1980 the American Alliance for Health, Physical Education, Recreation, and Dance (AAHPERD) published a separate *Health-Related Physical Fitness Test Manual* (1) to distinguish between "performance testing" (e.g., fifty-yard dash) and "fitness testing" (e.g., skinfold thickness). This health-related test battery is consistent with the direction of lifetime fitness programs, being concerned with obesity, cardiorespiratory fitness, and low-back function. AAHPERD's *Physical Best* contains the educational materials to go with this health-related fitness

test, and the Prudential Fitnessgram (developed by the Cooper Institute for Aerobic Research) provides the test, standards, and interpretation via computer analysis. For those readers interested in the history of fitness testing in schools we recommend Park's monograph in the Suggested Readings.

Paralleling this interest in the physical fitness of youth was the rising concern about the death rate from coronary heart disease in the middle-aged American male population. Epidemiological studies of the health status of the population underscored the fact that degenerative diseases related to poor health habits (e.g., high fat diet, smoking, inactivity) were responsible for more deaths than the classic infectious and contagious diseases. In 1966 a major symposium highlighted the need for more research in the area of physical activity and health (24). In the 1970s there was an increase in the use of exercise tests to diagnose heart disease and to aid in the prescription of exercise programs to improve cardiovascular health. Large corporations developed "executive" fitness programs to improve the health status of that high-risk group. While most Americans are now familiar with such programs and some students of exercise physiology seek careers in "Corporate Fitness," such programs are not new. The following photos, taken from the 1923 edition of McKensie's *Exercise in Education and Medicine* (19), show a group of businessmen in costume doing dance exercises (figure 1.2), and figure 1.3 shows fitness facilities on the roof of a large inner-city department store. In short, the idea that regular physical activity is an important part of a healthy life-style has been "rediscovered."

A Closer Look 1.1

For most of the twentieth century a primary driving force behind the need to have a physically active and fit society was war or the threat of war. Over the last twenty years the emphasis has shifted to physical activity and health. There is no question that being physically active and attaining a minimum level of fitness are essential ingredients to a healthy life (see chapters 14 and 16). The Healthy People 2000 Health Objectives for the Nation spell out clearly a variety of goals to achieve by the year 2000 to improve the health and well being of all Americans. The objectives deal with areas such as fitness and nutrition, tobacco use, and mental health, and focus on problems such as heart disease, cancer, accidents, and sexually transmitted diseases that claim so many lives each year. Examples of objectives include:

- Increase to at least 20 percent the proportion of people aged 18 and older and to at least 75 percent the proportion of children and adolescents aged 6 through 17 who engage in vigorous physical activity that promotes the development and maintenance of cardiorespiratory fitness 3 or more days per week for 20 or more minutes per occasion.
- Reduce dietary fat intake to an average of 30 percent of calories or less and average saturated fat intake to less than 10 percent of calories among people aged 2 and older.

These specific statements allow scientists to determine if we have achieved the objectives and if not, why not. The process of establishing goals, evaluating progress toward the goals, and redefining the goals provides direction for use of scarce health-care dollars. The process also helps identify the future needs for health-care providers to deliver the services.

Source: *Healthy People 2000: National Health Promotion and Disease Prevention Objectives.* U.S. Department of Health and Human Services, 1991.

in summary

- Fitness has been an issue in this country from the latter part of the nineteenth century until the present. War or the threat of war exerted a strong influence on fitness programs in the public schools.
- Recent interest in fitness is related to the growing concern over the high death rates from disease processes attributable to preventable factors, such as poor diet, lack of exercise, and smoking. The government and professional organizations have responded to this need by educating the public about these problems.
- Schools are now using health-related fitness tests such as the skinfold estimation of body fatness, rather than the more traditional performance tests, to evaluate a child's physical fitness.

Physical Education to Exercise Science

Undergraduate academic preparation in physical education has changed over the past two decades to represent the scientific knowledge base that is needed to deal with the issues related to fitness, performance, and skill acquisition. There has been an increase in the number of physical education programs requiring undergraduates to take one year of calculus, chemistry, and physics, and courses in organic chemistry, biochemistry, anatomy, physiology, and nutrition. In many colleges and universities, there is now little difference between the first two years of requirements in a pre-physical therapy or pre-medical track and the physical education track associated with fitness and exercise physiology. The differences among these tracks lie in the "application" courses that follow. Kinesiology, physiology of exercise, fitness assessment, exercise prescription, exercise leadership, and so on belong to the physical education track. However, it must again be pointed out that this new trend is but another example of a rediscovery of old roots rather than a revolutionary change. Kroll describes two four-year professional physical education programs in the 1890s, one at Stanford and the other at Harvard, that were the forerunners of today's programs (17, pp. 51–64). They included the detailed scientific work and application courses with clear prerequisites cited. Finally, considerable time was allotted for laboratory work. No doubt Lagrange's 1890 text, *Physiology of Bodily Exercise* (18), served as an important reference source for these students. The expectations and goals of those programs were almost identical to those specified for current exercise

Bruno Balke

Given the introduction to this chapter, it should be no surprise that some scientists who have had an impact on the present state of exercise physiology, fitness, and cardiac rehabilitation in the United States received their training in Europe. Dr. Bruno Balke received his training in medicine and physical education in Germany, and was invited to this country by Dr. Ulrich Luft in 1950. During the 1950s he did research on high-altitude tolerance and high-speed flight for the Civil Aeromedical Research Institute and the United States Air Force. His research on work-capacity testing on the treadmill led to the development of the exercise test protocols that bear his name. In addition, his distance-run field test to evaluate cardiovascular fitness (maximal aerobic power) was modified by Ken Cooper for use in the well-known *Aerobics* book (7).

Balke was active in the early days of the American College of Sports Medicine (ACSM), serving as its president in 1966. He was a prime mover in the development of the ACSM certifications for exercise leaders of fitness and cardiac rehabilitation programs (see later discussion) and was actively involved in the teaching and practical examinations associated with those certification workshops.

Balke left government service in 1963 to create the Biodynamics Laboratory at The University of Wisconsin, Madison. Francis J. Nagle followed in 1964, and both had joint appointments with the physical education and physiology departments. Balke's quantitative approach to human physiological questions, especially as they related to fitness and performance, set the standard for other graduate exercise physiology programs. Balke enjoyed teaching others how to do things and viewed as his greatest accomplishment the graduation of the Ph.D. students from his lab who would now teach others (15). As of 1987, fifty-two Ph.D. students were graduated from the Biodynamics Program (20). This is another example of how a scholar's work is multiplied by that of his or her students.

---

physiology undergraduate tracks. In fact, one of the aims of the Harvard program was to allow a student to pursue the study of medicine after completing two years of study (17, p. 61).

Graduate Study and Research in the Physiology of Exercise

While the Harvard Fatigue Laboratory was closing in 1947, the country was on the verge of a tremendous expansion in the number of universities offering graduate study and research opportunities in exercise physiology. A 1950 survey showed that only 16 colleges or universities had research laboratories in departments of physical education (13). By 1966, 151 institutions had research facilities, 58 of them in exercise physiology (28, p. 526). This expansion was due to the availability of more scientists trained in the research methodology of exercise physiology, the increased number of students attending college due to the GI Bill and student loans, and the increase in federal dollars to improve the research capabilities of universities.

"The scholar's work will be multiplied many fold through the contribution of his students." This quote, taken from Montoye and Washburn (21), expresses a view that has helped attract researchers and scholars to universities. Evidence to support this quote was presented in the form of genealogical charts of contributors to the *Research Quarterly* (22). These charts showed the tremendous influence a few people had through their students in the expansion of research in physical education. Probably the best example of this is Thomas K. Cureton, Jr., of the University of Illinois, a central figure in the training of productive researchers in exercise physiology and fitness. The Illinois Research Laboratory dates from 1944 (17, pp. 177–83) and it focused attention on the physiology of fitness. The *Proceedings* of a symposium honoring Cureton in 1969 listed the sixty-eight Ph.D. students who completed their work under his direction (10). While Cureton's scholarly record includes hundreds of research articles and dozens of books dealing with physical fitness, the publications of his students in the areas of epidemiology, fitness, cardiac rehabilitation, and exercise physiology represent the "multiplying effect" that students have on a scholar's productivity (see A Closer Look 1.2).

An example of a major university program that can trace its lineage to the Harvard Fatigue Laboratory is found at Pennsylvania State University. Dr. Ancel Keys, a staff member at the Harvard Fatigue Laboratory, brought Henry Longstreet Taylor back to the Laboratory for Physiological Hygiene at the University of Minnesota, where he received his Ph.D. in 1941 (4). Taylor subsequently advised the research work of

Elsworth R. Buskirk, who designed and directed the Laboratory for Human Performance Research (Noll Laboratory) at Pennsylvania State University. Noll Laboratory continues in the tradition of the Harvard Fatigue Laboratory with a comprehensive research program of laboratory and field research into basic exercise, environmental, and industrial research questions (3). However, it is clear that excellent research in exercise and environmental physiology is conducted in laboratories other than those that have a tie to the Harvard Fatigue Lab. Laboratories are found in physical education departments, physiology departments in medical schools, clinical medicine programs at hospitals, and in independent facilities like the Cooper Clinic. The proliferation and specialization of research involving exercise is discussed in the next section.

Professional Societies and Research Journals

The expansion of interest in exercise physiology and its application to fitness and rehabilitation resulted in an increase in the number of professional societies where scientists and clinicians could present their work. Prior to 1950 the two major societies concerned with physiology of exercise and its application were the American Physiological Society (APS) and the American Association of Health, Physical Education, and Recreation (AAHPER). The need to bring together physicians, physical educators, and physiologists interested in physical activity and health into one professional society resulted in the incorporation of the American College of Sports Medicine (ACSM) in 1955 (see Berryman's History of the ACSM in the Suggested Readings). The ACSM now has more than 15,000 members with regional chapters throughout the country, each holding its own annual meeting to present research, sponsor symposiums, and promote sports medicine. Since 1980 there has been an increase in the number of professional societies to meet the needs of practitioners involved in corporate wellness (e.g., Association for Worksite Health Promotion), and cardiopulmonary rehabilitation (e.g., American Association of Cardiovascular and Pulmonary Rehabilitation).

The growth of research journals has paralleled the increased number of professional societies. During the time of the Harvard Fatigue Laboratory much of the research was published in the following journals: *Journal of Biological Chemistry, American Journal of Physiology, Arbeitsphysiologie (European Journal of Occupational and Applied Physiology), Journal of Clinical Investigation, Journal of Aviation Medicine, Journal of Nutrition,* and *Journal of Physiology.* In 1948 the American Physiological Society published the *Journal of Applied Physiology* to bring together the research work in exercise and environmental physiology. In 1969 the American College of Sports Medicine published the research journal *Medicine and Science in Sports* to support

the growing productivity of its members. In the past ten years the *International Journal of Sports Medicine, Sports Medicine,* and *Journal of Cardiopulmonary Rehabilitation* have been introduced to report and review research.

One of the clear consequences of this increase in research activity is the degree to which scientists are having to specialize in order to be competitive for research grants and to manage the research literature. Laboratories may focus on neuromuscular physiology, cardiac rehabilitation, or the influence of exercise on bone structure. Graduate students are having to specialize earlier in their careers as researchers, and undergraduates must investigate graduate programs very carefully to make sure they meet their career goals (14).

This specialization in research has generated comments about the need to emphasize "basic" research examining the mechanisms underlying a physiological issue rather than "applied" research, which might describe responses of persons to exercise, environmental, or nutritional factors. It would appear that both types of research are needed and, to some extent, such a separation is arbitrary. For example, one scientist might study the interaction of exercise intensity and diet on muscle hypertrophy, another may characterize the changes in muscle cell size and contractile protein, a third might study changes in the energetics of muscle contraction relative to cytoplasmic enzyme activities, and a fourth might study gene expression needed to synthesize that contractile protein. Where does "applied" research begin and "basic" research end? In the introduction to his text *Human Circulation* (25), Loring Rowell provided a quote from T. H. Huxley that bears on this issue.

> I often wish that this phrase "applied science," had never been invented. For it suggests that there is a sort of scientific knowledge of direct practical use, which can be studied apart from another sort of scientific knowledge, which is of no practical utility, and which is termed "pure science." But there is no more complete fallacy than this. What people call applied science is nothing but the application of pure science to particular classes of problems. It consists of deductions from those principles, established by reasoning and observation, which constitute pure science. No one can safely make these deductions until he has a firm grasp of the principles; and he can obtain that grasp only by personal experience of the operations of observation and of reasoning on which they are found. (Huxley, 1948)

It is clear that we are moving along a continuum from the role of exercise in the prevention of disease in whole populations (epidemiology) to the domain of a cell biologist. We hope that all forms of inquiry are supported by fellow scientists such that present theories related to exercise physiology are continually questioned and modified. Lastly, we completely agree with the sentiments expressed in a statement ascribed to Arthur B. Otis: "Physiology is a good way to make a living and still have fun" (27).

in summary

- The growth and development of exercise physiology laboratories in the 1950s and 1960s increased the opportunities for graduate study and research.
- Graduates from these laboratories contributed to the increase in research productivity, and the number of research journals and professional societies.

Translation of Exercise Physiology to the Consumer

The practical implications of the "fitness boom" include an increase in the number of "health spas" offering fitness or weight-control programs, and an explosion in the number of diet and exercise books selling easy ways to shed pounds and inches. It is clear that there has been and continues to be a need to provide correct information to the consumer about the "facts" related to exercise and weight control, and to provide some guidelines about the qualities to look for in an instructor associated with health and fitness programs. Most readers are familiar with the videotapes and books based on fitness programs of movie stars and are also aware that some of what is offered may not be very sound. Fortunately, there are a number of well-known scientists and scholars in the area of exercise physiology and fitness who are now writing "popular" books related to fitness issues.

Concern over the qualifications of fitness instructors has been addressed by professional societies that offer "certification programs" for those interested in a career in fitness programming. The American College of Sports Medicine (ACSM) provided leadership in this area by initiating certification programs in 1975 for those involved in cardiac rehabilitation programs. These certifications include that of the Program Director$_{SM}$, Exercise Specialist$_{SM}$, and the Exercise Test Technologist$_{SM}$. Later, in response to the needs of those fitness personnel who conduct exercise programs for the apparently healthy individual, the ACSM developed the following certification programs: Exercise Leader$_{SM}$, Health/Fitness Instructor$_{SM}$, and Health/Fitness Director®. These certification programs are based on sets of behavioral objectives describing what the candidate must know. The exams are recognized nationwide by those involved in fitness programs as imparting a high standard of professional achievement (2).

Colleges and universities responded to this need for qualified personnel to direct exercise and weight-control programs. Many physical education departments offer undergraduate and graduate courses to train students for a career in fitness and cardiac rehabilitation programs, or for advanced graduate study leading to a career in research and teaching at the university level. The growth in these programs occurred at the same time that there was a glut in the job market for physical education positions in the public schools. The colleges and universities had simply overproduced physical education teachers at a time when teaching positions were decreasing. One can only hope that as more and more colleges and universities develop these undergraduate fitness tracks that the quality of the graduate will be maintained and the market will not be saturated. On the other hand, the increase in the number of well-educated people who can provide quality programming for the apparently healthy individual might be properly timed for the expected teacher shortage in the school systems in the late 1990s.

in summary

- In order to meet the needs of the consumer for correct information and programs about physical activity and health, university and college physical education departments have developed new areas of study in exercise physiology and fitness.
- Organizations like the American College of Sports Medicine have developed certification programs to establish a standard of knowledge and skill to be achieved by those who lead health-related exercise programs.

study questions

1. Name the three Nobel Prize winners whose research involved muscle or muscular exercise.
2. Who directed the Harvard Fatigue Laboratory? What kind of research questions did the laboratory investigate?
3. What were some of the forces driving the fitness movement in the first half of the twentieth century?
4. Compared to the first half of the twentieth century, what factors or events in the latter half triggered a renewed interest and concern about physical fitness?
5. Identify three professional organizations and four research journals that support the work of those in exercise physiology, fitness, and cardiac rehabilitation.

suggested readings

Berryman, J. W. 1995. *Out of Many, One: A History of the American College of Sports Medicine.* Champaign, IL: Human Kinetics.

Cannon, W. B. 1965. *The Way of an Investigator.* New York: Hafner.

Hill, A. V. 1966. *Trails and Trials in Physiology.* Baltimore: Williams & Wilkins.

Park, R. S. 1989. *Measurement of Physical Fitness: A Historical Perspective.* Washington, D.C.: ODPHP National Health Information Center.

references

1. American Alliance for Health, Physical Education, Recreation and Dance. 1980. *Lifetime Health Related Physical Fitness: Test Manual.* Reston, VA.

2. American College of Sports Medicine. 1995. *ACSM's Guidelines for Exercise Testing and Prescription,* 5th ed. Baltimore: Williams & Wilkins.

3. Buskirk, E. R. 1987. Personal communication based on "Our extended family: Graduates from the Noll Lab for Human Performance Research." Noll Laboratory, Pennsylvania State University, University Park, PA 16802.

4. Buskirk, E. R. 1992. From Harvard to Minnesota: Keys to our history. In *Exercise and Sport Sciences Reviews,* vol. 20, 1–26, ed. J. O. Holloszy. Baltimore: Williams & Wilkins.

5. Chapman, C. B., and J. H. Mitchell. 1965. The physiology of exercise. *Scientific American* 212:88–96.

6. Clarke, H. H., and D. H. Clarke. 1978. *Developmental and Adapted Physical Education.* Englewood Cliffs, NJ: Prentice-Hall.

7. Cooper, K. H. 1968. *Aerobics.* New York: Bantam Books.

8. Dill, D. B. 1938. *Life, Heat, and Altitude.* Cambridge, MA: Harvard University Press.

9. Fenn, W. O., and H. Rahn, eds. 1964. *Handbook of Physiology: Respiration,* vol. 1. American Physiological Society, Washington, D.C.

10. Franks, B. Don. 1969. *Exercise and Fitness 1969.* Chicago, IL: The Athletic Institute.

11. Hackensmith, C. W. 1966. *History of Physical Education.* New York: Harper & Row.

12. Horvath, S. M., and E. C. Horvath. 1973. *The Harvard Fatigue Laboratory: Its History and Contributions.* Englewood Cliffs, NJ: Prentice-Hall.

13. Hunsicker, P. A. 1950. A survey of laboratory facilities in college physical education departments. *Research Quarterly* 21:420–23.

14. Ianuzzo, D., and R. S. Hutton. 1987. A prospectus for graduate students in muscle physiology and biochemistry. *Sports Medicine Bulletin* 22:17–18. Indianapolis: The American College of Sports Medicine.

15. Jackson, M. A. 1977. Bruno Balke welcomes—and creates—avalanches. *Physician and Sportsmedicine* 7:93–98.

16. Kennedy, J. F. 1960. The soft American. *Sports Illustrated* 13:14–17.

17. Kroll, W. P. 1971. *Perspectives in Physical Education.* New York: Academic Press.

18. Lagrange, F. 1890. *Physiology of Bodily Exercise.* New York: D. Appleton and Company.

19. McKenzie, R. T. 1923. *Exercise in Education and Medicine.* Philadelphia: W. B. Saunders.

20. Montoye, H. J. 1987. Personal communication based on The University of Wisconsin Alumni Class Roster. Department of Physical Education and Dance, The University of Wisconsin, Madison.

21. Montoye, H. J., and R. Washburn. 1980. Genealogy of scholarship among academy members. *The Academy Papers,* vol. 13, 94–101. Washington, D.C.: AAHPERD.

22. Montoye, H. J., and R. Washburn. 1980. Research quarterly contributors: An academic genealogy. *Research Quarterly for Exercise and Sport* 51:261–66.

23. Powell, K. E., and R. S. Paffenbarger. 1985. Workshop on epidemiologic and public health aspects of physical activity and exercise: A summary. *Public Health Reports* 100:118–26.

24. Proceedings of the International Symposium on Physical Activity and Cardiovascular Health. 1967. *Canadian Medical Association Journal* 96:695–915.

25. Rowell, L. B. 1986. *Human Circulation: Regulation During Physical Stress.* New York: Oxford University Press.

26. Sargent, D. A. 1906. *Physical Education.* Boston: Ginn and Co.

27. Stainsby, W. N. 1987. Part two: "For what is a man profited?" *Sports Medicine Bulletin* 22:15. Indianapolis: The American College of Sports Medicine.

28. Van Dalen, D. B., and B. L. Bennett. 1971. *A World History of Physical Education: Cultural, Philosophical, Comparative,* 2d ed. Englewood Cliffs, NJ: Prentice-Hall.

Control of the Internal Environment

objectives

By studying this chapter, you should be able to do the following:

1. Define the terms *homeostasis* and *steady state*.
2. Diagram and discuss a biological control system.
3. Give an example of a biological control system.
4. Explain the term *negative feedback*.
5. Define what is meant by the gain of a control system.

outline

Homeostasis: Dynamic
    Constancy 14
Control Systems of the Body 15
Nature of the Control Systems 15
    Negative Feedback 16
    Gain of a Control System 16

Examples of Homeostatic
    Control 17
    Regulation of Arterial Blood
        Pressure 17
    Regulation of Blood Glucose 17

Exercise: A Test of Homeostatic
    Control 18

key terms

biological control system
effector
gain

homeostasis
integrating center
negative feedback

receptor
steady state

I f you had a body temperature of 104° F (40° C) while sitting at rest, you would know that something is wrong. As children we learned that normal body temperature is 98.6° F (37° C) and that values above or below normal signify a problem. How does the body manage to maintain core temperature within a narrow range? Further, how is it that during exercise, when the body is producing great amounts of heat, we generally do not experience overheating problems?

Over a hundred years ago the French physiologist Claude Bernard observed that the "milieu interior" (internal environment) of the body remained remarkably constant despite a changing external environment. The fact that the body manages to maintain a relatively constant internal environment in spite of various stressors such as exercise, heat, cold, or fasting is not an accident but the result of many complex control systems. Control mechanisms that are responsible for maintenance of a stable internal environment constitute a

Figure 2.1
Changes in body core temperature during sixty minutes of submaximal exercise in a thermoneutral environment. Note that body temperature reaches a plateau by approximately forty minutes of exercise.

Figure 2.2
Changes in arterial blood pressure across time during resting conditions. Notice that although the arterial pressure oscillates across time, the mean pressure remains unchanged.

major chapter in exercise physiology, and it is helpful to examine their function in light of simple control theory. Therefore, the purpose of this chapter is to introduce the concept of "control systems" and to discuss how the body maintains a rather constant internal environment during periods of stress.

Homeostasis: Dynamic Constancy

The term **homeostasis** was coined by Walter Cannon in 1932 and is defined as the maintenance of a constant or unchanging internal environment. A similar term, **steady state,** is often used by exercise physiologists to denote a steady physiological environment. Although the terms *steady state* and *homeostasis* are often used interchangeably, homeostasis generally refers to a relatively constant internal environment during unstressed conditions resulting from many compensating regulatory responses (1, 12, 16). In contrast, a steady state does not necessarily mean that the internal environment is completely normal, but simply that it is unchanging. In other words, a balance has been achieved between the demands placed on the body and the body's response to those demands. An example that is useful in distinguishing between these two terms is the case of body temperature during exercise. Figure 2.1 illustrates the changes in body core temperature during sixty minutes of constant-load submaximal exercise in a thermoneutral environment (i.e., low humidity and low temperature). Note that core temperature reaches a new and steady level within forty minutes after commencement of exercise. This plateau of core temperature represents a steady state since temperature is constant; however, this constant temperature is above the normal resting body temperature and thus does

not represent a true homeostatic condition. Therefore, the term homeostasis is generally reserved for describing normal resting conditions, and the term *steady state* is often applied to exercise where the physiological variable in question (i.e., body temperature) is unchanging but may not equal the "true" resting value.

Although the concept of homeostasis means that the internal environment is unchanging, this does not mean that the internal environment remains absolutely constant. In fact, most physiological variables vary around some "set" value and thus homeostasis represents a rather dynamic constancy. An example of this dynamic constancy is the arterial blood pressure. Figure 2.2 shows the change in mean (average) arterial blood pressure during eight minutes of rest. Note the oscillatory change in arterial pressure, but the mean (average) arterial pressure remains around 93 mm Hg. The reason such an oscillation occurs in physiological variables is related to the "feedback" nature of biological control systems (8, 9, 15). This will be discussed later in the chapter.

in summary

- Homeostasis is defined as the maintenance of a constant or unchanging "normal" internal environment.
- The term steady state is also defined as a constant internal environment but this does not necessarily mean that the internal environment is completely normal. When the body is in a steady state, a balance has been achieved between the demands placed on the body and the body's response to those demands.

Understanding How Biological Control Systems Operate During Exercise Is Important

An exciting area of research in exercise physiology centers around biological control systems. Indeed, many future investigations will be aimed at improving our understanding of how biological control systems regulate homeostasis during exercise. This type of research is termed "mechanistic" research because the goal of these studies is to determine the mechanism(s) of how a specific control system operates. For example, an important but unanswered question in physiology is, "How does the body regulate breathing during exercise to maintain constant blood levels of oxygen and carbon dioxide?" Given the importance of breathing to maintain homeostasis, it is not surprising that laboratories around the world continue to investigate how the body regulates breathing during exercise (see chapter 10). Mechanistic studies are critical to improving our understanding of both exercise physiology and how various diseases alter physiological function.

Control Systems of the Body

The body has literally hundreds of different control systems, and the overall goal of most is to regulate some physiological variable at or near a constant value (7, 12, 25). The most intricate of these control systems reside inside the cell itself. These cellular control systems act to regulate cell activities such as protein breakdown and synthesis, energy production, and maintenance of the appropriate amounts of stored nutrients (8, 22). Almost all organ systems of the body work to help maintain homeostasis (4, 9, 11, 15, 21). For example, the lungs (pulmonary system) and heart (circulatory system) work together to replenish oxygen and to remove carbon dioxide from the extracellular fluid. The fact that the cardiopulmonary system is usually able to maintain normal levels of oxygen and carbon dioxide even during periods of strenuous exercise is not an accident but the end result of a good control system.

Although much is known about how specific control systems of the body operate, the details of how many control systems work to maintain homeostasis remain a mystery. This is an active area of research in exercise physiology (see Research Focus 2.1).

Nature of the Control Systems

To develop a better understanding of how the body maintains a stable internal environment, let's begin with the analogy of a simple nonbiological control system such as a thermostat-regulated heating and cooling system in a home. Suppose the thermostat is set at 20° C. Any change in room temperature away from the 20° C "set point" results in the appropriate response by either the furnace or the air conditioner to return the room temperature back to 20° C. If the room temperature rises above the set point, the thermostat signals the air conditioner to start, which returns the room temperature to 20° C. In contrast, a decrease in temperature below the set point results in the thermostat signaling the heating system to begin operation (figure 2.3). In both cases the response by the heating or cooling systems was to correct the condition, low or high temperature, that initially turned it on.

A **biological control system** can be defined as a series of interconnected components that serve to maintain a physical or chemical parameter of the body at a near constant value (12, 26). The general components of a biological control system are as follows: (1) a receptor, (2) an integrating center, and (3) an effector. Figure 2.4 represents the schematic of such a control system. The signal to begin the operation of a control system is the stimulus (i.e., some detectable change in the environment), such as temperature, blood pressure, and so on. The stimulus excites a **receptor** (component capable of detecting change of the variable in question), which sends a message to the **integrating center,** which can be thought of as a control box. The integrating center assesses the strength of the stimulus and sends an appropriate output message to a component known as the **effector,** which is concerned with correcting the disturbance by responding in a manner that changes the internal environment back to normal. The return of the internal environment toward normal results in a decrease in the original stimulus that triggered the control system into action. This type of feedback is termed *negative feedback* and is discussed in detail in the next section.

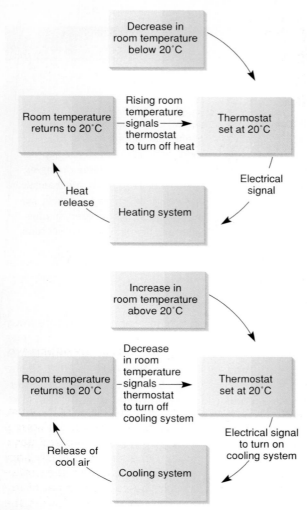

Figure 2.3
A thermostat-controlled heating/cooling system. An increase in temperature above the "set point" signals the air conditioner to turn on. In contrast, a decrease in room temperature below the set point results in turning on the furnace. This system illustrates a nonbiological control system.

Negative Feedback

Most control systems of the body operate via **negative feedback** (2, 8). An example of negative feedback can be seen in the respiratory system's regulation of the CO_2 concentration in extracellular fluid. In this case, an increase in extracellular CO_2 above normal levels triggers a receptor, which sends information to the respiratory control center (integrating center) to increase breathing. The effectors in this example are the respiratory muscles. This increase in breathing will lower extracellular CO_2 concentrations back to normal, thus reestablishing homeostasis. The reason that this type of feedback is termed negative is that the response of the control system is negative (opposite) to the stimulus.

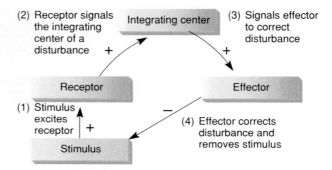

Figure 2.4
Schematic of the components that comprise a biological control system. The process begins with a change in the internal environment (stimulus), which excites a receptor to send information about the change to an integrating control center. The integrating center makes an assessment of the amount of response needed to correct the disturbance and sends the appropriate message to the effector. The effector is responsible for correcting the disturbance and thus the stimulus is removed.

Gain of a Control System

The precision with which a control system maintains homeostasis is termed the *gain* of the system. **Gain** can be thought of as the "capability" of the control system. A control system with a large gain is more potent and is therefore more capable of correcting alterations in homeostasis than a system with a low gain. The gain of a negative feedback control system is defined as the ratio of the amount of correction needed to maintain homeostasis to the amount of the abnormality that exists after correction by the system (8):

$$\text{Gain} = \frac{\text{Amount of correction needed}}{\text{Amount of abnormality that exists after correction}}$$

Consider the following example of the feedback gain of the temperature control system during exposure to cold. Suppose a person dressed in shorts leaves a comfortable room (i.e., 22° C) and enters a cold room (i.e., 0° C) for a twenty-minute stay. Upon entering the cold room the person's body temperature is 37° C, but after twenty minutes it has decreased to 36° C. During cold exposure, control systems automatically decrease skin blood flow to minimize heat loss and initiate shivering to increase heat production. Collectively these changes prevent body temperature from decreasing drastically. The feedback gain of this control system can be calculated as follows:

$$\text{Feedback gain} = \frac{22° \text{ C} - 0° \text{ C}}{37° \text{ C} - 36° \text{ C}} = \frac{22}{1} = 22$$

A high feedback gain of twenty-two means that for each degree change in body temperature that occurred during exposure to the cold room, there would

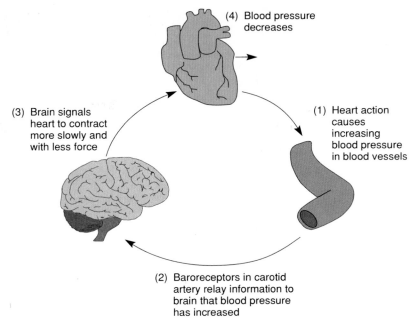

(4) Blood pressure decreases

(1) Heart action causes increasing blood pressure in blood vessels

(3) Brain signals heart to contract more slowly and with less force

(2) Baroreceptors in carotid artery relay information to brain that blood pressure has increased

Figure 2.5
Example of negative feedback mechanism to lower blood pressure. A similar mechanism helps to increase blood pressure if it decreases below normal.

have been a twenty-two times greater change in temperature if it were not for the control system! It is not surprising that the temperature control system has a high gain given the importance of maintaining a reasonably constant body temperature.

in summary

- A biological control system is composed of a receptor, an integrating center, and an effector.
- Most control systems act by way of negative feedback.
- The degree to which a control system maintains homeostasis is termed the gain of the system. A control system with a large gain is more capable of maintaining homeostasis than a system with a low gain.

Examples of Homeostatic Control

To better understand biological control systems, consider a few examples of homeostatic control.

Regulation of Arterial Blood Pressure

An excellent illustration of homeostatic control that uses negative feedback is the "baroreceptor system," which is responsible for the regulation of blood pressure. The baroreceptors are pressure-sensitive receptors

located in the carotid arteries and the arch of the aorta. When arterial blood pressure increases above normal levels, these baroreceptors are stimulated and nerve impulses are transmitted to the cardiovascular control center in the medulla of the brain. In turn, the cardiovascular control center decreases the number of impulses transmitted to the heart, which lowers the amount of blood pumped by the heart, and causes arterial pressure to return to normal (figure 2.5). In contrast, a reduction in arterial pressure reduces the number of impulses transmitted from the baroreceptors to the brain, which causes the cardiovascular control center to increase the number of impulses transmitted to the heart to produce an increase in blood pressure (6).

Regulation of Blood Glucose

Homeostasis is also a function of the endocrine system (chapter 5). The body contains eight major endocrine glands, which synthesize and secrete blood-borne chemical substances called hormones. Hormones are transported via the circulatory system throughout the body as an aid to regulate circulatory and metabolic functions (2, 10). An example of the endocrine system's role in the maintenance of homeostasis is the control of blood glucose levels. Indeed, in health, the blood glucose concentration is carefully regulated by the endocrine system. For example, the hormone insulin regulates cellular uptake and the metabolism of glucose and is therefore important in the regulation of the blood glucose concentration. After a large carbohydrate meal, the blood glucose level increases above

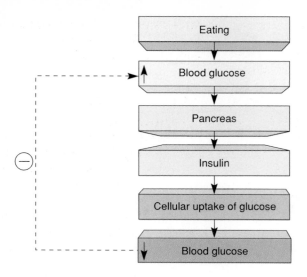

Figure 2.6

Illustration of the regulation of blood glucose concentration. Changes in blood glucose concentration from the normal range regulate insulin secretion. Insulin, in turn, acts to regulate blood glucose levels (completing the negative feedback loop) and to maintain homeostasis. In this system the pancreas is both the sensor and the effector organ. It senses the change in blood glucose from normal and releases insulin appropriately.

A Closer Look 2.1

Failure of a Biological Control System Results in Disease

Failure of any component of a biological control system results in a disturbance in homeostasis. A classic illustration of the failure of a biological control system is the disease, diabetes. Although there are two forms of diabetes (type I and type II), both types of the disease are characterized by abnormally high blood glucose levels (called hyperglycemia). In type I diabetes, the beta cells in the pancreas (beta cells produce insulin) become damaged. Hence, insulin is no longer produced and released into the blood to promote the transport of glucose into tissues. Therefore, damage to the pancreatic beta cells represents a failure of the "effector" component of this control system. If insulin cannot be released in response to an increase in blood glucose following a high carbohydrate meal, glucose cannot be transported into body cells and the end result is hyperglycemia and diabetes.

normal (figure 2.6). The rise in blood glucose signals the pancreas to release insulin, which then acts to lower blood glucose by increasing cellular uptake. Failure of the blood glucose control system results in disease (diabetes) and is discussed in A Closer Look 2.1.

Exercise: A Test of Homeostatic Control

Muscular exercise can be considered a dramatic test of the body's homeostatic control systems since exercise has the potential to disrupt many homeostatic variables. For example, during heavy exercise skeletal muscle produces large amounts of lactic acid, which causes an increase in intracellular and extracellular acidity (5, 18, 19, 20, 24, 27, 28). This increase in acidity represents a serious challenge to the body's acid-base control system (3, 6) (chapter 11). Additionally, heavy exercise results in large increases in muscle O_2 requirements and large amounts of CO_2 are produced. These changes must be countered by increases in breathing (pulmonary ventilation) and blood flow to increase O_2 delivery to the exercising muscle and remove metabolically produced CO_2. Further, during heavy exercise the working muscles produce large amounts of heat that must be removed to prevent overheating. The body's control systems must respond rapidly to prevent drastic alterations in the internal environment.

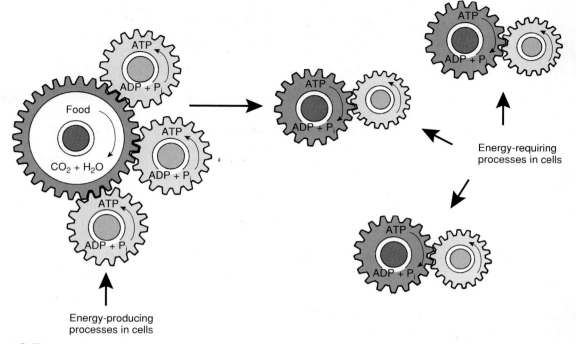

Figure 3.7
Model of ATP serving as the universal energy donor that drives the energy needs of the cell. On the left, the energy released from the breakdown of foodstuffs is used to form ATP. On the right, the energy released from the breakdown of ATP is used to "drive" the energy needs of the cell.

Therefore, energy-liberating reactions are linked to energy-requiring reactions like two meshed gears.

Bioenergetics

Muscle cells store limited amounts of ATP. Therefore, because muscular exercise requires a constant supply of ATP to provide the needed energy for contraction, metabolic pathways must exist in the cell with the capability to produce ATP rapidly. Indeed, muscle cells can produce ATP by any one or a combination of three metabolic pathways: (1) formation of ATP by **phosphocreatine (PC)** breakdown, (2) formation of ATP via the degradation of glucose or glycogen (called glycolysis), and (3) oxidative formation of ATP. Formation of ATP via the PC pathway and glycolysis does not involve the use of O_2 and are called **anaerobic** (without O_2) pathways. Oxidative formation of ATP by the use of O_2 is termed **aerobic** metabolism. A detailed discussion of the operation of the three metabolic pathways involved in the formation of ATP during exercise follows.

Anaerobic ATP Production

The simplest and consequently the most rapid method of producing ATP involves the donation of a phosphate group and its bond energy from PC to ADP to form ATP (4, 8a, 10, 18, 43):

$$PC + ADP \xrightarrow{\text{Creatine kinase}} ATP + C$$

The reaction is catalyzed by the enzyme creatine kinase. As rapidly as ATP is broken down to ADP + P_i at the onset of exercise, ATP is reformed via the PC reaction. However, muscle cells store only small amounts of PC and thus the total amount of ATP that can be formed via this reaction is limited. The combination of stored ATP and PC is called the **ATP-PC system** or the "phosphagen system" and provides energy for muscular contraction at the onset of exercise and during short-term, high-intensity exercise (i.e., lasting less than five seconds). PC reformation requires ATP and occurs only during recovery from exercise (8, 11).

The importance of the ATP-PC system in athletics can be appreciated by considering short-term intense exercise such as sprinting 50 meters, high jumping, performing a rapid weight-lifting move, or a football player racing 10 yards down field. All of these activities require only a few seconds to complete and thus need a rapid supply of ATP. The ATP-PC system provides a simple one-enzyme reaction to produce ATP for these types of activities. The fact that depletion of PC is likely to limit short-term, high-intensity exercise has led to the suggestion that ingestion of large amounts of creatine can improve exercise performance (see Research Focus 3.1).

A second metabolic pathway capable of producing ATP rapidly without the involvement of O_2 is termed **glycolysis.** Glycolysis involves the breakdown of glucose or glycogen to form two molecules of pyruvic acid or lactic

Research Focus 3.1

Creatine Supplementation and Exercise Performance

Depletion of phosphocreatine (PC) may limit exercise performance during short-term, high-intensity exercise (e.g., 60 meter dash) because the depletion of PC results in a reduction in the rate of ATP production by the ATP-PC system. Recent studies have shown that ingestion of large amounts of crea- tine (20 grams/day) over a 5-day period results in increased stores of muscle PC. This creatine supple- mentation has been shown to im- prove performance during short, high-intensity exercise (see refer- ences 16a and 25a for a review). Be- cause of these reports, creatine supplementation is now being practiced by many athletes and there are no reports of harmful side effects at the recommended dosage (i.e., 20 grams/day). At present, creatine supplementation does not violate doping regula- tions maintained by major athletic organizations. See chapter 25 for more details.

acid (figures 3.8 and 3.9). Simply stated, glycolysis is an anaerobic pathway used to transfer bond energy from glucose to rejoin P_i to ADP. This process involves a series of enzymatically catalyzed, coupled reactions. Glycolysis occurs in the sarcoplasm of the muscle cell and pro- duces a net gain of two molecules of ATP and two mol- ecules of pyruvic or lactic acid per glucose molecule.

Let's consider glycolysis in more detail. First, the reactions between glucose and pyruvate can be con- sidered as two distinct phases: (1) energy investment phase, and (2) energy generation phase (figure 3.8). The first five reactions make up the "energy investment phase" where stored ATP must be used to form sugar phosphates. Although the end result of glycolysis is energy producing (exergonic), glycolysis must be "primed" by the addition of ATP at two points at the be- ginning of the pathway (figure 3.9). The purpose of the ATP priming is to add phosphate groups (called phos- phorylation) to glucose and to fructose-6-phosphate. Note that if glycolysis begins with glycogen as the sub- strate, the addition of only one ATP is required (glyco- gen does not require phosphorylation by ATP, but is phosphorylated by inorganic phosphate instead). The last five reactions of glycolysis represent the "energy generation phase" of glycolysis. Figure 3.9 points out that two molecules of ATP are produced at each of two separate reactions near the end of the glycolytic path- way; thus, the net gain of glycolysis is two ATP if glu- cose is the substrate and three ATP if glycogen is the substrate.

Hydrogens are frequently removed from nutri- ent substrates in bioenergetic pathways and are transported by "carrier molecules." Two biologically important carrier molecules are **nicotinamide ade- nine dinucleotide (NAD)** and **flavin adenine dinu- cleotide (FAD).** Both NAD and FAD transport hydrogens and their associated energy to be used for later generation of ATP in the mitochondrion via aer- obic processes. In order for the chemical reactions in glycolysis to proceed, two hydrogens must be re- moved from glyceraldehyde-3-phosphate, which then

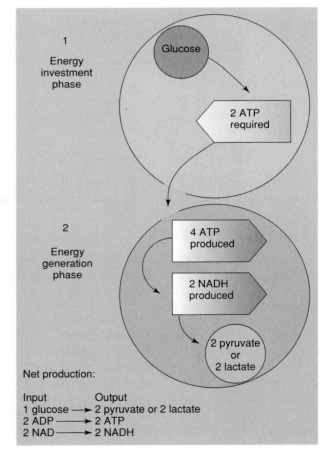

Figure 3.8

Illustration of the two phases of glycolysis and the products of glycolysis.

From *Biochemistry* by Mathews and vanHolde. Copyright © 1990 by The Benjamin/Cummings Publishing Company. Reprinted by permission.

forms 1,3, diphosphoglycerate. The hydrogen accep- tor in this reaction is NAD (figure 3.9). Here NAD ac- cepts one of the hydrogens while the remaining hydrogen is free in solution. Upon accepting the hy- drogen, NAD is converted to its reduced form, NADH

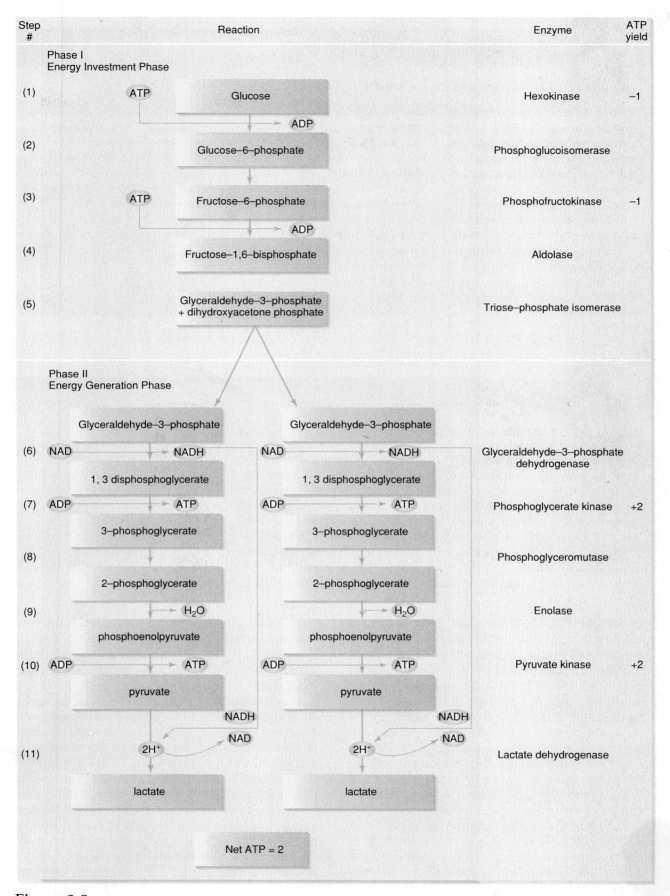

Figure 3.9

Summary of the anaerobic metabolism of glucose. Note that the end result of the anaerobic breakdown of one molecule of glucose is the production of two molecules of ATP and lactate.

A Closer Look 3.3

The Concept of Oxidation–Reduction Reactions

When a molecule accepts electrons from an electron donor it is said to become reduced; when a molecule gives up electrons the molecule has undergone a process called oxidation. Oxidation-reduction reactions are always linked together. In other words, a molecule cannot be reduced unless another molecule is oxidized first. The molecule that gives up the electrons is called a reducing agent, while the molecule that accepts the electrons is referred to as an oxidizing agent.

Oxidation does not mean oxygen is involved in this process. The term oxidation is derived from the fact that oxygen has the tendency to accept electrons. Hence, oxygen is a strong oxidizing agent. Cells make use of this fact by using oxygen as the final electron acceptor in the electron transport chain.

Two molecules that play an important role as oxidizing agents in cellular bioenergetics are nicotinamide adenine dinucleotide (NAD) and flavin adenine dinucleotide (FAD). Each NAD and FAD molecule can accept two electrons (see text for specific details). Examples of these reactions follow:

$$FAD + 2H^+ \longrightarrow FADH_2$$
and
$$NAD + 2H^+ \longrightarrow NADH + H^+$$

A Closer Look 3.4

NADH is "Shuttled" into Mitochondria

NADH generated during glycolysis must be converted back to NAD if glycolysis is to continue. As discussed in the text, the conversion of NADH to NAD can occur by pyruvic acid accepting the hydrogens (forming lactic acid) or "shuttling" the hydrogens from NADH across the mitochondrial membrane. The "shuttling" of hydrogens across the mitochondrial membrane requires a specific transport system. Figure 4.9 (chapter 4) illustrates this process. This transport system is located within the mitochondrial membrane and acts to transfer NADH-released hydrogens from the cytosol into the mitochondria where they can enter the electron transport chain.

(see A Closer Look 3.3). Adequate amounts of NAD must be available to accept the hydrogen atoms that must be removed from glyceraldehyde-3-phosphate if glycolysis is to continue (1, 8, 22). How is NAD reformed from NADH? There are two ways that the cell restores NAD from NADH. First, if sufficient oxygen (O_2) is available, the hydrogens from NADH can be "shuttled" into the mitochondria of the cell and can contribute to the aerobic production of ATP (see A Closer Look 3.4). Second, if O_2 is not available to accept the hydrogens in the mitochondria, pyruvic acid can accept the hydrogens to form **lactic acid** (figure 3.10). The enzyme that catalyzes this reaction is lactate dehydrogenase (LDH), with the end result being the formation of lactic acid and the reformation of NAD. Therefore, the reason for lactic acid formation is the "recycling" of NAD (i.e., NADH converted to NAD) so that glycolysis can continue.

Again, glycolysis is the breakdown of glucose into pyruvic acid or lactic acid with the net production of two or three ATP depending on whether the pathway began with glucose or glycogen, respectively. Figure 3.9 summarizes glycolysis in a simple flowchart. Glucose is a six-carbon molecule and pyruvic acid and lactic acid are three-carbon molecules. Thus, this explains the production of two molecules of pyruvic acid and lactic acid from one molecule of glucose. Since O_2 is not directly involved in glycolysis, the pathway is considered anaerobic. However, in the presence of O_2 in the mitochondria, pyruvate can participate in the aerobic production of ATP. Thus, in addition to being an anaerobic pathway capable of producing ATP without O_2, glycolysis can be considered the first step in the aerobic degradation of carbohydrates. This will be discussed in detail in the next section.

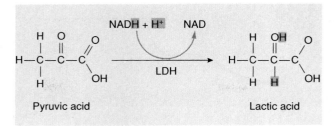

Figure 3.10

The addition of two hydrogen atoms to pyruvic acid forms lactic acid and NAD, which can be used again in glycolysis. The reaction is catalyzed by the enzyme lactate dehydrogenase (LDH).

in summary

- The immediate source of energy for muscular contraction is the high-energy phosphate ATP. ATP is degraded via the enzyme ATPase as follows:

$$ATP \xrightarrow[\text{ATPase}]{} ADP + P_i + energy$$

- Formation of ATP without the use of O_2 is termed anaerobic metabolism. In contrast, production of ATP using O_2 as the final electron acceptor is referred to as aerobic metabolism.
- Muscle cells can produce ATP by any one or combination of three metabolic pathways: 1) ATP-PC system, 2) glycolysis, and 3) oxidative phosphorylation.
- The ATP-PC system and glycolysis are two anaerobic metabolic pathways that are capable of producing ATP without O_2.

Aerobic ATP Production

Aerobic production of ATP occurs inside the mitochondria and involves the interaction of two cooperating metabolic pathways: (1) the Krebs cycle and (2) the electron transport chain. The primary function of the **Krebs cycle** (also called the citric acid cycle) is to complete the oxidation (hydrogen removal) of carbohydrates, fats, or proteins using NAD and FAD as hydrogen (energy) carriers. The importance of hydrogen removal is that hydrogens (by virtue of the electrons that they possess) contain the potential energy in the food molecules. This energy can be used in the electron transport chain to combine ADP + P_i to reform ATP. Oxygen does not participate in the reactions of the Krebs cycle but is the final hydrogen acceptor at the end of the electron transport chain (i.e., water is formed, $H_2 + O \rightarrow H_2O$). The process of aerobic production of ATP is termed **oxidative phosphorylation.** It

is convenient to think of aerobic ATP production as a three-stage process (figure 3.11). Stage 1 is the generation of a key two-carbon molecule, acetyl–CoA. Stage 2 is the oxidation of acetyl–CoA in the Krebs cycle. Stage 3 is the process of oxidative phosphorylation (i.e., ATP formation) in the electron transport chain (i.e., respiratory chain). A detailed look at the Krebs cycle and electron transport chain follows.

Krebs Cycle

The Krebs cycle is named after the biochemist Hans Krebs, whose pioneering research has increased our understanding of this rather complex pathway. Entry into the Krebs cycle requires preparation of a two-carbon molecule, acetyl-CoA. Acetyl-CoA can be formed from the breakdown of either carbohydrates, fats, or proteins (figure 3.11). For the moment let's focus on the formation of acetyl-CoA from pyruvate (pyruvate can be formed from both carbohydrates and proteins). Figure 3.12 depicts the cyclic nature of the reactions involved in the Krebs cycle. Note that pyruvate (three-carbon molecule) is broken down to form acetyl-CoA (two-carbon molecule) and the remaining carbon is given off as CO_2. Next, acetyl-CoA combines with oxaloacetate (four-carbon molecule) to form citrate (six carbons). What follows is a series of reactions to regenerate oxaloacetate and two molecules of CO_2, and the pathway begins all over again.

For every molecule of glucose entering glycolysis, two molecules of pyruvate are formed, and in the presence of O_2, they are converted to two molecules of acetyl-CoA. This means that each molecule of glucose results in two turns of the Krebs cycle. With this in mind let's examine the Krebs cycle in more detail. The primary function of the Krebs cycle is to remove hydrogens and the energy associated with those hydrogens from various substrates involved in the cycle. Figure 3.12 illustrates that during each turn of the Krebs cycle three molecules of NADH and one molecule of FADH are formed. For every pair of electrons passed through the electron transport chain from NADH to oxygen, enough energy is available to form three molecules of ATP (37, 41). For every FADH molecule that is formed, enough energy is available to produce two molecules of ATP. Thus, in terms of ATP production, FADH is not as energy rich as NADH.

In addition to the production of NADH and FADH, the Krebs cycle results in direct formation of an energy-rich compound, guanosine triphosphate (GTP) (37) (figure 3.12). GTP is a high-energy compound that can transfer its terminal phosphate group to ADP to form ATP. The direct formation of GTP in the Krebs cycle is called substrate-level phosphorylation and accounts for only a small amount of the total energy conversion in the Krebs cycle since most of the Krebs cycle energy yield (i.e., NADH and FADH) is taken to the electron transport chain to form ATP.

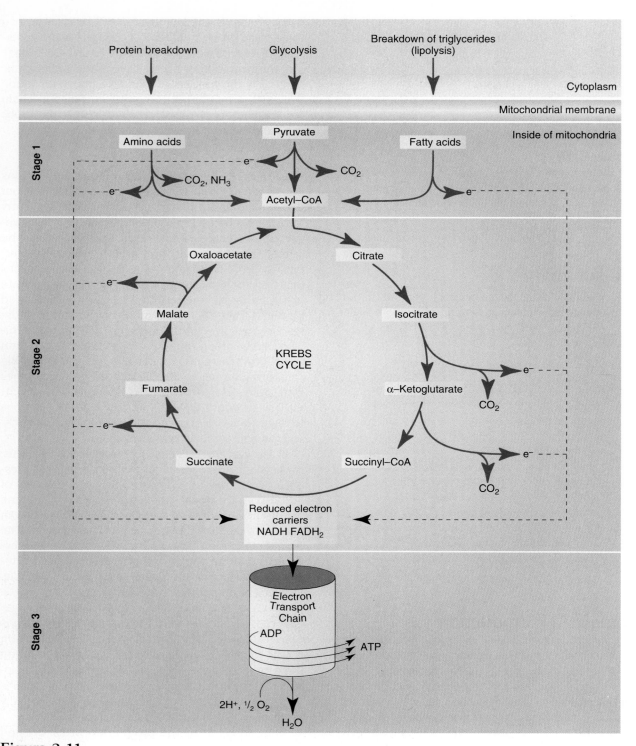

Figure 3.11

The three stages of oxidative phosphorylation.

From Mathews and vanHolde, *Biochemistry*, Diane Bowen, Ed. Copyright © 1990 Benjamin/Cummings Publishing Company, Menlo Park, CA. Reprinted by permission.

Up to this point we have focused on the role that carbohydrates play in producing acetyl-CoA to enter the Krebs cycle. How do fats and proteins undergo aerobic metabolism? The answer can be found in figure 3.13. Note that fats (triglycerides) are broken down to form fatty acids and glycerol. These fatty acids can then undergo a series of reactions to form acetyl-CoA (called beta oxidation; see A Closer Look 3.5 for details) and thus enter the Krebs cycle (37, 39). Although glycerol can be converted into an intermediate of glycolysis in the liver, this does not occur to a great extent in human skeletal muscle. Therefore, glycerol is not an important direct muscle fuel source during exercise (15, 19).

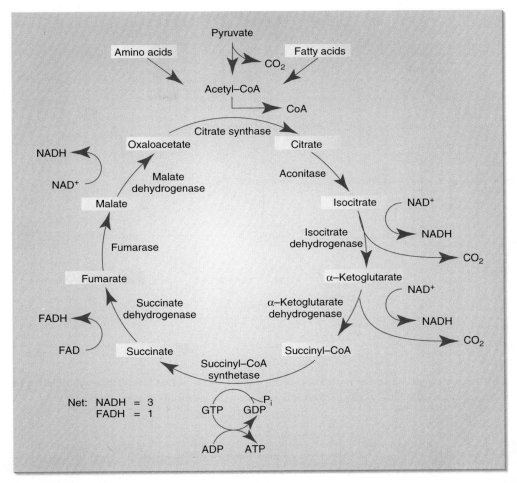

Figure 3.12
Compounds, enzymes, and reactions involved in the Krebs cycle. Note the formation of three molecules of NADH and one molecule of FADH per turn of the cycle.

As mentioned previously, protein is not considered a major fuel source during exercise since it contributes less than 2%–15% of the fuel utilized during exercise (12, 15, 23). Proteins can enter bioenergetic pathways in a variety of places. However, the first step is the breakdown of the protein into its amino acid subunits. What happens next depends on which amino acid is involved. For example, some amino acids can be converted to glucose or pyruvic acid, some to acetyl-CoA, and still others to Krebs-cycle intermediates. The role of proteins in bioenergetics is summarized in figure 3.13.

In summary, the Krebs cycle completes the oxidation of carbohydrates, fats, or proteins, produces CO_2, and supplies electrons to be passed through the electron transport chain to provide the energy for the aerobic production of ATP. Enzymes catalyzing Krebs-cycle reactions are located inside the mitochondria.

Electron Transport Chain
The aerobic production of ATP (called oxidative phosphorylation) occurs in the mitochondria. The pathway responsible for this process is called the **electron transport chain** (also called the respiratory chain or cytochrome chain). Aerobic production of ATP is possible due to a mechanism that uses the potential energy available in reduced hydrogen carriers such as NADH and FADH to rephosphorylate ADP to ATP. The reduced hydrogen carriers do not directly react with oxygen. Instead, electrons removed from the hydrogen atoms are passed down a series of electron carriers known as cytochromes. During this passage of electrons down the cytochrome chain enough energy is released to rephosphorylate ADP to form ATP at three different sites (35) (figure 3.14). Interestingly, as electrons pass down the electron transport chain, highly reactive molecules called free radicals are formed. Large quantities of free radicals may be harmful to the muscle and contribute to muscle fatigue (3) (see Research Focus 3.2).

The hydrogen carriers that bring the electrons to the electron transport chain come from a variety of sources. Recall that two NADH are formed per glucose molecule that is degraded via glycolysis (figure

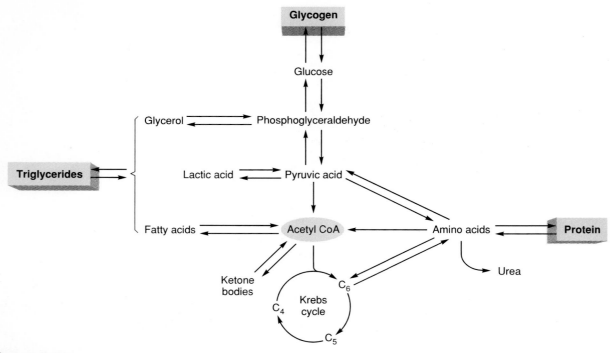

Figure 3.13
The relationship between the metabolism of proteins, carbohydrates, and fats. The overall interaction between the metabolic breakdown of these three foodstuffs is often referred to as the metabolic pool.

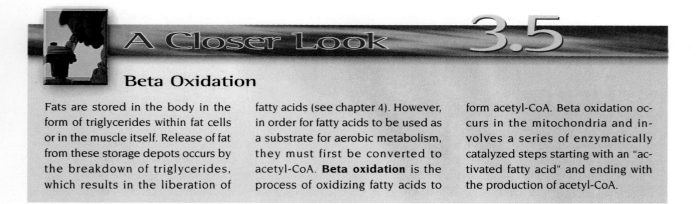

A Closer Look 3.5

Beta Oxidation

Fats are stored in the body in the form of triglycerides within fat cells or in the muscle itself. Release of fat from these storage depots occurs by the breakdown of triglycerides, which results in the liberation of fatty acids (see chapter 4). However, in order for fatty acids to be used as a substrate for aerobic metabolism, they must first be converted to acetyl-CoA. **Beta oxidation** is the process of oxidizing fatty acids to form acetyl-CoA. Beta oxidation occurs in the mitochondria and involves a series of enzymatically catalyzed steps starting with an "activated fatty acid" and ending with the production of acetyl-CoA.

3.9). These NADH are outside the mitochondria and their hydrogens must be transported across the mitochondrial membrane by special "shuttle" mechanisms. However, the bulk of the electrons that enter the electron transport chain come from those NADH and FADH molecules formed as a result of Krebs-cycle oxidation.

Figure 3.14 outlines the pathway for electrons entering the electron transport chain. Simply stated, pairs of electrons from NADH or FADH are passed down a series of compounds that undergo oxidation and reduction, with enough energy being released to synthesize ATP at three places along the way. Notice that FADH enters the cytochrome pathway at a point just below the entry level for NADH (figure 3.14). This is important because the level of FADH entry bypasses one of the sites of ATP formation and thus each molecule of FADH that enters the electron transport chain has enough energy to form only two ATP. In contrast, NADH entry into the electron transport chain results in the formation of three ATP (details will be mentioned later). At the end of the electron transport chain, oxygen accepts the electrons that are passed along, and combines with hydrogen to form water. If O_2 is not available to accept those electrons, oxidative phosphorylation is not possible and ATP formation in the cell must occur via anaerobic metabolism.

Again, note in figure 3.14 that ATP is formed at three points along the electron transport chain. How does this ATP formation occur? The mechanism to

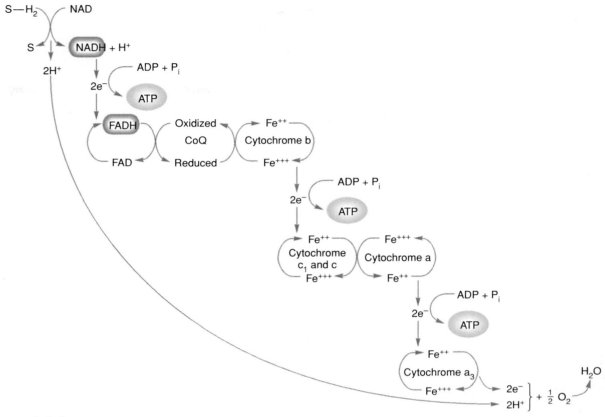

Figure 3.14
Simple representation of the formation of ATP at three sites in the electron transport chain. This process is known as oxidative phosphorylation.

Research Focus 3.2

Free Radicals Are Formed During Aerobic Metabolism

Although the passage of electrons down the electron transport chain performs an essential role in the process of aerobic ATP production, this pathway also forms a product that may negatively influence muscle during exercise. Recent research has shown that the activation of the electron transport chain results in the formation of free radicals (9). Free radicals are molecules that have an unpaired electron in their outer or-

bital which makes them highly reactive. That is, free radicals bind quickly to other molecules and this combination results in damage to the molecule combining with the radical. For example, free radical formation in muscle during exercise might contribute to muscle fatigue and a reduction in the activity of several Krebs cycle enzymes (2, 3, 22a, 33a).

What determines how many free radicals are formed during ex-

ercise? The number of free radicals produced during exercise is directly linked to the rate of aerobic metabolism. Therefore, radicals are formed at high rates during high-intensity or prolonged exercise. More will be said about free radicals and fatigue in chapter 19 and the potential roles of antioxidants in improving exercise performance will be addressed in chapter 25.

explain the aerobic formation of ATP is known as the **chemiosmotic hypothesis.** As electrons are transferred along the cytochrome chain, the energy released is used to "pump" hydrogens (protons; H^+) released from NADH and FADH from the inside of the mitochondria across the inner mitochondrial

membrane (figure 3.15). This results in an accumulation of H^+ within the space between the inner and outer mitochondrial membranes. The accumulation of H^+ is a source of potential energy which can be captured and used to recombine P_i with ADP to form ATP (19a). For example, this collection of H^+ is similar to

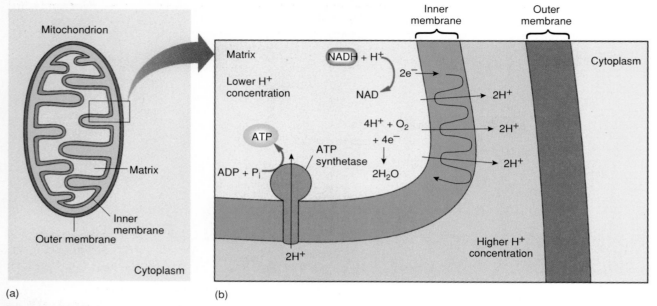

Figure 3.15

Illustration of the chemiosmotic hypothesis of aerobic ATP production. (*a*) Illustrates the location of the inner and outer mitochondrial membranes. (*b*) Illustrates how electron transport results in the pumping of protons (H^+) across the inner mitochondrial membrane; this results in a H^+ gradient across the inner and outer membranes. The energy released when the H^+ diffuse across the inner mitochondrial membrane results in the formation of ATP. See text for details.

the potential energy of water at the top of a dam; when the water accumulates and runs over the top of the dam, falling water becomes kinetic energy which can be used to do work (19a).

Now for the details of how the potential energy from H^+ accumulation is used to form ATP. The increase in H^+ concentration within the space between the inner and outer mitochondrial membranes results in a H^+ gradient; this gradient creates a strong drive for H^+ to diffuse back across the inner mitochondrial membrane. Since most of the inner mitochondrial membrane is not permeable to H^+, the H^+ can only cross the membrane through specialized "H^+" channels. This idea is illustrated in figure 3.15. The movement of two H^+ through these channels releases enough energy to form one molecule of ATP. This reaction, recombining ADP with P_i to form ATP, is catalyzed by the enzyme ATP synthetase. Where does oxygen enter this picture? After the H^+ pass through these channels they combine with oxygen to form water (H_2O). Why is oxygen essential to oxidative phosphorylation? In order for ATP to continue to be formed as H^+'s enter the inner membrane of the mitochondia, these H^+'s must be removed by combining with oxygen to form water. Therefore, oxygen is essential in aerobic production of ATP because it serves as the final acceptor of hydrogens.

As mentioned earlier, NADH and FADH differ in the amount of ATP that can be formed from each of these molecules. The explanation is as follows. Since each NADH results in the pumping of three pairs of H^+ across the inner mitochondrial membrane by the electron transport chain, three ATP are produced. Since each FADH results in the pumping of only two pairs of H^+, only two ATP are formed as the H^+ move back across the respiratory channels.

in summary

- Oxidative phosphorylation or aerobic ATP production occurs in the mitochondria as a result of a complex interaction between the Krebs cycle and the electron transport chain. The primary role of the Krebs cycle is to complete the oxidation of substrates and form NADH and FADH to enter the electron transport chain.
- The end result of the electron transport chain is the formation of ATP and water. Water is formed by oxygen-accepting electrons; hence, the reason we breathe oxygen is to use it as the final acceptor of electrons in aerobic metabolism.

Table 3.1   Aerobic ATP Tally from the Breakdown of One Molecule of Glucose

Metabolic Process	High-Energy Products	ATP from Oxidative Phosphorylation	ATP Subtotal
Glycolysis	2 ATP	—	2 (total if anaerobic)
	2 NADH	6	8 (if aerobic)
Pyruvic acid to acetyl-CoA	2 NADH	6	14
Krebs cycle	2 GTP	—	16
	6 NADH	18	34
	2 FADH	4	38
		Grand total:	38 ATP

Aerobic ATP Tally

It is now possible to compute the overall ATP production as a result of the aerobic breakdown of glucose or glycogen. Let's begin by counting the total energy yield of glycolysis. Recall that the net ATP production of glycolysis was two ATP per glucose molecule. Further, when O_2 is present in the mitochondria, two NADH produced by glycolysis can then be shuttled into the mitochondria with the energy used to synthesize an additional 6 ATP (table 3.1). Thus, glycolysis can produce two ATP directly via substrate-level phosphorylation and an additional 6 ATP by the energy contained in the two molecules of NADH.

How many ATP are produced as a result of the oxidation-reduction activities of the Krebs cycle? Table 3.1 shows that 2 NADH are formed when pyruvic acid is converted to acetyl-CoA which results in the formation of 6 ATP. Note that 2 GTP (similar to ATP) are produced via substrate-level phosphorylation. A total of 6 NADH and 2 FADH are produced in the Krebs cycle as a result of one glucose molecule. Hence, the 6 NADH formed via the Krebs cycle results in the production of a total of 18 ATP (6 NADH × 3 ATP per NADH = 18 ATP), with 4 ATP being produced from the 2 FADH. Therefore, the total ATP yield for the aerobic degradation of glucose is 38 ATP. The aerobic ATP yield for glycogen breakdown is 39 ATP since the net glycolytic production of ATP by glycogen is one ATP more than that of glucose.

Efficiency of Oxidative Phosphorylation

How efficient is oxidative phosphorylation as a system of converting energy from foodstuffs into biologically usable energy? This can be calculated by computing the ratio of the energy contained in the ATP molecules produced via aerobic respiration divided by the total potential energy contained in the glucose molecule. For example, a mole (a mole is one gram molecular weight) of ATP, when broken down, has an energy yield of 7.3 kcal. The potential energy released from the oxidation of a mole of glucose is 686 kcal. Thus, an efficiency figure for aerobic respiration can be computed as follows (21):

$$\text{Efficiency of respiration} = \frac{38 \text{ moles ATP/mole glucose} \times 7.3 \text{ kcal/mole ATP}}{686 \text{ kcal/mole glucose}} \times 100 = 40\%$$

Therefore, the efficiency of aerobic respiration is approximately 40%, with the remaining 60% of the free energy of glucose oxidation being released as heat.

in summary

- The aerobic metabolism of one molecule of glucose results in the production of 38 ATP molecules, whereas the aerobic ATP yield for glycogen breakdown is 39 ATP.
- The overall efficiency of aerobic respiration is approximately 40%, with the remaining 60% of the energy being released as heat.

Control of Bioenergetics

The biochemical pathways that result in the production of ATP are regulated by very precise control systems. Each of these pathways contains a number of reactions that are catalyzed by specific enzymes. In general, if ample substrate is available, an increase in the number of enzymes present results in an increased rate of chemical reactions. Therefore, regulation of one or more enzymes in a biochemical pathway would provide a means of controlling the rate of that particular pathway. Indeed, metabolism is regulated by control of enzymatic activity. Most metabolic pathways have one enzyme that is considered "rate limiting." This rate-limiting enzyme determines the speed of the particular metabolic pathway involved.

How does a rate-limiting enzyme work to control the speed of reactions? First, as a rule, rate-limiting

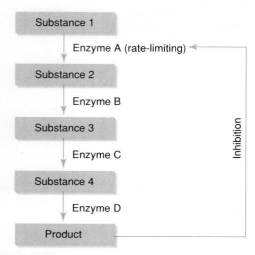

Figure 3.16
An example of a "rate-limiting" enzyme in a simple metabolic pathway. Here, a buildup of the product serves to inhibit the rate-limiting enzyme, which in turn slows down the reactions involved in the pathway.

enzymes are found early in a metabolic pathway. This position is important since products of the pathway might accumulate if the rate-limiting enzyme were located near the end of a pathway. Second, the activity of rate-limiting enzymes is regulated by modulators. Modulators are substances that increase or decrease enzyme activity. Enzymes that are regulated by modulators are called allosteric enzymes. In the control of energy metabolism, ATP is the classic example of an inhibitor, while ADP and P_i are examples of substances that stimulate enzymatic activity (6). The fact that large amounts of cellular ATP would inhibit the metabolic production of ATP is logical since large amounts of ATP would indicate that ATP usage in the cell is low. An example of this type of negative feedback is illustrated in figure 3.16. In contrast, an increase in cell levels of ADP and P_i (low ATP) would indicate that ATP utilization is high. Therefore, it makes sense that ADP and P_i stimulate the production of ATP to meet the increased energy need.

Control of ATP–PC System

Phosphocreatine breakdown is regulated by creatine kinase activity. Creatine kinase is activated when sarcoplasmic concentrations of ADP increase, and is inhibited by high levels of ATP. At the onset of exercise, ATP is split into ADP + P_i to provide energy for muscular contraction. This immediate increase in ADP concentrations stimulates creatine kinase to trigger the breakdown of PC to resynthesize ATP. If exercise is continued, glycolysis and finally aerobic metabolism begin to produce adequate ATP to meet the muscles' energy needs. The increase in ATP concentration, coupled with a reduction in ADP concentration, inhibits creatine kinase activity (table 3.2). Regulation of the ATP-PC system is an example of a "negative feedback" control system, which was introduced in chapter 2.

Control of Glycolysis

Although several factors serve to control glycolysis, the most important rate-limiting enzyme in glycolysis is **phosphofructokinase (PFK)** (33). Note that PFK is located near the beginning of glycolysis (figure 3.9). Table 3.2 lists known regulators of PFK. When exercise begins, ADP + P_i levels rise and enhance PFK activity, which serves to increase the rate of glycolysis. In contrast, at rest, when cellular ATP levels are high, PFK activity is inhibited and glycolytic activity is slowed. Further, high cellular levels of hydrogen ions, or citrate (produced via Krebs cycle) also inhibit PFK activity (36). Similar to the control of the ATP-PC system, regulation of PFK activity operates via negative feedback.

Another important regulatory enzyme in carbohydrate metabolism is phosphorylase, which is responsible for degrading glycogen to glucose. Although this enzyme is not technically considered a glycolytic enzyme, the reaction catalyzed by phosphorylase plays an important role in providing the glycolytic pathway with the necessary glucose at the origin of the pathway. With each muscle contraction, calcium (Ca^{++}) is released from the sarcoplasmic reticulum in muscle. This rise in sarcoplasmic Ca^{++} concentration indirectly activates phosphorylase, which immediately begins to break down glycogen to glucose for entry into glycolysis. Additionally, phosphorylase activity may be stimulated by high levels of the hormone epinephrine. Epinephrine is released at a faster rate during heavy exercise and results in the formation of the compound cyclic AMP (chapter 5). It is cyclic AMP, not epinephrine, that directly activates phosphorylase. Thus, the influence of epinephrine on phosphorylase is indirect.

Control of Krebs Cycle and Electron Transport Chain

The Krebs cycle, like glycolysis, is subject to enzymatic regulation. Although several Krebs cycle enzymes are regulated, the rate-limiting enzyme is **isocitrate dehydrogenase.** Isocitrate dehydrogenase, like PFK, is inhibited by ATP and stimulated by increasing levels of ADP + P_i (37, 39). Further, growing evidence suggests that increased levels of calcium (Ca^{++}) in the mitochondria also stimulates isocitrate dehydrogenase activity (26a). This is a logical signal to turn on energy metabolism in muscle cells since an increase in free calcium in muscle is the signal to begin muscular contraction (see chapter 8).

The electron transport chain is also regulated by the amount of ATP and ADP + P_i present (4, 37). When exercise begins, ATP levels decline, ADP + P_i levels increase, and cytochrome oxidase is stimulated to begin aerobic production of ATP. When exercise stops, cellular levels of ATP increase and ADP + P_i concentrations decline, and thus the electron transport activity is reduced when normal levels of ATP, ADP, and P_i are reached.

Table 3.2 Factors Known to Affect the Activity of Rate-Limiting Enzymes of Metabolic Pathways Involved in Bioenergetics

Pathway	Rate-Limiting Enzyme	Stimulators	Inhibitors
ATP-PC system	Creatine kinase	ADP	ATP
Glycolysis	Phosphofructokinase	AMP, ADP, P_i, pH$\uparrow$	ATP, CP, citrate, pH$\downarrow$
Krebs cycle	Isocitrate dehydrogenase	ADP, Ca^{++}, NAD	ATP, NADH
Electron transport chain	Cytochrome oxidase	ADP, P_i	ATP

Table 3.3 Contribution of Aerobic/Anaerobic Production of ATP During Maximal Exercise as a Function of the Duration of the Event

	Duration of Maximal Exercise								
	Seconds			Minutes					
	10	30	60	2	4	10	30	60	120
Percent aerobic	10	20	30	40	65	85	95	98	99
Percent anaerobic	90	80	70	60	35	15	5	2	1

Data from references 7 and 30.

in summary

- Metabolism is regulated by enzymatic activity. An enzyme that regulates a metabolic pathway is termed the "rate-limiting" enzyme.
- The rate-limiting enzyme for glycolysis is phosphofructokinase, while the rate limiting enzymes for the Krebs cycle and electron transport chain are isocitrate dehydrogenase and cytochrome oxidase, respectively.
- In general, cellular levels of ATP and ADP + P_i regulate the rate of metabolic pathways involved in the production of ATP. High levels of ATP inhibit further ATP production, while low levels of ATP and high levels of ADP + P_i stimulate ATP production. Evidence also exists that calcium may stimulate aerobic energy metabolism.

Interaction Between Aerobic/Anaerobic ATP Production

It is important to emphasize the interaction of anaerobic and aerobic metabolic pathways in the production of ATP during exercise. Although it is common to hear someone speak of aerobic versus anaerobic exercise, in reality the energy to perform most types of exercise comes from a combination of anaerobic/aerobic sources (7, 18, 26, 30). This point is illustrated in table 3.3. Notice that the contribution of anaerobic ATP production is greater in short-term, high-intensity activities, while aerobic metabolism predominates in longer activities. For example, approximately 90% of the energy to perform a 100-meter dash would come from anaerobic sources, with most of the energy coming via the ATP-PC system. Similarly, energy to run 400 meters (i.e., 55 seconds) would be largely anaerobic (70%–75%). However, ATP and PC stores are limited and thus glycolysis must supply much of the ATP during this type of an event (38).

On the other end of the energy spectrum, events like the marathon (i.e., 26.2-mile race) rely on aerobic production of ATP for the bulk of the needed energy. Where does the energy come from in events of moderate length (i.e., two to thirty minutes)? Table 3.3 provides an estimation of the percentage anaerobic/aerobic yield in events over a wide range of durations. Although these estimates are based on laboratory measurements of running or exercising on a cycle ergometer, they can be related to other athletic events that require intense effort by comparing the length of time spent in the activity.

In review, the shorter the duration of all-out activity, the greater the contribution of anaerobic energy production; conversely, the longer the duration, the greater the contribution of aerobic energy production. A more detailed discussion of the metabolic responses to various types of exercise is presented in chapter 4.

in summary

- Energy to perform exercise comes from an interaction of anaerobic and aerobic pathways.
- In general, the shorter the activity (high intensity), the greater the contribution of anaerobic energy production. In contrast, long-term activities (low to moderate intensity) utilize ATP produced from aerobic sources.

study questions

1. List and briefly discuss the function of the three major components of cell structure.
2. Briefly explain the concept of coupled reactions.
3. Define the following terms: (1) bioenergetics, (2) endergonic reactions, and (3) exergonic reactions.
4. Discuss the role of enzymes as catalysts. What is meant by the expression "energy of activation"?
5. Briefly, identify the common forms of carbohydrates, proteins, and fats. What role does each play as an energy source during exercise?
6. Define the terms glycogen, glycogenolysis, and glycolysis.
7. What are high-energy phosphates? Explain the statement that "ATP is the universal energy donor."
8. Define the terms aerobic and anaerobic.
9. Briefly discuss the function of glycolysis in bioenergetics. What role does NAD play in glycolysis?
10. Discuss the operation of the Krebs cycle and the electron transport chain in the aerobic production of ATP. What is the function of NAD and FAD in these pathways?
11. What is the efficiency of the aerobic degradation of glucose?
12. How is bioenergetics controlled? What are rate-limiting enzymes and how do they operate?
13. What enzyme regulates glycolysis? the Krebs cycle?
14. Briefly, discuss the interaction of anaerobic versus aerobic ATP production during exercise.
15. Discuss the chemiosmotic theory of ATP production.

suggested readings

Conley, K. 1994. Cellular energetics during exercise. *Advances in Veterinary Science and Comparative Medicine* 38a:1–39.

Houston, M. 1995. *Biochemistry Primer for Exercise Science.* Champaign, IL: Human Kinetics.

Kanter, M. 1994. Free radicals, exercise, and antioxidant supplementation. *International Journal of Sports Medicine* 4:205–20.

Maughan, R. 1995. Creatine supplementation and exercise performance. *International Journal of Sports Nutrition* 5:94–101.

references

1. Armstrong, R. 1979. Biochemistry: Energy liberation and use. In *Sports Medicine and Physiology*, ed. R. Strauss. Philadelphia: W. B. Saunders.
2. Balaban, R., and F. Heineman. 1989. Interaction of oxidative phosphorylation and work in the heart, In vivo. *News in Physiological Sciences* 4:215–18.
3. Barclay, J., and M. Hansel. 1991. Free radicals may contribute to oxidative skeletal muscle fatigue. *Canadian Journal of Physiology and Pharmacology* 69:279–84.
4. Bessman, S., and C. Carpender. 1985. The creatine phosphate shuttle. *Annual Review of Biochemistry* 54:831–62.
5. Booth, F. 1989. Application of molecular biology in exercise physiology. In *Exercise and Sport Sciences Reviews*, vol. 17, 1–28. Baltimore: Williams & Wilkins.
6. Brazy, P., and L. Mandel. 1986. Does availability of inorganic phosphate regulate cellular oxidative metabolism? *News in Physiological Sciences* 1:100–102.
7. Brooks, G., and T. Fahey. 1984. *Exercise Physiology: Human Bioenergetics and Its Applications.* New York: John Wiley & Sons.
8. Cerretelli, P., D. Rennie, and D. Pendergast. 1980. Kinetics of metabolic transients during exercise. *International Journal of Sports Medicine* 55:171–80.
8a. Conley, K. 1994. Cellular energetics during exercise. *Advances in Veterinary Science and Comparative Medicine* 38a:1–39.
9. Davies, K., A. Quintanilha, G. Brooks, and L. Packer. 1982. Free radical and tissue damage produced by exercise. *Biochemistry and Biophysics Research Communications* 107:1198–1205.
10. De Zwaan, A., and G. Thillard. 1985. Low and high power output modes of anaerobic metabolism: Invertebrate and vertebrate categories. In *Circulation, Respiration, and Metabolism*, ed. R. Giles, 166–92. Berlin: Springer-Verlag.
11. di Prampero, P., U. Boutellier, and P. Pietsch. 1983. Oxygen deficit and stores at the onset of muscular exercise in humans. *Journal of Applied Physiology* 55:146–53.
12. Dolny, D., and P. Lemon. 1988. Effect of ambient temperature on protein breakdown during prolonged exercise. *Journal of Applied Physiology* 64:550–55.
13. Fox, S. 1996. *Human Physiology.* Dubuque, IA: Wm. C. Brown.
14. Giese, A. 1979. *Cell Physiology.* Philadelphia: W. B. Saunders.
15. Gollnick, P. 1985. Metabolism of substrates: Energy substrate metabolism during exercise and as modified by training. *Federation Proceedings* 44:353–56.
16. Gollnick, P. et al. 1985. Differences in metabolic potential of skeletal muscle fibers and their significance for metabolic control. *Journal of Experimental Biology* 115:191–95.
16a. Greenhaff, P. 1995. Creatine and its application as an ergogenic aid. *International Journal of Sports Nutrition* 5: (supplement), s100–s110.
17. Hole, J. 1993. *Human Anatomy and Physiology.* Dubuque, IA: Wm. C. Brown.
18. Holloszy, J. 1982. Muscle metabolism during exercise. *Archives of Physical and Rehabilitation Medicine* 63:231–34.

19. Holloszy, J., and E. Coyle. 1984. Adaptations of skeletal muscle to endurance exercise and their metabolic consequences. *Journal of Applied Physiology* 56:831–38.

19a. Houston, M. 1995. *Biochemistry Primer for Exercise Science*. Champaign, IL: Human Kinetics.

20. Jain, M. 1972. *The Biomolecular Lipid Membrane: A System*. New York: Reinhold.

21. Jequier, E., and J. Flatt. 1986. Recent advances in human bioenergetics. *News in Physiological Sciences* 1:112–14.

22. Johnson, L. 1983. *Biology*. Dubuque, IA: Wm. C. Brown.

22a. Lawler, J., S. Powers, T. Visser, H. Van Dijk, M. Kordus, and L. Ji. Acute exercise and skeletal muscle antioxidant and metabolic enzymes: Effects of fiber type and age. *American Journal of Physiology* 265:R1344–R1350, 1993.

23. Lemon, P., and J. Mullin. 1980. Effect of initial muscle glycogen levels on protein catabolism during exercise. *Journal of Applied Physiology* 48:624–29.

24. MacLean, D., L. Spriet, E. Hultman, and T. Graham. 1991. Plasma and muscle amino acid and ammonia responses during exercise in humans. *Journal of Applied Physiology* 70:2095–2103.

25. Mathews, C., and K. van Holde. 1990. *Biochemistry*. Redwood City, CA: Benjamin-Cummings.

25a. Maughan, R. 1995. Creatine supplementation and exercise performance. *International Journal of Sports Nutrition* 5:94–101.

26. McArdle, W., F. Katch, and V. Katch. 1991. *Exercise Physiology*. Philadelphia: Lea & Febiger.

26a. McCormack, J., and R. Denton. 1994. Signal transduction by intramitochondrial calcium in mammalian energy metabolism. *News in Physiological Sciences*. 9:71–76.

27. McGilvery, R. 1983. *Biochemistry: A Functional Approach*. Philadelphia: W. B. Saunders.

28. McMurray, W. 1977. *Essentials of Human Metabolism*. New York: Harper & Row.

29. Miller, F. 1987. *College Physics*. New York: Harcourt Brace Jovanovich.

30. Mole, P. 1983. Exercise metabolism. In *Exercise Medicine: Physiological Principles and Clinical Application*. New York: Academic Press.

31. Nave, C., and B. Nave. 1985. *Physics of the Health Sciences*. Philadelphia: W. B. Saunders.

32. Newsholme, E. 1979. The control of fuel utilization by muscle during exercise and starvation. *Diabetes* 28 (Suppl.):1–7.

33. Newsholme E., and A. Leech. 1988. *Biochemistry for the Medical Sciences*. New York: J. Wiley & Sons.

33a. Reid, M., K. Haack, K. Franchek, P. Valberg, L. Kobzik, and M. West. 1992. Reactive oxygen in skeletal muscle. I. Intracellular oxidant kinetics and fatigue in vitro. *Journal of Applied Physiology* 73:1797–1804.

34. Sears, C., and C. Stanitski. 1983. *Chemistry for the Health-Related Sciences*. Englewood Cliffs, NJ: Prentice-Hall.

35. Senior, A. 1988. ATP synthesis by oxidative phosphorylation. *Physiological Reviews* 68:177–216.

36. Spriet L. 1991. Phosphofructokinase activity and acidosis during short-term tetanic contractions. *Canadian Journal of Physiology and Pharmacology* 69 298–304.

37. Stanley W., and R. Connett. 1991. Regulation of muscle carbohydrate metabolism during exercise. *FASEB Journal* 5:2155–59.

38. Stryer, L. 1988. *Biochemistry*. San Francisco: W. H. Freeman.

39. Suttie, J. 1977. *Introduction to Biochemistry*. New York: Holt, Rinehart & Winston.

40. Tulson, P., and R. Terjung. 1991. Adenine nucleotide metabolism in contracting skeletal muscle. *Exercise and Sport Science Reviews*, vol. 19, 507–37. Baltimore: Williams & Wilkins.

41. Weibel, E. 1984. *The Pathway for Oxygen*. Cambridge: Harvard University Press.

42. West, J. 1985. *Best's and Taylor's Physiological Basis of Medical Practice*. Baltimore: Williams & Wilkins.

43. Whipp, B., and M. Mahler. 1980. Dynamics of pulmonary gas exchange during exercise. In *Pulmonary Gas Exchange*, vol. 2, ed. J. West. New York: Academic Press.

4

Exercise Metabolism

objectives

By studying this chapter, you should be able to do the following:

1. Discuss the relationship between exercise intensity/duration and the bioenergetic pathways that are most responsible for production of ATP during various types of exercise.
2. Define the term oxygen deficit.
3. Define the term lactate threshold.
4. Discuss several possible explanations for the sudden rise in blood-lactate concentration during incremental exercise.
5. List the factors that regulate fuel selection during different types of exercise.
6. Explain why fat metabolism is dependent on carbohydrate metabolism.
7. Define the term oxygen debt.
8. Give the physiological explanation for the observation that the O_2 debt is greater following intense exercise when compared to the O_2 debt following light exercise.

outline

Rest-to-Exercise Transitions 46
Recovery from Exercise: Metabolic Responses 47
Metabolic Responses to Exercise: Influence of Duration and Intensity 49
   Short-Term Intense Exercise 49
   Prolonged Exercise 50
   Incremental Exercise 50

Estimation of Fuel Utilization During Exercise 53
Factors Governing Fuel Selection 53
   Exercise Intensity and Fuel Selection 54
   Exercise Duration and Fuel Selection 55

Interaction of Fat/Carbohydrate Metabolism 55
Body Fuel Stores 56

key terms

anaerobic threshold
Cori cycle
EPOC
free fatty acid (FFA)
gluconeogenesis

graded exercise test
incremental exercise test
lactate threshold
lipase
lipolysis

maximal oxygen uptake ($\dot{V}O_2$ max)
oxygen debt
oxygen deficit
respiratory exchange ratio (R)

Exercise poses a serious challenge to the bioenergetic pathways in the working muscle. For example, during heavy exercise the body's total energy expenditure may increase fifteen to twenty-five times above expenditure at rest. Most of this increase in energy production is used to provide ATP for contracting skeletal muscles, which may increase their energy utilization two hundred times over utilization at rest (1). Therefore, it is apparent that skeletal muscles have a great capacity to produce and use large quantities of ATP during exercise. This chapter will describe: (1) the metabolic responses at the beginning of exercise and during recovery from exercise; (2) the metabolic responses to high intensity, incremental, and prolonged exercise; (3) the selection of fuels used to produce ATP; and (4) how exercise metabolism is regulated. We begin with a discussion of which bioenergetic pathways are involved in energy production at the beginning of exercise.

Rest-to-Exercise Transitions

Suppose an individual steps onto a treadmill belt that is moving at 6 mph. Within one step the muscles must increase their rate of ATP production from that required for standing to that required for running at 6 mph. If not, the individual would exit off the back of the treadmill. What metabolic changes must occur in skeletal muscle at the beginning of exercise to provide the necessary energy to continue movement? Since the measurement of oxygen (O_2) consumption can be used as an index of aerobic ATP production, measurement of O_2 consumption during exercise can provide information about aerobic metabolism during exercise. For example, in the transition from rest to light or moderate exercise, O_2 consumption increases rapidly and reaches a steady state within one to four minutes (9, 16, 62) (figure 4.1). The fact that O_2 consumption does not increase instantaneously to a steady state value suggests that anaerobic energy sources contribute to the overall production of ATP at the beginning of exercise. Indeed, there is much evidence to suggest that at the onset of exercise the ATP-PC system is the first active bioenergetic pathway, followed by glycolysis and, finally, aerobic energy production (2, 12, 27, 50, 69). However, after a steady state is reached, the body's ATP requirement is met via aerobic metabolism. The major point to be emphasized concerning the bioenergetics of rest-to-work transitions is that several energy systems are involved. In other words, the energy needed for exercise is not provided by simply turning on a single bioenergetic pathway, but rather by a mixture of several metabolic systems operating with considerable overlap.

The term **oxygen deficit** applies to the lag in oxygen uptake at the beginning of exercise. Specifically, the oxygen deficit is defined as the difference between oxygen uptake in the first few minutes of exercise and an equal time period after steady state has been obtained (61, 67). This is represented as the shaded area in the left-hand portion of figure 4.1. Note in figure 4.2 that the time to reach steady state is shorter in trained subjects when compared to untrained subjects (44, 62). This difference in the time course of oxygen uptake at the onset of exercise between trained and untrained subjects results in the trained subjects having a lower oxygen deficit when compared to the untrained. What is the explanation for this difference? It seems likely that the trained subjects have a better developed aerobic bioenergetic capacity, resulting from either cardiovascular or muscular adaptations induced by endurance training (22, 44, 62, 67). Practically speaking, this means that aerobic ATP production is active earlier at the beginning of exercise and results in less production of lactic acid in the trained individual when compared to the untrained individual. Chapter 13 provides a detailed analysis of this adaptation to training.

Figure 4.2

Differences in the time course of oxygen uptake during the transition from rest to submaximal exercise between trained and untrained subjects. Note that the time to reach steady state is slower in untrained subjects. See text for details.

Figure 4.1

The time course of oxygen uptake ($\dot{V}O_2$) in the transition from rest to submaximal exercise.

in summary

- In the transition from rest to light or moderate exercise, oxygen uptake increases rapidly, generally reaching a steady state within one to four minutes.
- The term oxygen deficit applies to the lag in oxygen uptake at the beginning of exercise.
- The failure of oxygen uptake to increase instantly at the beginning of exercise suggests that anaerobic pathways contribute to the overall production of ATP early in exercise. After a steady state is reached, the body's ATP requirement is met via aerobic metabolism.

Recovery from Exercise: Metabolic Responses

Metabolism remains elevated for several minutes immediately following exercise. The magnitude and duration of this elevated metabolism is influenced by the intensity of the exercise (4, 37, 67). This point is illustrated in figure 4.3. Note that oxygen uptake is greater and remains elevated for a longer time period following high-intensity exercise when compared to exercise of light-to-moderate intensity (37, 38). The reason(s) for this observation will be discussed shortly.

Historically, the term **oxygen debt** has been applied to mean the excess oxygen uptake above rest following exercise. The prominent British physiologist A. V. Hill (45) first used the term O_2 debt and reasoned that the excess oxygen consumed (above rest) following exercise was repayment for the O_2 deficit incurred at the onset of exercise. Evidence collected in the 1920s and 1930s by Hill and other researchers in Europe and the United States suggested that the oxygen debt could be divided into two portions: the rapid portion immediately following exercise (i.e., approximately two to three minutes post exercise) and the slow portion, which persisted for greater than thirty minutes after exercise. The rapid portion is represented by the steep decline in oxygen uptake following exercise, and the slow portion is represented by the slow decline in O_2 across time following exercise (figure 4.3). The rationale for the two divisions of the O_2 debt was based on the belief that the rapid portion of the O_2 debt represented the oxygen that was required to resynthesize stored ATP and PC and replace tissue stores of O_2 (~20% of the O_2 debt), while the slow portion of the debt was due to the oxidative conversion of lactic acid to glucose in the liver (~80% of the O_2 debt).

Contradicting previous beliefs, recent evidence has shown that only about 20% of the oxygen debt is used to convert the lactic acid produced during exercise to glucose (the process of glucose synthesis from

(a) Light exercise

(b) Heavy exercise

Figure 4.3

Oxygen deficit and debt during light/moderate exercise (*a*) and during heavy exercise (*b*).

noncarbohydrate sources is called **gluconeogenesis**) (11, 13). Therefore, the notion that the "slow" portion of the O_2 debt is due entirely to oxidative conversion of lactic acid to glucose does not appear to be accurate. Several investigators have argued that the term oxygen debt be eliminated from the literature because the elevated oxygen consumption following exercise does not appear to be entirely due to the "borrowing" of oxygen from the body's oxygen stores (11, 13, 15, 30). In recent years several replacement terms have been suggested. One such term is **EPOC**, which stands for "excess post-exercise oxygen consumption" (15, 30).

If the EPOC is not exclusively used to convert lactic acid to glucose, why does oxygen consumption remain elevated post exercise? Several possibilities exist. First, at least part of the O_2 consumed immediately following exercise is used to restore PC in muscle and O_2 stores in blood and tissues (9, 30). Restoration of both PC and oxygen stores in muscle is completed within two to three minutes of recovery (41). This is consistent with the classic view of the rapid portion of the oxygen debt. Further, heart rate and breathing remain elevated above resting levels for several minutes following exercise; therefore, both of these activities require additional O_2 above resting levels. Other factors that may result in the EPOC are an elevated body temperature and specific

Removal of Lactic Acid Following Exercise

What happens to the lactic acid that is formed during exercise? Classical theory proposed that the majority of the post-exercise lactic acid was converted into glucose in the liver and resulted in an elevated post-exercise oxygen uptake (i.e., O_2 debt). However, recent evidence suggests that this is not the case and that lactic acid is mainly oxidized after exercise (11,13). That is, lactic acid is converted to pyruvic acid and used as a substrate by the heart and skeletal muscle. It is estimated that approximately 70% of the lactic acid produced during exercise is oxidized, while 20% is converted to glucose and the remaining 10% is converted to amino acids.

Figure 4.4 demonstrates the time course of lactic acid removal from the blood following strenuous exercise. Note that lactic acid removal is more rapid if continuous light exercise is performed as compared to a resting recovery. The explanation for these findings is linked to the fact that light exercise enhances oxidation of lactic acid by the working muscle (21, 32, 43). It is estimated that the optimum intensity of recovery exercise to promote blood lactic acid removal is

Figure 4.4

Blood lactate removal following strenuous exercise. Note that lactic acid can be removed more rapidly from the blood during recovery if the subject engages in continuous light exercise.

around 30%–40% of $\dot{V}O_2$ max (21). Higher exercise intensities would likely result in an increased muscle production of lactic acid and therefore hinder removal.

Due to the increase in muscle oxidative capacity observed with endurance training, some authors have speculated that trained subjects might have a greater capacity to remove lactic acid during recovery from

intense exercise (5, 7). Unfortunately, human studies examining the effects of training on the rate of blood lactate decline (following heavy exercise) have yielded conflicting results. However, two well-designed investigations have reported no differences in blood lactic acid disappearance between trained and untrained subjects during resting recovery from a maximal exercise bout (5, 28).

---

circulating hormones. Increases in body temperature result in an increased metabolic rate (called the Q_{10} effect) (14, 40, 65). Further, it has been argued that high levels of epinephrine or norepinephrine result in increased oxygen consumption after exercise (31). However, both of these hormones are rapidly removed from the blood following exercise and therefore may not exist long enough to have a significant impact on the EPOC.

Earlier it was mentioned that the EPOC was greater following high-intensity exercise when compared to the EPOC following light-to-moderate work. This difference in EPOC is due to differences in the amount of body heat gained, the total PC depleted, and the blood levels of epinephrine and norephinephrine

(37). First, assuming similar ambient conditions (i.e., room temperature/relative humidity) and equal exercise time, high-intensity exercise will result in greater body heat gain than light exercise. Secondly, depletion of PC is dependent on exercise intensity. Since high-intensity exercise would utilize more PC, additional oxygen would be required during recovery for resynthesis. Finally, intense exercise results in greater blood concentrations of lactic acid, epinephrine, and norepinephrine when compared to light work. All of these factors may contribute to the EPOC being greater following intense exercise than following light exercise. Figure 4.5 contains a summary of factors thought to contribute to the "excess post-exercise oxygen consumption."

Factors Contributing to Excess Post-Exercise Oxygen Consumption

Figure 4.5
A summary of factors that might contribute to excess post-exercise oxygen consumption (EPOC). See text for details.

in summary

- The oxygen debt (also called excess post-exercise oxygen consumption (EPOC)) is the O_2 consumption above rest following exercise.
- Several factors contribute to the EPOC. First, some of the O_2 consumed early in the recovery period is used to resynthesize stored PC in the muscle and replace O_2 stores in both muscle and blood. Other factors that contribute to the "slow" portion of the EPOC include an elevated body temperature, O_2 required to convert lactic acid to glucose (gluconeogenesis), and elevated blood levels of epinephrine and norepinephrine.

Metabolic Responses to Exercise: Influence of Duration and Intensity

The point was made in chapter 3 that short-term, high-intensity exercise lasting less than ten seconds utilizes primarily anaerobic metabolic pathways to produce ATP. In contrast, an event like the marathon makes primary use of aerobic ATP production to provide the needed ATP for work. However, events lasting longer than ten to twenty seconds and less than ten minutes generally produce the needed ATP for muscular contraction via a combination of both anaerobic/aerobic pathways. In fact, most sports use a combination of anaerobic/aerobic pathways for production of the needed ATP for muscular contraction. The next three sections consider which bioenergetic pathways are involved in energy production in specific types of exercise.

Short-Term Intense Exercise

The energy to perform short-term exercise of high intensity comes primarily from anaerobic metabolic pathways. Whether the ATP production is dominated by the ATP-PC system or glycolysis depends primarily on the length of the activity (1, 2, 50, 54). For example, the energy to run a 50-meter dash, or complete a single play in a football game comes principally from the ATP-PC system. In contrast, the energy to complete the 400-meter dash (i.e., fifty-five seconds) comes from a combination of the ATP-PC system, glycolysis, and aerobic metabolism, with glycolysis producing most of the ATP. In general, the ATP-PC system can supply almost all the needed ATP for work for events lasting one to five seconds; intense exercise lasting longer than five to six seconds begins to utilize the ATP-producing capability of glycolysis. It should be emphasized that the transition from the ATP-PC system to an increased dependence upon glycolysis during exercise is not an abrupt change but rather a gradual shift from one pathway to another.

Events lasting longer than forty-five seconds use a combination of all three energy systems (i.e., ATP-PC, glycolysis, and aerobic systems). This point was emphasized in table 3.3 in chapter 3. In general, intense exercise lasting approximately sixty seconds utilizes 70%/30% (anaerobic/aerobic) energy production, while events lasting two minutes utilize anaerobic and aerobic bioenergetic pathways almost equally to supply the needed ATP (see table 3.3).

in summary

- During high-intensity, short-term exercise (i.e., two to twenty seconds), the muscle's ATP production is dominated by the ATP-PC system.
- Intense exercise lasting more than twenty seconds relies more on anaerobic glycolysis to produce much of the needed ATP.
- Finally, high-intensity events lasting longer than forty-five seconds use a combination of the ATP-PC system, glycolysis, and the aerobic system to produce the needed ATP for muscular contraction.

Prolonged Exercise

The energy to perform long-term exercise (i.e., > ten minutes) comes primarily from aerobic metabolism. A steady state oxygen uptake can generally be maintained during submaximal exercise of moderate duration. However, two exceptions to this rule exist. First, prolonged exercise in a hot/humid environment results in a "drift" upward of oxgyen uptake; therefore, a steady state is not maintained in this type of exercise (65). Second, continuous exercise at a high relative work rate (i.e., >75% $\dot{V}O_2$ max) results in a slow rise in oxygen uptake across time (40) (figure 4.6). In each of these two types of exercise, the drift upward in $\dot{V}O_2$ is due principally to the effects of increasing body temperature and to a lesser degree to rising blood levels of the hormones epinephrine and norepinephrine (14, 30, 31, 40, 53). Both of these variables tend to increase the metabolic rate resulting in increased oxygen uptake across time.

in summary

- The energy to perform prolonged exercise (i.e., > ten minutes) comes primarily from aerobic metabolism.
- A steady state oxygen uptake can generally be maintained during prolonged low-intensity exercise. However, exercise in a hot/humid environment or exercise at a high relative work rate results in an upward "drift" in oxygen consumption over time; therefore a steady state is not obtained in these types of exercise.

Incremental Exercise

The maximal capacity to transport and utilize oxygen during exercise (**maximal oxygen uptake or $\dot{V}O_2$ max**) is considered by many exercise scientists to be the most valid measurement of cardiovascular fitness. Indeed, **incremental exercise tests** (also called **graded exercise tests**) are often employed by physicians to examine patients for possible heart disease and by exercise scientists to determine a subject's cardiovascular fitness. These tests are usually conducted on a treadmill or a cycle ergometer. However, an arm crank ergometer can be employed for testing paraplegics or athletes whose sport involves arm work (e.g., swimmers, rowers, etc.). The test generally begins with the subject performing a brief warm-up, followed by an increase in the work rate every one to three minutes until the subject cannot maintain the desired power output. This increase in work rate can be achieved on the treadmill by increasing either the speed of the treadmill or the incline. On the cycle or arm ergometer, the increase in power output is obtained by increasing the resistance against the flywheel.

Figure 4.7 illustrates the change in oxygen uptake during a typical incremental exercise test on a cycle ergometer. Oxygen uptake increases as a linear function

Figure 4.6
Comparison of oxygen uptake ($\dot{V}O_2$) across time during prolonged exercise in a hot and humid environment (*a*) and during prolonged exercise at a high relative work rate (>75% $\dot{V}O_2$ max) (*b*). Note that in both conditions there is a steady "drift" upward in $\dot{V}O_2$. See text for description.

Figure 4.7
Changes in oxygen uptake ($\dot{V}O_2$) during an incremental exercise test. The observed plateau in $\dot{V}O_2$ represents $\dot{V}O_2$ max.

of the work rate until $\dot{V}O_2$ max is reached. When $\dot{V}O_2$ max is reached, an increase in power output does not result in an increase in oxygen uptake; thus, $\dot{V}O_2$ max represents a "physiological ceiling" for the ability of the oxygen transport system to deliver O_2 to contracting muscles. The physiological factors that influence $\dot{V}O_2$ max include the following: (1) the maximum ability of

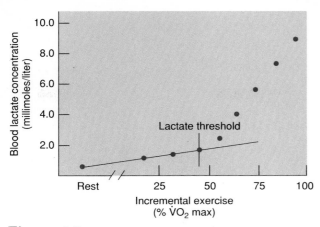

Figure 4.8

Changes in blood lactic acid concentrations during incremental exercise. The sudden rise in lactate is known as the lactate threshold.

Figure 4.9

Failure of the mitochondrial "hydrogen shuttle" system to keep pace with the rate of glycolytic production of NADH + H⁺ results in the conversion of pyruvic acid to lactic acid.

the cardiorespiratory system to deliver oxygen to the contracting muscle; and (2) the muscle's ability to take up the oxygen and produce ATP aerobically. Both genetics and exercise training are known to influence $\dot{V}O_2$ max and will be discussed in chapter 13.

Lactate Threshold

It is generally believed that most of the ATP production used to provide energy for muscular contraction during the early stages of an incremental exercise test comes from aerobic sources (59, 64, 72). However, as the exercise intensity increases, blood levels of lactic acid begin to rise in an exponential fashion (figure 4.8). This appears in untrained subjects around 50%–60% of $\dot{V}O_2$ max, while it occurs at higher work rates in trained subjects (i.e., 65%–80% $\dot{V}O_2$ max) (34). Although there is disagreement on the point, many investigators believe that this sudden rise in lactic acid during incremental exercise represents a point of increasing reliance on anaerobic metabolism (i.e., glycolysis) (19, 76–80). A common term used to describe the point of a systematic rise in blood lactic acid during exercise is the **anaerobic threshold** (10, 20, 26, 46, 52, 63, 78, 79, 83). However, arguments over terminology exist and this lactic acid inflection point has also been called the **lactate threshold** and the "onset of blood lactate accumulation" (OBLA) by some investigators (25, 42). To avoid confusion, we will refer to the sudden rise in blood lactic acid during incremental exercise as the "lactate threshold."

The basic argument against the term "anaerobic threshold" centers around the question of whether the rise in blood lactic acid during incremental exercise is due to a lack of oxygen (hypoxia) in the working muscle or occurs for other reasons. Historically, rising blood lactic acid levels have been considered an indication of increased anaerobic metabolism within the contracting muscle due to low levels of O_2

in the individual muscle cells (78, 79). However, whether the end product of glycolysis is pyruvic or lactic acid depends on a variety of factors. First, if the rate of glycolysis is rapid, then NADH production may exceed the transport capacity of the shuttle mechanisms that move hydrogens from the sarcoplasm into the mitochondria (73, 75, 82). Indeed, blood levels of epinephrine and norepinephrine begin to rise at 50%–65% of $\dot{V}O_2$ max during incremental exercise and have been shown to stimulate the glycolytic rate; this increase in glycolysis increases the rate of NADH production (75). Failure of the shuttle system to keep up with the rate of NADH production by glycolysis would result in pyruvic acid accepting some "unshuttled" hydrogens, and the formation of lactic acid could occur independent of whether the muscle cell had sufficient oxygen for aerobic ATP production (figure 4.9).

A second explanation for the formation of lactic acid in exercising muscle is related to the enzyme that catalyzes the conversion of pyruvate to lactate acid. The enzyme responsible for this reaction is lactate dehydrogenase (LDH) and exists in several forms (i.e., different forms of the same enzyme are called isozymes). Recall that the reaction is as follows:

$$\begin{array}{c} CH_3 \\ | \\ C = O \\ | \\ COO^- \end{array} + NADH + H^+ \xrightarrow{LDH} \begin{array}{c} CH_3 \\ | \\ H-C-OH \\ | \\ COO^- \end{array} + NAD$$

Pyruvate   Lactate

This reaction is reversible in that lactic acid can be converted back to pyruvic acid under the appropriate conditions. Human skeletal muscle can be classified into three different fiber types (chapter 8). One of these fiber types is labeled as "slow" fibers (sometimes called slow-twitch), whereas the remaining two are labeled as "fast" fibers (sometimes called fast-twitch). As the names imply, fast fibers are recruited during intense, rapid exercise, while slow fibers are used primarily during low-intensity activity. The LDH isozyme found in fast fibers has a greater affinity for attaching to pyruvic acid, promoting the formation of lactic acid (47, 72). In contrast, slow fibers contain an LDH form that promotes the conversion of lactic acid to pyruvic acid. Therefore, lactic acid formation might occur in fast fibers during exercise simply because of the type of LDH present. Thus, lactic acid production would again be independent of oxygen availability in the muscle cell. Early in an incremental exercise test it is likely that slow fibers are the first called into action. However, as the exercise intensity increases, the amount of muscular force developed must be increased. This increased muscular force is supplied by recruiting more and more fast fibers. Therefore, the involvement of more fast fibers may result in increased lactic acid production and thus be responsible for the lactate threshold.

A final explanation for the lactate threshold may be related to the rate of removal of lactic acid from the blood during incremental exercise. When a researcher removes a blood sample from an exercising subject the concentration of lactic acid in that sample is the difference between the amount of lactic acid entry into the blood and the rate of lactic acid removal from the blood. At any given time during exercise, some muscles are producing lactic acid and releasing it into the blood, and some tissues (e.g., liver, skeletal muscles, heart, etc.) are removing lactic acid. Therefore, the concentration of lactic acid in the blood at any given time can be expressed mathematically in the following way:

$$\text{Blood lactic acid concentration} = \text{lactic acid entry into the blood} - \text{blood lactic acid removal}$$

Thus a rise in the blood lactic acid concentration can occur due to either an increase in lactic acid production or a decrease in lactic acid removal. Recent evidence suggests that the rise in blood lactic acid levels in animals during incremental exercise may be the result of both an increase in lactic acid production and a decrease in the rate of lactic acid removal (12, 25). See chapter 13 for a discussion of how endurance training affects lactic acid production.

To summarize, controversy exists over both the terminology and the mechanism to explain the sudden rise in blood lactic acid concentrations during incremental exercise. It is possible that any one or a combination of the above explanations (including lack of O_2) might provide an explanation for the lactate threshold. Figure 4.10 contains a summary of possible mechanisms to explain the lactate threshold. The search for definitive evidence to explain the mechanism(s) altering the blood lactate concentration during incremental exercise will continue for years to come.

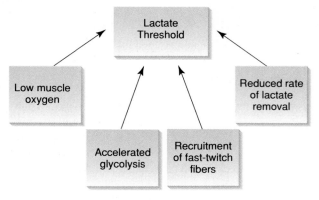

Potential causes of lactate threshold

Figure 4.10
Possible mechanisms to explain the lactate threshold during incremental exercise. See text for details.

Practical Use of the Lactate Threshold
Regardless of the physiological mechanism to explain the lactate threshold, the point of exponential rise in lactic acid during graded exercise has important implications for predicting sports performance and perhaps in planning training programs for endurance athletes. For example, several studies have demonstrated that the lactate threshold used in combination with other physiological measurements (e.g., $\dot{V}O_2$ max), is a useful predictor of success in distance running (29, 60). Further, the lactate threshold might serve as a guideline for coaches and athletes in planning the level of exercise intensity needed to optimize training results. This will be discussed in more detail in chapters 16 and 21.

in summary
- Oxygen uptake increases in a linear fashion during incremental exercise until $\dot{V}O_2$ max is reached.
- The point at which blood lactic acid rises systematically during graded exercise is termed the lactate threshold or anaerobic threshold.
- Controversy exists over the mechanism to explain the sudden rise in blood lactic acid concentrations during incremental exercise. It is possible that any one or a combination of the following factors might provide an explanation for the lactate threshold: (1) low muscle oxygen, (2) accelerated glycolysis, (3) recruitment of fast fibers, and (4) a reduced rate of lactate removal.
- The lactate threshold has practical uses such as in performance prediction and as a marker of training intensity.

Estimation of Fuel Utilization During Exercise

A noninvasive technique that is commonly used to estimate the percent contribution of carbohydrate or fat to energy metabolism during exercise is the ratio of carbon dioxide output ($\dot{V}CO_2$) to the volume of oxygen consumed ($\dot{V}O_2$). This ratio ($\dot{V}CO_2/\dot{V}O_2$) is called the **respiratory exchange ratio (R).** During steady state conditions the $\dot{V}CO_2/\dot{V}O_2$ ratio is often termed the respiratory quotient (RQ). For simplicity, we will refer to the $\dot{V}CO_2/\dot{V}O_2$ ratio as the respiratory exchange ratio (R). How can the R be used to estimate whether fat or carbohydrate is being used as a fuel? The answer is related to the fact that fat and carbohydrate differ in the amount of O_2 used and CO_2 produced during oxidation. When using R as a predictor of fuel utilization during exercise, the role that protein contributes to ATP production during exercise is ignored. This is reasonable since protein generally plays a small role as a substrate during physical activity. Therefore, the R during exercise is often termed a "nonprotein R."

Let's consider the R for fat first. When fat is oxidized, O_2 combines with carbon to form CO_2 and joins with hydrogen to form water. The chemical relationship is as follows:

> Fat (palmitic acid) $C_{16}H_{32}O_2$
> Oxidation : $C_{16}H_{32}O_2 + 23\ O_2 \rightarrow 16\ CO_2 + 16\ H_2O$
> Therefore the $R = \dot{V}CO_2 \div \dot{V}O_2 = 16\ CO_2 \div 23\ O_2$
> $= 0.70$

In order for R to be used as an estimate of substrate utilization during exercise, the subject must have reached a steady state. This is important because only during steady state exercise is the $\dot{V}CO_2$ and $\dot{V}O_2$ reflective of O_2 and CO_2 exchange in the tissues. For example, if a person is hyperventilating (i.e., breathing too much for a particular metabolic rate), excessive CO_2 loss could bias the ratio of $\dot{V}CO_2$ to $\dot{V}O_2$ and invalidate the use of R to estimate which fuel is being consumed.

Carbohydrate oxidation also results in a predictable ratio of the volume of oxygen consumed to the amount of CO_2 produced. The oxidation of carbohydrate results in an R of 1.0:

> Glucose $= C_6H_{12}O_6$
> Oxidation : $C_6H_{12}O_6 + 6\ O_2 \rightarrow 6\ CO_2 + 6\ H_2O$
> $R = \dot{V}CO_2 \div \dot{V}O_2 = 6\ CO_2 \div 6\ O_2 = 1$

Fat oxidation requires more O_2 than does carbohydrate oxidation. This is due to the fact that carbohydrate contains more O_2 than does fat (75).

It is unlikely that either fat or carbohydrate would be the singular substrate used during most types of submaximal exercise. Therefore, the exercise R would likely be somewhere between 1.0 and 0.70. Table 4.1 lists a range of R values and the percentage of fat or carbohydrate metabolism they represent. Note that a nonprotein R of 0.85 represents a condition where fat and carbohydrate contribute equally as energy substrates. Further, notice that the higher the R, the greater the role of carbohydrate as an energy source, and the lower the R, the greater the contribution of fat.

Table 4.1	Percentage of Fat and Carbohydrate Metabolized as Determined by a Nonprotein Respiratory Exchange Ratio (R)	
R	% Fat	% Carbohydrate
0.70	100	0
0.75	83	17
0.80	67	33
0.85	50	50
0.90	33	67
0.95	17	83
1.00	0	100

in summary

- The respiratory exchange ratio (R) is the ratio of carbon dioxide produced to the oxygen consumed ($\dot{V}CO_2/\dot{V}O_2$).
- In order for R to be used as an estimate of substrate utilization during exercise, the subject must have reached a steady state. This is important because only during steady state exercise is the CO_2 and O_2 reflective of metabolic exchange of gases in tissues.

Factors Governing Fuel Selection

Proteins contribute less than 2% of the substrate used during exercise of less than one hour duration. However, the role of proteins as a fuel source may increase slightly during prolonged exercise (i.e., three to five hours duration). During this type of exercise, the total contribution of protein to the fuel supply may reach 5%–15% during the final minutes of work (8, 15, 49, 56, 57, 68, 81). Therefore, proteins play only a minor role as a substrate during exercise, with fat and carbohydrate serving as the major sources of energy during activity in the healthy individual consuming a balanced diet. Whether fat or carbohydrate is the primary substrate during work is determined by several factors, including diet and the intensity and duration of exercise. For example, high-fat and low-carbohydrate diets promote a high rate of fat metabolism. In regard to exercise intensity, low-intensity exercise relies primarily on fat as fuel

A Closer Look 4.2

Regulation of Glycogen Breakdown During Exercise

Much of the carbohydrate broken down via glycolysis during moderate-to high-intensity exercise comes from intramuscular glycogen stores. Glycogen storage in muscle is dependent on the availability of glucose and the activity of the enzyme glycogen synthetase. Elevated blood levels of insulin and glucose along with high glycogen synthetase activity promotes glycogen storage in muscle.

Breakdown of glycogen (glycogenolysis) into individual glucose molecules is dependent on the enzyme phosphorylase (74). In nonworking muscle, phosphorylase is generally found in an inactive form and thus must be "activated" before glycogen breakdown can occur. This activation of phosphorylase is regulated by two mechanisms. First, the mechanism that best explains the activation of phosphorylase at the beginning of exercise and during low-intensity exercise is linked to the protein molecule, "calmodulin." Calmodulin is found in many tissues including muscle and is activated at the onset of exercise by the release of calcium from the sarcoplasmic reticulum (chapter 8). Active calmodulin then activates

phosphorylase, which promotes glycogenolysis (see chapter 5 for details of calmodulin activity).

The second system that can activate phosphorylase during exercise is controlled by the hormone epinephrine. Epinephrine binds to a receptor on the cell membrane, which results in the formation of "cyclic AMP," which then activates phosphorylase (chapter 5 contains additional information on cyclic AMP). This mechanism is operative during high-intensity or prolonged exercise, but is too slow to explain the immediate glycogenolysis at the onset of muscular contraction.

---

whereas carbohydrate is the primary energy source during high-intensity exercise. Fuel selection is also influenced by the duration of exercise. During low-intensity, prolonged exercise, there is a progressive increase in the amount of fat oxidized by the working muscles. In the next two sections we discuss the influence of exercise intensity and duration on fuel selection in detail.

Exercise Intensity and Fuel Selection

Again, fats are a primary fuel source for muscle during low-intensity exercise (i.e., <30% $\dot{V}O_2$ max) whereas carbohydrate is the dominant substrate during high-intensity exercise (i.e., >70% $\dot{V}O_2$ max (15a, 18a, 71). The influence of exercise intensity on muscle fuel selection is illustrated in figure 4.11. Note that as the exercise intensity increases, there is a progressive increase in carbohydrate metabolism and a decrease in fat metabolism. Also, notice that as the exercise intensity increases, there is an exercise intensity at which the energy derived from carbohydrate exceeds that of fat; this work rate has been labeled the "crossover" point (15a). That is, as the exercise intensity increases above the crossover point, there is a progressive shift from fat to carbohydrate metabolism.

What causes this shift from fat to carbohydrate metabolism as the exercise intensity increases? Two primary factors are involved: (1) recruitment of fast fibers and (2) increasing blood levels of epinephrine. As the exercise intensity increases, more and more fast muscle fibers are recruited (33). These fibers have a large abundance of

Figure 4.11

Illustration of the "crossover" concept. Note that as the exercise intensity increases, there is a progressive increase in the contribution of carbohydrate (CHO) as a fuel source.

glycolytic enzymes but few mitochondrial and lipolytic enzymes (enzymes responsible for fat breakdown). In short, this means that fast fibers are better equipped to metabolize carbohydrates than fats. Therefore, the increased recruitment of fast fibers results in greater carbohydrate metabolism and less fat metabolism (15a).

A second factor that regulates carbohydrate metabolism during exercise is epinephrine. As exercise intensity increases, there is a progressive rise in blood levels of epinephrine (see chapter 5). High levels of epinephrine increase muscle glycogen breakdown, carbohydrate metabolism (i.e., glycolysis increases) and lactate production (15a) (see A Closer Look 4.2).

This increased production of lactate inhibits fat metabolism by reducing the availability of fat as a substrate (75a). The lack of fat as a substrate for working muscles under these conditions dictates that carbohydrate will be the primary fuel.

Exercise Duration and Fuel Selection

During prolonged low-intensity exercise (i.e., > thirty minutes), there is a gradual shift from carbohydrate metabolism toward an increasing reliance on fat as a substrate (3, 35, 48, 55, 66). Figure 4.12 demonstrates this point.

What factors control the rate of fat metabolism during prolonged exercise? Fat metabolism is regulated by those variables that control the rate of fat breakdown (a process called **lipolysis**). Triglycerides are broken down into **free fatty acids (FFA)** and glycerol by enzymes called **lipases**. These lipases are generally inactive until stimulated by the hormones epinephrine, norepinephrine, and glucagon (48). For example, during low-intensity, prolonged exercise, blood levels of epinephrine rise, which increases lipase activity and thus promotes lipolysis. This increase in lipolysis results in an increase in blood and muscle levels of FFA and promotes fat metabolism. In general, lipolysis is a slow process and an increase in fat metabolism occurs only after several minutes of exercise. This point is illustrated in figure 4.12 by the slow increase in fat metabolism across time during prolonged submaximal exercise.

The mobilization of FFA into the blood is inhibited by the hormone insulin and high blood levels of lactic acid. Insulin inhibits lipolysis by direct inhibition of lipase activity. Normally, blood insulin levels decline during prolonged exercise (chapter 5). However, if a high-carbohydrate meal or drink is consumed thirty to sixty minutes prior to exercise, blood glucose levels rise and more insulin is released from the pancreas. This elevation in blood insulin results in diminished lipolysis and a reduction in fat metabolism.

Interaction of Fat/ Carbohydrate Metabolism

During short-term exercise it is unlikely that muscle stores of glycogen or blood glucose levels would be depleted. However, during prolonged exercise (e.g., > two hours) muscle and liver stores of glycogen can reach very low levels (15, 33, 39, 70). This is important because depletion of muscle and blood carbohydrate stores results in muscular fatigue (39). Why do low muscle glycogen levels produce fatigue? Recent evidence suggests the following answer. Depletion of available carbohydrate reduces the rate of

Figure 4.12
Shift from carbohydrate metabolism toward fat metabolism during prolonged exercise.

glycolysis, and therefore the concentration of pyruvic acid in the muscle is also reduced (39). This lowers the rate of aerobic production of ATP by reducing the number of Krebs cycle compounds (intermediates). In human muscle with adequate glycogen stores, submaximal exercise (i.e., 70% $\dot{V}O_2$ max) results in a nine-fold increase (above resting values) in the number of Krebs cycle intermediates (70). This elevated pool of Krebs cycle intermediates is required for the Krebs cycle to "speed up" in an effort to meet the high ATP demands during exercise. Pyruvic acid (produced via glycolysis) is important in providing this increase in Krebs cycle intermediates. For example, pyruvic acid is a precursor of several Krebs cycle intermediates (e.g., oxaloacetate, malate). When the rate of glycolysis is reduced due to the unavailability of substrate, pyruvic acid levels in the sarcoplasm decline and the levels of Krebs cycle intermediates decrease as well. This decline in Krebs cycle intermediates slows the rate of Krebs cycle activity, with the end result being a reduction in the rate of aerobic ATP production. This reduced rate of muscle ATP production limits muscular performance and may result in fatigue.

It is important to appreciate that a reduction in Krebs cycle intermediates (due to glycogen depletion) results in a diminished rate of ATP production from fat metabolism since fat can only be metabolized via Krebs-cycle oxidation. Hence, when carbohydrate stores are depleted in the body, the rate at which fat is metabolized is also reduced (70). Therefore, "fats burn in the flame of carbohydrates" (75). The role that depletion of body carbohydrate stores may play in limiting performance during prolonged exercise is introduced in Research Focus 4.1 and is further discussed in both chapters 19 and 23.

Does Carbohydrate Feeding Improve Exercise Performance?

Since depletion of muscle and blood carbohydrate stores results in muscular fatigue, can ingestion of carbohydrates during exercise improve performance? Studies investigating the potential ergogenic effects of carbohydrate feeding during low-intensity (i.e., <70% $\dot{V}O_2$ max) prolonged exercise (e.g., ≥ two hours) are numerous. Most studies using carbohydrate feedings of 30–60 grams · hour⁻¹ have demonstrated that carbohydrate feeding during exercise results in improved endurance performance in trained individuals (see references 18b and 60a for a review).

To date, few studies have been conducted to determine if carbohydrate feeding results in improved performance during short duration (i.e., < one hour) high- intensity exercise. However, a recent study by Below et al. (7a) demonstrated that carbohydrate ingestion improved performance by 6.5% during sixty minutes of cycle exercise at ~80% $\dot{V}O_2$ max. Based on these promising results, additional studies investigating the effects of carbohydrate feeding on performance during high-intensity exercise appear warranted.

Table 4.2	Principal Storage Sites of Carbohydrate and Fat in the Body of a Healthy, Nonobese (20% Body Fat), 70 kg Male Subject

Note that dietary intake of carbohydrate influences the amount of glycogen stored in both the liver and muscle. Mass units for storage are grams (g) and kilograms (kg). Energy units are kilocalories (kcal) and kilojoules (kJ). Data are from references 21, 20, and 47.

	Carbohydrate (CHO)		
Storage Site	Mixed Diet	High CHO Diet	Low CHO Diet
Liver glycogen	60g (240 kcal or 1,005 kJ)	90g (360 kcal or 1,507 kJ)	<30g (120 kcal or 502 kJ)
Glucose in blood and extracellular fluid	10g (40 kcal or 167 kJ)	10g (40 kcal or 167 kJ)	10g (40 kcal or 167 kJ)
Muscle glycogen	350g (1,400 kcal or 5,860 kJ)	600g (2,400 kcal or 10,046 kJ)	300g (1,200 kcal or 5,023 kJ)

	Fat		
Storage Site	Mixed Diet		
Adipocytes	14 kg (107,800 kcal or 451,251 kJ)		
Muscle	0.5 kg (3,850 kcal or 16,116 kJ)		

Body Fuel Sources

In this section we outline the storage sites in the body for carbohydrates, fats, and proteins. Further, we will define the role that each of these fuel storage sites plays in providing energy during exercise. Finally, we will discuss the use of lactate as a fuel source during work.

Sources of Carbohydrate During Exercise

Carbohydrate is stored as glycogen in both the muscle and the liver (see table 4.2). Muscle glycogen stores provide a direct source of carbohydrate for muscle energy metabolism whereas liver glycogen stores serve as a means of replacing blood glucose. For example, when blood glucose levels decline during prolonged

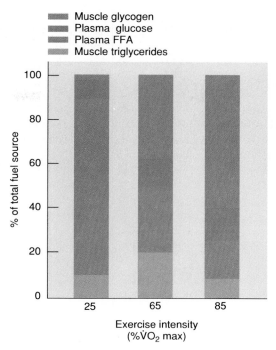

Figure 4.13
Influence of exercise intensity on muscle fuel source. Data are from highly trained endurance athletes.

Figure 4.14
Percentage of energy derived from the four major sources of fuel during submaximal exercise (i.e., 65%–75% $\dot{V}O_2$ max). Data are from trained endurance athletes.

exercise, liver glycogenolysis is stimulated and glucose is released into the blood. This glucose can then be transported to the contracting muscle and used as fuel.

Carbohydrate used as a substrate during exercise comes from both glycogen stores in muscle and from blood glucose (17, 18c, 33, 51, 74). The relative contribution of muscle glycogen and blood glucose to energy metabolism during exercise varies as a function of the exercise intensity and duration. Blood glucose plays the greater role during low-intensity exercise whereas muscle glycogen is the primary source of carbohydrate during high-intensity exercise (see figure 4.13). As mentioned earlier, the increased glycogen usage during high-intensity exercise can be explained by the increased rate of glycogenolysis that occurs due to recruitment of fast-twitch fibers and elevated blood epinephrine levels.

During the first hour of submaximal prolonged exercise, much of the carbohydrate metabolized by muscle comes from muscle glycogen. However, as muscle glycogen levels decline across time, blood glucose becomes an increasingly important source of fuel (see figure 4.14).

Sources of Fat During Exercise

When an individual consumes more energy (i.e., food) than he or she expends, this additional energy is stored in the form of fat. A gain of 3,500 kcal of energy results in the storage of one pound of fat. Most fat is stored in the form of triglycerides in adipocytes (fat cells), but some is stored in muscle cells as well (see

table 4.2). As mentioned earlier, the major factor that determines the role of fat as a substrate during exercise is its availability to the muscle cell. In order to be metabolized, triglycerides must be degraded to FFA (three molecules) and glycerol (one molecule). When triglycerides are split, FFA can be converted into acetyl-CoA and enter the Krebs cycle.

Which fat stores are used as a fuel source varies as a function of the exercise intensity and duration. For example, plasma FFA's (i.e., FFA from adipocytes) are the primary source of fat during low-intensity exercise. At higher work rates, metabolism of muscle triglycerides increases (see figure 4.13). At exercise intensities between 65%–85% $\dot{V}O_2$ max, the contribution of fat as a muscle fuel source is approximately equal between plasma FFA and muscle triglycerides (18a, 40a, 69a).

The contribution of plasma FFA and muscle triglycerides to exercise metabolism during prolonged exercise is summarized in figure 4.14. Note that at the beginning of exercise, the contribution of plasma FFA and muscle triglycerides is equal. However, as the duration of exercise increases, there is a progressive rise in the role of plasma FFA as a fuel source.

Sources of Protein During Exercise

To be used as a fuel source, proteins must first be degraded into amino acids. Amino acids can be supplied to muscle from the blood or from the amino acid pool in the fiber itself. Again, the role that protein plays as a substrate during exercise is small and is principally dependent on the availability of branch-chained amino acids and the amino acid alanine (6, 38a). Skeletal muscle can directly metabolize certain types of amino acids (e.g., valine, leucine, isoleucine) to produce ATP (36, 49). Further, in the liver, alanine can be converted to glucose and returned via the blood to skeletal muscle to be utilized as a substrate.

A Closer Look 4.3

The Cori Cycle: Lactate as a Fuel Source

During exercise some of the lactic acid that is produced by skeletal muscles is transported to the liver via the blood. Upon entry into the liver, lactate can be converted to glucose via gluco-neogensis. This "new" glucose can be released into the blood and transported back to skeletal muscles to be used as an energy source during exercise. The cycle of lactate-to-glucose between the muscle and liver is called the **Cori cycle** and is illustrated in figure 4.15

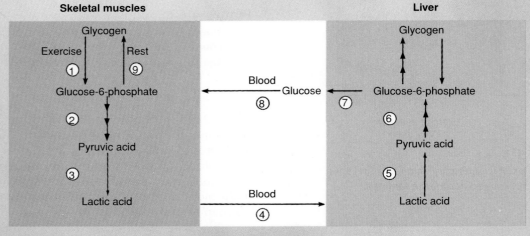

Figure 4.15
The Cori cycle. The sequence of steps is indicated by the numbers 1–9, beginning with exercise.

Any factor that increases the amino acid pool (amount of available amino acids) in the liver or in skeletal muscle can theoretically enhance protein metabolism (49, 58). One such factor is prolonged exercise (i.e., > two hours). Dohm and associates (23, 24) have demonstrated that enzymes capable of degrading muscle proteins (proteases) are activated during long-term exercise. The mechanism to explain activation of these proteases during prolonged exercise is not currently known. However, the practical aspect of this finding is that during the course of prolonged exercise, proteases become active and amino acids are liberated from their parent proteins. This rise in the amino acid pool results in a small increase in the use of amino acids as fuel for exercise.

Lactate as a Fuel Source During Exercise

For many years, lactate was considered to be a waste product of glycolysis with limited metabolic use. However, new evidence has shown that lactate is not necessarily a waste product but can play a beneficial role during exercise by serving as both a substrate for the liver to synthesize glucose (see A Closer Look 4.3) and as a direct fuel source for skeletal muscle and the heart (12, 13, 40a). That is, in slow skeletal muscle fibers and the heart, lactate removed from the blood can be converted to pyruvate which can then be transformed to acetyl-CoA. This acetyl-CoA can then enter the Krebs cycle and contribute to oxidative metabolism. The concept that lactate can be produced in one tissue and then transported to another to be used as an energy source has been termed the "lactate shuttle" (10–13).

in summary

- Regulation of fuel selection during exercise is under complex control and is dependent upon several factors including diet and the intensity and duration of exercise.
- In general, carbohydrates are used as the major fuel source during high-intensity exercise.
- During prolonged exercise, there is a gradual shift from carbohydrate metabolism toward fat metabolism.
- Proteins contribute less than 2% of the fuel used during exercise of less than one hour duration. During prolonged exercise (i.e., three to five hours duration), the total contribution of protein to the fuel supply may reach 5%–15% during the final minutes of prolonged work.

study questions

1. Identify the predominant energy systems used to produce ATP during the following types of exercise:
   a. short-term intense exercise (i.e., < ten seconds duration).
   b. 400-meter dash
   c. 20-kilometer race (i.e., 12.4 miles)
2. Graph the change in oxygen uptake during the transition from rest to steady state submaximal exercise. Label the oxygen deficit. Where does the ATP come from during the transition period from rest to steady state?
3. Graph the change in oxygen uptake and blood lactate concentration during incremental exercise. Label the point on the graph that might be considered the lactate threshold or lactate inflection point.
4. Discuss several possible reasons why blood lactate begins to rise rapidly during incremental exercise.
5. Briefly, explain how the respiratory exchange ratio is used to estimate which substrate is being utilized during exercise. What is meant by the term *nonprotein* R?
6. List two factors that play a role in the regulation of carbohydrate metabolism during exercise.
7. List those variables that regulate fat metabolism during exercise.
8. Define the following terms: (a) *triglyceride*, (b) *lipolysis*, and (c) *lipases*.
9. Graph the change in oxygen uptake during recovery from exercise. Label the oxygen debt.
10. How does modern theory of EPOC differ from the classical oxygen debt theory proposed by A. V. Hill?
11. Discuss the influence of exercise intensity on muscle fuel selection.
12. How does the duration of exercise influence muscle fuel selection?

suggested readings

Bowers, R., and E. Fox. 1992. *Sports Physiology*. Dubuque, IA: Wm. C. Brown.

Brooks, G., and J. Mercier. 1994. Balance of carbohydrate and lipid utilization during exercise: The "crossover" concept. *Journal of Applied Physiology* 76:2253–61.

Conley, K. 1994. Cellular energetics during exercise. *Advances in Veterinary Science and Comparative Medicine*. 38A:1–39.

Coyle, E. 1995. Substrate utilization during exercise in active people. *American Journal of Clinical Nutrition*. 61:(Suppl.) S968–S979.

Hargreaves, M. (Ed.) 1995. *Exercise Metabolism*. Champaign, IL: Human Kinetics.

references

1. Armstrong, R. 1979. Biochemistry: Energy liberation and use. In *Sports Medicine and Physiology*, ed. R. Strauss. Philadelphia: W. B. Saunders.
2. Åstrand, P., and K. Rodahl. 1986. *Textbook of Work Physiology*. New York: McGraw-Hill.
3. Ball-Burnett, M., H. Green, and M. Houston. 1991. Energy metabolism in human slow and fast twitch fibers during prolonged cycle exercise. *Journal of Physiology* (London) 437:257–67.
4. Barnard, R., and M. Foss. 1969. Oxygen debt: Effect of beta adrenergic blockade on the lactacid and alactacid components. *Journal of Applied Physiology* 27:813–16.
5. Bassett, D. et al. 1991. Rate of decline in blood lactate after cycling exercise in endurance-trained and untrained subjects. *Journal of Applied Physiology* 70:1816–20.
6. Bates, P. et al. 1980. Exercise and protein turnover in the rat. *Journal of Physiology* (London) 303:41P.
7. Belcastro, A., and A. Bonen. 1975. Lactic acid removal rates during controlled and uncontrolled recovery exercise. *Journal of Applied Physiology* 39:932–36.
7a. Below, P., R. Mora-Rodriguez, J. Gonzalez-Alonso, and E. Coyle. 1995. Fluid and carbohydrate ingestion independently improve performance during 1 hour of intense exercise. *Medicine and Science in Sports and Exercise*. 27:200–210.
8. Berg, A., and J. Keul. 1980. Serum alanine during long-lasting exercise. *International Journal of Sports Medicine* 1:199–202.
9. Boutellier, U. et al. 1984. Aftereffects of chronic hypoxia on O_2 kinetics and on O_2 deficit and debt. *European Journal of Applied Physiology* 53:87–91.
10. Brooks, G. 1985. Anaerobic threshold: Review of the concept and directions for future research. *Medicine and Science in Sports and Exercise* 17:22–23.
11. ———. 1985. Lactate: Glycolytic end product and oxidative substrate during sustained exercise in mammals—the lactate shuttle. In *Circulation, Respiration, and Metabolism*, ed. R. Giles. Berlin: Springer-Verlag.
12. ———. 1986. Lactate production under fully aerobic conditions: The lactate shuttle during rest and exercise. *Federation Proceedings* 45:2924–29.
13. ———. 1986. The lactate shuttle during exercise and recovery. *Medicine and Science in Sports and Exercise* 18:360–68.
14. Brooks, G. et al. 1971. Temperature, skeletal muscle, mitochondrial functions, and oxygen debt. *American Journal of Physiology* 220:1053–59.
15. Brooks, G., and T. Fahey. 1984. *Exercise Physiology: Human Bioenergetics and Its Applications*. New York: John Wiley & Sons.
15a. Brooks, G., and J. Mercier. 1994. Balance of carbohydrate and lipid utilization during exercise: The "crossover" concept. *Journal of Applied Physiology* 76:2253–61.
16. Cerretelli, P. et al. 1977. Oxygen uptake transients at the onset and offset of arm and leg work. *Respiration Physiology* 30:81–97.

17. Coggin, A. 1991. Plasma glucose metabolism during exercise in humans. *Sports Medicine* 11:102–24.

18. Coyle, E. 1986. Muscle glycogen utilization during prolonged strenuous exercise when fed carbohydrate. *Journal of Applied Physiology* 61:165–72.

18a. ———. 1995. Substrate utilization during exercise in active people. *American Journal of Clinical Nutrition* 61:(Suppl.) 968s–979s.

18b. Coyle, E. and S. Montain. 1992. Carbohydrate and fluid ingestion during exercise: Are there tradeoffs? *Medicine and Science in Sports and Exercise* 24:671–78.

18c. Coyle, E. F. et al. 1991. Carbohydrate metabolism during intense exercise when hyperglycemic. *Journal of Applied Physiology* 70:834–40.

19. Davis, J. 1985. Anaerobic threshold: Review of the concept and directions for future research. *Medicine and Science in Sports and Exercise* 17:6–18.

20. Davis, J. et al. 1976. Anaerobic threshold and maximal aerobic power for three modes of exercise. *Journal of Applied Physiology* 41:544–50.

21. Dodd, S. et al. 1984. Blood lactate disappearance at various intensities of recovery exercise. *Journal of Applied Physiology* 57:1462–65.

22. Dodd, S. et al. 1988. Effects of beta-blockade on ventilation and gas exchange during the rest-to-work transition. *Aviation, Space, and Environmental Medicine* 59:255–58.

23. Dohm, G. et al. 1978. Changes in tissue protein levels as a result of endurance exercise. *Life Sciences* 23:845–50.

24. Dohm, G. et al. 1981. Influence of exercise on free amino acid concentrations in rat tissues. *Journal of Applied Physiology* 50:41–44.

25. Donovan, C., and G. Brooks. 1983. Endurance training affects lactate clearance, not lactate production. *American Journal of Physiology* 244:E83–E92.

26. England, P. et al. 1985. The effect of acute thermal dehydration on blood lactate accumulation during incremental exercise. *Journal of Sports Sciences* 2:105–11.

27. Essen, B., and L. Kaijser. 1978. Regulation of glycolysis in intermittent exercise in man. *Journal of Physiology* 281:499–511.

28. Evans, B., and K. Cureton. 1983. Effect of physical conditioning on blood lactate disappearance after supramaximal exercise. *British Journal of Sports Medicine* 17:40–45.

29. Farrell, P. et al. 1979. Plasma lactate accumulation and distance running performance. *Medicine and Science in Sports* 11:338–44.

30. Gaesser, G., and G. Brooks. 1984. Metabolic bases of excess post-exercise oxygen consumption: A review. *Medicine and Science in Sports and Exercise* 16:29–43.

31. Gladden, B., W. Stainsby, and B. MacIntosh. 1982. Norepinephrine increases canine muscle O_2 during recovery. *Medicine and Science in Sports and Exercise* 14:471–76.

32. Gladden, L. B. 1991. Net lactate uptake during progressive steady-level contractions in canine muscle. *Journal of Applied Physiology* 71:514–20.

33. Gollnick, P. 1985. Metabolism of substrates: Energy substrate metabolism during exercise and as modified by training. *Federation Proceedings* 44:353–56.

34. Gollnick, P., W. Bayly, and D. Hodgson. 1986. Exercise intensity, training, diet, and lactate concentration in muscle and blood. *Medicine and Science in Sports and Exercise* 18:334–40.

35. Gollnick, P., and B. Saltin. 1988. Fuel for muscular exercise: Role of fat. In *Exercise, Nutrition, and Energy Metabolism*, eds. E. Horton and R. Terjung, 72–88. New York: Macmillan.

36. Goodman, M. 1988. Amino acid and protein metabolism. In *Exercise, Nutrition, and Energy Metabolism*, eds. E. Horton and R. Terjung, 89–99. New York: Macmillan.

37. Gore, C., and R. Withers. 1990. Effect of exercise intensity and duration on post-exercise metabolism. *Journal of Applied Physiology* 68:2362–68.

38. ———. 1990. The effect of exercise intensity and duration on the oxygen deficit and excess post-exercise oxygen consumption. *European Journal of Applied Physiology* 60:169–74.

38a. Graham, T. et al. 1995. Skeletal muscle amino acid metabolism and ammonia production during exercise. In *Exercise Metabolism*, 131–75. Champaign, IL: Human Kinetics.

39. Green, H. 1991. How important is endogenous muscle glycogen to fatigue during prolonged exercise? *Canadian Journal of Physiology and Pharmacology* 69:290–97.

40. Hagberg, J., J. Mullin, and F. Nagle. 1978. Oxygen consumption during constant load exercise. *Journal of Applied Physiology* 45:381–84.

40a. Hargreaves, M. 1995. Skeletal muscle carbohydrate metabolism during exercise. In *Exercise Metabolism*, 41–72. Champaign, IL: Human Kinetics.

41. Harris, R. et al. 1976. The time course of phosphocreatine resynthesis during recovery of the quadriceps muscle in man. *Pflugers Archives* 367:137–42.

42. Heck, H., and A. Mader. 1985. Justification of the 4-mmol/l lactate threshold. *International Journal of Sports Medicine* 6:117–30.

43. Hermanson, L., and I. Stensvold. 1972. Production and removal of lactate during exercise in man. *Acta Physiologica Scandinavica* 86:191–201.

44. Hickson, R., H. Bomze, and J. Holloszy. 1978. Faster adjustment of O_2 uptake to the energy requirement of exercise in the trained state. *Journal of Applied Physiology* 44:877–81.

45. Hill, A. 1914. The oxidative removal of lactic acid. *Journal of Physiology* (London) 48:x–xi.

46. Hollman, W. 1985. Historical remarks on the development of the aerobic-anaerobic threshold up to 1966. *International Journal of Sports Medicine* 6:109–16.

47. Holloszy, J. 1982. Muscle metabolism during exercise. *Archives of Physical and Rehabilitation Medicine* 63:231–34.

48. ———. 1990. Utilization of fatty acids during exercise. In *Biochemistry of Exercise VII*, eds. A. W. Taylor et al., 319–28. Champaign, IL: Human Kinetics.

49. Hood, D., and R. Terjung. 1990. Amino acid metabolism during exercise and following endurance training. *Sports Medicine* 9:23–35.

50. Hultman, E. 1973. Energy metabolism in human muscle. *Journal of Physiology* (London) 231:56.

51. Hultman, E., and H. Sjoholm. 1983. Substrate availability. In *Biochemistry of Exercise*, eds. H. Knuttgen, J. Vogel, and J. R. Poortmans. Champaign, IL: Human Kinetics.

52. Jones, N., and R. Ehrsam. 1982. The anaerobic threshold. *Exercise and Sports Science Review* 10:49–83.

Section One Physiology of Exercise

53. Kalis, J. et al. 1988. Effects of beta blockade on the drift in O_2 consumption during prolonged exercise. *Journal of Applied Physiology* 64:753–58.

54. Knuttgen, H., and B. Saltin. 1972. Muscle metabolites and oxygen uptake in short-term submaximal exercise in man. *Journal of Applied Physiology* 32:690–94.

55. Ladu, M., H. Kapsas, and W. Palmer. 1991. Regulation of lipoprotein lipase in muscle and adipose tissue during exercise. *Journal of Applied Physiology* 71:404–9.

56. Lemon, P., and F. Mullin. 1980. Effect of initial glycogen levels on protein metabolism during exercise. *Journal of Applied Physiology* 48:624–29.

57. Lemon, P., and R. Nagle. 1980. Effects of exercise on protein and amino acid metabolism. *Medicine and Science in Sports and Exercise* 13:141–49.

58. MacLean, D. et al. 1991. Plasma and muscle amino acid and ammonia responses during prolonged exercise. *Journal of Applied Physiology* 70:2095–2103.

59. Mader, A., and H. Heck. 1986. A theory of the metabolic origin of the anaerobic threshold. *International Journal of Sports Medicine* 7:45–65.

60. Marti, B., T. Abelin, and H. Howald. 1987. A modified fixed blood lactate threshold for estimating running speed for joggers in 16-Km races. *Scandavian Journal of Sports Sciences* 9:41–45.

60a. Maughan, R. 1991. Carbohydrate-electrolyte solutions during prolonged exercise. Perspectives in exercise science and sports medicine. In *Ergogenics: Enhancements of Performance in Exercise and Sport*, vol. 4, eds. D. Lamb and M. Williams, 35–76. Dubuque, IA: Brown and Benchmark Publishers.

61. Medbo, J. et al. 1988. Anaerobic capacity determined maximal accumulated O_2 deficit. *Journal of Applied Physiology* 64:50–60.

62. Powers, S., S. Dodd, and R. Beadle. 1985. Oxygen uptake kinetics in trained athletes differing in O_2 max. *European Journal of Applied Physiology* 39:407–15.

63. Powers, S., S. Dodd, and R. Garner. 1984. Precision of ventilatory and gas exchange alterations as a predictor of the anaerobic threshold. *European Journal of Applied Physiology* 52:173–77.

64. Powers, S. et al. 1983. Effects of caffeine ingestion on metabolism and performance during graded exercise. *European Journal of Applied Physiology* 560:301–7.

65. Powers, S., E. Howley, and R. Cox. 1982. Ventilatory and metabolic reactions to heat stress during prolonged exercise. *Journal of Sports Medicine and Physical Fitness* 22:32–36.

66. Powers, S., W. Riley, and E. Howley. 1980. A comparison of fat metabolism in trained men and women during prolonged aerobic work. *Research Quarterly for Exercise and Sport* 52:427–31.

67. Powers, S. et al. 1987. Oxygen deficit-debt relationships in ponies during submaximal treadmill exercise. *Respiratory Physiology* 70:251–63.

68. Refsum, H., L. Gjessing, and S. Stromme. 1978. Changes in plasma amino acid distribution and urine amino acid excretion during prolonged heavy exercise. *Scandinavian Journal of Clinical and Laboratory Investigation* 39:407–13.

69. Riley, W., S. Powers, and H. Welch. 1981. The effect of two levels of muscular work on urinary creatinine excretion. *Research Quarterly for Exercise and Sport* 52:339–47.

69a. Romijin, J. et al. 1993. Regulation of endogenous fat and carbohydrate metabolism in relation to exercise intensity. *American Journal of Physiology* 265:E380–E391.

70. Sahlin, K., A. Katz, and S. Broberg. 1990. Tricarboxylic acid cycle intermediates in human muscle during prolonged exercise. *American Journal of Physiology* 259:C834–C841.

71. Saltin, B., and P. Gollnick. 1988. Fuel for muscular exercise: Role of carbohydrate. In *Exercise, Nutrition, and Energy Metabolism*, ed. E. Horton and R. Terjung, 45–71. New York: Macmillan.

72. Skinner, J., and T. McLellan. 1980. The transition from aerobic to anaerobic exercise. *Research Quarterly* 51:234–48.

73. Stainsby, W. 1986. Biochemical and physiological bases for lactate production. *Medicine and Science in Sports and Exercise* 18:341–43.

74. Stanley, W., and R. Connett. 1991. Regulation of muscle carbohydrate metabolism during exercise. *FASEB Journal* 5:2155–59.

75. Stryer, L. 1988. *Biochemistry*. San Francisco: W. H. Freeman.

75a. Turcotte, L. et al. 1995. Lipid metabolism during exercise. In *Exercise Metabolism*, 99–130. Champaign, IL: Human Kinetics.

76. Wasserman, K. 1986. Anaerobiosis, lactate, and gas exchange during exercise: The issues. *Federation Proceedings* 45:2904–09.

77. Wasserman, K., W. Beaver, and B. Whipp. 1986. Mechanisms and pattern of blood lactate increase during exercise in man. *Medicine and Science in Sports and Exercise* 18:344–52.

78. Wasserman, K., and M. McIlroy. 1964. Detecting the threshold of anaerobic metabolism. *American Journal of Cardiology* 14:844–52.

79. Wasserman, K. et al. 1973. Anaerobic threshold and respiratory gas exchange during exercise. *Journal of Applied Physiology* 35:236–43.

80. Wasserman, K., B. Whipp, and J. Davis. 1981. Respiratory physiology of exercise: Metabolism, gas exchange, and ventilatory control. In *International Review of Physiology, Respiratory Physiology III*, ed. J. Widdicombe. Baltimore: University Park Press.

81. White, T., and G. Brooks. 1981. (C^{14}) Glucose, alanine, and leucine oxidation in rats at rest and two intensities of running. *Journal of Physiology* 240:R147–R152.

82. Wilson, D. et al. 1977. Effect of oxygen tension on cellular energetics. *American Journal of Physiology* 233:C135–C140.

83. Yoshida, T. 1986. Effect of dietary modifications on the anaerobic threshold. *Sports Medicine* 3:4–9.

CHAPTER 5

Hormonal Responses to Exercise

objectives

By studying this chapter, you should be able to do the following:

1. Describe the concept of hormone-receptor interaction.
2. Identify the four factors influencing the concentration of a hormone in the blood.
3. Describe the mechanism by which steroid hormones act on cells.
4. Describe the "second messenger" hypothesis of hormone action.
5. Describe the role of the hypothalamus-releasing factors in the control of hormone secretion from the anterior pituitary gland.
6. Describe the relationship of the hypothalamus to the secretion of hormones from the posterior pituitary gland.
7. Identify the site of release, stimulus for release, and the predominant action of the following hormones: epinephrine, norepinephrine, glucagon, insulin, cortisol, aldosterone, thyroxine, growth hormone, estrogen, and testosterone.
8. Discuss the use of testosterone (an anabolic steroid) and growth hormone on muscle growth and their potential side effects.
9. Contrast the role of plasma catecholamines with intracellular factors in the mobilization of muscle glycogen during exercise.
10. Graphically describe the changes in the following hormones during graded and prolonged exercise and discuss how those changes influence the four mechanisms used to maintain the blood glucose concentration: insulin, glucagon, cortisol, growth hormone, epinephrine, and norepinephrine.
11. Describe the effect of changing hormone and substrate levels in the blood on the mobilization of free fatty acids from adipose tissue.

outline

Neuroendocrinology   64
  Blood Hormone Concentration   65
  Hormone-Receptor
    Interaction   66
Hormones: Regulation and
    Action   68
  Hypothalamus and the Pituitary
    Gland   68
  Thyroid Gland   71

Parathyroid Gland   72
Adrenal Gland   72
Pancreas   75
Testes and Ovaries   76
Hormonal Control of Substrate
    Mobilization During
    Exercise   80
  Muscle-Glycogen Utilization   81

Blood Glucose Homeostasis During
    Exercise   82
Hormone-Substrate Interaction   89

acromegaly
adenylate cyclase
adrenal cortex
adrenocorticotrophic hormone (ACTH)
aldosterone
alpha receptors
anabolic steroid
androgenic steroid
androgens
angiotensin I and II
anterior pituitary
antidiuretic hormone (ADH)
beta receptors
calcitonin
calmodulin
catecholamines
cortisol
cyclic AMP
diabetes mellitus

diacylglycerol
endocrine gland
endorphin
epinephrine (E)
estrogens
follicle-stimulating hormone (FSH)
G protein
glucagon
glucocorticoids
growth hormone (GH)
hormone
hypothalamic somatostatin
hypothalamus
inositol triphosphate
insulin
luteinizing hormone (LH)
mineralocorticoids
neuroendocrinology
norepinephrine (NE)

pancreas
phosphodiesterase
phospholipase C
pituitary gland
posterior pituitary gland
prolactin
protein kinase C
releasing hormone
renin
second messenger
sex steroids
somatomedins
somatostatin
steroids
testosterone
thyroid gland
thyroid-stimulating hormone (TSH)
thyroxine (T_4)
triiodothyronine (T_3)

 s presented in the last chapter, the fuels for muscular exercise include muscle glycogen and fat, plasma glucose and free fatty acids, and to a lesser extent, amino acids. These fuels must be provided at an optimal rate for activities as diverse as the 400-meter run and the 26-mile, 385-yard marathon, or performance will suffer. What controls the mixture of fuel used by the muscles? What stimulates the adipose tissue to release more FFA? How is the liver made aware of the need to replace the glucose that is being removed from the blood by exercising muscles? If glucose is not replaced, a hypoglycemic (low-blood glucose) condition will occur. Hypoglycemia is a topic of crucial importance in discussing exercise as a challenge to homeostasis. Blood glucose is the primary fuel for the central nervous system (CNS), and without optimal CNS function during exercise, the chance of fatigue and risk of serious injury are increased. While blood glucose was used as an example, it should be noted that sodium, calcium, potassium, and water concentrations, as well as blood pressure and pH are also maintained within narrow limits during exercise. It should be no surprise then that there are a variety of automatic control systems maintaining these variables within these limits. Chapter 2 presented an overview of automatic control systems that maintain homeostasis. This chapter will expand on that by providing information on **neuroendocrinology,** a branch of physiology dedicated to the systematic study of control systems. The first part of the chapter will present a brief introduction to each hormone, indicate the factors controlling its secretion, and discuss its role in homeostasis.

Following that, we will discuss how hormones control the delivery of carbohydrates and fats during exercise.

Neuroendocrinology

The two major homeostatic systems involved in the control and regulation of various functions (cardiovascular, renal, metabolic, etc.) are the nervous and endocrine systems. Both are structured to sense information, organize an appropriate response, and then deliver the message to the proper organ or tissue. Often the two systems work together to maintain homeostasis, and the term "neuroendocrine response" is reflective of that interdependence. The two systems differ in the way the message is delivered: the endocrine system releases hormones into the blood to circulate to tissues, while nerves use neurotransmitters to relay messages from one nerve to the other, or from a nerve to a tissue.

Endocrine glands release **hormones** (chemical messengers) directly into the blood, which carries the hormone to a tissue to exert an effect. It is the binding of the hormone to a specific protein receptor that allows the hormone to exert its effect. In that way the hormone can circulate to all tissues while affecting only a few—those with the specific receptor.

Hormones can be divided into several classes based on chemical makeup: amino acid derivatives, peptides/protein, and **steroids.** The chemical structure influences the way in which the hormone is transported in the blood and the manner in which it exerts its effect on the tissue. For example, while steroid hormones' lipid-like structure requires that they be transported bound to plasma protein (to "dissolve" in the plasma), that same lipid-like structure allows them to diffuse through cell membranes to exert their effects. This will be discussed in detail in a later section. Hormones exist in very small quantities in the blood and are measured in microgram (10^{-3} g), nanogram (10^{-9} g), and picogram (10^{-12} g) amounts. It wasn't until the 1950s that analytical techniques were improved to the point of monitoring these low plasma concentrations (67).

Blood Hormone Concentration

The effect a hormone exerts on a tissue is directly related to the concentration of the hormone in the plasma and the number of active receptors to which it can bind. The hormone concentration in the plasma is dependent upon the following factors:

- the rate of secretion of the hormone from the endocrine gland,
- the rate of metabolism or excretion of the hormone,
- the quantity of transport protein (for some hormones), and
- changes in the plasma volume.

Control of Hormone Secretion

The rate at which a hormone is secreted from an endocrine gland is dependent on the magnitude of the input and whether it is stimulatory or inhibitory in nature. The input in every case is a chemical one, be it an ion (e.g., Ca^{++}) or substrate (e.g., glucose) in the plasma, a neurotransmitter such as acetylcholine or norepinephrine, or another hormone. Most endocrine glands are under the direct influence of more than one type of input, which may either reinforce or interfere with each other's effect. An example of this interaction is found in the control of insulin release from the pancreas. Figure 5.1 shows that the pancreas, which produces insulin, responds to changes in plasma glucose and amino acids, norepinephrine released from sympathetic neurons as well as circulating epinephrine, parasympathetic neurons, which release acetylcholine, and a variety of hormones. Elevations of plasma glucose and amino acids increase insulin secretion (+), while an increase in sympathetic nervous system activity (epinephrine and norepinephrine) decreases (−) insulin secretion. It is this magnitude of inhibitory versus excitatory input that determines whether there will be an increase or decrease in the secretion of insulin.

Metabolism and Excretion of Hormones

The concentration of a hormone in the plasma is also influenced by the rate at which it is metabolized (inactivated) and/or excreted. Inactivation can take place at or near the receptor, or in the liver, the major site for hormone metabolism. In addition, the kidneys

Figure 5.1
The secretion of a hormone can be modified by a number of factors, some exerting a positive influence and others, a negative influence.

From A. J. Vander, et al., *Human Physiology: The Mechanisms of Body Function*, 4th ed. Copyright © 1985 McGraw-Hill, Inc., New York. Reprinted by permission.

can metabolize a variety of hormones, or excrete them in their free (active) form. In fact, the rate of excretion of a hormone in the urine has been used as an indicator of its rate of secretion during exercise (6, 27, 50, 51). Since blood flow to the kidneys and liver decreases during exercise, the rate at which hormones are inactivated or excreted decreases. This results in an elevation of the plasma level of the hormone over and above that due to higher rates of secretion.

Transport Protein

The concentration of some hormones is influenced by the quantity of transport protein in the plasma. Steroid hormones and thyroxine are transported bound to plasma proteins. In order for a hormone to exert its effect on a cell it must be "free" to interact with the receptor, and not "bound" to the transport protein. The amount of free hormone is dependent on the quantity of transport protein and the capacity and affinity of the protein to bind the hormone molecules. Capacity refers to the maximal quantity of hormone that can be bound to the transport protein, and affinity refers to the tendency of the transport protein to bind to the hormone. An increase in the quantity, capacity, or affinity of transport protein would reduce the amount of free hormone and its effect on tissue (36, 60). For example, high levels of estrogen during pregnancy increase the quantity of thyroxine's transport protein, causing a reduction in free thyroxine. The thyroid gland produces more thyroxine to correct this problem.

Plasma Volume

Changes in plasma volume will change the hormone concentration independent of changes in the rate of secretion or inactivation of the hormone. During exercise, plasma volume decreases due to the movement of water out of the cardiovascular system. This causes an increase in the concentration of hormones in the plasma.

Hormone–Receptor Interaction

Hormones are carried by the circulation to all tissues, but affect only certain tissues. Tissues responsive to specific hormones have specific protein receptors capable of binding those hormones. These protein receptors should not be viewed as static fixtures associated with cells, but like any cellular structures, are subject to change. The number of receptors varies from 500 to 100,000 per cell, depending on the receptor. Receptor number may decrease when exposed to a chronically elevated level of a hormone (*down-regulation*), resulting in a diminished response for the same hormone concentration. The opposite case, chronic exposure to a low concentration of a hormone, may lead to an increase in receptor number (*up-regulation*), with the tissue becoming very responsive to the available hormone. Since there is a finite number of receptors on or in a cell, a situation can arise in which the concentration of a hormone is so high that all receptors are bound to the hormone; this is called *saturation*. Any additional increase in the plasma hormone concentration will have no additional effect (30). Further, since the receptors are specific to a hormone, any chemical similar in "shape" will compete for the limited receptor sites. A major way in which endocrine function is studied is to use chemicals (drugs) to block receptors and observe the consequences. For example, patients with heart disease may receive a drug that blocks the receptors to which epinephrine (adrenaline) binds; this prevents the heart rate from getting too high during exercise. After the hormone binds to a receptor, cellular activity is altered by a variety of mechanisms.

Mechanisms of Hormone Action

Mechanisms by which hormones modify cellular activity include:

- alteration of membrane transport mechanisms,
- stimulation of DNA in the nucleus to initiate the synthesis of a specific protein, and
- activation of special proteins in the cells by "second messengers."

Membrane Transport After binding to a receptor on a membrane, the major effect of some hormones is to activate carrier molecules in or near the membrane to increase the movement of substrates or ions from outside to inside the cell. For example, insulin binds to receptors on the surface of the cell and mobilizes glucose transporters located in the membrane of the cell. The transporters link up with glucose on the outside of the cell membrane where the concentration of glucose is high, and the glucose-transporter diffuses to the inside of the membrane to release glucose for use in the cell (56a). If an individual does not have adequate insulin, as exists in uncontrolled diabetes, glucose accumulates in the plasma because the glucose transporters in the membrane are not activated.

Stimulation of DNA in the Nucleus Due to their lipid-like nature, steroid hormones diffuse easily through cell membranes where they become bound to a protein receptor in the cytoplasm of the cell. Figure 5.2 shows that the steroid-receptor complex enters the nucleus and binds to a specific protein linked to DNA, which contains the instruction codes for protein synthesis. This initiates the steps leading to the synthesis of a specific messenger RNA (mRNA) that carries the codes from the nucleus to the cytoplasm where the specific protein is synthesized. While thyroid hormones are not steroid hormones, they act in a similar manner. These processes—the activation of DNA and the synthesis of specific protein—take time to turn on (making the hormones involved "slow acting" hormones), but their effects are longer lasting than those generated by "second messengers" (41).

Second Messengers Many hormones, because of their size or highly charged structure, cannot easily cross cell membranes. These hormones exert their effects by binding to a receptor on the membrane surface and activating a **G protein** located in the membrane of the cell. The G protein is the link between the hormone-receptor interaction on the surface of the membrane and the subsequent events inside the cell. The G protein may open an ion channel to allow Ca^{++} to enter the cell, or it may activate an enzyme in the membrane. If the G protein activates **adenylate cyclase,** then **cyclic AMP** (cyclic 3', 5'-adenosine monophosphate) is formed from ATP (see figure 5.3). In turn, the cyclic AMP concentration increases in the cell and activates proteins, which directly alter cellular activity. For example, this mechanism is used to convert glycogen to glucose in the muscle, and triglycerides to free fatty acids and glycerol in adipose tissue. The cyclic AMP is inactivated by **phosphodiesterase,** an enzyme which converts cyclic AMP to 5'AMP. Factors that interfere with phosphodiesterase activity, such as caffeine, would increase the effect of the hormone by allowing cyclic AMP to exert its effect for a longer period of time. For example, caffeine exerts this effect on adipose tissue, causing free fatty acids to be mobilized at a faster rate (see chapter 25).

If the G protein activates a Ca^{++} ion channel, then Ca^{++} enters the cell and binds to and activates a

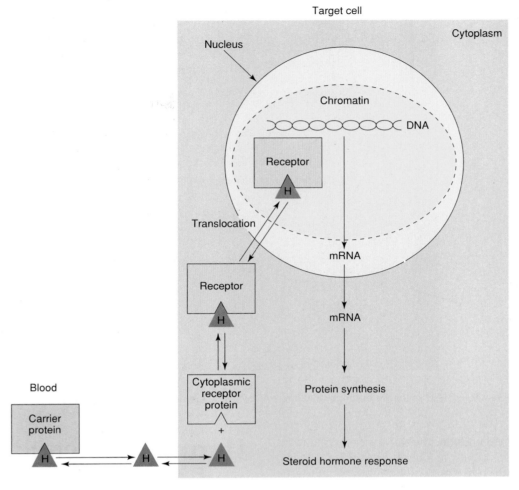

Figure 5.2

The mechanism by which steroid hormones act on target cells. The steroid hormone, represented by the triangle with the letter "H," binds to a cytoplasmic receptor to be transported to the nucleus where it stimulates DNA to bring about a change in cellular activity.

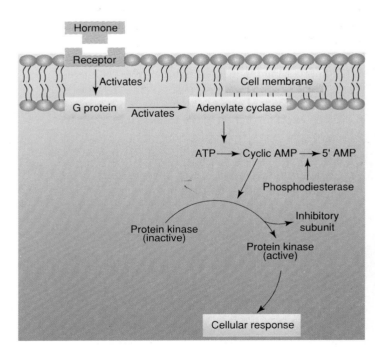

Figure 5.3

The cyclic AMP "second messenger" mechanism by which hormones act on target cells.

Figure 5.4
Calcium and phospholipase C second messenger mechanisms by which hormones act on target cells.

protein called **calmodulin.** The activated calmodulin influences cellular activity in much the same way as cyclic AMP does (see figure 5.4). Lastly, a G protein may activate a membrane-bound enzyme **phospholipase C.** When this occurs, a phospholipid in the membrane, phosphatidylinositol, is hydrolyzed into two intracellular molecules, **inositol triphosphate,** which causes Ca^{++} release from intracellular stores, and **diacylglycerol.** The diacylglycerol activates **protein kinase C** that, in turn; activates proteins in the cell (see figure 5.4). Cyclic AMP, Ca^{++}, inositol triphosphate, and diacylglycerol are viewed as **second messengers** in the events following the hormone's binding to a receptor on the cell membrane. These second messengers should not be viewed as being independent of one another, because changes in one can affect the action of the others (105).

in summary

- The hormone-receptor interaction triggers events at the cell, and changing the concentration of the hormone, the number of receptors on the cell, or the affinity of the receptor for the hormone will all influence the magnitude of the effect.
- Hormones bring about their effects by altering membrane transport, stimulating DNA to increase protein synthesis, and activating second messengers (cyclic AMP, Ca^{++}, inositol triphosphate, and diacylglycerol).

Hormones: Regulation and Action

This section will present the major endocrine glands, their hormones and how they are regulated, the effects the hormones have on tissues, and how some of the hormones respond to exercise. This information is essential in order to discuss the role of the neuroendocrine system in the mobilization of fuel for exercise.

Hypothalamus and the Pituitary Gland

The **pituitary gland** is located at the base of the brain, attached to the **hypothalamus.** The gland has two lobes, the anterior lobe (adenohypophysis), which is a true endocrine gland, and the posterior lobe (neurohypophysis), which is neural tissue extending from the hypothalamus. Both lobes are under the direct control of the hypothalamus. In the case of the **anterior pituitary,** hormone release is controlled by chemicals (**releasing hormones** or factors) that originate in neurons located in the hypothalamus. These releasing hormones stimulate or inhibit the release of specific hormones from the anterior pituitary. The posterior pituitary gland receives its hormones from special neurons originating in the hypothalamus. The hormones move down the axon to blood vessels in the posterior hypothalamus where they are discharged into the general circulation (60).

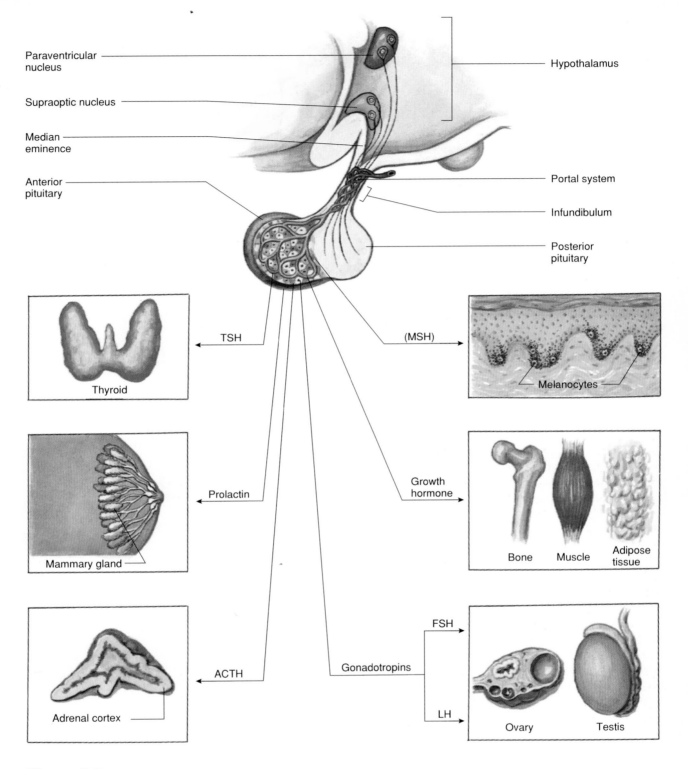

Paraventricular nucleus

Supraoptic nucleus

Median eminence

Anterior pituitary

Hypothalamus

Portal system

Infundibulum

Posterior pituitary

TSH

Thyroid

(MSH)

Melanocytes

Prolactin

Mammary gland

Growth hormone

Bone   Muscle   Adipose tissue

ACTH

Adrenal cortex

FSH

Gonadotropins

LH

Ovary   Testis

Figure 5.5
Summary of the hormones released from the anterior pituitary gland, and their target tissues.

Anterior Pituitary Gland
The anterior pituitary hormones include **adrenocorticotrophic hormone (ACTH), follicle-stimulating hormone (FSH), luteinizing hormone (LH), thyroid-stimulating hormone (TSH), growth hormone (GH),** and **prolactin.** Figure 5.5 shows each hormone and its target tissue. While prolactin directly stimulates the breast to produce milk, the majority of the hormones secreted from the anterior pituitary control the release of other hormones. TSH controls the rate of thyroid hormone formation and secretion from the thyroid gland; ACTH stimulates the production and

A Closer Look 5.1

Growth Hormone and Performance

An excess of growth hormone (GH) during childhood is tied to gigantism, while an inadequate secretion causes dwarfism. The latter condition requires the administration of GH (along with other growth-promoting hormones) during the growing years if the child is to regain his or her normal position on the growth chart. GH was originally obtained by extracting it from the pituitary glands of cadavers—an expensive and time-consuming proposition. Due to the success of genetic engineering, human GH is now available in large quantities.

If an excess of GH occurs during adulthood, a condition called **acromegaly** occurs. The additional GH during adulthood does not affect growth in height since the epiphyseal growth plates at the ends of the long bones have closed. Unfortunately, the excess GH causes permanent deformities as seen in a thickening of the bones in the face, hands, and feet. Until recently, the usual cause of acromegaly was a tumor in the anterior pituitary gland that resulted in excess secretion of

secretion of cortisol in the adrenal cortex; LH stimulates the production of testosterone in the testes and estrogen in the ovary; and, GH stimulates the release of **somatomedins** from the liver. However, as we will see, growth hormone exerts important effects on protein, fat, and carbohydrate metabolism (60).

Growth Hormone Growth hormone (GH) is secreted from the anterior pituitary gland and exerts profound effects on the growth of all tissues. Growth hormone secretion is controlled by releasing hormones secreted from the hypothalamus. Growth hormone releasing hormone (GHRH) stimulates GH release from the anterior pituitary, while another factor, **hypothalamic somatostatin,** inhibits it. The GH and somatomedin levels in blood exert a negative feedback effect on the continued secretion of GH. As shown in figure 5.6, additional input to the hypothalamus that can influence the secretion of GH includes exercise, stress (broadly defined), a low plasma-glucose concentration, and sleep (104).

GH stimulates tissue uptake of amino acids, the synthesis of new protein, and long bone growth. In addition, GH opposes the action of insulin to reduce the use of plasma glucose, increases the synthesis of new glucose in the liver (gluconeogenesis), and increases the mobilization of fatty acids from adipose tissue to spare plasma glucose. Given these characteristics, it should be no surprise that GH increases with exercise to help maintain the plasma glucose concentration (this will be covered in detail in a later section). Some of these effects are due to the direct effect of GH on tissues, while others are due to somatomedins, which are growth factors released from the liver in response to GH. Growth hormone, because of its role in protein synthesis, is being used by some athletes to enhance muscle mass. However, there are problems with this approach to better performance through chemistry (see A Closer Look 5.1).

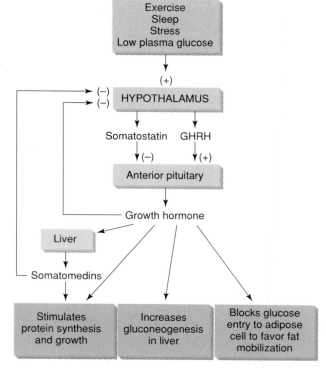

Figure 5.6

Summary of the positive and negative input to the hypothalamus, influencing growth hormone secretion.

From A. J. Vander, et al., *Human Physiology: The Mechanisms of Body Function*, 4th ed. Copyright © 1985 McGraw-Hill, Inc., New York. Reprinted by permission.

in summary

- The hypothalamus controls the activity of both the anterior pituitary and posterior pituitary glands.
- GH is released from the anterior pituitary gland and is essential for normal growth.
- GH increases during exercise to mobilize fatty acids from adipose tissue and aid in the maintenance of blood glucose.

GH. This is no longer the case. In an unfortunate drive to take advantage of the muscle-growth-stimulating effects of GH, body builders and strength trainers are injecting the now readily available human GH, along with other hormones (see A Closer Look 5.3). Evidence exists showing that GH increases protein synthesis in muscle; however, it is connective tissue protein (collagen) that is increased more than contractile protein. Consistent with these observations is the fact that strength gains do not parallel gains in muscle size (73). Similar observations have been made in studies involving GH-deficient adults who were injected with GH during a resistance-training program (97a, 113a). As with all hormones that have multiple effects, the user can't have one effect without the other. Chronic use of GH may lead to diabetes, carpal tunnel compression, muscle disease, and shortened life span (73, 112, 113a). Concern over the use of GH is so great that some people are recommending that it be reclassified as a "controlled substance" to reduce its availability (19, 98).

Posterior Pituitary Gland

The **posterior pituitary gland** releases two hormones, oxytocin and **antidiuretic hormone (ADH),** which is also called *vasopressin*. Oxytocin is a powerful stimulator of smooth muscle, especially at the time of childbirth, and is also involved in the milk "let down" response needed for the release of milk from the breast.

Antidiuretic Hormone Antidiuretic hormone (ADH) does what its name implies: it reduces water loss from the body. ADH favors the reabsorption of water from the kidney tubules back into the capillaries to maintain body fluid. There are two major stimuli that result in an increased secretion of ADH:

- high plasma osmolality (a low water concentration) that can be caused by excessive sweating without water replacement, and
- a low plasma volume, which can be due either to the loss of blood, or to inadequate fluid replacement.

There are osmoreceptors in the hypothalamus that sense the water concentration in the interstitial fluid. When the plasma has a high concentration of particles (low water concentration) the osmoreceptors shrink, and a neural reflex to the hypothalamus stimulates ADH release, which causes a reduction in water loss at the kidney. If the osmolality of the plasma is normal, but the volume of plasma is low, stretch receptors in the left atrium initiate a reflex leading to ADH release to attempt to maintain body fluid. During exercise, plasma volume decreases and osmolality increases, and for exercise intensities in excess of 60% of $\dot{V}O_2$ max, ADH secretion is increased as shown in figure 5.7 (17). This favors the conservation of water to maintain plasma volume (107).

Thyroid Gland

The **thyroid gland** is stimulated by TSH to synthesize two iodine-containing hormones: **triiodothyronine (T$_3$)** and **thyroxine (T$_4$).** T$_3$ contains three iodine atoms

Figure 5.7
Percent change in the plasma antidiuretic hormone (ADH) concentration with increasing exercise intensity.

and T$_4$ contains four. TSH is also the primary stimulus for release of T$_3$ and T$_4$ into the circulation where they are bound to plasma proteins. Remember, it is the "free" hormone concentration (that which is not bound to plasma proteins) that is important in bringing about an effect on tissue.

Thyroxine

Thyroid hormones are central in establishing the overall metabolic rate (i.e., a hypothyroid (low T$_3$) individual would be characterized as being lethargic and hypokinetic). It is this effect of the hormone that has been linked to weight-control problems, however, only a small percentage of obese individuals are hypothyroid. T$_3$ and T$_4$ act as permissive hormones in that they permit other hormones to exert their full effect. There is a relatively long latent period between the time T$_3$ and T$_4$ are elevated and when their effects are observed. The latent period is six to twelve hours for T$_3$ and two to three days for T$_4$. However, once initiated, their effects are long lasting (41). The control of T$_3$ and

T_4 secretion is another example of the negative feedback mechanism introduced in chapter 2. As the plasma concentrations of T_3 and T_4 increase, they inhibit the release of TSH-releasing hormone from the hypothalamus as well as TSH itself. This self-regulating system insures the necessary level of T_3 and T_4 for the maintenance of a normal metabolic rate. During exercise the "free" hormone concentration increases due to changes in the binding characteristic of the transport protein, and the hormones are taken up at a faster rate by tissues. In order to counter the higher rate of removal of T_3 and T_4, TSH secretion increases and causes an increased secretion of these hormones from the thyroid gland (100). Recent evidence suggests that resistance training has little effect on the pituitary (TSH)-thyroid (T_3, T_4) function (2).

in summary

- Thyroid hormones, T_3 and T_4, are important for maintaining the metabolic rate and allowing other hormones to bring about their full effect.

Calcitonin

The thyroid gland also secretes **calcitonin,** which is involved in a minor way in the regulation of plasma calcium (Ca^{++}), a crucial ion for normal muscle and nerve function. The secretion of this hormone is controlled by another negative feedback mechanism. As the plasma Ca^{++} concentration increases, calcitonin release is increased. Calcitonin blocks the release of Ca^{++} from bone to lower the plasma Ca^{++} concentration. As the Ca^{++} concentration is decreased, the rate of calcitonin secretion is reduced.

Parathyroid Gland

Parathyroid hormone is the primary hormone involved in plasma Ca^{++} regulation. The parathyroid gland releases parathyroid hormone in response to a low plasma Ca^{++} concentration. The hormone stimulates bone to release Ca^{++} into the plasma, and simultaneously increases the renal absorption of Ca^{++}; both raise the plasma Ca^{++} level. Parathyroid hormone also stimulates the kidney to convert a form of Vitamin D (vitamin D_3) into a hormone that increases the absorption of Ca^{++} from the gastrointestinal tract. Exercise increases the concentration of parathyroid hormone in the plasma (68, 69).

Adrenal Gland

The adrenal gland is really two different glands, the adrenal medulla, which secretes the **catecholamines, epinephrine (E),** and **norepinephrine (NE),** and the **adrenal cortex,** which secretes steroid hormones.

Adrenal Medulla

The adrenal medulla is part of the sympathetic nervous system. Eighty percent of the gland's hormonal secretion is epinephrine, which affects receptors in the cardiovascular and respiratory systems, gastrointestinal (GI) tract, liver, other endocrine glands, muscle, and adipose tissue. E and NE are involved in the maintenance of blood pressure and the plasma glucose concentration. Their role in the cardiovascular system is discussed in chapter 9 and their involvement in the mobilization of substrate for exercise is discussed later in this chapter. E and NE also respond to strong emotional stimuli, and are the bases of Cannon's "fight or flight" hypothesis of how the body responds to challenges from the environment (11). Cannon's view was that the activation of the sympathetic nervous system prepared you either to confront a danger, or to flee from it. Statements by broadcasters such as "The adrenalin must really be pumping now" is a rough translation of this hypothesis.

E and NE bind to adrenergic (from adrenaline, the European name for epinephrine) receptors on target tissues. The receptors are divided into two major classes: **alpha** (α) and **beta** (β), with subgroups (α_1 and α_2; β_1 and β_2). E and NE bring about their effects via the second messenger mechanisms mentioned earlier. The response generated in the target tissue, both size and direction (inhibitory or excitatory), is dependent on the receptor type and whether E or NE is involved. This is an example of how important the receptors are in determining the cell's response to a hormone. Table 5.1 summarizes the effects of E and NE relative to the type of adrenergic receptor involved (93). The different receptors cause changes in the cell's activity by increasing or decreasing the cyclic AMP or Ca^{++} concentrations. From this table it can be seen that if a cell experienced a loss of β_1 receptors and gain in α_2 receptors the same epinephrine concentration would bring about very different effects in the cell.

in summary

- The adrenal medulla secretes the catecholamines epinephrine (E) and norepinephrine (NE). E is the adrenal medulla's primary secretion (80%), while NE is primarily secreted from the adrenergic neurons of the sympathetic nervous system.
- Epinephrine and norepinephrine bind to α and β adrenergic receptors and bring about changes in cellular activity (e.g., increased heart rate, mobilization of fatty acids from adipose tissue) via second messengers.

Table 5.1   Physiological Responses to Catecholamines: Role of Receptor Type

Receptor Type	Effect of E/NE	Membrane-bound Enzyme	Intracellular Mediator	Effects on Various Tissues
β_1	E = NE	Adenylate clyclase	↑ cAMP	↑Heart rate ↑Glycogenolysis ↑Lipolysis
β_2	E >>> NE	Adenylate clyclase	↑ cAMP	↑Bronchodilation ↑Vasodilation
α_1	E ≥ NE	Phospholipase C	↑ Ca^{++}	↑Phosphodiesterase ↑Vasoconstriction
α_2	E ≥ NE	Adenylate clyclase	↓ cAMP	Opposes action of β_1 and β_2 receptors

Adapted from J. Tepperman and H. M. Tepperman. 1987. *Metabolic and Endocrine Physiology*, 5th ed. Chicago: Year Book Medical Publishers.

Adrenal Cortex

The adrenal cortex secretes a variety of steroid hormones having rather distinct physiological functions. The hormones can be grouped into three different categories:

- **mineralocorticoids** (aldosterone), involved in the maintenance of the Na^+ and K^+ concentrations in plasma,
- **glucocorticoids** (cortisol), involved in plasma glucose regulation, and
- **sex steroids (androgens** and **estrogens),** which support prepubescent growth, with androgens being associated with postpubescent sex drive in women.

The chemical precursor common to all of these steroid hormones is cholesterol, and while the final active hormones possess minor structural differences, their physiological functions differ greatly.

Aldosterone **Aldosterone** (mineralocorticoid) is an important regulator of Na^+ reabsorption and K^+ secretion at the kidney. Aldosterone is directly involved in Na^+/H_2O balance and, consequently, plasma volume and blood pressure (chapter 9). There are two levels of control over aldosterone secretion. The release of aldosterone from the adrenal cortex is controlled directly by the plasma K^+ concentration. An increase in K^+ concentration increases aldosterone secretion, which stimulates the kidney's active transport mechanism to secrete K^+ ions. This control system uses the negative feedback loop we have already seen. Aldosterone secretion is also controlled by another more complicated mechanism. A decrease in plasma volume, a fall in blood pressure at the kidney, or an increase in sympathetic nerve activity to the kidney stimulates special cells in the kidney to secrete an enzyme called **renin.** Renin enters the plasma and converts renin substrate

Figure 5.8
Parallel increases in renin activity, angiotensin II, and aldosterone with increasing intensities of exercise. Data are expressed as the percent change from resting values.

to **angiotensin I,** which is, in turn, converted to **angiotensin II** by a "converting enzyme" in the lung. Angiotensin II stimulates aldosterone release, which increases Na^+ reabsorption. The stimuli for aldosterone and ADH secretion are also the signals that stimulate thirst, a necessary ingredient to restore body fluid volume. During light exercise there is little or no change in plasma renin activity or aldosterone (74), however, when a heat load is imposed during light exercise, both renin and aldosterone secretion are increased (32). When exercise intensity approaches 50% $\dot{V}O_2$ max (figure 5.8) renin, angiotensin, and aldosterone increase in parallel, showing the linkage within this homeostatic system (74, 100). Further, liver production of renin substrate increases to maintain the plasma concentration (76).

A Closer Look 5.2

Endorphins and Exercise

The reader may be familiar with the expression "runner's high" as a description of the good feeling some individuals experience during long-distance runs. This experience has been linked to **endorphins**, endogenous morphine-like substances that interact with opiate receptors in the brain areas involved in the transmission of information about pain. β-endorphin is formed in the anterior pituitary from β-lipotrophin, which is itself generated during the formation of adrenocorticotrophic hormone (ACTH) (104). Given the close relationship between these substances and ACTH, which is the cornerstone of Selye's General Adaptation Syndrome, investigators became interested in how plasma levels of β-lipotrophin and β-endorphin would respond to exercise stress. Studies conducted in the early 1980s found that exercise caused parallel changes in plasma ACTH and β-endorphin (31). A summary of the early work in this area supported this observation, showing an elevation in β-lipotrophin/β-endorphin with exercise in men (28) and women (75). As chemical techniques improved to separate β-endorphin from β-lipotrophin, other studies

---

Cortisol The primary glucocorticoid secreted by the adrenal cortex is **cortisol**. Cortisol contributes to the maintenance of plasma glucose during long-term fasting and exercise by a variety of mechanisms:

- promoting the breakdown of tissue protein (by inhibiting protein synthesis) to form amino acids, which are then used by the liver to form new glucose (gluconeogenesis),
- stimulating the mobilization of free fatty acids from adipose tissue,
- stimulating liver enzymes involved in the metabolic pathway leading to glucose synthesis, and
- blocking the entry of glucose into tissues, forcing those tissues to use more fatty acids as fuel (41, 104).

A summary of cortisol's actions and its regulation is presented in figure 5.9. Cortisol secretion is controlled in the same manner as thyroxine. The hypothalamus secretes corticotrophic-releasing hormone (CRH), which causes the anterior pituitary gland to secrete more ACTH into the general circulation. ACTH binds to receptors on the adrenal cortex and increases cortisol secretion. As the cortisol level increases, CRH and ACTH are inhibited in another negative feedback system. However, the hypothalamus, like any brain center, receives neural input from other areas of the brain. This input can influence the secretion of hypothalamic-releasing hormones beyond the level seen in a negative feedback system. Over fifty years ago Hans Selye observed that a wide variety of stressful events such as burns, bone breaks, and heavy

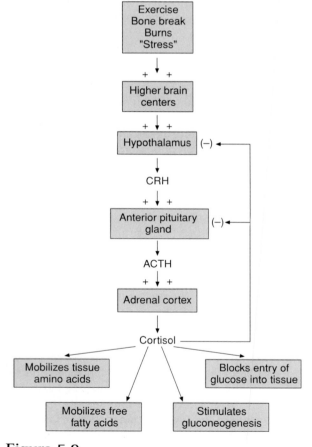

Figure 5.9

Control of cortisol secretion, showing the balance of positive and negative input to the hypothalamus, and cortisol's influence on metabolism.

were conducted. One study found no changes in β-endorphin in subjects who exercised at 60% $\dot{V}O_2$ max for one hour (66). This has been confirmed in both trained and untrained subjects who showed elevated plasma β-endorphin levels only when the exercise intensity exceeded 70% $\dot{V}O_2$ max. Further, the higher the intensity, the shorter the duration needed to cause the elevation (37, 38). While there is support for the change in β-endorphin to be linked to lactate levels above 4 mM (lactate threshold), trained subjects had the same β-endorphin response as untrained subjects, even though lactate levels were lower in the trained subjects (38, 89). The results support the proposition that β-endorphins may be related to changes in mood and pain threshold during endurance exercise. However, the plasma levels may not adequately reflect the influence of these substances on neuroendocrine function in the brain (101). Consistent with this cautious interpretation, Morgan (80) emphasizes the need to explore alternative hypotheses in studying the effect of exercise on mood changes. The reader is referred to a paper that does just that (101).

exercise led to predictable increases in ACTH and cortisol; he called this response the *General Adaptation Syndrome* (GAS). A key point in this response was the release of ACTH and cortisol to aid in the adaptation. His GAS had three stages: (a) *the alarm reaction*, involving cortisol secretion, (b) *stage of resistance*, where repairs are made, and (c) *stage of exhaustion*, in which repairs are not adequate, and sickness or death results (91). The usefulness of the GAS is seen in times of "stress" caused by tissue damage. Cortisol stimulates the breakdown of tissue protein to form amino acids, which can then be used at the site of the tissue damage for repair. While it is clear that muscle tissue is a primary source of amino acids, the functional overload of muscle with resistance or endurance training can prevent the muscle atrophy the glucocorticoids can cause (3, 47, 47a). Could the GAS be linked to the "runner's high" experienced during long-term exercise? See A Closer Look 5.2 for details.

in summary

- The adrenal cortex secretes aldosterone (mineralocorticoid), cortisol (glucocorticoid), and estrogens and androgens (sex steroids).
- Aldosterone regulates Na$^+$ and K$^+$ balance. Aldosterone secretion increases with strenuous exercise, driven by the renin-angiotensin system.
- Cortisol responds to a variety of stressors including exercise to insure that fuel (glucose and free fatty acids) are available, and to make amino acids available for tissue repair.

Pancreas

The **pancreas** is both an exocrine and endocrine gland. The exocrine secretions include digestive enzymes and bicarbonate, which are secreted into ducts leading to the small intestine. The hormones, released from groups of cells in the endocrine portion of the pancreas called the islets of Langerhans, include **insulin, glucagon,** and **somatostatin.**

Insulin

Insulin is secreted from beta cells of the islets of Langerhans. Insulin is the most important hormone during the absorptive state, when nutrients are entering the blood from the small intestine. Insulin stimulates tissues to take up nutrient molecules such as glucose and amino acids and store them as glycogen, proteins, and fats. Insulin's best-known role is in the facilitated diffusion of glucose across cell membranes. A lack of insulin causes an accumulation of glucose in the plasma since the tissues cannot take it up. The plasma glucose concentration can become so high that reabsorption mechanisms in the kidney are overwhelmed and glucose is lost to the urine, taking large volumes of water with it. This condition is called **diabetes mellitus.**

As mentioned earlier in this chapter, insulin secretion is influenced by a wide variety of factors: plasma glucose concentration, plasma amino acid concentration, sympathetic and parasympathetic nerve stimulation, and various hormones. The rate of secretion of insulin is dependent on the level of excitatory and inhibitory input to the beta cells of the pancreas (see figure 5.1). The blood glucose concentration is a major source of input that is part of a simple negative feedback loop; as the plasma glucose concentration increases (following a meal), the beta cells directly monitor this increase and secrete additional insulin to enhance tissue uptake of glucose. This increased uptake lowers the plasma glucose concentration, and insulin secretion is reduced (41, 67).

Glucagon

Glucagon, secreted from the alpha cells in the islets of Langerhans, exerts an effect opposite that of insulin. Glucagon secretion increases in response to a low plasma glucose concentration, which is monitored by the alpha cells. Glucagon stimulates both the mobilization of glucose from liver stores (glycogenolysis) and free fatty acids from adipose tissue (to spare blood glucose as a fuel). Lastly, along with cortisol, glucagon stimulates gluconeogenesis in the liver. Glucagon secretion is also influenced by factors other than the glucose concentration, notably, the sympathetic nervous system (99). A complete description of the role of insulin and glucagon in the maintenance of blood glucose during exercise is presented later in this chapter.

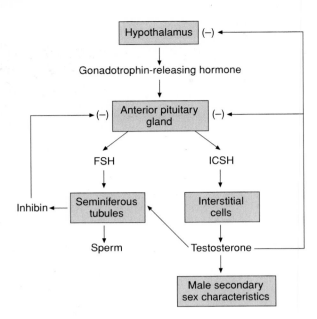

Figure 5.10
Control of testosterone secretion and sperm production by hypothalamus and anterior pituitary.

in summary

- Insulin is secreted by the β cells of the islets of Langerhans in the pancreas and promotes the storage of glucose, amino acids, and fats.
- Glucagon is secreted by the α cells of the islets of Langerhans in the pancreas and promotes the mobilization of glucose and fatty acids.

Somatostatin

Pancreatic somatostatin is secreted by the delta cells of the islets of Langerhans. Pancreatic somatostatin secretion is increased during the absorptive state and modifies the activity of the GI tract to control the rate of entry of nutrient molecules into the circulation. It may also be involved in the regulation of insulin secretion (99).

Testes and Ovaries

Testosterone and estrogen are the primary sex steroids secreted by the testis and ovary, respectively. These hormones are not only important in establishing and maintaining reproductive function, they determine the secondary sex characteristics associated with masculinity and femininity.

Testosterone

Testosterone is secreted by the interstitial cells of the testes and is controlled by interstitial cell stimulating hormone (ICSH—also known as LH), produced in the anterior pituitary. LH is, in turn, controlled by a releasing

hormone secreted by the hypothalamus. Sperm production from the seminiferous tubules of the testes requires follicle-stimulating hormone (FSH) from the anterior pituitary and testosterone. Figure 5.10 shows testosterone secretion to be controlled by a negative feedback loop involving the anterior pituitary gland and the hypothalamus. Sperm production is controlled, in part, by another negative feedback loop involving the hormone inhibin (67, 104).

Testosterone is both an **anabolic** (tissue building) and **androgenic** (promoter of masculine characteristics) **steroid** because it stimulates protein synthesis and is responsible for the characteristic changes in boys at adolescence that lead to the high muscle-mass to fat-mass ratio. The plasma testosterone concentration is increased 10%–37% during prolonged submaximal work (106), exercise taken to maximum levels (20), and during endurance or strength training workouts (58). Some feel that these small changes are due to a reduction in plasma volume, or to a decrease in the rate of inactivation and removal of testosterone (100). However, others have concluded on the basis of a parallel increase in the LH concentration, that the increase in plasma testosterone is due to an increased rate of production (20). While the testosterone response to exercise is small, and returns to resting values two hours after exercise (58), there is evidence that the resting plasma concentration is lower in both endurance-trained and resistance-trained males (4a, 43). In a recent study, high-mileage (108 km · wk^{-1}) runners had lower levels of testosterone, sperm count, and sperm motility compared to moderate-mileage (54 km · wk^{-1}) runners (23). Most readers probably recognize testosterone or one of its synthetic analogs

A Closer Look 5.3

Anabolic Steroids and Performance

Testosterone, as both an anabolic and androgenic steroid, causes size changes as well as male secondary sexual characteristics, respectively. Due to these combined effects, scientists developed steroids to maximize the anabolic effects and minimize the androgenic effects. These synthetic steroids were developed to promote tissue growth in patients who had experienced atrophy as a result of prolonged bed rest. Before long the thought occurred that these anabolic steroids might be helpful in developing muscle mass and strength in athletes.

Numerous studies were conducted to determine whether or not these steroids would bring about the desired changes, but a consensus was not achieved (4, 111, 112). The variation in results in published studies was related to the different tests used to measure body composition and strength, the study participants (novice or experienced), the length of the study, and training methods (114). In most of these studies the scientists used the recommended therapeutic dosage, as required by committees approving research with human subjects. Unfortunately, the "results" of many personal studies conducted in various gyms and weight training facilities throughout the world disagreed with these scientific results. Why the disagreement in results between the controlled scientific studies and these latter "studies"? In the weight room it was not uncommon for a person looking for greater "strength through chemistry" to take 10 to 100 times the recommended dosage! In effect, it was impossible to compare the results of the controlled scientific studies with those done in the gym.

By the mid-1980s, the steroid problem had reached a level that prompted both professional and college sport teams to institute testing of athletes to control drug use. Olympic and Pan-American athletes were also tested to disqualify those who used the steroid. The problem escalated when athletes started to take pure testosterone rather than the anabolic steroid. Part of the reason for the switch was to reduce the chance of detection when drug testing was conducted, and part was related to the availability of testosterone. The loss of the gold medal by Canadian sprinter Ben Johnson in the 1988 Olympic Games indicates that testing has caught up with some of those who break the rules.

Like the GH example presented in A Closer Look 5.1, the use of testosterone or synthetic anabolic steroids can bring about undesirable effects. Females taking anabolic steroids experience an increase in male secondary sex characteristics, (including deepening of voice and beard growth), clitoral enlargement, and a disruption in menstrual function (114a). Adverse reactions to chronic anabolic steroid use in males include (a) a decrease in testicular function, including a reduction in sperm production, (b) gynaecomastia—breast development, (c) liver dysfunction, and (d) mood or behavioral changes (2a, 5, 114a). Given that the use of anabolic steroids has a detrimental effect on ventricular wall mass (22, 102), blood lipids (2a, 65, 79, 114a), and glucose tolerance (2a, 114a), the risk of heart disease is also increased. These changes can be invoked by short-term use, but they revert to normal values upon discontinuance of the drug (2a, 114a). Although special attention has been directed at the habitual long-term user, there are questions about the validity of extrapolating from short-term studies to long-term consequences (114).

---

as one of the most abused drugs in the drive to increase muscle mass and performance. Such use is not without its problems (see A Closer Look 5.3).

Estrogen

Estrogen is a group of hormones that exerts similar physiological effects. These hormones include estradiole, estrone, and estriol. Estrogen stimulates breast development, female fat deposition, and other secondary sex characteristics (see figure 5.11). During the early part of the menstrual cycle called the *follicular phase*, LH stimulates the production of androgens in the follicle, which are subsequently converted to estrogens under the influence of FSH. Following ovulation, the *luteal phase* of the menstrual cycle begins, and both estrogens and progesterone are produced by the corpus luteum, a secretory structure occupying the space where the ovum was located (104). How does exercise affect these hormones, and vice versa? In one study (59) the plasma levels of LH, FSH, estradiole, and progesterone were measured at rest and at three different work rates during both the follicular and luteal phases of the menstrual cycle. The patterns of response of these hormones during graded exercise were very similar in the two phases of the menstrual cycle (59). Figure 5.12 shows only small changes in progesterone and estradiole with increasing intensities of work. Given that LH and FSH changed little or not at all during the luteal phase, the small increases in progesterone and estradiole were

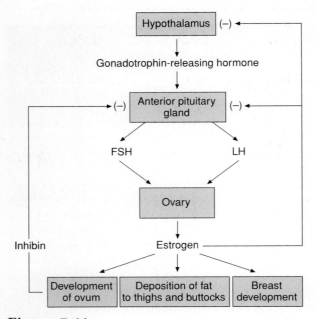

Figure 5.11
Role of estrogen in the development of female secondary sex characteristics and maturation of the ovum.

Figure 5.12
Percent change (from resting values) in the plasma FSH, LH, progesterone, and estradiole concentrations during graded exercise in the follicle and luteal phases of the menstrual cycle.

believed to be due to changes in plasma volume and to a decreased rate of removal rather than an increased rate of secretion (8, 100).

The effect of the phase of the menstrual cycle on exercise metabolism is not clear cut. Some have shown that the pattern of substrate use (7) and the respiratory exchange ratio (23a) are the same for the two phases of the menstrual cycle. Further, amenorrheic subjects (23a) or those taking oral contraceptives (7) responded similarly to eumenorrheic control subjects. In contrast, there is evidence that estradiole decreases glycogen use and increases lipid use to result in an increase in performance (9, 61). Other studies support this observation. Investigators report lower rates of carbohydrate oxidation for exercise at 35% and 60% $\dot{V}O_2$ max (but not at 75% $\dot{V}O_2$ max) during the midluteal phase of the menstrual cycle, compared to the midfollicular phase (43a). Consistent with the role that estrogen might play in this process, women who were matched for maximal aerobic power and training with men, had a lower rate of glycogen use during a moderate-intensity, prolonged treadmill run test (97). The lack of agreement across the studies makes this an exciting area of inquiry (87b).

Although the changes in estrogen and progesterone during an acute exercise bout are small, concern is being raised about the effect of chronic heavy exercise on the menstrual cycle of distance runners, gymnasts, and ballet dancers. For example, it has been shown that 29% of endurance athletes have primary (delay of menarche until age sixteen) or secondary (absence of menstruation in women who have had normal menstrual cycles) amenorrhea (109).

Special attention is now being directed at the issue of secondary amenorrhea (24, 71). Athletic amenorrhea is associated with chronically low estradiole levels, which can have a deleterious effect on bone mineral content. Osteoporosis, usually associated with the elderly (see chapter 17), is common in athletes with amenorrhea (48). Interested readers are referred to recent reviews of the possible causes of exercise-induced menstrual cycle alterations (4b, 60, 70), and the effect of the phase of the menstrual cycle on athletic performance (67a).

Table 5.2 contains a summary of the information on each of the endocrine glands, their secretion(s), actions, controlling factors, the stimuli that elicit a response, and the effect of exercise on the hormonal response. This would be a good place to stop and review before proceeding to the discussion of the hormonal control of muscle glycogen mobilization, and the maintenance of the plasma glucose concentration during exercise.

Endocrine Gland	Hormone	Action	Controlling Factors	Stimuli	Exercise Effect
Anterior pituitary	Growth hormone (GH)	Increases growth, FFA mobilization, and gluconeogenesis; decreases glucose uptake	Hypothalamic GH-releasing hormone; hypothalamic somatostatin	Exercise; "stress"; low blood glucose	↑
	Thyroid-stimulating hormone (TSH)	Increases T_3 and T_4 production and secretion	Hypothalamic TSH-releasing hormone	Low plasma T_3 and T_4	↑
	Adrenocorticotrophic hormone (ACTH)	Increases cortisol synthesis and secretion	Hypothalamic ACTH-releasing hormone	"Stress"; bone breaks; heavy exercise; burns etc.	?
	Gonadotrophins: Follicle-stimulating hormone (FSH); luteinizing hormone (LH)	Female: estrogen and progesterone production and ovum development Male: testosterone production and sperm development	Hypothalamic gonadotrophic-releasing hormone Females: plasma estrogen and progesterone Males: plasma testosterone	Cyclic or intermittent firing of neurons in the hypothalamus	Small or no change
	Prolactin	Increases breast milk production	Prolactin-inhibiting hormone (dopamine)	Sucking of nipple	?
	Endorphins	Blocks pain by acting on opiate receptors in brain	ACTH-releasing hormone ???	"Stress"	↑ for exercise ≥ 70% $\dot{V}O_2$ max
Posterior pituitary	Antidiuretic hormone (ADH) (vasopressin)	Decreases water loss at kidney; increases peripheral resistance	Hypothalamic neurons	Plasma volume; plasma osmolality	↑
	Oxytocin	Decreases uterine contractions; milk "let down"	Hypothalamic neurons	Uterine receptors; sucking of nipple	?
Thyroid	Triiodothyronine (T_3); thyroxine (T_4)	Increases metabolic rate, mobilization of fuels, growth	TSH; plasma T_3 and T_4	Low T_3 and T_4	↑ "Free" T_3 and T_4
	Calcitonin	Decreases plasma calcium	Plasma calcium	Elevated plasma calcium	?
Parathyroid	Parathyroid hormone	Increases plasma calcium	Plasma calcium	Low plasma calcium	↑
Adrenal cortex	Cortisol	Increases gluconeogenesis, FFA mobilization and protein synthesis; decreases glucose utilization	ACTH	See ACTH, above	↑ Heavy exercise; ↓ light exercise

Continued

Table 5.2   Continued

Endocrine Gland	Hormone	Action	Controlling Factors	Stimuli	Exercise Effect
	Aldosterone	Increases potassium secretion and sodium reabsorption at kidney	Plasma potassium concentration and renin-angiotensin system	Low blood pressure and plasma volume; elevated plasma potassium and sympathetic activity to kidney	↑
Adrenal medulla	Epinephrine (80%); norepinephrine (20%)	Increases glycogenolysis, FFA mobilization, heart rate, stroke volume, and peripheral resistance	Output of baroreceptors; glucose receptor in hypothalamus; brain and spinal centers	Low blood pressure, and blood glucose; too much "stress"; emotion	↑
Pancreas	Insulin	Increases glucose, amino acid, and FFA uptake into tissues	Plasma glucose and amino acid concentrations; autonomic nervous system	Elevated plasma glucose and amino acid concentrations; decreased epinephrine and norepinephrine	↓
	Glucagon	Increases glucose and FFA mobilization; gluconeo-genesis	Plasma glucose and amino acid concentrations; autonomic nervous system	Low plasma glucose and amino acid concentrations; elevated epinephrine and norepinephrine	↑
Testes	Testosterone	Protein synthesis; secondary sex characteristics; sex drive; sperm production	FSH and LH (ICSH)	Increased FSH and LH	Small ↑
Ovaries	Estrogen	Fat deposition; secondary sex characteristics; ovum development	FSH and LH	Increased FSH and LH	Small ↑

in summary

- Testosterone and estrogen establish and maintain reproductive function and determine secondary sex characteristics.
- Chronic exercise (training) can decrease testosterone levels in males and estrogen levels in females. The latter adaptation has potentially negative consequences related to osteoporosis.

Hormonal Control of Substrate Mobilization During Exercise

The type of substrate and the rate at which it is utilized during exercise depend to a large extent on the intensity and duration of the exercise. While diet and the training state of the person are important (chapters 21 and 23), the factors of intensity and duration of

Figure 5.13
Glycogen depletion in the quadriceps muscle during bicycle exercise of increasing exercise intensities.

Figure 5.14
Changes in the plasma epinephrine concentration during exercises of different intensities and durations.

exercise ordinarily have prominence. Because of this, our discussion of the hormonal control of substrate mobilization during exercise will be divided into two parts. The first part will deal with control of muscle glycogen utilization, and the second part with the control of glucose mobilization from the liver and free fatty acids (FFA) from adipose tissue.

Muscle–Glycogen Utilization

At the onset of most types of exercise, and for the entire duration of very strenuous exercise, muscle glycogen is the primary carbohydrate fuel for muscular work (88). The intensity of exercise, which is inversely related to exercise duration, determines the rate at which muscle glycogen is used as a fuel. Figure 5.13 shows a series of lines describing the rates of glycogen breakdown for various exercise intensities expressed as a percent of $\dot{V}O_2$ max. (88). The heavier the exercise, the faster glycogen is broken down. This process of glycogen breakdown (glycogenolysis) is initiated by second messengers, which activate protein kinases in the muscle cell (described in figure 5.3). Plasma epinephrine, a powerful stimulator of cyclic AMP formation when bound to β-adrenergic receptors on a cell, was believed to be primarily responsible for glycogenolysis. Figure 5.14 also shows a family of lines, the slopes of which describe how fast plasma E changes with increasing intensities of exercise (62). Clearly, the data presented in figures 5.13 and 5.14 are consistent with the view that there is a linkage between changes in plasma E during exercise and the increased rate of glycogen degradation. However, there is more to this story.

In order to test the hypothesis that glycogenolysis in muscle is controlled by circulating E during exercise, investigators had subjects take propra-nolol,

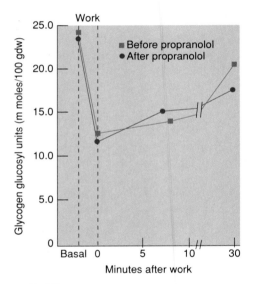

Figure 5.15
Changes in muscle glycogen due to two minutes of work at 1,200 kpm/min, before and after propranolol administration. Blocking the beta-adrenergic receptors had no effect on glycogen breakdown.

a drug that blocks both β_1 and β_2 adrenergic receptors on the cell membrane. This procedure should block glycogenolysis since cyclic AMP formation would be affected. In the control experiment, subjects worked for two minutes at an intensity of exercise that caused the muscle glycogen to be depleted to half its initial value, and the muscle lactate concentration to be elevated tenfold. Surprisingly, as shown in figure 5.15, when the subjects took the propranolol and repeated the test, there was no difference in glycogen depletion or lactate formation (44).

Figure 5.16

The breakdown of muscle glycogen, glycogenolysis, can be initiated by either the Ca^{++}-calmodulin mechanism or the cyclic AMP mechanism. When a drug blocks the β-receptor, glycogenolysis can still occur.

Other experiments have also shown that β-adrenergic blocking drugs have little effect on slowing the rate of glycogen breakdown during exercise (103). How can this be?

As mentioned in chapter 3, enzymatic reactions in a cell are under the control of both intracellular and extracellular factors. In the aforementioned example with propranolol, plasma E may not have been able to activate adenylate cyclase to form the cyclic AMP needed to activate the protein kinases to initiate glycogen breakdown. However, when a muscle cell is stimulated to contract, Ca^{++}, which is stored in the sarcoplasmic reticulum, floods the cell. Some Ca^{++} ions are used to initiate contractile events (chapter 8), but other Ca^{++} ions bind to calmodulin, which, in turn, activates the protein kinases needed for glycogenolysis (see figure 5.4). In this case, the increased intracellular Ca^{++} (rather than cAMP) is the initial event stimulating muscle glycogen breakdown. Figure 5.16 summarizes these events. Experiments in which the increased secretion of catecholamines was blocked during exercise confirmed the propranolol experiments, showing that an intact sympathoadrenal system was not necessary to initiate glycogenolysis in skeletal muscle (13).

Observations of glycogen depletion patterns support this view. Individuals who do heavy exercise with one leg will cause elevations in plasma E, which circulates to all muscle cells. The muscle glycogen, however, is depleted only from the exercised leg (53), suggesting that intracellular factors (e.g., Ca^{++}) are more responsible for these events. Further, in experiments in which individuals engaged in intermittent intense exercise interspersed with a rest period (interval work), the glycogen was depleted faster from fast-twitch fibers (25, 26, 39). The plasma E concentration should be the same outside both fast- and slow-twitch muscle fibers, but the glycogen was depleted at a faster rate from the fibers used in the activity. This is reasonable since a "resting" muscle fiber should not be using glycogen (or any other fuel) at a high rate.

The rate of glycogenolysis would be expected to parallel the rate at which ATP is used by the muscle, and this has been shown to be the case, independent of E (85). This discussion does not mean that E cannot or does not cause glycogenolysis (14, 113). There is ample evidence to show that a surge of E will in fact cause this to occur (57, 93, 94, 95).

in summary

- Glycogen breakdown to glucose in muscle is under the dual control of epinephrine-cyclic AMP and Ca^{++}-calmodulin. The latter's role is enhanced during exercise due to the increase in Ca^{++} from the sarcoplasmic reticulum. In this way the delivery of fuel (glucose) parallels the activation of contraction.

Blood Glucose Homeostasis During Exercise

As mentioned in the introduction, a focal point of hormonal control systems is the maintenance of the plasma glucose concentration during times of inadequate carbohydrate intake (fasting/starvation) and accelerated glucose removal from the circulation (exercise). In both cases body energy stores are used to meet the challenge, and the hormonal response to these two different situations, exercise and starvation, is quite similar.

The plasma glucose concentration is maintained through four different processes:

- mobilization of glucose from liver glycogen stores,
- mobilization of plasma FFA from adipose tissue to spare plasma glucose,
- synthesis of new glucose in the liver (gluconeogenesis) from amino acids, lactic acid, and glycerol, and
- blocking of glucose entry into cells to force the substitution of FFA as a fuel.

The overall aim of these four processes is to provide fuel for work while maintaining the plasma glucose concentration. This is a major task when you consider that the liver may have only 80 grams of glucose before exercise begins and the rate of blood glucose oxidation approaches 1 gm/min in heavy exercise or in prolonged (≥3 hours) moderate exercise (16, 19a).

While the hormones will be presented separately, keep in mind that each of the above processes is controlled by more than one hormone, and all four processes are involved in the adaptation to exercise. Some hormones act in a "permissive" way, or are "slow acting," while others are "fast acting" controllers of substrate mobilization. For this reason, this discussion of the hormonal control of plasma glucose will be divided into two sections, one dealing with permissive and slow-acting hormones, and the other dealing with fast-acting hormones.

Permissive and Slow-Acting Hormones

Thyroxine, cortisol, and growth hormone are involved in the regulation of carbohydrate, fat, and protein metabolism. These hormones are discussed in this section because they act either to facilitate the actions of other hormones, or to respond to stimuli in a slow manner. Remember, that to act in a permissive manner the hormone concentration doesn't have to change. However, as you will see, there are certain stressful situations in which permissive hormones can achieve such elevated plasma concentrations that they act directly to influence carbohydrate and fat metabolism rather than to simply facilitate the actions of other hormones.

Thyroxine The discussion of substrate mobilization during exercise must include thyroxine, a hormone whose concentration doesn't change dramatically from resting to the exercise state. As mentioned earlier, the thyroid hormones T_3 and T_4 are important in establishing the overall metabolic rate, and in allowing other hormones to exert their full effect (permissive hormone). Thyroxine accomplishes this latter function by influencing either the number of receptors on the surface of a cell (for other hormones to interact with), or the affinity of the receptor for the hormone. For example, without thyroxine, epinephrine has little effect on the mobilization of free fatty acids from adipose tissue. During exercise there is an increase in "free" thyroxine due to changes in the binding characteristics of the transport protein (100). T_3 and T_4 are removed from the plasma by tissues during exercise at a greater rate than at rest. In turn, TSH secretion from the anterior pituitary is increased to stimulate the secretion of T_3 and T_4 from the thyroid gland to maintain the plasma level (35). A low thyroxine (hypothyroid) state would interfere with the ability of other hormones to mobilize fuel for exercise (81, 100).

Cortisol The primary glucocorticoid in humans is cortisol. As figure 5.17 shows, cortisol stimulates FFA mobilization from adipose tissue, mobilizes tissue protein to yield amino acids for glucose synthesis in the liver (gluconeogenesis), and decreases the rate of glucose utilization by cells (41). There are problems, however, when attempting to describe the cortisol response to exercise. Given the GAS of Selye, events other than exercise can influence the cortisol response. Imagine how a naive subject might view a treadmill test on first exposure. The wires, noise, nose clip, mouthpiece, and blood sampling could all influence the level of arousal of the subject and result in a cortisol response that is not related to a need to mobilize additional substrate. Results supporting such a proposition were reported in the following study (84).

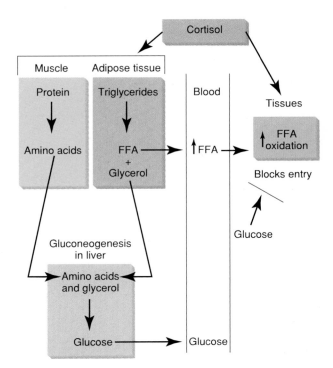

Figure 5.17
Role of cortisol in the maintenance of plasma glucose.

Twelve subjects walked on a treadmill at five times their resting metabolic rate (5 METs) for thirty minutes, and blood samples were taken for cortisol analysis. Ten of the twelve subjects showed a decrease in cortisol due to the exercise, while the other two, who were anxious, had an increase. Clearly, the perception of the subject can influence the cortisol response to mild exercise.

As exercise intensity increases, one might expect the cortisol secretion to increase. This is true, but only within certain limits. For example, Bonen (6) showed that the urinary excretion of cortisol was not changed by exercise at 76% $\dot{V}O_2$ max for ten minutes, but was increased about twofold when the duration was extended to thirty minutes. Davies and Few (21) extended our understanding of the cortisol response to exercise when they studied subjects who completed several one-hour exercise bouts. Each test was set at a constant intensity between 40%–80% $\dot{V}O_2$ max. Exercise at 40% $\dot{V}O_2$ max resulted in a decrease in plasma cortisol over time, while the response was considerably elevated for exercise at 80% $\dot{V}O_2$ max. Figure 5.18 shows the plasma cortisol concentration measured at sixty minutes into each of the above exercise tests plotted against % $\dot{V}O_2$ max. When the exercise intensity exceeded 60% $\dot{V}O_2$ max, the cortisol concentration increased; below that, the cortisol concentration decreased. What caused these changes? Using radioactive cortisol as a tracer, the researchers found that during light exercise cortisol was removed faster than the adrenal cortex secreted it, and during intense

Figure 5.18

Percent change (from resting values) in the plasma cortisol concentration with increasing exercise intensity.

Figure 5.19

Role of plasma growth hormone in the maintenance of plasma glucose.

Figure 5.20

(*a*) Percent change (from resting values) in the plasma growth hormone concentration with increasing exercise intensity. (*b*) Percent change (from resting values) in the plasma growth hormone concentration during exercise at 60% $\dot{V}O_2$ max for runners and nonrunners (controls).

exercise the increase in plasma cortisol was due to a higher rate of secretion that could more than match the rate of removal, which had doubled.

What is interesting is that for low-intensity, long-duration exercise where the effects of cortisol would go a long way in maintaining the plasma glucose concentration, the concentration of cortisol does not change very much. Even if it did, the effects on metabolism would not be immediately noticeable. The direct effect of cortisol is mediated through the stimulation of DNA and the resulting mRNA formation which leads to protein synthesis, a slow process. In essence, cortisol, like thyroxine, exerts a permissive effect on substrate mobilization during acute exercise, allowing other fast-acting hormones such as epinephrine and glucagon to deal with glucose and FFA mobilization. Given that athletic competitions (triathlon, ultra marathon, most team sports) can result in tissue damage, the reason for changes in the plasma cortisol concentration might not be for the mobilization of fuel for exercising muscles. In these situations cortisol's role in dealing with tissue repair might come to the forefront.

Growth Hormone Growth hormone plays a major role in the synthesis of tissue protein, acting either directly, or through the enhanced secretion of somatomedins from the liver. However, GH can also influence fat and carbohydrate metabolism. Figure 5.19 shows that growth hormone supports the action of cortisol: it decreases glucose uptake by tissue, increases FFA mobilization, and enhances gluconeogenesis in the liver. The net effect is to preserve the plasma glucose concentration.

Describing the plasma GH response to exercise is as difficult as describing cortisol's response to exercise since GH can also be altered by a wide variety of stresses: physical, chemical, and psychological (18, 40, 96). Given that, the earlier comments about cortisol should be kept in mind. Figure 5.20a shows plasma GH to increase with increasing intensities of exercise, achieving, at maximal work, values twenty-five times those at rest (96). Figure 5.20b shows the plasma GH concentration to increase over time during sixty minutes of exercise at 60% $\dot{V}O_2$ max (10). What is interesting, compared to other hormonal responses, is that the trained runners had a higher response compared to a group of nonrunners (see later discussion). By sixty minutes, values for both groups were about five to six times those measured at rest. In conclusion, GH, a hormone primarily concerned with protein synthesis, can achieve plasma concentrations during exercise that can exert a direct but "slow-acting" effect on carbohydrate and fat metabolism.

in summary

- The hormones thyroxine, cortisol, and growth hormone act in a permissive manner to support the actions of other hormones during exercise.
- Growth hormone and cortisol also provide a "slow-acting" effect on carbohydrate and fat metabolism during exercise.

Fast-Acting Hormones

In contrast to the aforementioned "permissive" and slow-acting hormones, there are very fast responding hormones whose actions quickly return the plasma glucose to normal. Again, while each will be presented separately, they behave collectively and in a predictable way during exercise to maintain the plasma glucose concentration (15).

Epinephrine and Norepinephrine Epinephrine and norepinephrine have already been discussed relative to muscle glycogen mobilization. However, as figure 5.21 shows, they are also involved in the mobilization of glucose from the liver, FFA from adipose tissue, and may interfere with the uptake of glucose by tissues (87). Although plasma NE can increase ten- to twentyfold during exercise and can achieve a plasma concentration that can exert a physiological effect (92), the primary means by which NE acts is when released from sympathetic neurons onto the surface of the tissue under consideration. The plasma level of NE is usually taken as an index of overall sympathetic nerve activity, but there is evidence that muscle sympathetic nerve activity during exercise may be a better indicator than that of plasma NE (90). Epinephrine, released from the adrenal medulla, is viewed as the primary catecholamine in the mobilization of glucose from the liver.

Figure 5.22 shows plasma E and NE to increase linearly with duration of exercise (52, 82). These changes are related to cardiovascular adjustments to exercise, as well as to the mobilization of fuel. These responses favor the mobilization of glucose and FFA to maintain the plasma glucose concentration. While it is sometimes difficult to separate the effect of E from NE, E seems to be more responsive to changes in the

Figure 5.21
Role of catecholamines in substrate mobilization.

Figure 5.22
Percent change (from resting values) in the plasma epinephrine and norepinephrine concentrations during exercise at ~60% $\dot{V}O_2$ max.

plasma glucose concentration. A low plasma glucose concentration stimulates a receptor in the hypothalamus to increase E secretion while having only a modest effect on plasma NE. In contrast, when the blood pressure is challenged, as during an increased heat load, the primary catecholamine involved is norepinephrine (82). Epinephrine binds to β-adrenergic receptors on the liver and stimulates the breakdown of liver glycogen to form glucose for release into the plasma. For example, when arm exercise is added to existing leg exercise, the adrenal medulla secretes a large amount of E. This causes the liver to release more glucose than muscles are using, and the blood glucose concentration actually increases (64). What happens if we block the effects of E and NE? If β-adrenergic receptors are blocked with propranolol (a β-adrenergic receptor blocking drug), the plasma glucose concentration is more difficult to maintain during exercise, especially if the subject has fasted (103). In addition, since the propranolol blocks β-adrenergic receptors on adipose tissue cells, less FFA are released and the muscles have to rely more on the limited carbohydrate supply for fuel (34).

Figure 5.23

Changes in plasma epinephrine and norepinephrine responses to a fixed work load over seven weeks of endurance training.

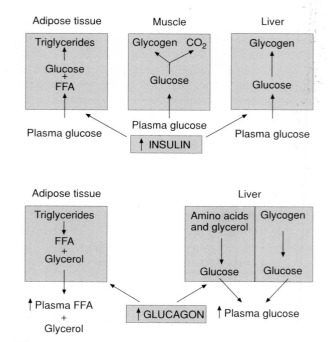

Figure 5.24

Effect of insulin and glucagon on glucose and fatty-acid uptake and mobilization.

Figure 5.23 shows that endurance training causes a very rapid decrease in the plasma E and NE responses to a fixed exercise bout. Within three weeks the concentration of both catecholamines is greatly reduced (110). Paralleling this rapid decrease in E and NE with endurance exercise training is a reduction in glucose mobilization (75a). In spite of this, the plasma glucose concentration is maintained, indicating the complexity of the control over the mobilization of fuel (see later discussion on hormone/substrate interaction). Interestingly, during a very stressful event a trained individual has a greater capacity to secrete E than an untrained individual (63). This suggests that physical training, which stimulates the sympathetic nervous system on a regular basis, increases the capacity of the adrenal medulla to respond to extreme challenges.

Insulin and Glucagon These two hormones will be discussed together since they respond to the same stimuli but exert opposite actions relative to the mobilization of liver glucose and adipose tissue FFA. In fact, it is the ratio of glucagon to insulin that provides control over the mobilization of these fuels (15, 105). Figure 5.24 shows insulin to be the primary hormone involved in the uptake and storage of glucose and FFA, and glucagon to cause the mobilization of those fuels from storage, as well as increase gluconeogenesis.

Given that insulin is directly involved in the uptake of glucose into tissue, and that glucose uptake by muscle can increase seven- to twentyfold during exercise (29), what should happen to the insulin concentration during exercise? Figure 5.25a shows that the insulin concentration decreases during exercise of increasing intensity (33, 45, 83); this of course is an appropriate response. If exercise were associated with an increase in insulin, the plasma glucose would be taken up into all tissues (including adipose tissue) at a faster rate, leading to an immediate hypoglycemia. The lower insulin concentration during exercise favors the mobilization of glucose from the liver and FFA from adipose tissue, both of which are necessary to maintain the plasma glucose concentration. Figure 5.25b shows that plasma insulin decreases during moderate-intensity, long-term exercise (42).

With plasma insulin decreasing with long-term exercise, it should be no surprise that the plasma glucagon concentration increases (42). This increase in plasma glucagon (shown in figure 5.26) favors the mobilization of FFA from adipose tissue and glucose from the liver, as well as an increase in gluconeogenesis. Overall, the reciprocal responses of insulin and glucagon favor the maintenance of the plasma glucose concentration at a time when the muscle is using plasma glucose at a high rate. Figure 5.26 also shows that following an endurance training program the glucagon response to a fixed exercise task is diminished to the point that there is no increase during exercise. In effect, endurance training allows the plasma glucose concentration to be maintained with little or no change in insulin and glucagon. The increased ability of

(a)

(b)

Figure 5.25

(*a*) Percent change (from resting values) in the plasma insulin concentration with increasing intensities of exercise. (*b*) Percent change (from resting values) in the plasma insulin concentration during prolonged exercise at 60% $\dot{V}O_2$ max showing the effect of endurance training on that response.

Figure 5.26

Percent change (from resting values) in the plasma glucagon concentration during prolonged exercise at 60% $\dot{V}O_2$ max showing the effect of endurance training on that response.

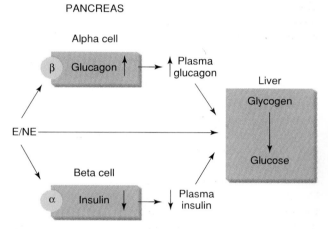

Figure 5.27

Effect of epinephrine and norepinephrine on insulin and glucagon secretion from the pancreas during exercise.

a trained person to use fat as a fuel is consistent with this reduction in the glucagon response to submaximal exercise because less liver glycogen is required to maintain the plasma glucose concentration (15).

These findings raise several questions. If the plasma glucose concentration is relatively constant during exercise, and the plasma glucose concentration is a primary stimulus for insulin and glucagon secretion, what causes the insulin secretion to decrease and glucagon secretion to increase? The answer lies in the multiple levels of control over hormonal secretion mentioned earlier in the chapter (see figure 5.1). There is no question that changes in the plasma glucose concentration provide an important level of control over the secretion of glucagon and insulin (34). However, when the plasma glucose concentration is relatively constant, the sympathetic nervous system can modify the secretion of insulin and glucagon. Figure 5.27 shows that E and NE stimulate α-adrenergic receptors on the beta cells of the pancreas to decrease insulin secretion during exercise when the plasma glucose concentration is normal. Figure 5.27

also shows that E and NE stimulate β-adrenergic receptors on the alpha cells of the pancreas to increase glucagon secretion when the plasma glucose concentration is normal. These effects have been confirmed through the use of adrenergic receptor blocking drugs. When phentolamine, an α-adrenergic receptor blocker, is given, insulin secretion increases with exercise. When propranolol, a β-adrenergic receptor blocker is given, the glucagon concentration remains the same or decreases with exercise (72). Figure 5.28 summarizes the effect the sympathetic nervous system has on the mobilization of fuel for muscular work. Endurance training decreases the sympathetic nervous system response to a fixed exercise bout, resulting in less stimulation of adrenergic receptors on the pancreas, and less change in insulin and glucagon.

During Submaximal Exercise

Figure 5.28
Effect of increased sympathetic nervous system activity on free-fatty-acid and glucose mobilization during submaximal exercise.

The observation that plasma insulin decreases with prolonged submaximal exercise raises another question. How can exercising muscle take up glucose seven to twenty times faster than at rest if the insulin concentration is decreasing? Part of the answer lies in the large increase in blood flow to muscle during exercise. Glucose delivery is the product of muscle blood flow and the blood glucose concentration. Therefore, during exercise more glucose and insulin are delivered to muscle than at rest, and because the muscle is using glucose at a higher rate, a gradient for its facilitated diffusion is created (55). Another part of the answer relates to exercise-induced changes in the number of glucose transporters in the membrane. It has been known for some time that acute (a single bout) and chronic (training program) exercise increase a muscle's sensitivity to insulin such that less insulin is needed to have the same effect on glucose uptake into tissue (46, 56). The effects of insulin and exercise on glucose transport are additive, suggesting that two separate pools of glucose transporters are activated or translocated in the membrane (56, 108). Interestingly, hypoxia brings about the same effect as exercise, but it is not an additive effect, suggesting that hypoxia and exercise recruit the same transporters (12). What is there about exercise that could cause these changes in glucose transporters?

The answer lies in the high intramuscular Ca^{++} concentration that exists during exercise. The Ca^{++} appears to recruit inactive glucose transporters such that more glucose is transported for the same concentration of insulin (12, 49, 55). This improved glucose

(a) Hormonal responses to graded exercise

(b) Hormonal responses to prolonged exercise

Figure 5.29
(a) Summary of the hormonal responses to exercise of increasing intensity. (b) Summary of the hormonal responses to moderate exercise of long duration.

transport remains following exercise and facilitates the filling of muscle glycogen stores (see chapter 23). Repeated exercise bouts (training) reduces whole body insulin resistance and makes it an important part of therapy for the diabetic (55, 78, 115). Consistent with this, bed rest (77) and limb immobilization (86) increase insulin resistance.

In summary, figures 5.29a and 5.29b show the changes in epinephrine, norepinephrine, growth hormone, cortisol, glucagon and insulin to exercise of varying intensity and duration. The decrease in insulin and the increase in all the other hormones favor the mobilization of glucose from the liver, FFA from adipose tissue, gluconeogenesis in the liver, while inhibiting the uptake of glucose. These combined actions maintain homeostasis relative to the plasma glucose concentration so that the central nervous system and the muscles can have the fuel they need.

Hormone–Substrate Interaction

In the examples mentioned above, insulin and glucagon responded as they did during exercise with a normal plasma glucose concentration due to the influence of the sympathetic nervous system. It must be mentioned that if there were a sudden change in the plasma glucose concentration during exercise, these hormones would respond to that change. For example, if the ingestion of glucose before exercise caused an elevation of plasma glucose, the plasma concentration of insulin would increase. This hormonal change would reduce FFA mobilization and force the muscle to use additional muscle glycogen (1).

During intense exercise, plasma glucagon, GH, cortisol, E, and NE are elevated and insulin is decreased. These hormonal changes favor the mobilization of FFA from adipose tissue that would spare carbohydrate and help maintain the plasma glucose concentration. If this is the case, why does plasma FFA use decrease with increasing intensities of exercise (87a)? Part of the answer seems to be that there is an upper limit in the adipose cell's ability to deliver FFA to the circulation during exercise. For example, in trained subjects, the rate of release of FFA from adipose tissue was the highest at 25% $\dot{V}O_2$ max, and decreased at 65% and 85% $\dot{V}O_2$ max (87a). Given the fact that the adipose cell is under stronger hormonal stimulation at the higher work rates, the FFA actually appears to be "trapped" in the adipose cell (48a, 87a). This may be due to a variety of factors, one of which is lactate. Figure 5.30a shows that as the blood lactate concentration increases, the

(a)

(b)

Figure 5.30

(a) Changes in plasma free fatty acids due to increases in lactic acid. (b) Effect of lactic acid on the mobilization of free fatty acids from the adipose cell.

plasma FFA concentration decreases (54). The elevated lactate has been linked to an increase in alpha glycerol phosphate, the activated form of glycerol needed to make triglycerides. In effect, as fast as the FFA become available from the breakdown of triglycerides, the alpha glycerol phosphate recycles the FFA to generate a new triglyceride molecule (see figure 5.30b). The result is that the FFA are not released from the adipose cell (80a). Other explanations of the reduced availability of adipose tissue FFA during heavy exercise include a reduced blood supply to adipose tissue resulting in less FFA to transport to muscle (87a), and an inadequate amount of albumin, the plasma protein needed to transport the FFA in the plasma (48a). The result is that FFA are not released from the adipose cell, the plasma FFA level falls, and the muscle must use more carbohydrate as a fuel. One of the effects of endurance training is to decrease the lactate concentration at any fixed work rate. Such an adaptation would reduce the inhibition of this mobilization of FFA from adipose tissue and allow the trained person to use more fat as a fuel, thus sparing the limited carbohydrate stores and improving performance.

in summary

- The plasma FFA concentration decreases during heavy exercise even though the adipose cell is stimulated by a variety of hormones to increase triglyceride breakdown to FFA and glycerol. This may be due to (a) the high levels of lactate during heavy exercise that promotes the resynthesis of triglycerides, (b) an inadequate blood flow to adipose tissue, or (c) insufficient albumin needed to transport the FFA in the plasma.

study questions

1. Draw and label a diagram of a negative feedback mechanism for hormonal control using cortisol as an example.
2. List the factors that can influence the blood concentration of a hormone.
3. Discuss the use of testosterone and growth hormone as aids to increase muscle size and strength, and discuss the potential long-term consequences of such use.
4. List each endocrine gland, the hormone(s) secreted from that gland, and its (their) action(s).
5. Describe the two mechanisms by which muscle glycogen is broken down to glucose (glycogenolysis) for use in glycolysis. Which one is activated at the same time as muscle contraction?
6. Identify the four mechanisms involved in maintaining the blood glucose concentration.
7. Draw a summary graph of the changes in the following hormones with exercise of increasing intensity or duration: epinephrine, norepinephrine, cortisol, growth hormone, insulin, and glucagon.
8. What is the effect of training on the responses of epinephrine, norepinephrine, and glucagon to the same exercise task?
9. Briefly explain how glucose can be taken into the muscle at a high rate during exercise when plasma insulin is reduced. Include the role of glucose transporters.
10. Explain how free fatty acid mobilization from the adipose cell decreases during maximal work in spite of the cell being stimulated by all the hormones to break down triglycerides.
11. Discuss the effect of glucose ingestion on the mobilization of free fatty acids during exercise.

references

1. Ahlborg, G., and P. Felig. 1976. Influence of glucose ingestion on fuel-hormone response during prolonged exercise. *Journal of Applied Physiology* 41:683–88.
2. Alen, M., A. Pakarinen, and K. Hakkinen. 1993. Effects of prolonged training on serum thyrotropin and thyroid hormones in elite strength athletes. *Journal of Sports Science* 11:493–97.
2a. Alen, M., and P. Rahkila. 1988. Anabolic-androgenic steroid effects on endocrinology and lipid metabolism in athletes. *Sports Medicine* 6:327–32.
3. Almon, R. R., and D. C. Dubois. 1990. Fiber-type discrimination in disuse and glucocorticoid-induced atrophy. *Medicine and Science in Sports and Exercise* 22(3):304–11.
4. American College of Sports Medicine. 1984. The use of anabolic-androgenic steroids in sports. In *Position Stands and Opinion Statements*. Indianapolis: The American College of Sports Medicine.
4a. Arce, J. C., M. M. De Souza, L. S. Pescatello, and A. A. Luciano. 1993. Subclinical alterations in hormone and semen profile in athletes. *Fertility-Sterility* 59:398–404.
4b. Arena, B., N. Maffulli, F. Maffulli, and M. A. Morleo. 1995. Reproductive hormones and menstrual changes with exercise in female athletes. *Sports Medicine* 19:278–87.
5. Bahrke, M. S., C. E. Yesalis III, and J. E. Wright. 1990. Psychological and behavioural effects of endogenous testosterone levels and anabolic-androgenic steroids among males: A review. *Sports Medicine* 10(5):303–37.
6. Bonen, A. 1976. Effects of exercise on excretion rates of urinary free cortisol. *Journal of Applied Physiology* 40:155–58.
7. Bonen, A., F. W. Haynes, and T. E. Graham. 1991. Substrate and hormonal responses to exercise in women using oral contraceptives. *Journal of Applied Physiology* 70(5):1917–27.
8. Bunt, J. C. 1986. Hormonal alterations due to exercise. *Sports Medicine* 3:331–45.
9. ———. 1990. Metabolic actions of estradiol: Significance for acute and chronic exercise responses. *Medicine and Science in Sports and Exercise* 22(3):286–90.
10. Bunt, J. C. et al. 1986. Sex and training differences in human growth hormone levels during prolonged exercise. *Journal of Applied Physiology* 61:1796–1801.
11. Cannon, W. B. 1953. *Bodily Changes in Pain, Hunger, Fear and Rage*. 2d ed. Boston: Charles T. Branford Company.
12. Cartee, G. D., A. G. Douen, T. Ramlal, A. Klip, and J. O. Holloszy. 1991. Stimulation of glucose transport in skeletal muscle by hypoxia. *Journal of Applied Physiology* 70(4):1593–1600.

13. Cartier, L., and P. D. Gollnick. 1985. Sympathoadrenal system and activation of glycogenolysis during muscular exercise. *Journal of Applied Physiology* 58:1122–27.

14. Christensen, N. J., and H. Galbo. 1983. Sympathetic nervous activity during exercise. *Annual Review of Physiology* 45:139–53.

15. Coggan, A. R. 1991. Plasma glucose metabolism during exercise in humans. *Sports Medicine* 11:102–24.

16. Coggan, A. R., and E. F. Coyle. 1991. Carbohydrate ingestion during prolonged exercise: Effects on metabolism and performance. In *Exercise and Sport Sciences Reviews*, vol. 19, ed. J. Holloszy, 1–40. Philadelphia: Williams & Wilkins.

17. Convertino, V. A., L. C. Keil, and J. E. Greenleaf. 1983. Plasma volume, renin and vasopressin responses to graded exercise after training. *Journal of Applied Physiology: Respiratory, Environmental and Exercise Physiology* 54:508–14.

18. Copinschi, G. et al. 1967. Effect of various blood-sampling procedures on serum levels of immunoreactive human growth hormone. *Metabolism: Clinical and Experimental* 16:402–9.

19. Cowart, V. S. 1988. Human growth hormone: The latest ergogenic aid. *Physician and Sportsmedicine* 16(3):175–85.

19a. Coyle, E. F. 1995. Substrate utilization during exercise in active people. *American Journal of Clinical Nutrition* 61(suppl.):968S–979S.

20. Cumming, D. C. et al. 1986. Reproductive hormone increases in response to acute exercise in men. *Medicine and Science in Sports and Exercise* 18:369–73.

21. Davies, C. T. M., and J. D. Few. 1973. Effects of exercise on adrenocorticol function. *Journal of Applied Physiology* 35:887–91.

22. De Piccoli, B., F. Giada, A. Benettin, F. Sartori, and E. Piccolo. 1991. Anabolic steroid use in body builders: An echocardiographic study of left ventricle morphology and function. *Journal of Sports Medicine* 12(4):408–12.

23. De Souza, M. J., J. C. Arce, L. S. Pescatello, H. S. Scherzer, and A. A. Luciano. 1994. Gonadal hormones and semen quality in male runners. *International Journal of Sports Medicine* 15:383–91.

23a. De Souza, M. J., M. S. Maguire, K. R. Rubin, and C. M. Maresh. 1990. Effects of menstrual phase and amenorrhea on exercise performance in runners. *Medicine and Science in Sports and Exercise* 22(5):575–80.

24. De Souza, M. J., and D. A. Metzger. 1991. Reproductive dysfunction in amenorrheic athletes and anorexic patients: A review. *Medicine and Science in Sports and Exercise* 23(9):995–1007.

25. Edgerton, V. R. et al. 1975. Glycogen depletion in specific types of human skeletal muscle fibers in intermittent and continuous exercise. In *Metabolic Adaptation to Prolonged Physical Exercise*, ed. H. Howald and J. R. Poortmans, 402–15. Verlag Basel, Switzerland: Birkhauser.

26. Essen, B. 1978. Glycogen depletion of different fibre types in human skeletal muscle during intermittent and continuous exercise. *Acta Physiologica Scandinavica* 103:446–55.

27. Euler, U. S. von. 1969. Sympatho-adrenal activity and physical exercise. In *Biochemistry of Exercise, Medicine and Sport 3*, ed. J. R. Poortmans, 170–81. New York: Karger, Basal.

28. Farrell, P. A. 1985. Exercise and endorphins—male responses. *Medicine and Science in Sports and Exercise* 17:89–93.

29. Felig, P., and J. Wahren. 1975. Fuel homeostasis in exercise. *The New England Journal of Medicine* 293:1078–84.

30. Fox, S. I. 1984. *Human Physiology*. Dubuque, IA: Wm. C. Brown.

31. Fraioli, F. et al. 1980. Physical exercise stimulates marked concomitant release of β-endorphin and adrenocorticotrophic hormone (ACTH) in peripheral blood in man. *Experientia* 36:987–89.

32. Francesconi, R. P., M. Sawka, and K. B. Pandolf. 1983. Hypohydration and heat acclimatization: Plasma renin and aldosterone during exercise. *Journal of Applied Physiology: Respiratory, Environmental and Exercise Physiology* 55:1790–94.

33. Galbo, H., J. J. Holst, and N. J. Christensen. 1975. Glucagon and plasma catecholamine responses to graded and prolonged exercise in man. *Journal of Applied Physiology* 38:70–76.

34. Galbo, H. et al. 1976. Glucagon and plasma catecholamines during beta-receptor blockade in exercising man. *Journal of Applied Physiology* 40:855–63.

35. Galbo, H. et al. 1977. Thyroid and testicular hormone responses to graded and prolonged exercise in man. *European Journal of Applied Physiology* 36:101–6.

36. Ganong, W. F. 1979. *Review of Medical Physiology*. Los Altos, CA: Lange Medical Publications.

37. Goldfarb, A. H., B. D. Hatfield, D. Armstrong, and J. Potts. 1990. Plasma beta-endorphin concentration: Response to intensity and duration of exercise. *Medicine and Science in Sports and Exercise* 22(2):241–44.

38. Goldfarb, A. H., B. D. Hatfield, J. Potts, and D. Armstrong. 1991. Beta-endorphin time course response to intensity of exercise: Effect of training status. *Journal of Sports Medicine* 12(3):264–68.

39. Gollnick, P. D. et al. 1975. Glycogen depletion patterns in human skeletal muscle fibers after varying types and intensities of exercise. In *Metabolic Adaptation to Prolonged Physical Exercise*, ed. H. Howald and J. R. Poortmans, 416–21. Verlag Basel, Switzerland: Birkhauser.

40. Greenwood, F. C., and J. Landon. 1966. Growth hormone secretion in response to stress in man. *Nature* 210:540–41.

41. Guyton, A. C. 1986. *Textbook of Medical Physiology*, 7th ed. Philadelphia: W. B. Saunders.

42. Gyntelberg, F. et al. 1977. Effect of training on the response of plasma glucagon to exercise. *Journal of Applied Physiology: Respiratory, Environmental and Exercise Physiology* 43:302–5.

43. Hackney, A. C. 1989. Endurance training and testosterone levels. *Sports Medicine* 8(2):117–27.

43a. Hackney, A. C., M. A. McCracken-Compton, and B. Ainsworth. 1994. Substrate responses to submaximal exercise in the midfollicular and midluteal phases of the menstrual cycle. *International Journal of Sport Nutrition* 4:299–308.

44. Harris, R. C., J. Bergström, and E. Hultman. 1971. The effect of propranolol on glycogen metabolism during exercise. In *Muscle Metabolism During Exercise*, ed. B. Pernow and B. Saltin, 301–5. New York: Plenum Press.

45. Hartley, L. H. et al. 1972. Multiple hormonal responses to graded exercise in relation to physical training. *Journal of Applied Physiology* 33:602–6.

46. Heath, G. W. et al. 1983. Effect of exercise and lack of exercise on glucose tolerance and insulin sensitivity. *Journal of Applied Physiology: Respiratory, Environmental and Exercise Physiology* 55:512–17.

47. Hickson, R. C., S. M. Czerwinski, M. T. Falduto, and A. P. Young. 1990. Glucocorticoid antagonism by exercise and androgenic-anabolic steroids. *Medicine and Science in Sports and Exercise* 22(3):331–40.

47a. Hickson, R. C. and J. R. Marone. 1993. Exercise and inhibition of glucocorticoid-induced muscle atrophy. In *Exercise and Sport Sciences Reviews*, vol. 21, ed. J. O. Holloszy, 135–68, Baltimore: Williams & Wilkins.

48. Highet, R. 1989. Athletic amenorrhea: An update on aetiology, complications and management. *Sports Medicine* 7:82–108.

48a. Hodgetts, V., S. W. Coppack, K. N. Frayn, and T. D. R. Hockaday. 1991. Factors controlling fat mobilization from human subcutaneous adipose tissue during exercise. *The American Physiological Society*, 445.

49. Holloszy, J. O., and H. T. Narahara. 1967. Enhanced permeability of sugar associated with muscle contraction: Studies of the role of Ca^{++}. *Journal of General Physiology* 50:551–62.

50. Howley, E. T. 1976. The effect of different intensities of exercise on the excretion of epinephrine and norepinephrine. *Medicine and Science in Sports* 8:219–22.

51. ———. 1980. The excretion of catecholamines as an index of exercise stress. In *Exercise in Health and Disease*, ed. F. J. Nagle and H. J. Montoye, 171–83. Springfield, IL: Charles C Thomas.

52. Howley, E. T. et al. 1983. Effect of hyperoxia on metabolic and catecholamine responses to prolonged exercise. *Journal of Applied Physiology: Respiratory, Environmental and Exercise Physiology* 54:54–63.

53. Hultman, E. 1967. Physiological role of muscle glycogen in man with special reference to exercise. In *Circulation Research XX and XXI*, ed. C. B. Chapman, 1–99 and 1–114. New York: The American Heart Association.

54. Issekutz, B., and H. Miller. 1962. Plasma free fatty acids during exercise and the effect of lactic acid. *Proceedings of the Society of Experimental Biology and Medicine* 110:237–39.

55. Ivy, J. 1987. The insulin-like effects of muscle contraction. In *Exercise and Sport Sciences Reviews*, ed. K. B. Pandolf, vol. 15, 29–51. New York: Macmillan.

56. Ivy, J. L. et al. 1983. Exercise training and glucose uptake by skeletal muscle in rats. *Journal of Applied Physiology: Respiratory, Environmental and Exercise Physiology* 55:1393–96.

56a. James, D. E. 1995. The mammalian facilitative glucose transporter family. *International Union Physiology of Science/American Physiology Society* 10:67–71.

57. Jasson, E., P. Hjemdahl, and L. Kaijser. 1986. Epinephrine-induced changes in carbohydrate metabolism during exercise in male subjects. *Journal of Applied Physiology* 60:1466–70.

58. Jensen, J., H. Oftebro, B. Breigan, A. Johnsson, K. Ahlin, H. D. Meen, S. B. Stromme, and H. A. Dahl. 1991. Comparison of changes in testosterone concentrations after strength and endurance exercise in well trained men. *European Journal of Applied Physiology and Occupational Physiology* 63:467–71.

59. Jurkowski, J. E. et al. 1978. Ovarian hormonal responses to exercise. *Journal of Applied Physiology: Respiratory, Environmental and Exercise Physiology* 44:109–14.

60. Keizer H. A., and A. D. Rogol. 1990. Physical exercise and menstrual cycle alterations: What are the mechanisms? *Sports Medicine* 10(4):218–35.

61. Kendrick, Z. V., and G. S. Ellis. 1991. Effect of estradiol on tissue glycogen metabolism and lipid availability in exercised male rats. *Journal of Applied Physiology* 71(5):1694–99.

62. Kjaer, M. 1989. Epinephrine and some other hormonal responses to exercise in man: With special reference to physical training. *International Journal of Sports Medicine* 10:2–15.

63. Kjaer, M., and H. Galbo. 1988. Effects of physical training on the capacity to secrete epinephrine. *Journal of Applied Physiology* 64:11–16.

64. Kjaer, M., B. Kiens, M. Hargreaves, and E. A. Richter. 1991. Influence of active muscle mass on glucose homeostasis during exercise in humans. *Journal of Applied Physiology* 71(2):552–57.

65. Kuipers, H., J. A. G. Wijnen, F. Hartgens, and S. M. M. Willems. 1991. Influence of anabolic steroids on body composition, blood pressure, lipid profile and liver functions in body builders. *International Journal of Sports Medicine* 12(4):413–18.

66. Langenfeld, M. E., L. S. Hart, and P. C. Kao. 1987. Plasma β-endorphin responses to one-hour bicycling and running at 60% max. *Medicine and Science in Sports and Exercise* 19:83–86.

67. Laycock, J. F., and P. H. Wise. 1983. *Essential Endocrinology*. New York: Oxford University Press.

67a. Lebrun, C. M. 1994. The effect of the phase of the menstrual cycle and the birth control pill on athletic performance. *Clinical Sports Medicine* 13:419–41.

68. Ljunghall, S. et al. 1986. Prolonged low-intensity exercise raises the serum parathyroid hormone levels. *Clinical Endocrinology* 25:535–42.

69. Ljunghall, S. et al. 1988. Increase in serum parathyroid hormone levels after prolonged exercise. *Medicine and Science in Sports and Exercise* 20:122–25.

70. Loucks, A. B. 1990. Effects of exercise training on the menstrual cycle: Existence and mechanisms. *Medicine and Science in Sports and Exercise* 22:275–80.

71. Loucks, A. B., and S. M. Horvath. 1985. Athletic amenorrhea: A review. *Medicine and Science in Sports and Exercise* 17:56–72.

72. Luyckx, A. S., and P. J. Lefebvre. 1974. Mechanisms involved in the exercise-induced increase in glucagon secretion in rats. *Diabetes* 23:81–93.

73. Macintyre, J. G. 1987. Growth hormone and athletes. *Sports Medicine* 4:129–42.

74. Maher, J. T. et al. 1975. Aldosterone dynamics during graded exercise at sea level and high altitude. *Journal of Applied Physiology* 39:18–22.

75. McArthur, J. W. 1985. Endorphins and exercise in females: Possible connection with reproductive dysfunction. *Medicine and Science in Sports and Exercise* 17:82–88.

75a. Mendenhall, L. A., S. C. Swanson, D. L. Habash, and A. R. Coggan. 1994. Ten days of exercise training reduces glucose production and utilization during moderate-intensity exercise. *American Journal of Physiology* 266(1 Pt 1):E136–E143.

76. Metsrinne, K. 1988. Effect of exercise on plasma renin substrate. *International Journal of Sports Medicine* 9:267–69.

77. Mikines, K. J., E. A. Richter, F. Dela, and H. Galbo. 1991. Seven days of bed rest decrease insulin action on glucose uptake in leg and whole body. *Journal of Applied Physiology* 70(3):1245–54.

78. Mikines, K. J., B. Sonne, B. Tronier, and H. Galbo. 1989. Effects of acute exercise and detraining on insulin action in trained men. *Journal of Applied Physiology* 66(2):704–11.

79. Moffatt, R. J., M. B. Wallace, and S. P. Sady. 1990. Effects of anabolic steroids on lipoprotein profiles of female weight lifters. *Physician and Sportsmedicine* 18(9):106–15.

80. Morgan, W. P. 1985. Affective beneficence of vigorous physical activity. *Medicine and Science in Sports and Exercise* 17:94–100.

80a. Paul, P. 1970. FFA metabolism of normal dogs during steady-state exercise at different work loads. *Journal of Applied Physiology* 28:127–32.

81. ———. 1971. Uptake and oxidation of substrates in the intact animal during exercise. In *Muscle Metabolism during Exercise*, ed. B. Pernow and B. Saltin, 225–48. New York: Plenum Press.

82. Powers, S. K., E. T. Howley, and R. H. Cox. 1982. A differential catecholamine response during prolonged exercise and passive heating. *Medicine and Science in Sports and Exercise* 14:435–39.

83. Pruett, E. D. R. 1970. Glucose and insulin during prolonged work stress in men living on different diets. *Journal of Applied Physiology* 28:199–208.

84. Raymond, L. W., J. Sode, and J. R. Tucci. 1972. Adrenocorticotrophic response to non-exhaustive muscular exercise. *Acta Endocrinologica* 70:73–80.

85. Ren, J. M., and E. Hultman. 1990. Regulation of phosphorylase a activity in human skeletal muscle. *Journal of Applied Physiology* 69(3):919–23.

86. Richter, E. A., B. Kiens, M. Mizuno, and S. Strange. 1989. Insulin action in human thighs after one-legged immobilization. *Journal of Applied Physiology* 67(1):19–23.

87. Rizza, R. et al. 1979. Differential effects of epinephrine on glucose production and disposal in man. *American Journal of Physiology* 237: E356–E362.

87a. Romijn, J. A., E. F. Coyle, L. S. Sidossis, A. Gastaldelli, J. F. Horowitz, E. Endert, and R. R. Wolfe. 1993. Regulation of endogenous fat and carbohydrate metabolism in relation to exercise intensity and duration. *The American Physiological Society* E380–E391.

87b. Ruby, B. C., and R. A. Roberges. 1994. Gender differences in substrate utilisation during exercise. *Sports Medicine* 17:393–410.

88. Saltin, B., and J. Karlsson. 1971. Muscle glycogen utilization during work of different intensities. In *Muscle Metabolism During Exercise*, ed. B. Pernow and B. Saltin, 289–99. New York: Plenum Press.

89. Schwarz, L., and W. Kindermann. 1992. Changes in β-endorphin levels in response to aerobic and anaerobic exercise. *Sports Medicine* 13(1):25–36.

90. Seals, D. R., R. G. Victor, and A. L. Mark. 1988. Plasma norepinephrine and muscle sympathetic discharge during rhythmic exercise in humans. *Journal of Applied Physiology* 65(2):940–44.

91. Selye, H. 1976. *The Stress of Life*. New York: McGraw-Hill.

92. Silverberg, A. B. et al. 1978. Norepinephrine: Hormone and neurotransmitter in man. *American Journal of Physiology* 234:E252–E256.

93. Spriet, L. L., J. M. Ren, and E. Hultman. 1988. Epinephrine infusion enhances muscle glycogenolysis during prolonged electrical stimulation. *Journal of Applied Physiology* 64:1439–44.

94. Stainsby, W. N., C. Sumners, and G. M. Andrew. 1984. Plasma catecholamines and their effect on blood lactate and muscle lactate output. *Journal of Applied Physiology* 57:321–25.

95. Stainsby, W. N., C. Sumners, and P. D. Eitzman. 1985. Effects of catecholamines on lactic acid output during progressive working contractions. *Journal of Applied Physiology* 59:1809–14.

96. Sutton, J., and L. Lazarus. 1976. Growth hormone in exercise: Comparison of physiological and pharmacological stimuli. *Journal of Applied Physiology* 41:523–27.

97. Tarnopolsky, L. J., J. D. MacDougall, S. A. Atkinson, M. A. Tarnopolsky, and J. R. Sutton. 1990. Gender differences in substrate for endurance exercise. *Journal of Applied Physiology* 68(1):302–8.

97a. Taafe, D. R., L. Pruitt, J. Reim, R. L. Hintz, G. Butterfield, A. R. Hoffman, and R. Marcus. 1994. Effect of recombinant human growth hormone on the muscle strength response to resistance exercise in elderly men. *Journal of Clinical Endocrinology Metabolism* 79:1361–66.

98. Taylor, W. M. 1988. Synthetic human growth hormone: A call for federal control. *Physician and Sportsmedicine* 16(3):189–92.

99. Tepperman, J., and H. M. Tepperman. 1987. *Metabolic and Endocrine Physiology*, 5th ed. Chicago: Year Book Medical Publishers.

100. Terjung, R. 1979. Endocrine response to exercise. In *Exercise and Sport Sciences Reviews*, vol. 7, ed. R. S. Hutton and D. I. Miller, 153–79. New York: Macmillan.

101. Thorn, P., J. S. Floras, P. Hoffmann, and D. R. Seals. 1990. Endorphins and exercise: Physiological mechanisms and clinical implications. *Medicine and Science in Sports and Exercise* 22(4):417–28.

102. Urhausen, A., R. Holpes, and W. Kindermann. 1989. One- and two-dimensional echocardiography in bodybuilders using anabolic steroids. *European Journal of Applied Physiology* 58:633–40.

103. Van Baak, M. A. 1988. β-adrenoceptor blockade and exercise: An update *Sports Medicine* 4:209–25.

104. Vander, A. J., J. H. Sherman, and D. S. Luciano. 1985. *Human Physiology: The Mechanisms of Body Function*, 4th ed. New York: McGraw-Hill.

105. Voet, D., and J. G. Voet. 1990. *Biochemistry*. New York: John Wiley & Sons.

106. Vogel, R. B. et al. 1985. Increase of free and total testosterone during submaximal exercise in normal males. *Medicine and Science in Sports and Exercise* 17:119–23.

107. Wade, C. E. 1984. Response, regulation, and actions of vasopressin during exercise: A review. *Medicine and Science in Sports and Exercise* 16:506–11.

108. Wallberg-Henriksson, H., S. H. Constable, D. A. Young, and J. O. Holloszy. 1988. Glucose transport into rat skeletal muscle: Interaction between exercise and insulin. *Journal of Applied Physiology* 65(2):909–13.

109. Weicker, H. et al. 1984. Changes in sexual hormones with female top athletes. *International Journal of Sports Medicine* 5:200–202.

110. Winder, W. W. et al. 1978. Time course of sympathoadrenal adaptation to endurance exercise training in man. *Journal of Applied Physiology: Respiratory, Environmental and Exercise Physiology* 45:370–74.

111. Wright, J. E. 1980. Anabolic steroids and athletics. In *Exercise and Sport Sciences Reviews*, vol. 8, ed. R. S. Hutton and D. I. Miller, 149–202. New York: Macmillan.

112. ———. 1982. *Anabolic Steroids and Sports*, vol. 2. New York: Sports Science Consultants.

113. Yakovlev, N. N., and A. A. Viru. 1985. Adrenergic regulation of adaptation to muscular activity. *International Journal of Sports Medicine* 6:255–65.

113a. Yarasheski, K. E. 1994. Growth hormone effects on metabolism, body composition, muscle mass, and strength. *Exercise Sports Science Review* 22:285–312.

114. Yesalis, C. E., and M. S. Bahrke. 1995. Anabolic-androgenic steroids: Current issues. *Sports Medicine* 19:341–57.

114a. Yesalis, C. E., J. E. Wright, and M. S. Bahrke. 1989. Epidemiological and policy issues in the measurement of the long term health effects of anabolic-androgenic steroids. *Sports Medicine* 8(3):129–38.

115. Young, J. C., J. Enslin, and B. Kuca. 1989. Exercise intensity and glucose tolerance in trained and nontrained subjects. *Journal of Applied Physiology* 67(1):39–43.

Measurement of Work, Power, and Energy Expenditure

objectives

By studying this chapter, you should be able to do the following:

1. Define the terms *work, power, energy,* and *net efficiency.*
2. Give a brief explanation of the procedure used to calculate work performed during: (a) cycle ergometer exercise and (b) treadmill exercise.
3. Describe the concept behind the measurement of energy expenditure using: (a) direct calorimetry and (b) indirect calorimetry.
4. Discuss the procedure used to estimate energy expenditure during horizontal treadmill walking and running.
5. Define the following terms: (a) kilogram-meter, (b) relative $\dot{V}O_2$, (c) MET, and (d) open-circuit spirometry.

6. Describe the procedure used to calculate net efficiency during steady state exercise.

outline

Units of Measure   96
 Metric System   96
 SI Units   96
Work and Power Defined   96
 Work   96
 Power   97
Measurement of Work and Power   97

 Bench Step   97
 Cycle Ergometer   98
 Treadmill   98
Measurement of Energy Expenditure   99
 Direct Calorimetry   99
 Indirect Calorimetry   100

Estimation of Energy Expenditure   101
Calculation of Exercise Efficiency   102
 Factors That Influence Exercise Efficiency   103
Running Economy   104

key terms

cycle ergometer
direct calorimetry
ergometer
ergometry
indirect calorimetry

kilocalorie (kcal)
MET
net efficiency
open-circuit spirometry
percent grade

power
relative $\dot{V}O_2$
SI units
work

easurement of energy expenditure and power output has many applications in exercise science. For example, adequate knowledge of the energy requirements of physical activities (e.g., running) is important to a coach in planning a training and dietary program for athletes. This same information can be used by an exercise specialist to prescribe exercise for adults entering a fitness program. Therefore, an understanding of human energy expenditure, how it is measured, and its practical significance is critical for the physical therapist, coach, physical educator, exercise specialist, or exercise physiologist. It is the purpose of this chapter to discuss those concepts necessary for understanding the measurement of human work output and the associated energy expenditure.

Units of Measure

Metric System

In the United States, the English system of measurement remains in common use. In contrast, the metric system is used in many other countries, is the standard system of measurement for scientists, and is used by many scientific journals. In the metric system, the basic units of length, volume, and mass are the meter, the liter, and the gram, respectively. The main advantage of the metric system is that subdivisions or multiples of its basic units are expressed in factors of 10 using prefixes attached to the basic unit. Students not familiar with the metric system should refer to table 6.1 for a list of the basic prefixes used in metric measurements.

SI Units

An ongoing problem in exercise science is the failure of scientists to standardize units of measurement employed in presenting research data. In an effort to eliminate this problem, a uniform system of reporting scientific measurement has been developed through international cooperation. This system, known as System International units or **SI units,** has been endorsed by numerous exercise and sports medicine journals for the publication of research data (17, 18). The SI system ensures standardization in the reporting of scientific data and makes comparison of published values easy. Table 6.2 contains SI units of importance in the measurement of exercise performance.

Table 6.1	Common Metric Prefixes
mega: one million (1,000,000)	
kilo: one thousand (1,000)	
centi: one-hundredth (0.01)	
milli: one-thousandth (0.001)	
micro: one-millionth (0.000001)	
nano: one-billionth (0.000000001)	
pico: one-trillionth (0.000000000001)	

Table 6.2	SI Units of Importance in the Measurement of Human Exercise Performance
Units for Quantifying Human Exercise	**SI Unit**
Mass	kilogram (kg)
Distance	meter (m)
Time	second (s)
Force	Newton (N)
Work	joule (J)
Energy	joule (J)
Power	watt (W)
Velocity	meters per second (m · s^{-1})
Torque	newton-meter (N · m)

in summary

- The metric system is the system of measurement used by scientists to express mass, length, and volume.
- In an effort to standardize terms for the measurement of energy, force, work, and power, scientists have developed a common system of terminology called System International (SI units).

Work and Power Defined

Work

Work is defined by the physicist as the product of force times distance:

$$\text{Work} = \text{Force} \times \text{distance}$$

If you lift a 5-kilogram (kg) weight (1 kg = 2.2 lbs) upward over the vertical distance of 2 meters (m), the work performed would be:

$$\text{Work} = 5 \text{ kp} \times 2 \text{ m}$$
$$= 10 \text{ kpm}$$

Here the force exerted by the 5-kg weight is 5 kiloponds (kp), and the distance traveled is 2 meters, with the resulting amount of work performed being expressed in kilopond-meters (kpm). The explanation for the shift from kg to kp in the example just given is that kg is a measure of mass, not force. That is, one kp is the force acting upon the mass of one kg at the normal acceleration of gravity.

Although SI units are the preferred units for quantifying exercise performance, note that there are a number of traditional units that can be used to express both work and energy expenditure. Table 6.3 contains a list of

Table 6.3 — Common Units Used to Express the Amount of Work Performed or Energy Expended

Term	Abbreviation	Conversion Table
Kilogram-meter	kgm	1 kgm = 9.81 joules
		1 kgm = 7.23 ft-lbs
		1 kgm = 9.81 × 10 ergs
		1 kgm = 2.34 × 10^{-3} kcal
Kilopond-meter	kpm	1 kpm = 1 kgm
Kilocalorie	kcal	1 kcal = 4,186 joules
		1 kcal = 426.8 kpm
		1 kcal = 3,087 ft-lbs
Joule*	J	1 J = 2.38 × 10^{-4} kcal
		1 J = 0.737 ft-lbs
		1 J = 0.101 kgm
Foot-pounds	ft-lbs	1 ft-lb = 0.1383 kgm

*The joule is the basic unit adopted by the System International (called SI unit) for expression of energy expenditure or work.

Table 6.4 — Common Terms and Units Used to Express Power

Term	Abbreviation	Conversion Table
Watt*	W	1 W = 0.001 kilowatt
		1 W = 1 J · s^{-1}
		1 W = 6.12 kpm · min^{-1}
Horsepower	hp	1 hp = 745.1 W
		1 hp = 745.7 J · s^{-1}
		1 hp = 10.69 kcal · min^{-1}
Kilopond-meter · min^{-1}	kpm · min^{-1}	1 kpm · min^{-1} = 0.163 W

*The watt is the basic unit adopted by the System International (called SI units) for expression of power.

terms that are in common use today. The SI unit for work is joules where 1 kpm of work is equal to 9.81 joules. Therefore, in the above example, 10 kpm is equal to 98.1 joules (see table 6.3 for other unit conversions).

It is often difficult to compute how much work is performed during sporting events. For instance, a shot-putter performs work since the shot has mass and is moved vertically; however, the exact amount of vertical displacement of the shot is difficult to measure without sophisticated photographic equipment, and thus computation of work performed is not a simple problem. In contrast, a weight lifter performing a clean and jerk is lifting a known amount of weight over a fixed vertical distance, making calculation of work quite easy.

Power

Power is the term used to describe how much work is accomplished per unit of time. The SI unit for power is the watt (W) and is defined as 6.12 kpm · min^{-1}. Power can be calculated as:

Power = Work ÷ time

The concept of power is important since it describes the rate at which work is being performed (work rate). It is the work rate or power output that describes the intensity of exercise. Given enough time, any healthy adult could perform a total work output of 2,000 kpm (19.6 kilojoules). However, only a few highly trained athletes could perform this amount of work in sixty seconds (s). Calculation of power output using this example can be done as follows:

Power = 2,000 kpm ÷ 60 s
= 33.33 kpm · s^{-1}

Expressed in SI units, the above power output is 326.8 W (e.g., 1 W = 0.102 kpm · s^{-1}). Table 6.4 contains a list of traditional ways that power can be expressed other than in SI units.

Measurement of Work and Power

Bench Step

The term **ergometry** pertains to the measurement of work output. The word **ergometer** refers to the apparatus or device used to measure a specific type of work.

One of the earliest ergometers employed to measure work capacity in humans was the bench step. This ergometer is still in use today and simply involves the subject stepping up and down on a bench at a specified rate. Calculation of the work performed during bench stepping is very easy. Suppose a 70-kg man steps up and down on a 50-centimeter (0.5 meter) bench for ten minutes at a rate of thirty steps per minute. The amount of work performed during this ten-minute task can be computed as follows:

Force = 70 kp (i.e., body weight = 70 kg)
Distance = 0.5 m · step^{-1} × 30 steps · min^{-1}
    × 10 min = 150 m
Therefore, total work performed = 70 kp × 150 m
    = 10,500 kpm or
    ~103 kilojoules
    (see table 6.3 for
    conversions)

The power output can be calculated as:

Power = 10,500 kpm ÷ 10 min
    = 1,050 kpm · min^{-1} or 171.6 W

Cycle Ergometer

One of the most popular ergometers is the **cycle ergometer** (19). This type of ergometer is a stationary exercise bicycle that permits accurate measurement of the amount of work performed. The most common type of cycle ergometer is the Monark® friction-braked cycle, which incorporates a belt wrapped around the wheel (called a flywheel). The belt can be loosened or tightened to provide a change in resistance. Distance traveled can be determined by computing the distance covered per revolution of the pedals (6 meters per revolution on a standard Monark® cycle) times the number of pedal revolutions. Consider the following example for computation of work and power using the cycle ergometer. Calculate work given:

Duration of exercise = 10 min
Resistance against flywheel = 1.5 kp
Distance traveled per pedal revolution = 6 m
Pedalling speed = 60 rev · min^{-1}
Therefore the total revolutions in 10 min
    = 10 min × 60 rev · min^{-1}
Hence, total work = 1.5 kp × (6 m · rev^{-1} × 600 rev)
    = 5,400 kpm or 52.97 kilojoules

Calculation of the power output in the above example is computed by dividing the total work performed by time:

Power = 5,400 kpm ÷ 10 min
    = 540 kpm · min^{-1} or 88.2 W

Treadmill

Calculation of the work performed while a subject runs or walks on a treadmill is not generally possible when the treadmill is horizontal. Although running horizontally on a treadmill requires energy, the vertical dis-

Table 6.5	Determination of Percent Grade from Angles of Incline	
Degrees	**Sine**	**Percent Grade**
1	0.0175	1.75
2	0.0349	3.49
3	0.0523	5.23
4	0.0698	6.98
5	0.0872	8.72
6	0.1045	10.45
7	0.1219	12.19
8	0.1392	13.92
9	0.1564	15.64
10	0.1736	17.36

placement of the body's center of gravity is not easily measured. Therefore, measurement of work performed during horizontal walking or running is complicated. However, quantifiable work is being performed when walking or running up a slope, and calculation of the amount of work done is a simple task. The incline of the treadmill is expressed in units called "percent grade." **Percent grade** is defined as the amount of vertical rise per 100 units of belt travel. For instance, a subject walking on a treadmill at a 10% grade travels 10 meters vertically for every 100 meters of the belt travel. Percent grade is calculated by multiplying the sine of the treadmill angle by 100. Examples of this calculation are presented in table 6.5. In practice, the treadmill angle (expressed in degrees) can be determined by simple trigometric computations, or by using a measurement device called an inclinometer (7).

To calculate the work output during treadmill exercise, you must know both the subject's body weight and the distance traveled vertically. Vertical travel can be computed by multiplying the distance the belt traveled (D) by the percent grade. This can be written as:

Vertical displacement = % grade × D

where percent grade is expressed as a fraction and the value of D is calculated by multiplying the treadmill speed (m · min^{-1}) by the total minutes of exercise (figure 6.1). Consider the following sample calculation of work output during treadmill exercise. Calculate work given:

Subject's body weight = 70 kg (i.e., force = 70 kp)
Treadmill speed = 200 m · min^{-1}
Treadmill angle = 7.5% grade (7.5% ÷ 100 = 0.075 as
    fractional grade)
Exercise time = 10 min
Total vertical distance traveled = 200 m · min^{-1}
    × 0.075 × 10 min
    = 150 m
Therefore, total work performed = 70 kp × 150 m
    = 10,500 kpm or
    ~103 kilojoules

Fixed rear-axle treadmill
Grade = Sine θ = Rise ÷ Hypotenuse

Figure 6.1

Determination of the "percent grade" on an inclined treadmill. Theta (θ) represents the angle of inclination. Percent grade is computed as the sine of angle θ × 100.

in summary

- An understanding of the terms *work* and *power* is necessary in order to compute human work output and the associated exercise efficiency.
- Work is defined as the product of force times distance:

  Work = Force × distance

- Power is defined as work divided by time:

  Power = Work ÷ time

Measurement of Energy Expenditure

Measurement of an individual's energy expenditure at rest or during a particular activity has many practical applications. One direct application applies to exercise-assisted weight loss programs. Clearly, knowledge of the energy cost of walking, running, or swimming at various speeds is useful to individuals who use these modes of exercise as an aid in weight loss. Further, an industrial engineer might measure the energy cost of various tasks around a job site and use this information to assist in making the appropriate job assignments to workers (13, 27). In this regard, the engineer might recommend that the supervisor assign those jobs that demand large energy requirements to workers that are physically fit and possess high work capacities. In general, there are two techniques employed in the measurement of human energy expenditure: (1) direct calorimetry and (2) indirect calorimetry.

Direct Calorimetry

When the body uses energy to do work, heat is liberated. This production of heat by cells occurs via both cellular respiration (bioenergetics) and cell work. The general process can be drawn schematically as (3, 28, 29):

Foodstuff + O_2 → ATP + heat
↓ cell work
Heat

Direct calorimetry

Figure 6.2

Diagram of a simple calorimeter used to measure metabolic rate via measurement of production of body heat. This method of determining metabolic rate is called direct calorimetry.

The process of cellular respiration was discussed in detail in chapter 3. Note that the rate of heat production in an animal is directly proportional to the metabolic rate. Therefore, measuring heat production (calorimetry) by an animal gives a direct measurement of metabolic rate.

The SI unit to measure heat energy is the joule. However, a common unit employed to measure heat energy is the calorie (table 6.3). A calorie is defined as the amount of heat required to raise the temperature of one gram of water by one degree Celsius. Since the calorie is very small, the term **kilocalorie (kcal)** is generally used to express energy expenditure and the energy value of foods. One kcal is equal to 1,000 calories. In converting kcal's to SI units, one kcal is equal to 4,186 joules or 4.186 Kilojoules(kJ) (see table 6.3 for conversions). The process of measuring an animal's metabolic rate via measurement of heat production is called **direct calorimetry,** and has been used by scientists since the eighteenth century. This technique involves placement of the animal in a tight chamber (called a calorimeter), which is insulated from the environment (usually by a jacket of water surrounding the chamber), and allowance is made for free exchange of O_2 and CO_2 from the chamber (figure 6.2). The animal's body heat raises the temperature of the water circulating around the chamber. Therefore, by measuring the volume of water flowing through the chamber per minute and the temperature change of the water per unit of time, the amount of heat production can be computed. In addition, heat is lost from the animal by evaporation of water from the skin and respiratory passages. This heat loss can be measured and added back to the total heat picked up by the water to yield an estimate of the rate of energy utilization by the animal (3, 7).

Figure 6.3

Modern open-circuit spirometry utilizing electronic gas analyzers and computer technology. Computerized open-circuit spirometer for measurement of oxygen consumption and carbon dioxide production. Courtesy of Sensor-medics, Inc.

Indirect Calorimetry

Although direct calorimetry is considered to be a precise technique for measurement of metabolic rate, construction of a chamber that is large enough for humans is expensive. Also, use of direct calorimetry to measure metabolic rate during exercise is complicated since the ergometer used may produce heat. Fortunately, another procedure can be used to measure metabolic rate. This technique is termed **indirect calorimetry** because it does not involve the direct measurement of heat production. The principle of indirect calorimetry can be explained by the following relationship:

$$\text{Foodstuffs} + O_2 \longrightarrow \text{Heat} + CO_2 + H_2O$$
(Indirect calorimetry)   (Direct calorimetry)

Since a direct relationship exists between O_2 consumed and the amount of heat produced in the body, measurement of O_2 consumption provides an estimate of metabolic rate (2, 3, 11). In order to convert the amount of O_2 consumed into heat equivalents, it is necessary to know the type of nutrient (i.e., carbohydrate, fat, or protein) that was metabolized. The energy liberated when fat is the only foodstuff metabolized is 4.7 kcal (or 19.7 kJ) $\cdot$ l O_2^{-1}, while the energy released when only carbohydrates are used is 5.05 kcal (or 21.13 kJ) $\cdot$ l O_2^{-1}. Although it is not exact, the caloric expenditure of exercise is often estimated to be approximately 5 kcal (or 21 kJ) per liter of O_2 consumed (16). Therefore, a person exercising at an oxygen consumption of 2.0 $\ell \cdot$ min^{-1} would expend approximately 10 kcal (or 42 kJ) of energy per minute.

The most common technique used to measure oxygen consumption today is termed **open-circuit spirometry.** Modern-day open-circuit spirometry employs computer technology and is shown diagrammatically in figure 6.3 (24). The laboratory equipment used to measure oxygen consumption is illustrated in the accompanying photo. The volume of air inspired is measured via a device that is capable of measuring gas volumes. The expired gas from the subject is channeled to a small mixing chamber to be analyzed for O_2 and CO_2 content by electronic gas analyzers. Information concerning the volume of air inspired and the fraction of O_2 and CO_2 in the expired gas is sent to a digital computer by way of a device called an analog-to-digital converter (converts a voltage signal to a digital signal). The computer is programmed to perform the necessary calculations of $\dot{V}O_2$ (volume of O_2 consumed per min) and the volume of carbon dioxide produced ($\dot{V}CO_2$). In short, $\dot{V}O_2$ is calculated in the following way:

$$\dot{V}O_2 = [\text{volume of } O_2 \text{ inspired}] - [\text{volume of } O_2 \text{ expired}]$$

See appendix A for details of $\dot{V}O_2$ and $\dot{V}CO_2$ calculations.

in summary

- Measurement of energy expenditure at rest or during exercise is possible using either direct or indirect calorimetry.
- Direct calorimetry uses the measurement of heat production as an indication of metabolic rate.
- Indirect calorimetry estimates metabolic rate via measurement of oxygen consumption.

Estimation of the O_2 Requirement of Treadmill Walking

The O_2 requirement of horizontal treadmill walking can be estimated with reasonable accuracy for speeds between 50 and 100 m · min^{-1} using the following formula (1):

$\dot{V}O_2$ (ml · kg^{-1} · min^{-1}) = 0.1 ml · kg^{-1} · min^{-1}/(m · min^{-1}) × speed (m · min^{-1}) + 3.5 ml · kg^{-1} · min^{-1} (resting $\dot{V}O_2$)

This equation tells us that the O_2 requirement of walking increases as a linear function of walking speed. The slope of the line is 0.1 and the Y intercept is 3.5 ml · kg^{-1} · min^{-1} (resting $\dot{V}O_2$). The O_2 cost of grade walking is:

$\dot{V}O_2$ (ml · kg^{-1} · min^{-1}) = 1.8 ml · kg^{-1} · min^{-1} × speed (m · min^{-1}) × % grade (expressed as a fraction)

The total O_2 requirement of graded treadmill walking is the sum of the horizontal O_2 cost and the vertical O_2 cost. For example, the O_2 cost of walking at 80 m · min^{-1} at 5% grade would be:

Horizontal O_2 cost = 0.1 ml · kg^{-1} · min^{-1} × 80 m min^{-1} + 3.5 ml · kg^{-1} · min^{-1}
= 11.5 ml · kg^{-1} · min^{-1}

Vertical O_2 cost = 1.8 ml · kg^{-1} · min^{-1} × (0.05 × 80) = 7.2 ml · kg^{-1} · min^{-1}

Hence, the total O_2 requirement of walking would amount to:

11.5 ml · kg^{-1} · min^{-1} + 7.2 ml · kg^{-1} · min^{-1} = 18.7 ml · kg^{-1} · min^{-1}

This O_2 requirement can be expressed in METs by dividing the measured (or estimated) $\dot{V}O_2$ (ml · kg^{-1} · min^{-1}) by 3.5 ml · kg^{-1} · min^{-1} per MET:

18.7 ml · kg^{-1} · min^{-1} ÷ 3.5 ml · kg^{-1} · min^{-1} per MET = 5.3 METs

Formulas are taken from reference 1.

Estimation of Energy Expenditure

Researchers studying the oxygen cost (O_2 cost = $\dot{V}O_2$ at steady state) of exercise have demonstrated that it is possible to estimate the energy expended during physical activity with reasonable precision (6, 8, 9, 15, 23). Walking and running are two activities that have been studied in detail. The O_2 requirements of walking and running graphed as a function of speed are presented in figure 6.4. Note that the relationship between the relative O_2 requirement (ml · kg^{-1} · min^{-1}) and walking/running speed is a straight line (1, 15). The fact that this relationship is linear over a wide range of speeds is convenient and makes the calculation of the O_2 cost (or energy cost) very easy (see A Closer Look 6.1 and A Closer Look 6.2 for examples). Estimation of the energy expenditure of other types of activities is more complex. For example, estimation of energy expenditure during tennis is dependent on whether the match is singles or doubles, and is also influenced by the participants' skill level. Nonetheless, a gross estimate of the energy expended during a tennis match is possible. Appendix B contains a list of activities and their estimated energy costs.

The need to express the energy cost of exercise in simple units has led to the development of the

Figure 6.4
The relationship between speed and $\dot{V}O_2$ cost is linear for both walking and running. Note that x equals the walking/running speed in meters · min^{-1}.

term, metabolic equivalent (MET). The concept of a MET is simple. One **MET** is equal to resting $\dot{V}O_2$, which is approximately 3.5 ml · kg^{-1} · min^{-1} (1,2). Thus, the energy cost of exercise can be described in multiples of resting $\dot{V}O_2$ (i.e., METs), which will simplify the quantification of exercise energy requirement.

Estimation of the O_2 Requirement of Treadmill Running

The O_2 requirements of horizontal treadmill running for speeds greater than 134 m · min^{-1} can be estimated in a manner similar to the procedure used to estimate the O_2 requirement for treadmill walking. It is also possible to estimate the O_2 requirement for running up a grade. This calculation is done in two parts:

1. First, the O_2 cost of the horizontal component is calculated using the following formula:

$$\dot{V}O_2 \text{ (ml · kg}^{-1} \cdot \text{min}^{-1}) = 0.2 \text{ ml · kg}^{-1} \cdot \text{min}^{-1}/\text{m · min}^{-1} \times \text{speed (m · min}^{-1}) + 3.5 \text{ ml · kg}^{-1} \cdot \text{min}^{-1} \text{ (resting } \dot{V}O_2)$$

2. Second, the O_2 requirement of the vertical component is computed using the relationship that running 1 m/min vertically requires 0.9 ml · kg^{-1} · min^{-1}. The vertical velocity is computed by multiplying running speed by the fractional grade. Therefore, the formula to estimate the O_2 cost of vertical treadmill work while running is as follows:

$$\dot{V}O_2 \text{ (ml · kg}^{-1} \cdot \text{min}^{-1}) = 0.9 \text{ ml · kg}^{-1} \text{ per m · min}^{-1} \times \text{vertical velocity (m · min}^{-1})$$

Formulas are taken from reference 1.

For example, a physical activity requiring a 10-MET energy expenditure (i.e., 10 times resting metabolic rate) represents a $\dot{V}O_2$ of 35 ml · kg^{-1} · min^{-1} (10 METs × 3.5 ml · kg^{-1} · min^{-1} per MET = 35 ml · kg^{-1} · min^{-1}). The absolute oxygen requirement of an activity requiring 10 METs can be calculated by multiplying the individual's body weight times the $\dot{V}O_2$ (ml · kg^{-1} · min^{-1}). Therefore, the oxygen requirement for a 60-kg individual performing a 10-MET activity would be:

$$\dot{V}O_2 \text{ (ml · min}^{-1}) = 35 \text{ ml · kg}^{-1} \cdot \text{min}^{-1} \times 60 \text{ kg}$$
$$= 2,100 \text{ ml · min}^{-1}$$

in summary

- The energy cost of horizontal treadmill walking or running can be estimated with reasonable accuracy since the O_2 requirements of both walking and running increase as a linear function of speed.
- The need to express the energy cost of exercise in simple terms has led to the development of the term MET. One MET is equal to the resting $\dot{V}O_2$ (3.5 ml · kg^{-1} · min^{-1}).

Calculation of Exercise Efficiency

Exercise physiologists have long searched for ways to mathematically describe the efficiency of human movement. Although disagreement exists as to the most valid technique of calculating efficiency, the efficiency of exercise is often described by the term **net efficiency** (4, 5, 9, 23, 30, 31). Net efficiency is defined as the mathematical ratio of work output divided by the energy expended above rest:

$$\% \text{ net efficiency} = \frac{\text{Work output}}{\text{Energy expended above rest}} \times 100$$

No machine is 100% efficient since some energy is lost due to friction of the moving parts. Likewise, the human machine is not 100% efficient because energy is lost as heat. It is estimated that the gasoline automobile engine operates with an efficiency of approximately 20%–25%. Similarly, net efficiency for humans exercising on a cycle ergometer ranges from 15%–27%, depending on work rate (10, 12, 23, 26, 31).

To compute net efficiency during cycle ergometer or treadmill exercise requires measurement of work output and an appraisal of the subject's energy expenditure during the exercise and at rest. It should be emphasized that $\dot{V}O_2$ measurements must be made during steady state conditions. The work rate on the cycle ergometer or treadmill is calculated as discussed earlier and is generally expressed in kpm · min^{-1}. The energy expenditure during these types of exercise is usually estimated by first measuring $\dot{V}O_2$ (liter · min^{-1}) using open-circuit spirometry, and then converting it to either kcal or kJ (i.e., 5 kcal or 21 kJ = 1 liter O_2). In order to do the computation using the net-efficiency formula, both numerator and denominator must be expressed in similar terms. Since the numerator (work output) is expressed in kJ and energy expenditure is also expressed in kJ, no conversion of units is required. Consider the following sample calculation of

Figure 6.5
Changes in net efficiency during arm crank ergometry as a function of work rate.

Figure 6.6
Relationship between energy expenditure and work rate. Note that energy expenditure increases as a curvilinear function of work rate.

net efficiency during submaximal steady state cycle ergometer exercise using kJ as both work and energy units. Given:

Resistance against the cycle flywheel = 2 kp
Cranking speed = 50 rpm
Steady state resting $\dot{V}O_2$ = $0.25\ell \cdot min^{-1}$
Steady state exercise $\dot{V}O_2$ = $1.5\ell \cdot min^{-1}$
Distance traveled per revolution = 6 m
Therefore:
Work rate = [(2 kp) × (50 rpm × 6 m/rev)]
= 600 kpm · min⁻¹ or 5.89 kJ
Energy expenditure = [$\dot{V}O_2(\ell \cdot min^{-1})$ × 21kJ · ℓ^{-1}]
= 26.25 kJ
note: $\dot{V}O_2$ = (1.5ℓ · min⁻¹ − 0.25ℓ · min⁻¹)
Hence, net efficiency = $\dfrac{5.89 kJ \cdot min^{-1}}{26.25 kJ \cdot min^{-1}}$ × 100%
= 22.4%

Factors That Influence Exercise Efficiency

The efficiency of exercise is influenced by several factors: (1) the exercise work rate, (2) the speed of movement, and (3) the fiber composition of the muscles performing the exercise. A brief discussion of each of these factors follows.

Work Rate and Exercise Efficiency

Figure 6.5 depicts the changes in net efficiency during cycle ergometry exercise as a function of work rate. Note that efficiency decreases as the work rate increases (10, 23). This is because the relationship between energy expenditure and work rate is curvilinear rather than linear (see figure 6.6) (12, 23). That is, as the work rate increases, total body energy expenditure increases out of proportion to the work rate; this results in a lowered efficiency.

Figure 6.7
Effects of decreasing or increasing speed of movement on exercise efficiency. Note an optimum speed of movement for maximum efficiency at any given work rate.

Movement Speed and Efficiency

Research has shown that there is an "optimum" speed of movement for any given work rate. Recent evidence suggests that the optimum speed of movement increases as the power output increases (6). In other words, at higher power outputs, a greater speed of movement is required to obtain optimum efficiency. At low-to-moderate work rates, a pedaling speed of 40–60 rpm is generally considered optimum during arm or cycle ergometry (12, 21, 23, 25). Note that any change in the speed of movement away from the optimum results in a decrease in efficiency (figure 6.7). This decline in efficiency at low speeds of movement is probably due to inertia (23). That is, there may be an increased energy cost of performing work when movements are slow and the limbs involved must repeatedly stop and start. The decline in efficiency associated with high-speed movement (low work rates) may be because increasing speeds might augment muscular friction and thus increase internal work (4, 23).

Fiber Type and Efficiency

People differ greatly in their net efficiency during cycle ergometer exercise. Why? Recent evidence suggests that subjects with a high percentage of slow muscle fibers display a higher exercise efficiency compared to subjects with a high percentage of fast muscle fibers (see chapter 8 for a discussion of muscle fiber types) (15a). The physiological explanation for this observation is that slow muscle fibers are more efficient than fast fibers. That is, slow fibers require less ATP per unit of work performed compared to fast fibers.

The significance of a high exercise efficiency is that superior efficiency can improve exercise performance. Indeed, studies have shown that endurance performance is improved by a high exercise efficiency (15a). This can be explained by the fact that, compared to subjects with a relatively low efficiency, subjects with high efficiency can generate a greater power output at any rate of energy expenditure. In other words, a high exercise efficiency improves endurance performance by increasing the power output produced for a given amount of ATP used.

in summary

- Net efficiency is defined as the mathematical ratio of work performed divided by the energy expenditure above rest, and is expressed as a percent:

  % Net efficiency =
  $$\frac{\text{Work output}}{\text{Energy expended above rest}} \times 100$$

- The efficiency of exercise decreases as the exercise work rate increases. This occurs because the relationship between work rate and energy expenditure is curvilinear.
- To achieve maximal efficiency at any work rate, there is an optimal speed of movement.
- Exercise efficiency is greater in subjects that possess a high percentage of slow muscle fibers compared to subjects with a high percentage of fast fibers. This is due to the fact that slow muscle fibers are more efficient than fast fibers.

Running Economy

As discussed previously, computation of work is not generally possible during horizontal treadmill running, and thus a calculation of exercise efficiency cannot be performed. However, the measurement of the steady state $\dot{V}O_2$ requirement (O_2 cost) of running at various speeds offers a means of comparing running economy (not efficiency) between two runners or groups of runners (14, 15, 20). Figure 6.8 compares the O_2 cost of running between a group of highly trained male and female distance runners at slow running speeds (i.e., slower than race pace). A runner who exhibits poor running economy would require a higher $\dot{V}O_2$ (ml · kg^{-1} · min^{-1}) at any given running speed than an economical runner. Notice that the O_2 cost of running labeled on the ordinate (y-axis) is expressed as $\dot{V}O_2$ in ml · kg^{-1} · min^{-1}. Expressing $\dot{V}O_2$ as a function of the body weight is referred to as **relative $\dot{V}O_2$**, and is appropriate when describing the O_2 cost of weight-bearing activities such as running, climbing steps, walking, or ice skating.

Do gender differences exist in running economy? This issue has been studied by numerous investigators, with mixed findings. Figure 6.8 illustrates the results of one of these studies (15). This study compared the oxygen cost of running between highly trained men and women distance runners. The runners were matched for maximal aerobic power and the number of years of training experience. The similar slopes of the two lines suggests that running economy is comparable for highly trained men and women distance runners at slow running speeds (15). However, recent evidence suggests that at fast "race pace" speeds, male runners may be more economical than females (9). The reason for this apparent gender variation in running economy is unclear and requires further study (22).

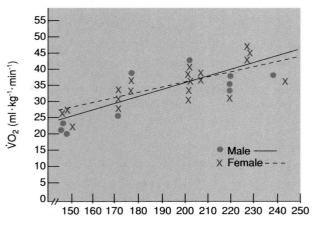

Figure 6.8
Comparison of the oxygen cost of horizontal treadmill running between highly trained men and women distance runners.

in summary

- Although it is not possible to compute efficiency during horizontal running, the measurement of the O_2 cost of running $(ml \cdot kg^{-1} \cdot min^{-1})$ at any given speed offers a measure of running economy.
- Running economy does not differ between highly trained men and women distance runners at slow running speeds. However, at fast "race pace" speeds, male runners may be more economical than females. The reasons for these differences are unclear.

study questions

1. Define the following terms:
   a. work
   b. power
   c. percent grade
   d. relative $\dot{V}O_2$
   e. net efficiency
   f. metric system
   g. SI units

2. Calculate the total amount of work performed in five minutes of exercise on the cycle ergometer, given the following:

   Resistance on the flywheel = 2.5 kp
   Cranking speed = 60 rpm
   Distance traveled per revolution = 6 meters

3. Compute total work and power output per minute for ten minutes of treadmill exercise, given the following:

   Treadmill grade = 15%
   Horizontal speed = 200 m $\cdot$ min^{-1}
   Subject's weight = 70 kg

4. Briefly, describe the procedure used to estimate energy expenditure using (a) direct calorimetry and (b) indirect calorimetry.

5. Compute the estimated energy expenditure during horizontal treadmill walking for the following examples:
   a. Treadmill speed = 50 m $\cdot$ min^{-1}
      Subject's weight = 62 kg
   b. Treadmill speed = 100 m $\cdot$ min^{-1}
      Subject's weight = 75 kg
   c. Treadmill speed = 80 m $\cdot$ min^{-1}
      Subject's weight = 60 kg

6. Calculate the estimated O_2 cost of horizontal treadmill running for a 70-kg subject at 150, 200, and 235 m $\cdot$ min^{-1}.

7. Calculate net efficiency, given the following:

   Exercise $\dot{V}O_2$ = 3.0$\ell \cdot$ min^{-1}
   Resting exercise $\dot{V}O_2$ = 0.3$\ell \cdot$ min^{-1}
   Work rate = 1200 kpm $\cdot$ min^{-1} (196 Watts)

8. Calculate the power output during one minute of cycle ergometer exercise, given the following:

   Resistance on the flywheel = 5.0 kp
   Cranking speed = 50 rpm
   Distance traveled per revolution = 6 meters

9. Calculate the total work performed during ten minutes of cycle ergometer exercise, given the following:

   Resistance on the flywheel = 2.0 kp
   Cranking speed = 70 rpm
   Distance traveled per revolution = 6 meters

10. Calculate net efficiency, given the following:

    Resting $\dot{V}O_2$ = 0.3$\ell \cdot$ min^{-1}
    Exercise $\dot{V}O_2$ = 2.1$\ell \cdot$ min^{-1}
    Work rate = 900 kpm $\cdot$ min^{-1}

11. Compute the power output for three minutes of treadmill exercise, given the following:

    Treadmill grade = 10%
    Horizontal speed = 100 m $\cdot$ min^{-1}
    Subject's weight = 60 kg

12. Calculate the power output (expressed in watts) for a subject who performed ten minutes of cycle ergometer exercise at:

    Resistance on the flywheel = 2.0 kp
    Cranking speed = 60 rpm
    Distance traveled per revolution = 6 meters

suggested readings

American College of Sports Medicine. 1991. *Guidelines for Graded Exercise Testing and Exercise Prescription.* Philadelphia: Lea & Febiger.

Horowitz, J. et al. 1994. High efficiency of type I muscle fibers improves performance. *International Journal of Sports Medicine.* 15:152–157.

Knuttgen, H., and P. Komi. 1992. Basic definitions for exercise. In *Strength and Power in Sport,* ed. P. Komi. Oxford: Blackwell Scientific Publications.

Morgan, D., and M. Craib. 1992. Physiological aspects of running economy. *Medicine and Science in Sports and Exercise* 24:456–61.

references

1. American College of Sports Medicine. 1991. *Guidelines for Graded Exercise Testing and Exercise Prescription.* Philadelphia: Lea & Febiger.
2. Åstrand, P., and K. Rodahl. 1986. *Textbook of Work Physiology.* New York: McGraw-Hill.
3. Brooks, G., and T. Fahey. 1984. *Exercise Physiology: Human Bioenergetics and Its Applications.* New York: Macmillan.
4. Cavanagh, P., and R. Kram. 1985. Mechanical and muscular factors affecting the efficiency of human movement. *Medicine and Science in Sports and Exercise* 17:326–31.
5. ———. 1985. The efficiency of human movement—a statement of the problem. *Medicine and Science in Sports and Exercise* 17:304–8.
6. Coast, J., and H. G. Welch. 1985. Linear increase in optimal pedal rate with increased power output in cycle ergometry. *European Journal of Applied Physiology* 53:339–42.
7. Consolazio, C., R. Johnson, and L. Pecora. 1963. *Physiological Measurements of Metabolic Function in Man.* New York: McGraw-Hill.
8. Daniels, J. 1985. A physiologist's view of running economy. *Medicine and Science in Sports and Exercise* 17:332–38.
9. Daniels, J., and N. Daniels. 1992. Running economy of elite male and elite female distance runners. *Medicine and Science in Sports and Exercise* 24:483–89.
10. Donovan, C., and G. Brooks. 1977. Muscular efficiency during steady-rate exercise: Effects of speed and work rate. *Journal of Applied Physiology* 43:431–39.
11. Fox, E., and D. Mathews. 1981. *The Physiological Basis of Physical Education and Athletics.* Philadelphia: Saunders College Publishing.
12. Gaesser, G., and G. Brooks. 1975. Muscular efficiency during steady-rate exercise: Effects of speed and work rate. *Journal of Applied Physiology* 38:1132–39.
13. Grandjean, E. 1982. *Fitting the Task to the Man: An Ergonomic Approach.* New York: International Publications Service.
14. Hagan, R. et al. 1980. Oxygen uptake and energy expenditure during horizontal treadmill running. *Journal of Applied Physiology* 49:571–75.
15. Hopkins, P., and S. Powers. 1982. Oxygen uptake during submaximal running in highly trained men and women. *American Corrective Therapy Journal* 36:130–32.
15a. Horowitz, J. et al. 1994. High efficiency of type I muscle fibers improves performance. *International Journal of Sports Medicine.* 15:152–57.
16. Howley, E., and B. D. Franks. 1992. *Health/Fitness Instructor's Handbook.* Champaign, IL: Human Kinetics.
17. Knuttgen, H. 1978. Force, power, and exercise. *Medicine and Science in Sports and Exercise* 10:227–28.
18. Knuttgen, H., and P. Komi. 1992. Basic definitions for exercise. In *Strength and Power in Sport,* ed. P. Komi. Oxford: Blackwell Scientific Publications.
19. Lakomy, H. 1986. Measurement of work and power output using friction-loaded cycle ergometers. *Ergonomics* 29:509–17.
20. Margaria, R. et al. 1963. Energy cost of running. *Journal of Applied Physiology* 18:367–70.
21. Michielli, D., and M. Stricevic. 1977. Various pedalling frequencies at equivalent power outputs. *New York State Medical Journal* 77:744–46.
22. Morgan, D., and M. Craib. 1992. Physiological aspects of running economy. *Medicine and Science in Sports and Exercise* 24:456–61.
23. Powers, S., R. Beadle, and M. Mangum. 1984. Exercise efficiency during arm ergometry: Effects of speed and work rate. *Journal of Applied Physiology* 56:495–99.
24. Powers, S. et al. 1987. Measurement of oxygen uptake in the non-steady state. *Aviation, Space, and Environmental Medicine* 58:323–27.
25. Seabury, J., W. Adams, and M. Ramey. 1977. Influence of pedalling rate and power output on energy expenditure during bicycle ergometry. *Ergonomics* 20:491–98.
26. Shephard, R. 1982. *Physiology and Biochemistry of Exercise.* New York: Praeger.
27. Singleton, W. 1982. *The Body at Work.* London: Cambridge University Press.
28. Spence, A., and E. Mason. 1992. *Human Anatomy and Physiology.* Menlo Park, CA: Benjamin-Cummings.
29. Stegeman, J. 1981. *Exercise Physiology: Physiological Bases of Work and Sport.* Chicago: Year Book Publishers.
30. Stuart, M. et al. 1980. Efficiency of trained subjects differing in maximal oxygen uptake and type of training. *Journal of Applied Physiology* 50:444–49.
31. Whipp, B., and K. Wasserman. 1969. Efficiency of muscular work. *Journal of Applied Physiology* 26:644–48.

CHAPTER 7

The Nervous System

Structure and Control
of Movement

objectives

*By studying this chapter, you should be able to do
the following:*

1. Discuss the general organization of the
   nervous system.
2. Describe the structure and function of a nerve.
3. Draw and label the pathways involved in a
   withdrawal reflex.
4. Define depolarization, action potential,
   and repolarization.
5. Discuss the role of position receptors in the control
   of movement.
6. Describe the role of the vestibular apparatus in
   maintaining equilibrium.
7. Discuss the brain centers involved in voluntary
   control of movement.
8. Describe the structure and function of the
   autonomic nervous system.

outline

General Nervous System
    Functions 108
Organization of the Nervous
    System 108
  Structure of the Neuron 109
  Electrical Activity in Neurons 111
Sensory Information and
    Reflexes 115
  Proprioceptors 115
  Muscle Chemoreceptors 115
  Reflexes 116

Somatic Motor Function 117
Vestibular Apparatus and
    Equilibrium 117
Motor Control Functions of the
    Brain 118
  Brain Stem 118
  Cerebrum 119
  Cerebellum 119

Motor Functions of the Spinal
    Cord 119
Control of Motor Functions 120
Autonomic Nervous System 121

action potential	dendrites	proprioceptors
afferent fibers	efferent fibers	reciprocal inhibition
autonomic nervous system	EPSP	resting membrane potential
axon	IPSP	Schwann cell
brain stem	irritability	spatial summation
cell body	kinesthesia	sympathetic nervous system
central nervous system (CNS)	motor cortex	synapses
cerebellum	neuron	temporal summation
cerebrum	parasympathetic nervous system	vestibular apparatus
conductivity	peripheral nervous system (PNS)	

T he nervous system provides the body with a rapid means of internal communication that allows us to move about, talk, and coordinate the activity of billions of cells. Thus, neural activity is critically important in the body's ability to maintain homeostasis. The purpose of this chapter is to present an overview of the nervous system, with emphasis on neural control of voluntary movement. We will begin with a brief discussion of the functions of the nervous system.

General Nervous System Functions

The nervous system is the body's means of perceiving and responding to events in the internal and external environments. Receptors capable of sensing touch, pain, temperature changes, and chemical stimuli send information to the **central nervous system (CNS)** concerning changes in our environment. The CNS may respond to these stimuli in several ways. The response may be involuntary movement (e.g., rapid removal of a hand from a hot surface), or alteration in the rate of release of some hormone from the endocrine system (chapter 5). In addition to integrating body activities and controlling voluntary movement, the nervous system is responsible for storing experiences (memory) and establishing patterns of response based on previous experiences (learning). A summary of the functions of the nervous system follows (9, 28):

1. Control of the internal environment (nervous system works with endocrine system).
2. Voluntary control of movement.
3. Programming of spinal cord reflexes.
4. Assimilation of experiences necessary for memory and learning.

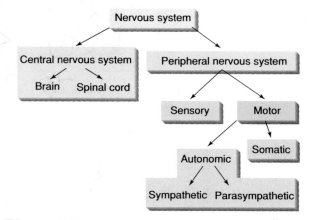

Figure 7.1
Anatomical divisions of the nervous system.

Organization of the Nervous System

Anatomically, the nervous system can be divided into two main parts: the CNS and the **peripheral nervous system (PNS).** The CNS is that portion of the nervous system contained in the skull (brain) and the spinal cord; the PNS consists of nerve cells **(neurons)** outside the CNS (see figure 7.1).

The PNS can be further subdivided into two sections: (1) the sensory portion and (2) the motor portion. The sensory division is responsible for transmission of neuron impulses from sense organs (receptors) to the CNS. These sensory nerve fibers, which conduct information toward the CNS, are called **afferent fibers.** The motor portion of the PNS can be further subdivided into the somatic motor (which innervates skeletal muscle) and autonomic motor (which innervates involuntary effector organs like smooth muscle in the gut, cardiac muscle, and glands). Motor nerve fibers, which conduct impulses away from the CNS, are referred to as

Figure 7.2
The relationship between the motor and sensory fibers of the peripheral nervous system (PNS) and the central nervous system (CNS).

efferent fibers. The relationships between the CNS and the PNS are visualized in figure 7.2.

in summary

- The nervous system is the body's means of perceiving and responding to events in the internal and external environments. Receptors capable of sensing touch, pain, temperature, and chemical stimuli send information to the CNS concerning changes in our environment. The CNS responds by either voluntary movement or a change in the rate of release of some hormone from the endocrine system, depending on which response is appropriate.
- The nervous system is divided into two major divisions: (1) the central nervous system and (2) the peripheral nervous system. The central nervous system includes the brain and the spinal cord, whereas the peripheral nervous system includes the nerves outside the central nervous system.

Structure of the Neuron

The functional unit of the nervous system is the neuron. Anatomically, neurons can be divided into three regions: (1) **cell body,** (2) **dendrites,** and (3) **axon** (see figure 7.3). The center of operation for the neuron is the cell body, or soma, which contains the nucleus. Narrow, cytoplasmic attachments extend from the cell body and are called dendrites. Dendrites serve as a receptive area that can conduct electrical impulses toward the cell body. The axon (also called the nerve fiber) carries the electrical message away from the cell body toward another neuron or effector organ. Axons vary in length from a few millimeters to a meter (9, 14). Each neuron has only one axon; however, the axon can divide into several collateral branches that terminate at other neurons, muscle cells, or glands (figure 7.3). Contact points between an axon of one neuron and the dendrite of another neuron are called **synapses** (see figure 7.4).

In large nerve fibers like those innervating skeletal muscle, the axons are covered with an insulating layer of cells called **Schwann cells.** The membranes of Schwann cells contain a large amount of a lipid-protein

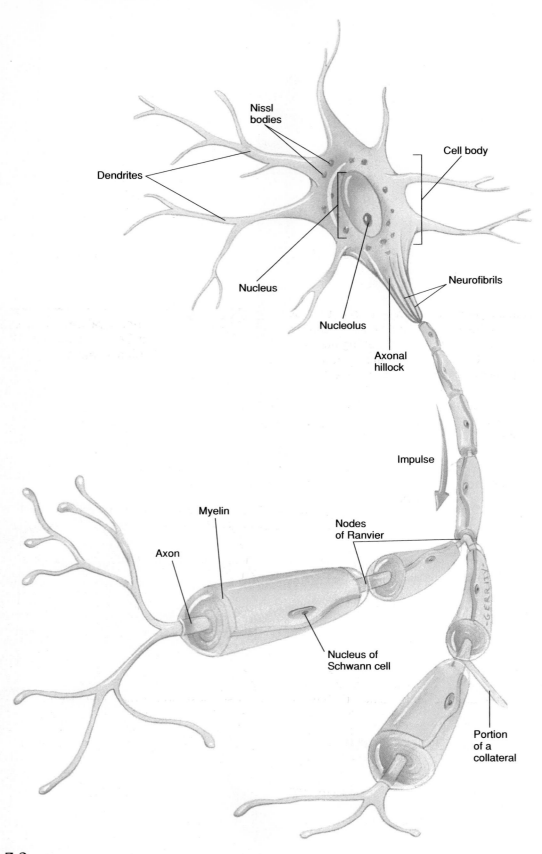

Figure 7.3
The parts of a neuron.

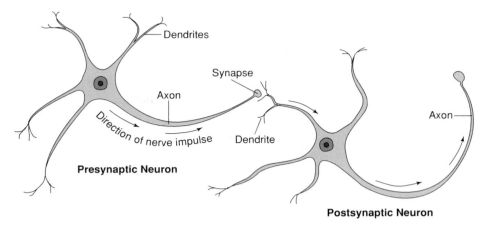

Figure 7.4

An illustration of synaptic transmission. For a nerve impulse to continue from one neuron to another, it must cross the synaptic cleft at a synapse.

substance called myelin, which forms a discontinuous sheath that covers the outside of the axon. The gaps or spaces between the myelin segments along the axon are called nodes of Ranvier and play an important role in neural transmission. In general, the larger the diameter of the axon, the greater the speed of neural transmission (9, 14). Thus, those axons with large myelin sheaths conduct impulses more rapidly than small nonmyelinated fibers.

Electrical Activity in Neurons

Neurons are considered "excitable tissue" because of their specialized properties of irritability and conductivity. **Irritability** is the ability of the dendrites and neuron cell body to respond to a stimulus and convert it to a neural impulse. **Conductivity** refers to the transmission of the impulse along the axon. A nerve impulse can be thought of as an electrical signal carried the length of the axon. This electrical signal is initiated via some stimulus that causes a change in the normal electrical charge of the neuron.

Resting Membrane Potential

At rest, all cells (including neurons) are negatively charged on the inside of the cell with respect to the charge on the exterior of the cell. This negative charge is the result of an unequal distribution of charged ions (ions are elements with a positive or negative charge) across the cell membrane. Thus, a neuron is said to be polarized and this electrical charge difference is called the **resting membrane potential.** The magnitude of the resting membrane potential varies from –5 to –100 mv depending upon the cell type; in neurons, the resting membrane potential is generally in the range of –40 mv to –75 mv (35).

Let's discuss the resting membrane potential in more detail. Cellular proteins, phosphate groups, and

Table 7.1	Concentration of Ions Across the Cell Membrane of a Typical Neuron	
Concentration (millimoles/liter)		
Ion	Extracellular	Intracellular
Sodium (Na$^+$)	150	15
Chloride (Cl$^-$)	110	10
Potassium (K$^+$)	5	150

other nucleotides are negatively charged (anions) and are fixed inside the cell because they cannot penetrate the cell membrane. Since these negatively charged molecules are unable to leave the cell, they attract positively charged ions (cations) from the extracellular fluid. This results in an accumulation of a net positive charge on the outside surface of the membrane and a net negative charge on the inside surface of the membrane (9, 15).

The magnitude of the resting membrane potential is determined mainly by two factors: (1) the permeabilities of the plasma membrane to the different ion species and (2) the difference in ion concentrations of the intracellular and extracellular fluid (35). Although numerous intracellular and extracellular ions exist, sodium, potassium, and chloride ions are present in the greatest concentrations and therefore play the most important roles in generating the resting membrane potential (29, 35). The concentrations of sodium, potassium, and chloride in the extracellular and intracellular fluid are listed in table 7.1. Note that the sodium concentration is much greater outside the cell compared to inside, and the potassium concentration is greater inside the cell than outside.

The permeability of the neuron membrane to potassium, sodium, and other ions is regulated by proteins within the membrane that function as gates. Since the concentration of potassium (+ charge) is high inside the cell and the concentration of sodium (+ charge) is high outside the cell, an alteration of the membrane's permeability to either potassium or sodium would result in a movement of these charged ions down their concentration gradients. That is, sodium would enter the cell and potassium would leave the cell. At rest, almost all of the sodium gates are closed whereas a few potassium gates are open. This means that more potassium ions are leaving the cell compared to the number of sodium ions "leaking" into the cell. This results in a net loss of positive charges from the inside of the membrane, thus, making the resting membrane potential negative. In short, the negative membrane potential in a resting neuron is due primarily to the diffusion of potassium out of the cell, caused by: (1) the higher permeability of the membrane for potassium than sodium and (2) the concentration gradient for potassium from inside to outside the cell.

As mentioned above, a small number of ions are always moving across the cell membrane. If potassium ions continued to diffuse out of the cell and the sodium ions continued to diffuse into the cell, the concentration gradients for these ions would decrease. This would result in a loss of the negative membrane potential. What prevents this from happening? The cell membrane has a sodium/potassium pump that uses energy from ATP to maintain the intracellular/extracellular concentrations by pumping sodium out of the cell and potassium into the cell. Interestingly, this pump not only maintains the concentration gradients that are needed to maintain the resting membrane potential, but it also helps to generate the potential since it exchanges three sodium ions for every two potassium ions (35).

Action Potential

A neural message is generated when a stimulus of sufficient strength reaches the neuron membrane and opens sodium gates, which allows sodium ions to diffuse into the neuron, making the inside more and more positive (depolarizing the cell). When depolarization reaches a critical value called "threshold," the sodium gates open wide and an **action potential** or nerve impulse is formed (see figures 7.5 and 7.6a). Once an action potential has been generated, a sequence of ionic exchanges occurs along the axon to propagate the nerve impulse. This ionic exchange along the neuron occurs in a sequential fashion at the nodes of Ranvier (figure 7.3).

Repolarization occurs immediately following depolarization, resulting in a return of the resting membrane potential with the nerve ready to be stimulated

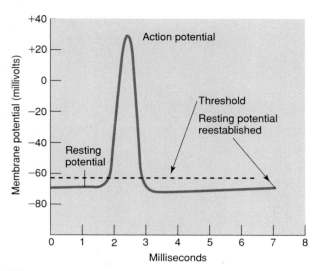

Figure 7.5

An action potential is produced by an increase in sodium conductance into the neuron. As sodium enters the neuron the change becomes more and more positive and an action potential is generated.

again (figure 7.5). How does repolarization occur? Depolarization, with a slight time delay, causes a brief increase in membrane permeability to potassium. As a result, potassium leaves the cell rapidly, making the inside of the membrane more negative (see figure 7.6b). Secondly, after the depolarization stimulus is removed, the sodium gates within the cell membrane close and sodium entry into the cell is slowed (therefore, few positive charges are entering the cell). The combined result of these activities quickly restores the resting membrane potential back to the original negative charge.

All-or-None Law

The development of a nerve impulse is considered to be an "all-or-none" response and is referred to as the "all-or-none" law of action potentials. This means that if a nerve impulse is initiated, the impulse will travel the entire length of the axon without a decrease in voltage. In other words, the neural impulse is just as strong after traveling the length of the axon as it was at the initial point of stimulation.

A mechanical analogy of the all-or-none law is the firing of a gun (35). That is, the speed of the bullet leaving the gun does not depend upon how hard you pulled the trigger. Indeed, firing a gun is all or none; you cannot fire a gun halfway.

Neurotransmitters and Synaptic Transmission

As mentioned previously, neurons communicate with other neurons at junctions called synapses. A synapse is a small gap (20–30 nanometers) between the synaptic endfoot of the presynaptic neuron and a dendrite of

Figure 7.6

(a) When a polarized nerve fiber is stimulated, sodium channels open, some sodium ions diffuse inward, and the membrane is depolarized. (b) When the potassium channels open, potassium ions diffuse outward, and the membrane is repolarized.

a postsynaptic neuron (see figure 7.7). Communication between neurons occurs via a process called synaptic transmission, and happens when sufficient amounts of a specific neurotransmitter (a neurotransmitter is a chemical messenger that neurons use to communicate with each other) are released from synaptic vesicles contained in the presynaptic neuron. The nerve impulse results in the synaptic vesicles releasing stored neurotransmitter into the synaptic cleft. Neurotransmitters that cause depolarization of membranes are termed *excitatory transmitters*. After release into the synaptic cleft, these neurotransmitters bind to "receptors" on the target membrane, which produces a series of graded depolarizations in the dendrites and cell body (1, 2, 15, 19, 23, 27). These graded depolarizations are known as excitatory postsynaptic potentials **(EPSPs).** If sufficient amounts of the neurotransmitter are released, the postsynaptic neuron is depolarized to threshold and an action potential is generated.

There are two ways in which EPSPs can bring the postsynaptic neuron to threshold: (1) temporal summation and (2) spatial summation. The summing of several EPSPs from a single presynaptic neuron over a short time period is termed **temporal summation** ("temporal" refers to time). The number of EPSPs required to bring the postsynaptic neuron to threshold varies, but it is estimated that the addition of up to fifty EPSPs might be required to produce an action potential

within some neurons (29). Nonetheless, one means by which an action potential can be generated is through rapid, repetitive excitation from a single excitatory presynaptic neuron.

A second means of achieving an action potential at the postsynaptic membrane is to sum EPSPs from several different presynaptic inputs (i.e., different points in space) and is known as **spatial summation.** In spatial summation, concurrent EPSPs come into a postsynaptic neuron from numerous different excitatory inputs. As with temporal summation, up to fifty EPSPs arriving simultaneously on the postsynaptic membrane may be required to produce an action potential (29).

A common neurotransmitter, which also happens to be the transmitter at the nerve/muscle junction, is acetylcholine. Upon release into the synaptic cleft, acetylcholine binds to receptors on the postsynaptic membrane and opens "channels," which allow sodium to enter the nerve or muscle cell. When enough sodium enters the postsynaptic membrane of a neuron or muscle, depolarization results. In order to prevent chronic depolarization of the postsynaptic neuron, the neurotransmitter must be broken down into less active molecules via enzymes found in the synaptic cleft. In the case of acetylcholine, the degrading enzyme is called acetylcholinesterase. This enzyme breaks down acetylcholine into acetyl and choline and thus removes the stimulus for depolarization (9). Following breakdown

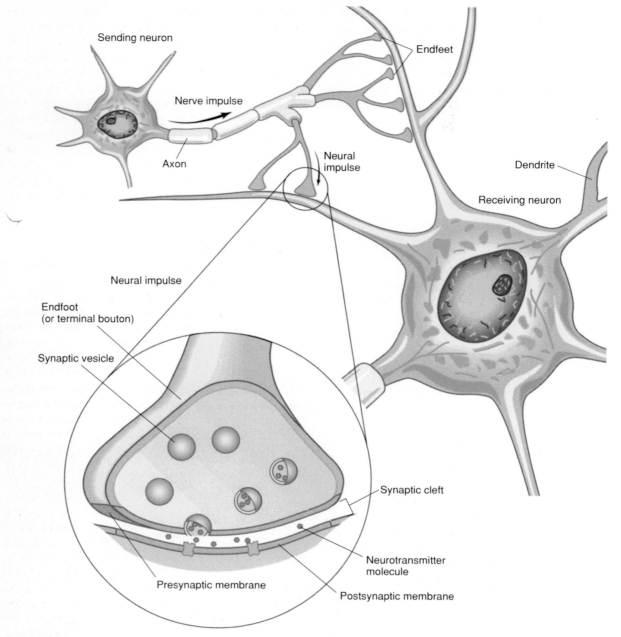

Figure 7.7

The basic structure of a chemical synapse. In this idealized drawing, the essential elements of the synapse may be seen: the endfoot of the axon containing synaptic vesicles, the synaptic cleft, and the postsynaptic membrane.

of the neurotransmitter, the postsynaptic membrane repolarizes and is prepared to receive additional neurotransmitters and generate a new action potential. Note that not all neurotransmitters are excitatory. In fact, some neurotransmitters have just the opposite effect of excitatory transmitters (23). These inhibitory transmitters cause a hyperpolarization (increased negativity) of the postsynaptic membrane. This hyperpolarization of the membrane is called an inhibitory postsynaptic potential, or **IPSP.** The end result of an IPSP is that the neuron develops a more negative resting membrane potential, is pushed further

from threshold, and thus resists depolarization. In general, whether a neuron reaches threshold or not is dependent on the ratio of the number of EPSPs to the number of IPSPs. For example, a neuron that is simultaneously bombarded by an equal number of EPSPs and IPSPs will not reach threshold and generate an action potential. On the other hand, if the EPSPs outnumber the IPSPs, the neuron is moved toward threshold and an action potential may be generated.

An interesting example of a neurotransmitter that can be both inhibitory and excitatory is acetylcholine. While acetylcholine produces depolarization of skeletal muscle, it causes a hyperpolarization of the heart, slowing the heart rate. This occurs because the combination of acetylcholine with receptors in the heart causes the opening of membrane channels that allow potassium to diffuse out of the cell. Therefore, an outward diffusion of potassium produces a hyperpolarization of heart tissue and the membrane potential is moved further away from the threshold valve.

in summary

- Nerve cells are called neurons and are divided anatomically into three parts: (1) the cell body, (2) dendrites, and (3) the axon. Axons are generally covered by Schwann cells, with gaps between these cells called nodes of Ranvier.
- Neurons are specialized cells that respond to physical or chemical changes in their environment. At rest, neurons are negatively charged in the interior with respect to the electrical charge outside the cell. This difference in electrical charge is called the resting membrane potential.
- A neuron "fires" when a stimulus changes the permeability of the membrane, allowing sodium to enter at a high rate, which depolarizes the cell. When the depolarization reaches threshold, an action potential or nerve impulse is initiated. Repolarization occurs immediately following depolarization due to an increase in membrane permeability to potassium, and a decreased permeability to sodium.
- Neurons communicate with other neurons at junctions called synapses. Synaptic transmission occurs when sufficient amounts of a specific neurotransmitter are released from the presynaptic neuron. Upon release, the neurotransmitter binds to a receptor on the postsynaptic membrane.
- Neurotransmitters can be excitatory or inhibitory. An excitatory transmitter increases neuronal permeability to sodium and results in excitatory postsynaptic potentials (EPSPs). Inhibitory neurotransmitters cause the neuron to become more negative (hyperpolarized). This hyperpolarization of the membrane is called an inhibitory postsynaptic potential (IPSP).

Sensory Information and Reflexes

The CNS receives a constant bombardment of messages from receptors throughout the body about changes in both the internal and external environment. These receptors are "sense organs" that "change" forms of energy in the "real world" into the energy of nerve impulses, which are conducted to the CNS by sensory neurons. Van De Graaff (34) has called these sense organs "windows for the brain." A complete discussion of sense organs is beyond the scope of this chapter, so we will limit our discussion to those receptors responsible for position sense and muscle chemoreceptors (i.e., receptors that are sensitive to changes in the chemical environment of muscles). Receptors that provide the CNS with information about body position are called **proprioceptors,** or kinesthetic receptors, and include muscle spindles, Golgi tendon organs, and joint receptors. Muscle spindles and Golgi tendon organs are discussed in chapter 8, so our discussion will center around joint receptors, chemoreceptors, and neural reflexes.

Proprioceptors

The term **kinesthesia** means conscious recognition of the position of body parts with respect to one another as well as recognition of limb-movement rates (20, 21, 24). These functions are accomplished by extensive sensory devices in and around joints. There are three principle types of proprioceptors: (1) free nerve endings, (2) Golgi-type receptors, and (3) pacinian corpuscles. The most abundant of these are free nerve endings, which are sensitive to touch and pressure. These receptors are stimulated strongly at the beginning of movement; they adapt (i.e., become less sensitive to stimuli) slightly at first, but then transmit a steady signal until the movement is complete (4, 10). A second type of position receptor, Golgi-type receptors (not to be confused with Golgi tendon organs found in muscle tendons), are found in ligaments around joints. These receptors are not as abundant as free nerve endings, but function in a similar manner (9, 28). Pacinian corpuscles are found in the tissues around joints and adapt rapidly following the initiation of movement. This rapid adaptation presumably helps detect the rate of joint rotation (9, 28). To summarize, the joint receptors work together to provide the body with a conscious means of recognition of the orientation of body parts as well as feedback relative to the rates of limb movement.

Muscle Chemoreceptors

Numerous studies have demonstrated the existence of muscle chemoreceptors (16, 17, 18, 22). These receptors are sensitive to changes in the chemical environment surrounding muscle and send information to the CNS via slow conducting fibers classified as group III (myelinated) and group IV (unmyelinated) fibers. Scientific debate continues about the complete list of factors that stimulate muscle chemoreceptors. However, changes in the concentration of hydrogen ions, carbon dioxide, and/or potassium around muscle are known to be potent stimulators of these receptors. The physiological role of muscle chemoreceptors is to provide the CNS with information concerning the

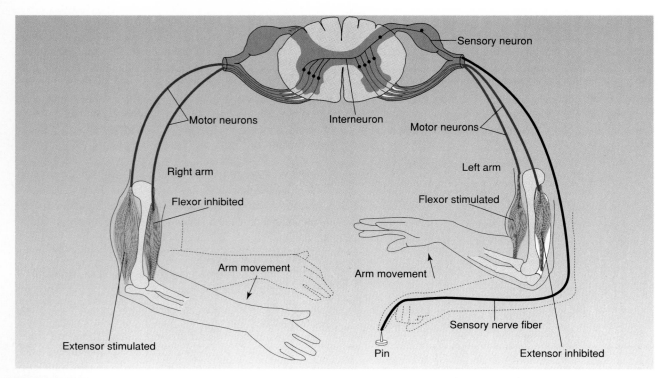

Figure 7.8
When the flexor muscle on one side of the body is stimulated to contract via a withdrawal reflex, the extensor on the opposite side also contracts.

metabolic rate of muscular activity. This information may be important in the regulation of the cardiovascular and pulmonary responses to exercise (3, 18, 22) and will be discussed in chapters 9 and 10.

Reflexes
A reflex arc is the nerve pathway from the receptor to the CNS and from the CNS along a motor pathway back to the effector organ. Reflex contraction of skeletal muscles can occur in response to sensory input, and is not dependent on activation of higher brain centers. One purpose of a reflex is to provide a rapid means of removing a limb from a source of pain. Consider the case of a person touching a sharp object. The obvious reaction to this painful stimulus is to quickly remove the hand from the source of pain. This rapid removal is accomplished via reflex action. Again, the pathways for this neural reflex are as follows (14): (1) first, a sensory nerve (pain receptor) sends a nerve impulse to the spinal column; (2) secondly, interneurons within the spinal cord are excited and in turn stimulate motor neurons; (3) finally, the excited interneurons cause depolarization of specific motor neurons, which control the flexor muscles necessary to withdraw the limb from the point of injury. The antagonistic muscle group (e.g., extensors) are simultaneously inhibited via IPSPs. This simultaneous excitatory and inhibitory activity is known as **reciprocal inhibition** (see figure 7.8).

Another interesting feature of the withdrawal reflex is that the opposite limb is extended to support the body during the removal of the injured limb. This event is called the crossed-extensor reflex and is illustrated by the left portion of figure 7.8. Notice that the extensors are contracting as the flexors are inhibited.

in summary
- Proprioceptors are position receptors located in joint capsules, ligaments, and muscles. The three most abundant joint and ligament receptors are free nerve endings, Golgi-type receptors, and pacinian corpuscles. These receptors provide the body with a conscious means of recognizing the orientation of body parts as well as feedback relative to the rates of limb movement.
- Muscle chemoreceptors are sensitive to changes in the chemical environment surrounding muscle and send information back to the CNS regarding the metabolic rate of muscular activity.
- Reflexes provide the body with a rapid unconscious means of reacting to some stimuli.

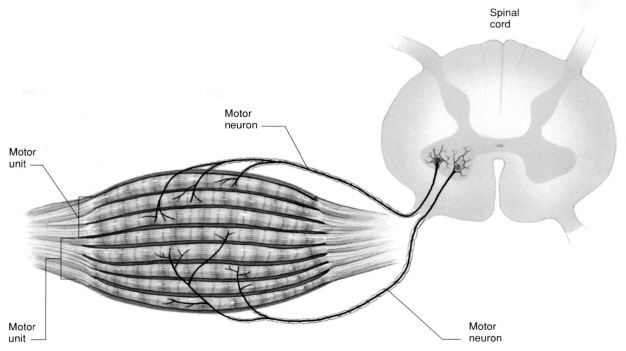

Spinal
cord

Motor
neuron

Motor
unit

Motor
unit

Motor
neuron

Figure 7.9
Illustration of a motor unit. A motor unit is defined as a motor neuron and all the muscle fibers it innervates.

Somatic Motor Function

The term *somatic* refers to the outer (i.e., nonvisceral) regions of the body. The somatic motor portion of the peripheral nervous system is responsible for carrying neural messages from the spinal cord to skeletal muscle fibers. These neural messages are the signals for muscular contraction to occur. Muscular contraction will be discussed in detail in chapter 8.

The organization of the somatic motor nervous system is illustrated in figure 7.9. The somatic neuron that innervates skeletal muscle fibers is called a motor neuron (also called an alpha motor neuron). Note (figure 7.9) that the cell body of motor neurons is located within the spinal cord. The axon of the motor neuron leaves the spinal cord as a spinal nerve and extends to the muscle that it is responsible for innervating. Once the axon reaches the muscle, the axon splits into collateral branches; each collateral branch innervates a single muscle fiber. Each motor neuron and all the muscle fibers that it innervates is known as a motor unit.

When a single motor neuron is activated, all of the muscle fibers that it innervates are stimulated to contract. However, note that the number of muscle fibers that a motor neuron innervates is not constant and varies from muscle to muscle. The number of muscle fibers innervated by a single motor neuron is called the innervation ratio (i.e., number of muscle fibers/motor neuron). In muscle groups that require fine motor control the innervation ratio is low. For

example, the innervation ratio of the extraocular muscles (i.e., muscles that regulate eye movement) is 23/1. In contrast, innervation ratios of large muscles that are not involved in fine motor control (e.g., leg muscles) may range from 1,000/1 to 2,000/1.

in summary

- The somatic motor portion of the peripheral nervous system is responsible for carrying neural messages from the spinal cord to skeletal muscle fibers.
- A motor neuron and all the muscle fibers that it innervates is known as a motor unit.
- The number of muscle fibers innervated by a single motor neuron is called the innervation ratio (i.e., number of muscle fibers/motor neuron).

Vestibular Apparatus and Equilibrium

The **vestibular apparatus,** an organ located in the inner ear, is responsible for maintaining general equilibrium. Although a detailed discussion of the anatomy of the vestibular apparatus will not be presented here, a brief discussion of the function of the vestibular apparatus is appropriate. The receptors contained within the vestibular apparatus are sensitive to any change in head position or movement direction (15, 25). Movement of the

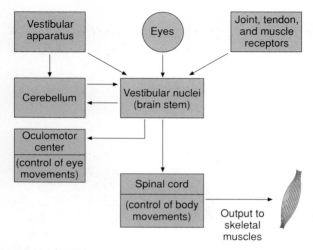

Figure 7.10
The role of the vestibular apparatus in maintenance of equilibrium and balance.

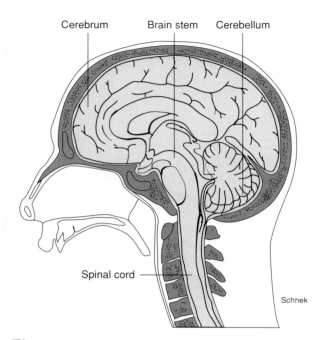

Figure 7.11
The anatomical relationship between the cerebrum, the cerebellum, and the brainstem.

head excites these receptors, and nerve impulses are sent to the CNS regarding this change in position. Specifically, these receptors provide information about linear acceleration and angular acceleration. This mechanism allows us to have a sense of acceleration or deceleration when running or traveling by car. Further, a sense of angular acceleration helps us maintain balance when the head is turning or spinning (e.g., performing gymnastics or diving).

The neural pathways involved in control of equilibrium are outlined in figure 7.10. Any head movement results in stimulation of receptors in the vestibular apparatus, which transmits neural information to the cerebellum and the vestibular nuclei located in the brain stem. Further, the vestibular nuclei relay a message to the oculomotor center (controls eye movement) and to neurons in the spinal cord that control movements of the head and limbs. Thus, the vestibular apparatus controls head and eye movement during physical activity, which serves to maintain balance and visually track the events of movement. In summary, the vestibular apparatus is sensitive to the position of the head in space and to sudden changes in the direction of body movement. Its primary function is to maintain equilibrium and preserve a constant plane of head position. Failure of the vestibular apparatus to function properly would prevent accurate performance of any athletic task that requires head movement. Since most sporting events require at least some head movement, the importance of the vestibular apparatus is obvious.

in summary

- The vestibular apparatus is responsible for maintaining general equilibrium and is located in the inner ear. Specifically, these receptors provide information about linear and angular acceleration.

Motor Control Functions of the Brain

The brain can be conveniently subdivided into three parts: the brain stem, cerebrum, and cerebellum. Figure 7.11 demonstrates the anatomical relationship of these components. Each of these structures makes important contributions to the regulation of movement. The next several paragraphs will outline the brain's role in regulating performance of sports skills.

Brain Stem

The **brain stem** is located inside the base of the skull just above the spinal cord. It consists of a complicated series of nerve tracts and nuclei (clusters of neurons), and is responsible for many metabolic functions, cardiorespiratory control, and some highly complex reflexes. The major structures of the brain stem are the medulla, pons, and midbrain. In addition, there is a series of complex neurons scattered throughout the brain stem that are collectively called the *reticular formation*. The reticular formation receives and integrates information from all regions of the CNS and works with higher brain centers in controlling muscular activity (6, 35).

In general, the neuronal circuits in the brain stem are thought to be responsible for the control of eye movement and muscle tone, equilibrium, support of the body against gravity, and many special reflexes. One of the most important roles of the brain stem in control of locomotion is that of maintaining postural

Section One Physiology of Exercise

tone. That is, centers in the brain stem provide the nervous activity necessary to maintain normal upright posture and therefore support the body against gravity. It is clear that the maintainence of upright posture requires that the brain stem receive information from several sensory modalities (e.g., vestibular receptors, pressure receptors of the skin, vision). Damage to any portion of the brain stem results in impaired movement control (8, 15) (see A Closer Look 7.1).

Cerebrum

The **cerebrum** is the large dome of the brain that is divided into right and left cerebral hemispheres. The outermost layer of the cerebrum is called the *cerebral cortex* and is composed of tightly arranged neurons. Although the cortex is only about one-fourth an inch thick, it contains over eight million neurons. The cortex performs three very important motor behavior functions (9, 28): (1) organization of complex movement, (2) storage of learned experiences, and (3) the reception of sensory information. We will limit our discussion to the role of the cortex in the organization of movement. The portion of the cerebral cortex that is most concerned with voluntary movement is the **motor cortex.** Although the motor cortex plays a significant role in motor control, it appears that input to the motor cortex from subcortical structures (i.e., cerebellum, etc.) is absolutely essential for coordinated movement to occur (12, 28). Thus, the motor cortex can be described as the final relay point upon which subcortical inputs are focused. After the motor cortex sums these inputs, the final movement plan is formulated and the motor commands are sent to the spinal cord. This "movement plan" can be modified by both subcortical and spinal centers, which supervise the fine details of the movement.

Cerebellum

The **cerebellum** lies behind the pons and medulla and has a convoluted appearance (figure 7.11). Although complete knowledge about cerebellar function is not presently available, much is known about the role of this structure in movement control. It is clear that the cerebellum plays an important role in coordinating and monitoring complex movement. This work is accomplished via connections leading from the cerebellum to the motor cortex, the brain stem, and the spinal cord. Evidence exists to suggest that the primary role of the cerebellum is to aid in the control of movement in response to feedback from proprioceptors (28). Further, the cerebellum may initiate fast, ballistic movements via its connection with the motor cortex (12). Damage to the cerebellum results in poor movement control and muscular tremor that is most severe during rapid movement.

in summary

- The brain can be subdivided into three parts: (1) the brain stem, (2) the cerebrum, and (3) the cerebellum.
- The motor cortex controls motor activity with the aid of input from subcortical areas.

Motor Functions of the Spinal Cord

One motor function of the spinal cord has already been discussed (withdrawal reflex). The precise role of spinal reflexes in the control of movement is still being debated. However, there is increasing evidence that normal motor function is influenced by spinal reflexes. In fact, some authors claim that reflexes play a major role in control of voluntary movements. These investigators believe that the events that underlie volitional movement are built on a variety of spinal reflexes (12, 32). Support for this idea comes from the demonstration that spinal reflex neurons are directly affected by descending neural traffic from the brain stem and cortical centers.

The spinal cord makes a major contribution in the control of movement by the preparation of spinal centers to perform the desired movement. The spinal mechanism by which a voluntary movement is translated into appropriate muscle action is termed *spinal tuning*. Spinal tuning appears to operate in the following way. Higher brain centers of the motor system are concerned with only the general parameters of movement. The specific details of the movement are refined at the spinal cord level via interaction of spinal cord neurons and high brain centers. In other words, although the general pattern of the anticipated movement is controlled by higher motor centers, additional refinement of this movement may occur by a complex interaction of spinal cord neurons and higher centers (7, 28, 32). Thus, it appears that spinal centers play an important role in volitional movement.

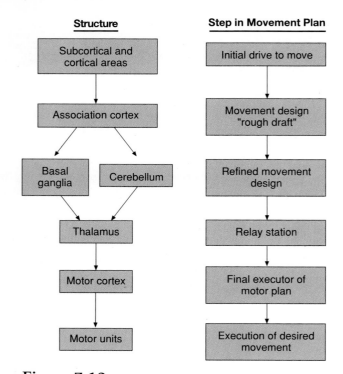

Figure 7.12
Block diagram of the structures and processes leading to voluntary movement.

in summary

- Evidence exists that the spinal cord plays an important role in voluntary movement due to groups of neurons capable of controlling certain aspects of motor activity.
- The spinal mechanism by which a voluntary movement is translated into appropriate muscle action is termed spinal tuning.

Control of Motor Functions

Watching a highly skilled athlete perform a sports skill is exciting, but really does not give the observer an appreciation of the complex integration of many parts of the nervous system required to perform this act. A pitcher throwing a baseball seems to the observer to be accomplishing a simple act, but in reality this movement consists of a complex interaction of higher brain centers with spinal reflexes performed together with precise timing. How the nervous system produces a coordinated movement has been one of the major unresolved mysteries facing neurophysiologists for many decades. Although progress has been made toward answering the basic question of "How do humans control voluntary movement?" much is still unknown about this process. Our purpose here

will be to provide the reader with a simplistic overview of the brain and control of movement.

Traditionally, it was believed that the motor cortex controlled voluntary movement with little input from subcortical areas (26, 30). Recent evidence suggests that this is not the case (12, 28). Although the motor cortex is the final executor of movement programs, it appears that the motor cortex does not give the initial signal to move, but rather is at the end of the chain of neurophysiological events involved in volitional movement (12). The first step in performing a voluntary movement occurs in subcortical and cortical motivational areas, which play a key role in consciousness. This conscious "prime drive" sends signals to the so-called association areas of the cortex (not motor cortex), which forms a "rough draft" of the planned movement from a stock of stored subroutines (7). Information concerning the nature of the plan of movement is then sent to both the cerebellum and the basal ganglia (clusters of neurons located in the cerebral hemispheres) (see figure 7.12). These structures cooperate to convert the "rough draft" into precise temporal (timing) and spatial excitation programs (12). The cerebellum is possibly more important for making fast movements, while the basal ganglia is more responsible for slow or deliberate movements. From the cerebellum and basal ganglia the precise program is sent through the thalamus to the motor cortex, which forwards the message down to spinal neurons for "spinal tuning" and finally to skeletal muscle (11). Feedback to the CNS from muscle receptors and proprioceptors allows for modification of motor programs if necessary. The ability to change movement patterns allows the individual to correct "errors" in the original movement plan.

To summarize, control of voluntary movement is complex and requires the cooperation of many areas of the brain as well as several subcortical areas. Recent evidence suggests that the motor cortex does not by itself formulate the signals required to initiate voluntary movement. Instead the motor cortex receives input from a variety of cortical and subcortical structures. Feedback to the CNS from muscle and joint receptors allows for adjustments to improve the movement pattern. Much is still unknown about the details of the control of complex movement, and this topic provides an exciting frontier for future research.

in summary

- Control of voluntary movement is complex and requires the cooperation of many areas of the brain as well as several subcortical areas.
- The first step in performing a voluntary movement occurs in subcortical and cortical motivational areas which sends signals to the association cortex which forms a "rough draft" of the planned movement.
- The movement plan is then sent to both the cerebellum and the basal ganglia. These structures cooperate to convert the "rough draft" into precise temporal (timing) and spatial excitation programs.
- The cerebellum is important for making fast movements, while the basal ganglia are more responsible for slow or deliberate movements.
- From the cerebellum and basal ganglia the precise program is sent through the thalamus to the motor cortex, which forwards the message down to spinal neurons for "spinal tuning" and finally to skeletal muscle.
- Feedback to the CNS from muscle receptors and proprioceptors allows for modification of motor programs if necessary.

Autonomic Nervous System

The **autonomic nervous system** plays an important role in maintaining the constancy of the body's internal environment. In contrast to somatic motor nerves, autonomic motor nerves innervate effector organs (e.g., smooth muscle, cardiac muscle), which are not usually under voluntary control. Autonomic motor nerves innervate cardiac muscle, glands, and smooth muscle found in airways, the gut, and blood vessels. In general, the autonomic nervous system operates below the conscious level, although some individuals apparently can learn to control some portions of this system. Although involuntary, it appears that the function of the autonomic nervous system is closely linked to emotion. For example, all of us have experienced an increase in heart rate following extreme excitement or fear. Further, secretions of digestive glands and sweat glands are affected by periods of excitement. It should not be surprising that participation in intense exercise results in an increase in autonomic activity.

The autonomic nervous system can be separated both functionally and anatomically into two divisions: (1) **sympathetic** division and (2) **parasympathetic** division (see figure 7.13). Most organs receive dual innervation, by both the parasympathetic and sympathetic branches of the autonomic nervous system (35). In general, the sympathetic portion of the autonomic nervous system tends to activate an organ (e.g., increases heart rate), while parasympathetic impulses tend to inhibit it (e.g., slows heart rate). Therefore, the activity of a particular organ can be regulated according to the ratio of sympathetic/parasympathetic impulses to the tissue. In this way, the autonomic nervous system may regulate the activities of involuntary muscles and glands in accordance with the needs of the body (see chapter 5).

The sympathetic division of the autonomic nervous system has its cell bodies of the preganglionic neurons (a ganglion is a group of cell bodies outside of the CNS) in the thoracic and lumbar regions of the spinal cord. These fibers leave the spinal cord and enter the sympathetic ganglia (figure 7.13). The neurotransmitter between the preganglionic neurons and postganglionic neurons is acetylcholine. Postganglionic sympathetic fibers leave these sympathetic ganglia and innervate a wide variety of tissues. The neurotransmitter released at the effector organ is primarily norepinephrine. Recall from chapter 5 that norepinephrine exerts its action on the effector organ by binding to either an alpha or beta receptor on the membrane of the target organ (5). Following sympathetic stimulation, norepinephrine is removed in a variety of ways. First, much of the norepinephrine is taken back up into the postganglionic fiber, while the remaining portion will be broken down into nonactive byproducts (5, 13, 31, 33).

The parasympathetic division of the autonomic nervous system has its cell bodies located within the brain stem and the sacral portion of the spinal cord. Parasympathetic fibers leave the brain stem and the spinal cord and converge on ganglia in a wide variety of

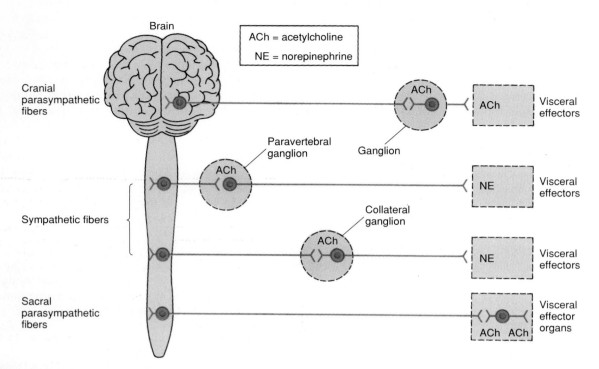

Figure 7.13
A simple schematic demonstrating the neurotransmitters of the autonomic nervous system. ACh = acetylcholine; NE = norepinephrine.

anatomical areas. Acetylcholine is the neurotransmitter in both preganglionic and postganglionic fibers. After parasympathetic nerve stimulation, acetylcholine is released and rapidly degraded by the enzyme acetylcholinesterase.

in summary

- The autonomic nervous system is responsible for maintaining the constancy of the body's internal environment.
- Anatomically and functionally, the autonomic nervous system can be divided into two divisions: (1) the sympathetic division and (2) the parasympathetic division.
- In general, the sympathetic portion (releasing norepinephrine) tends to excite an organ, while the parasympathetic portion (releasing acetylcholine) tends to inhibit the same organ.

study questions

1. Identify the location and functions of the central nervous system.
2. Draw a simple chart illustrating the organization of the nervous system.
3. Define synapses.
4. Define membrane potential and action potential.
5. Discuss an IPSP and an EPSP. How do they differ?
6. What are proprioceptors? Give some examples.
7. Describe the location and function of the vestibular apparatus.
8. What is meant by the term *spinal tuning*?
9. List the possible motor functions played by the brain stem, the motor cortex, and the cerebellum.
10. Describe the divisions and functions of the autonomic nervous system.
11. Define the terms, motor unit and innervation ratio.

suggested readings

Fox, S. I. 1996. *Human Physiology*. Dubuque, IA: Wm. C. Brown.

Henatsch, H., and H. Langer. 1985. Basic neurophysiology of motor skills in sport: A review. *International Journal of Sports Medicine* 6:2–14.

Hole, J. W. 1992. *Human Anatomy and Physiology*. Dubuque, IA: Wm. C. Brown.

Ito, M. 1986. Where are neurophysiologists going? *News in Physiological Sciences* 1:30–31.

Vander, A., J. Sherman, and D. Luciano. 1994. *Human Physiology*. New York: McGraw-Hill.

references

1. Barchas, J. D. et al. 1978. Behavioral neurochemistry: Neuroregulators and behavioral states. *Science* 200:964.

2. Barde, Y. A., D. Edgar, and H. Thoen. 1983. New neurotropic factors. *Annual Review of Physiology* 45:601.

3. Busse, M., N. Maassen, and H. Konrad. 1991. Relation between plasma K^+ and ventilation during incremental exercise after glycogen depletion and repletion in man. *Journal of Physiology* (London) 443:469–76.

4. Clark, F., and P. Burgess. 1975. Slowly adapting receptors in the cat knee joint: Can they signal joint angle? *Journal of Neurophysiology* 38:1448–63.

5. Collins, S., M. Caron, and R. Lefkowitz. 1991. Regulation of adrenergic receptor responsiveness through modulation of receptor gene expression. *Annual Review of Physiology* 53:497–508.

6. Delong, M., and P. Strick. 1974. Relation of the basal ganglia, cerebellum, and motor cortex units to ramp and ballistic limb movements. *Brain Research* 71:327–35.

7. Dietz, V. 1992. Human neuronal control of automatic functional movements interaction between central programs and afferent input. *Physiological Reviews* 72:33–69.

8. Eccles, J. C. 1977. *The Understanding of the Brain*. New York: McGraw-Hill.

9. Fox, S. I. 1996. *Human Physiology*. Dubuque, IA: Wm. C. Brown.

10. Goodwin, G., D. McCloskey, and P. Mathews. 1972. The contribution of muscle afferents to kinesthesia shown by vibration-induced illusions of movement and by the effects of paralyzing joint afferents. *Brain* 95:705–48.

11. Grillner, S. 1981. Control of locomotion in bipeds, tetrapods, and fish. In *Handbook of Physiology. The Nervous System. Motor Control.* Section 1, vol. II, part 2, 1179–1236. Washington, D.C.: American Physiological Society.

12. Henatsch, H., and H. Langer. 1985. Basic neurophysiology of motor skills in sport: A review. *International Journal of Sports Medicine* 6:2–14.

13. Hoffman, B., and R. Lefkowitz. 1980. Alpha and beta receptor subtypes. *New England Journal of Medicine* 302:1390.

14. Hole, J. W. 1992. *Human Anatomy and Physiology.* Dubuque, IA: Wm. C. Brown.

15. Kandel, E., and J. Schwartz, eds. 1991. *Principles of Neural Science*. New York: Elsevier-North Holland.

16. Kaufman, M., K. Rybicki, T. Waldrop, and G. Ordway. 1984. Effect of ischemia on responses of group III and IV afferents to contraction. *Journal of Applied Physiology* 57:644–50.

17. Kaufman, M., K. Rybicki, T. Waldrop, G. Ordway, and J. Mitchell. 1984. Effects of static and rhythmic twitch contractions on the discharge of group III and IV muscle afferents. *Cardiovascular Research* 18:663–68.

18. Kniffki, K., S. Mense, and R. Schmidt. 1981. Muscle receptors with fine afferent fibers which may evoke circulatory reflexes. *Circulation Research* 48 (Suppl.):25–31.

19. Krieger, D. T., and J. B. Martin. 1981. Brain peptides. *New England Journal of Medicine* 304:876.

20. Mathews, P. 1977. Muscle afferents and kinesthesia. *British Medical Bulletin* 33:137–42.

21. ———. 1982. Where does Sherrington's muscle sense originate? *Annual Review of Neuroscience* 5:189–218.

22. McCloskey, D., and J. Mitchell. 1972. Reflex cardiovascular and respiratory responses originating in exercising muscle. *Journal of Physiology* (London) 224:173–86.

23. Nicoll, R., R. Malenka, and J. Kauer. 1990. Functional comparison of neurotransmitter receptor subtypes in mammalian central nervous system. *Physiological Reviews* 70:513–65.

24. O'Donovan, M. 1985. Developmental regulation of motor function. *Medicine and Science in Sports and Exercise* 17:35–43.

25. Pozzo, T., A. Berthoz, L. Lefort, and E. Vittle. 1991. Head stabilization during various locomotor tasks in humans. II. Patients with bilateral peripheral vestibular deficits. *Brain Research* 85:208–17.

26. Prochazka, A. 1989. Sensorimotor gain control: A basic strategy of motor systems. *Progressive Neurobiology* 33:281–307.

27. Redman, S. 1986. Monosynaptic transmission in the spinal cord. *News in Physiological Sciences* 1:171–74.

28. Sage, G. H. 1984. *Motor Learning and Control: A Neuropsychological Approach*. Dubuque, IA: Wm. C. Brown.

29. Sherwood, L. 1993. *Fundamentals of Physiology*. St. Paul, MN.: West.

30. Smith, J. C., J. Feldman, and B. Schmidt. 1988. Neural mechanisms generating locomotion studied in mammalian brain stem-spinal cord in vitro. *FASEB Journal* 2:2283–88.

31. Snyder, S. H. 1980. Brain peptides as neurotransmitters. *Science* 209:976.

32. Soechting, J., and M. Flanders. 1991. Arm movements in three-dimensional space: Computation, theory, and observation. In *Exercise and Sport Science Reviews*, vol. 19, ed. J. Holloszy, 389–418. Baltimore: Williams & Wilkins.

33. Stjarne, L. 1986. New paradigm: Sympathetic neurotransmission by lateral interaction between secretory units? *News in Physiological Sciences* 1:103–6.

34. Van De Graaff, K. 1995. *Human Anatomy*. Dubuque, IA: Wm. C. Brown.

35. Vander, A., J. Sherman, and D. Luciano. 1994. *Human Physiology*. New York: McGraw-Hill.

CHAPTER 8

Skeletal Muscle

Structure and Function

objectives

By studying this chapter, you should be able to do the following:

1. Draw and label the microstructure of skeletal muscle.
2. Outline the steps leading to muscle contraction.
3. Define the terms *isotonic* and *isometric*.
4. Discuss the following terms: (1) *twitch*, (2) *summation*, and (3) *tetanus*.
5. Discuss the major biochemical and mechanical properties of human skeletal fiber types.
6. Discuss the relationship between skeletal muscle fiber types and performance.
7. List and discuss those factors that regulate the amount of force exerted during muscular contraction.
8. Graph the relationship between movement velocity and the amount of force exerted during muscular contraction.
9. Discuss the structure and function of a muscle spindle.
10. Describe the function of a Golgi tendon organ.

outline

Structure of Skeletal Muscle   126
Neuromuscular Junction   128
Muscular Contraction   129
    Overview of the Sliding Filament Model   129
    Energy for Contraction   131
    Regulation of Excitation-Contraction Coupling   131
Fiber Types   135
    Biochemical and Contractile Characteristics of Skeletal Muscle   135

Characteristics of Individual Fiber Types   136
    Fiber Types and Performance   139
Alteration of Muscle Fiber Types by Exercise Training   139
Age-Related Changes in Skeletal Muscle   140
Isometric and Isotonic Contractions   141
Speed of Muscle Contraction and Relaxation   142

Force Regulation in Muscle   142
Force-Velocity/Power-Velocity Relationships   144
Receptors in Muscle   145
    Muscle Spindle   146
    Golgi Tendon Organs   146

actin	isometric	sliding filament model
concentric contraction	isotonic	slow-twitch fibers
dynamic	lateral sac	static
eccentric contraction	motor neurons	summation
endomysium	motor unit	terminal cisternae
end-plate potential (EPP)	muscle spindle	tetanus
epimysium	myofibrils	transverse tubules
extensors	myosin	tropomyosin
fascicle	neuromuscular junction	troponin
fast-twitch fibers	perimysium	Type I fibers
flexors	sarcolemma	Type IIa fibers
Golgi tendon organs (GTOs)	sarcomeres	Type IIb fibers
intermediate fibers	sarcoplasmic reticulum	twitch

The human body contains over four hundred skeletal muscles, which constitute 40%–50% of the total body weight (25, 36, 37). Skeletal muscle performs three important functions: (1) force generation for locomotion and breathing, (2) force generation for postural support, and (3) heat production during periods of cold stress. The most obvious function of skeletal muscle is to enable an individual to move freely and breathe. Skeletal muscles are attached to bones by tough connective tissue called tendons. One end of the muscle is attached to a bone that does not move (origin), while the opposite end is fixed to a bone (insertion) that is moved during muscular contraction. A variety of different movements are possible, depending on the type of joint and muscles involved. Muscles that decrease joint angles are called **flexors,** while muscles that increase joint angles are called **extensors.**

Given the role of skeletal muscles in determining sports performance, a thorough understanding of muscle structure and function is important to the exercise scientist, physical educator, physical therapist, and coach. It is the purpose of this chapter to discuss the structure and function of skeletal muscle.

Structure of Skeletal Muscle

Skeletal muscle is composed of several kinds of tissue. These include muscle cells themselves, nerve tissue, blood, and various types of connective tissue. Figure 8.1 displays the relationship between muscle and the various connective tissues. Individual muscles are separated from each other and held in position by connective tissue called *fascia*. There are three separate layers of connective tissue found in skeletal muscle. The outermost layer that surrounds the entire muscle is called the **epimysium.** As we move inward from the epimysium, connective tissue called the **perimysium** surrounds individual bundles of muscle fibers (note: for muscle, the terms *cell* and *fiber* are often interchangeably). These individual bundles of muscle fibers are called a **fascicle.** Each muscle fiber within the fasciculus is surrounded by connective tissue called the **endomysium.**

Despite their unique shape, muscle cells have many of the same organelles that are present in other cells. That is, they contain mitochondria, lysosomes, and so on. However, unlike most other cells in the body, muscle cells are multinucleated (i.e., have many nuclei). One of the most distinctive features of the microscopic appearance of skeletal muscles is their striated appearance (see figure 8.2). These stripes are produced by alternating light and dark bands that appear across the length of the fiber.

Each individual muscle fiber is a thin, elongated cylinder that generally extends the length of the muscle. The cell membrane surrounding the muscle cell is called the **sarcolemma.** Beneath the sarcolemma lies the sarcoplasm (also called cytoplasm), which contains the cellular proteins, organelles, and myofibrils. **Myofibrils** are numerous threadlike structures that contain the contractile proteins (figure 8.2). In general, myofibrils are composed of two major types of protein filaments: (1) thick filaments composed of the protein **myosin** and (2) thin filaments composed primarily of the protein **actin.** The arrangement of these two protein filaments give skeletal muscle its striated appearance (figure 8.2). Located on the actin molecule itself are two additional proteins, **troponin** and **tropomyosin.** These proteins make up a small portion of the muscle, but play an important role in regulation of the contractile process.

Myofibrils can be further subdivided into individual segments called **sarcomeres.** Sarcomeres are divided from each other by a thin sheet of structural proteins called a Z *line.* Myosin filaments are located primarily within the dark portion of the sarcomere, which is called the A *band*, while actin filaments occur

Figure 8.1
Connective tissue surrounding skeletal muscle.

Bone

Tendon

Fascia

Muscle

Epimysium

Perimysium

Endomysium

Fascicle

Axon of
motor neuron

Muscle fibers

Sarcolemma

Myofibrils

Blood vessel

Filaments

Sarcoplasmic
reticulum

Nucleus

Figure 8.2
The microstructure of muscle. Note that a skeletal muscle
fiber contains numerous myofibrils, each consisting of
units called sarcomeres.

Myofibril

Skeletal
muscle fiber

Z line

Z line

Sarcomere

Filaments
of actin

(a)

H zone

M line

Z line

(b)

I band

A band

I band

A band

Myosin (thick)
filaments

Actin (thin)
filaments

(c)

Sarcolemma

Triad of the reticulum:

Terminal cisternae

Transverse tubule

Sarcoplasmic reticulum

Mitochondria

Waldrop

Myofibrils

A band

I band

Z line

Nucleus

Figure 8.3
Within the sarcoplasm of muscle is a network of channels called the sarcoplasmic reticulum and the transverse tubules.

principally in the light region of the sarcomere called I *bands* (figure 8.2). In the center of the sarcomere there is a portion of the myosin filament with no overlap of the actin. This is the H *zone*.

Within the sarcoplasm of muscle is a network of membranous channels that surround each myofibril and run parallel with it. These channels are called the **sarcoplasmic reticulum** and are storage sites for calcium, which plays an important role in muscular contraction (see figure 8.3). Another set of membranous channels called the **transverse tubules** extends inward from the sarcolemma and passes completely through the fiber. These transverse tubules pass between two enlarged portions of the sarcoplasmic reticulum called the **terminal cisternae.** All of these parts serve a function in muscular contraction and will be discussed in further detail later in this chapter.

Neuromuscular Junction

Each skeletal muscle cell is connected to a nerve fiber branch coming from a nerve cell. These nerve cells are called **motor neurons** and extend outward from the spinal cord. The motor neuron and all the muscle fibers it innervates is called a **motor unit.** Stimulation from motor neurons initiates the contraction process. The site where the motor neuron and muscle cell meet is called the **neuromuscular junction.** At this junction the sarcolemma forms a pocket that is called the *motor end plate* (see figure 8.4).

The end of the motor neuron does not physically make contact with the muscle fiber, but is separated by a short gap called the *neuromuscular cleft*. When a nerve

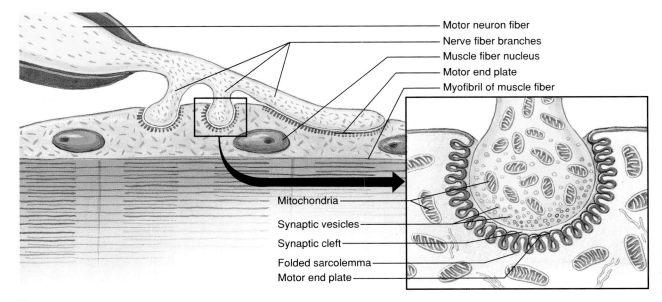

Motor neuron fiber
Nerve fiber branches
Muscle fiber nucleus
Motor end plate
Myofibril of muscle fiber

Mitochondria
Synaptic vesicles
Synaptic cleft
Folded sarcolemma
Motor end plate

Figure 8.4

The connecting point between a motor neuron and a single muscle fiber is called the neuromuscular junction. The neurotransmitter acetylcholine is stored in synaptic vesicles at the end of the nerve fiber.

impulse reaches the end of the motor nerve, the neurotransmitter acetylcholine is released and diffuses across the synaptic cleft to bind with receptor sites on the motor end plate. This causes an increase in the permeability of the sarcolemma to sodium, resulting in a depolarization called the **end-plate potential (EPP).** The EPP is always large enough to exceed threshold and is the signal to begin the contractile process.

in summary

- The human body contains over four hundred voluntary skeletal muscles, which constitute 40%–50% of the total body weight. Skeletal muscle performs three major functions: (1) force production for locomotion and breathing, (2) force production for postural support, and (3) heat production during cold stress.
- Individual muscle fibers are composed of hundreds of threadlike protein filaments called myofibrils. Myofibrils contain two major types of contractile protein: (1) actin (part of the thin filaments) and (2) myosin (major component of the thick filaments).
- Motor neurons extend outward from the spinal cord and innervate individual muscle fibers. The site where the motor neuron and muscle cell meet is called the neuromuscular junction. Acetylcholine is the neurotransmitter that stimulates the muscle fiber to depolarize, which is the signal to start the contractile process.

Muscular Contraction

Muscular contraction is a complex process involving a number of cellular proteins and energy production systems. The final result is a sliding of actin over myosin, which causes the muscle to shorten and therefore develop tension. Although complete details of muscular contraction at the molecular level continues to be debated, the basic process of muscular contraction is well defined. The process of muscular contraction is best explained by the **sliding filament model** of contraction (18, 19, 57b, 69a).

Overview of the Sliding Filament Model

The general process of muscular contraction is illustrated in figure 8.5. Muscle fibers contract by a shortening of their myofibrils due to actin sliding over the myosin. This results in a reduction in the distance from Z line to Z line. Understanding the details of how muscular contraction occurs requires an appreciation of the microscopic structure of the myofibril. Note that the "heads" of the myosin cross-bridges are oriented toward the actin molecule (see figure 8.6). The actin and myosin filaments slide across each other during muscular contraction due to the action of the numerous cross-bridges extending out as "arms" from myosin and attaching to actin in a "strong binding state." It was previously believed that the myosin cross-bridges were not attached to actin when skeletal muscle is not contracting. However, recent evidence shows that myosin cross-bridges are

Figure 8.5

The sliding filament theory of contraction. As contraction occurs, the Z lines are brought closer together. The A bands remain the same length, but the I and H bands get progressively narrower as shortening continues.

Figure 8.6

Proposed relationships between troponin, tropomyosin, myosin cross-bridges, and calcium. Note that when Ca^{++} binds to troponin, tropomyosin is removed from the active sites on actin and cross-bridge attachment can occur.

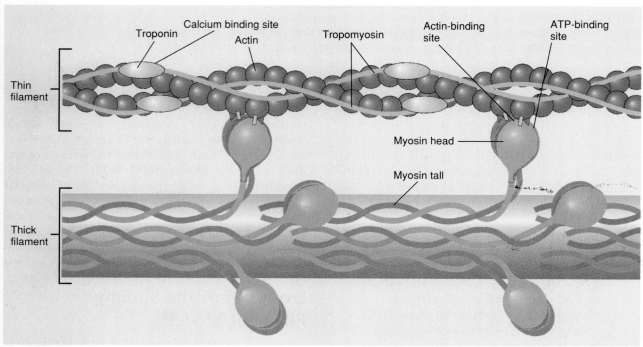

always attached to actin but the strength of the attachment varies from a "weak" bond to a "strong" bond. These two states of myosin-actin bonding are referred to as the: (1) weak binding state and (2) strong binding state. Force development and muscular contraction occur only when the cross-bridges are in the strong binding state. The development of this strong binding state results in an orientation of cross-bridges so that when they attach to actin on each side of the sarcomere they can pull the actin from each side toward the center. This "pulling" of actin over the myosin molecule results in muscle shortening and the generation of force.

The term *excitation-contraction coupling* refers to the sequence of events in which a nerve impulse (action potential) reaches the muscle membrane and leads to muscle shortening by cross-bridge activity. This process will be discussed step-by-step in the next several paragraphs. Let's begin with a discussion of the energy source for contraction.

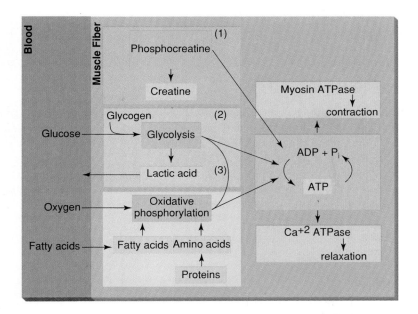

Figure 8.7
The three sources of ATP production in muscle during contraction: (1) phosphocreatine, (2) glycolysis, and
(3) oxidative phosphorylation.

From A. J. Vander, et al., *Human Physiology: The Mechanisms of Body Function*, 4th ed. Copyright © 1985 McGraw-Hill, Inc., New York. Reprinted by permission.

Energy for Contraction

The energy for muscular contraction comes from the breakdown of ATP by the enzyme myosin ATPase (16a, 28, 33, 38). This enzyme is located on the "head" of the myosin cross-bridge. Recall that the bioenergetic pathways responsible for synthesis of ATP were discussed earlier in chapter 3 and are summarized in figure 8.7. The breakdown of ATP to ADP + P_i and the release of energy serves to energize the myosin cross-bridges, which in turn pull the actin molecules over myosin and thus shorten the muscle (19, 45, 57b, 58, 69a).

Note that a single contraction cycle or "power stroke" of all the cross-bridges in a muscle would shorten the muscle by only one percent of its resting length (58). Since some muscles can shorten up to 60% of their resting length, it is clear that the contraction cycle must be repeated over and over again (58).

Regulation of Excitation–Contraction Coupling

Relaxed muscles are easily stretched, which demonstrates that at rest, actin and myosin are not firmly attached and therefore exist in the weak binding state. What regulates the interaction of actin and myosin and thus regulates muscle contraction? The first step in the process of muscular contraction begins with a nerve impulse arriving at the neuromuscular junction. The action potential from the motor neuron causes the release of acetylcholine into the synaptic cleft of the neuromuscular junction; acetylcholine binds to receptors on the motor end-plate, producing an end-plate potential that leads to depolarization of the muscle cell (58). This depolarization (i.e., excitation) is conducted down the transverse tubules deep into the muscle fiber. When the action potential reaches the sarcoplasmic reticulum, calcium is released and diffuses into the muscle to bind to a protein called *troponin*. This is the "trigger" step in the control of muscular contraction since the regulation of contraction is a function of two regulatory proteins, troponin and tropomyosin, which are located on the actin molecule. Troponin and tropomyosin regulate muscular contraction by controlling the interaction of actin and myosin.

To understand how troponin and tropomyosin control muscular contraction, one needs to appreciate the anatomical relationship between actin, troponin, and tropomyosin (see figure 8.6). Notice that the actin filament is formed from many protein subunits arranged in a double row and twisted. Tropomyosin is a thin molecule that lies in a groove between the double rows of actin. Attached directly to the tropomyosin is the protein troponin. This arrangement allows troponin and tropomyosin to work together to regulate the attachment of the actin and myosin cross-bridges. In a relaxed muscle, tropomyosin blocks the active sites on the actin molecule where the myosin cross-bridges must attach to form a strong binding state to produce a contraction. The trigger for contraction to occur is linked to the release of stored calcium (Ca++) from a region of the sarcoplasmic reticulum termed the **lateral sac** or

A Closer Look 8.1

Muscle Fatigue

Short-term, high-intensity exercise or prolonged submaximal exercise can result in a decline in muscle force production. This decrease in muscle force production is known as fatigue. Specifically, muscular fatigue is defined as a reduction in maximal force production of the muscle and is characterized by a reduced ability to perform work (see figure 8.8).

What factors contribute to muscular fatigue? The cause of muscle fatigue varies and depends upon the type of exercise performed. For example, fatigue resulting from high-intensity exercise (e.g., sprinting 400 meters) appears to be due to an accumulation of inorganic phosphate and hydrogen ions within the muscle fiber. Accumulation of these metabolites interact with the contractile proteins and reduce muscle force production (24b).

In contrast, fatigue resulting from prolonged exercise (e.g., running a marathon) may involve the failure of excitation-contraction coupling; this is likely due to a reduction in the release of calcium from the sarcoplasmic reticulum (24b). Reduced calcium release results in fewer myosin cross-bridges in the strong binding state (i.e., force generating state) and therefore reduced muscle force production. Fatigue and limiting factors to exercise performance are discussed in detail in chapter 19.

Figure 8.8
Muscular fatigue is characterized by a reduced ability to generate force.

---

sometimes called the *terminal cisternae* (46a, 66). In a resting (relaxed) muscle the concentration of Ca^{++} in the sarcoplasm is very low. However, when a nerve impulse arrives at the neuromuscular junction, it travels down the transverse tubules to the sarcoplasmic reticulum and causes the release of Ca^{++}. Much of this Ca^{++} binds to troponin (figure 8.6), which causes a position change in tropomyosin such that the active sites on the actin are uncovered. This permits the strong binding of a "cocked or energized" myosin cross-bridge on the actin molecule. The strong cross-bridge binding initiates the release of energy stored within the myosin molecule; this produces an angular movement of each cross-bridge, resulting in muscle shortening. Attachment of "fresh" ATP to the myosin cross-bridges breaks the strong binding state of the myosin cross-bridge bound

to actin and results in a weak binding state. The enzyme, ATPase, again hydrolyzes (i.e., breaks down) the ATP attached to the myosin cross-bridge and provides the energy necessary for cocking (i.e., energizing) the myosin cross-bridge for reattachment to another active site on an actin molecule. This contraction cycle can be repeated as long as free Ca^{++} is available to bind to troponin and ATP can be hydrolyzed to provide the energy. Failure of the muscle to maintain adequate Ca^{++} levels or to hydrolyze ATP results in a disturbance of muscle homeostasis and fatigue occurs (see A Closer Look 8.1).

The signal to stop contraction is the absence of the nerve impulse at the neuromuscular junction. When this occurs, an energy-requiring Ca^{++} *pump* located within the sarcoplasmic reticulum begins to move Ca^{++} back into the sarcoplasmic reticulum. This

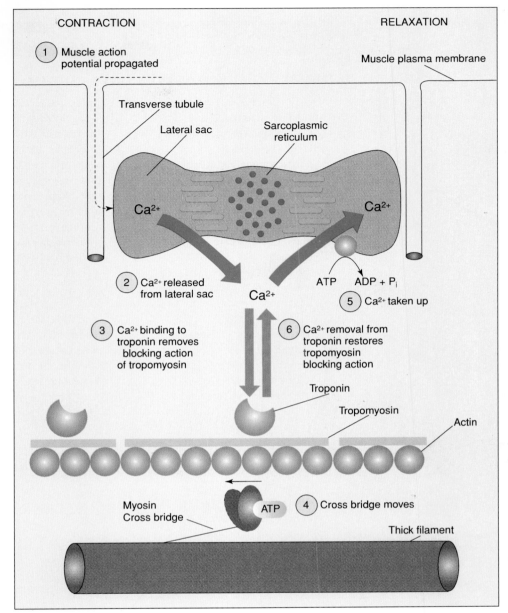

Figure 8.9

Illustration of the steps involved in muscle excitation, contraction, and relaxation.

From A. J. Vander, et al., *Human Physiology: The Mechanisms of Body Function*, 4th ed. Copyright © 1985 McGraw-Hill, Inc., New York. Reprinted by permission.

removal of Ca^{++} from troponin causes tropomyosin to move back to cover the binding sites on the actin molecule and cross-bridge interaction ceases. Figure 8.9 illustrates the basic steps involved in muscle contraction and relaxation.

A Closer Look 8.2 contains a step-by-step summary of the events that occur during excitation and muscular contraction. For a detailed discussion of molecular events involved in skeletal muscle contraction, see references 8, 19, 22, 57b, 58 and 69a. Time spent learning the microstructure of muscle and the events that lead to contraction will pay dividends later, as this material is important to a thorough understanding of exercise physiology.

Step–by–Step Summary of Excitation Contraction–Coupling

Excitation

The process of excitation is illustrated in steps 1 and 2 in figure 8.9 and involves two processes:

1. The generation of an action potential in a motor neuron causes the release of acetylcholine into the synaptic cleft of the neuromuscular junction.
2. Acetylcholine binds with receptors on the motor endplate, producing an end-plate potential which leads to a depolarization that is conducted down the transverse tubules deep into the muscle fiber. This depolarization results in calcium being released from the sarcoplasmic reticulum.

Contraction

The steps involved in muscular contraction are illustrated in figure 8.10 and are listed in sequential order below (57b, 69a):

1. In the resting state the myosin cross-bridges remain connected to actin in a weak binding state (no force generation; step 1, figure 8.10).
2. When the depolarization (i.e., neural stimulation) reaches the sarcoplasmic reticulum, Ca^{++} is released into the sarcoplasm. The Ca^{++} then binds to troponin, which causes a shift in the position of tropomyosin to uncover the "active sites" on the actin. The "energized" or "cocked" myosin cross-bridge then forms a strong bond (i.e., strong binding state) at the active site on actin (step 2, figure 8.10).
3. Inorganic phosphate is now released from the myosin cross-bridge and the energized cross-bridge pulls the actin molecule (step 3, figure 8.10).
4. Cross-bridge movement is completed by the release of ADP from the myosin cross-bridge. Note, at this point within the contraction cycle, the myosin cross-bridge remains in the strong binding state with actin (step 4, figure 8.10).
5. Attachment of ATP to the myosin cross-bridge allows the myosin cross-bridge to break the strong binding state and form a weak binding state. In this weak binding state, ATP is broken down to $ADP + P_i +$ energy, and the released energy is used to "energize" the myosin cross-bridge (step 5, figure 8.10). This contraction cycle can be repeated as long as Ca^{++} and ATP are present (i.e., step 5 moves to step 2 and the cycle continues). The contraction cycle is broken when action potentials stop and the sarcoplasmic reticulum actively removes Ca^{++} from the sarcoplasm (i.e., step 5 moves to step 1).

in summary

- The process of muscular contraction can be best explained by the sliding filament model which proposes that muscle shortening occurs due to movement of the actin filament over the myosin filament.
- The steps leading to muscular contraction are: (see figure 8.10 for a detailed step-by-step illustration):
  a. The nerve impulse travels down the transverse tubules and reaches the sarcoplasmic reticulum and Ca^{++} is released.
  b. Ca^{++} binds to the protein troponin.
  c. Ca^{++} binding to troponin causes a position change in tropomyosin away from the "active sites" on the actin molecule and permits a strong binding state between actin and myosin.
  d. Muscular contraction occurs by multiple cycles of cross-bridge activity. Shortening will continue as long as energy is available and Ca^{++} is free to bind to troponin.
- When neural activity ceases at the neuromuscular junction, Ca^{++} is removed from the sarcoplasm and actively pumped into the sarcoplasmic reticulum by the Ca^{++} pump. This results in tropomyosin moving to cover the active site on actin and the muscle relaxes.

Figure 8.10
Steps leading to muscular contraction. See text for details.

The figure shows the following labels:

Key
- Troponin (Ca++ binding site)
- Tropomyosin
- Actin
- Myosin cross bridge (cocked)
- Weak binding state: Cocked cross bridge (no Ca++ bound to troponin)
- Strong binding state: Cocked cross bridge (Ca++ bound to troponin)

(1) Without calcium (Ca++) bound to troponin (weak binding state)

Neural Stimulation Stops: Sarcoplasmic reticulum removes Ca++

Neural Stimulation Begins: Ca++ released from sarcoplasmic reticulum

ADP + Pi

ATP hydrolyzed and myosin cross bridge cocked

Neural Stimulation Continues: Ca++ remains bound to troponin

(2) Formation of strong binding state

ADP + Pi

(5) ATP binds to cross bridge. Formation of weak binding state

ATP

release of Pi

(3) Cross bridge movement begins

(4) Cross bridge movement completed (myosin no longer cocked)

release of ADP

Fiber Types

Human skeletal muscle can be divided into several different classes based on the histochemical or biochemical characteristics of the individual fibers (How fibers are "typed" is discussed later in A Closer Look 8.4). Although some confusion exists concerning the nomenclature of fiber types, historically, muscle fibers have been classified into two general categories: (1) fast (also called fast-twitch) fibers or (2) slow (also called slow-twitch) fibers (14, 15, 20, 21). Though some muscle groups are known to be composed of predominantly fast or slow fibers, most muscle groups in the body contain an equal mixture of both slow and fast fiber types. The percentage of the respective fiber types contained in skeletal muscles can be influenced by genetics, blood levels of hormones, and the exercise habits of the individual. From a practical standpoint, the fiber composition of skeletal muscles plays an important role in performance in both power and endurance events (10, 62).

Biochemical and Contractile Characteristics of Skeletal Muscle

Prior to discussing the specific characteristics of muscle fiber types, a brief discussion of the key biochemical and contractile properties of skeletal muscle is warranted.

Biochemical Properties of Muscle

In general, the two key biochemical characteristics of muscle that are important to muscle function are the

(1) oxidative capacity and (2) the type of ATPase isoform. The oxidative capacity of a muscle fiber is determined by the number of mitochondria, the number of capillaries surrounding the fiber, and the amount of myoglobin within the fiber. A large number of mitochondria provides a greater capacity to produce ATP aerobically. A high number of capillaries surrounding a muscle fiber insures that the fiber will receive adequate oxygen during periods of contractile activity. Finally, myoglobin is similar to hemoglobin in the blood in that it binds O_2, and it also acts as a "shuttle" mechanism for O_2 between the cell membrane and the mitochondria. Therefore, a high myoglobin concentration improves the delivery of oxygen from the capillary to the mitochondria where it will be used. Collectively, the significance of these biochemical characteristics is that a muscle fiber with a high concentration of myoglobin along with a high number of mitochondria and capillaries will have a high aerobic capacity and therefore will be fatigue resistant.

The second important biochemical characteristic of muscle fiber is the ATPase activity. Numerous isoforms of ATPase exist and the various isoforms differ in their activities (i.e., speed that they degrade ATP). Muscle fibers that contain ATPase isoforms with high ATPase activity will degrade ATP rapidly; this results in a high speed of muscle shortening. Conversely, muscle fibers with low ATPase activities shorten at slow speeds.

Contractile Properties of Skeletal Muscle

In comparing the contractile properties of muscle fiber types, three performance characteristics are important: (1) maximal force production, (2) speed of contraction, and (3) muscle fiber efficiency. Let's discuss each of these characteristics briefly.

First, maximal force production of a muscle fiber is compared by expressing how much force the fiber produces per unit of fiber cross-sectional area (specific tension). In other words, specific tension is the force production divided by the size of the fiber (e.g., specific force = force/fiber cross-sectional area).

The contraction speed of muscle fibers is compared by measuring the maximal shortening velocity (called Vmax) of individual fibers. Vmax represents the highest speed that a fiber can shorten. Since muscle fibers shorten by cross-bridge movement (called cross-bridge cycling), Vmax is determined by the rate of cross-bridge cycling. Again, a key biochemical factor that regulates fiber Vmax is the myosin ATPase activity. Fibers with high myosin ATPase activities (e.g., fast fibers) possess a high Vmax whereas fibers with low myosin ATPase activities possess a low Vmax (e.g., slow fibers).

The efficiency of a muscle fiber is a measure of the muscle fiber's economy. That is, an efficient fiber would require less energy to perform a certain amount of work compared to a less efficient fiber. In practice, this measurement is made by dividing the amount of energy used (i.e., ATP used) by the amount of force produced.

Characteristics of Individual Fiber Types

It is generally agreed that three individual human skeletal muscle fibers exist (two subtypes of fast fibers—identified as Type IIb and IIa; and a slow fiber—identified as Type I). However, recent evidence has identified the existence of two new skeletal muscle fibers in rats (see Research Focus 8.1). While it seems possible that human skeletal muscles may contain more than three fiber types, we will discuss only the three fiber types that have been carefully studied in man. Let's begin our discussion of muscle fiber types by examining the biochemical and contractile properties of both slow and fast fibers.

Slow Fibers

One type of slow fiber has been identified in humans—type I. **Type I fibers** (also called slow-oxidative or **slow-twitch fibers**) contain large numbers of oxidative enzymes (i.e., high mitochondrial volume) and are surrounded by more capillaries than any of the fibers. In addition, Type I fibers contain higher concentrations of myoglobin than fast fibers. The high concentration of myoglobin, the large number of capillaries, and the high mitochondrial enzyme activities provide Type I fibers with a large capacity for aerobic metabolism and a high resistance to fatigue.

In terms of contractile properties, Type I fibers possess a slower Vmax compared to fast fibers (see figure 8.11). Further, it appears that Type I fibers produce a lower specific tension compared to fast fibers (see A Closer Look 8.3). Finally, Type I fibers are more efficient than fast fibers.

Fast Fibers

Two subtypes of fast fibers exist in humans: (1) Type IIb, and (2) Type IIa. **Type IIb fibers** (sometimes called **fast-twitch fibers** or fast-glycolytic fibers) have a relatively small number of mitochondria, a limited capacity for aerobic metabolism, and are less resistant to fatigue than slow fibers (29, 49). However, these fibers are rich in glycolytic enzymes, which provide them with a large anaerobic capacity (47).

The specific tension of Type IIb fibers is similar to Type IIa fibers but is greater than Type I fibers. Further, the myosin ATPase activity in Type IIb fibers is higher than other fiber types, resulting in the highest Vmax of all fiber types. The speed of contraction differences between slow and fast fibers is illustrated in figure 8.11.

Discovery of Two "New" Skeletal Muscle Fiber Types in Rodents

Recent research has demonstrated the existence of two new muscle fibers in rats: (1) Type IId (fast fiber), and (2) Type Ia (slow fiber). Two teams of researchers, working independently, have provided positive identification of the new fast fiber in rat skeletal muscle. Although limited data exist, it seems possible that this new fast fiber also exists in human skeletal muscle (61a, 61c). German researchers, lead by Dr. Dirk Pette, reported the existence of this new fast

fiber in 1988 in rats (7a). Because this fiber is found in large numbers in the rat diaphragm, the German investigators called the new fast fiber, Type IId. In 1989, an Italian research team lead by Dr. Stefano Schiaffino also identified this new fast fiber in rat skeletal muscle (61b); the Italian scientists called this fiber, Type IIx. Unfortunately, to date, scientists have not agreed upon whether the fiber should be called a Type IId or Type IIx.

In 1993, Dr. Simon Hughes and colleagues (34a) at Stanford University reported the existence of a "new" slow muscle fiber in rat skeletal muscle. Researchers at Boston University (24a) have also reported the existence of two slow fibers in rat skeletal muscle. However, while these studies suggest that rat skeletal muscle may contain at least two slow fiber types, additional research is required to confirm their findings.

Do Fast Fibers Exert More Force Than Slow Fibers?

The question, "Do fast muscle fibers exert more force than slow fibers?" has been a topic of research for many years. Although controversial, recent research using single rat muscle fibers demonstrates that the maximal specific force production (force per cross-sectional area) of fast muscle fibers (Types IIb, and IIa) is

10%–20% greater than the force produced by slow (Type I) fibers (11b).

What is the physiological explanation for the observation that fast fibers exert more force than slow fibers? The amount of force generated by a muscle fiber is directly related to the number of myosin cross-bridges in the strong binding

state (i.e., force generating state) at any given time. That is, the more cross-bridges generating force, the greater the force production. Therefore, it appears that fast fibers exert more force than slow fibers because they contain more myosin cross-bridges per cross-sectional area of fiber than slow fibers.

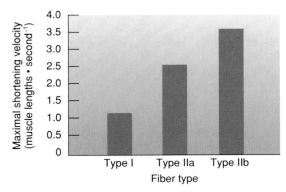

Figure 8.11

Comparison of maximal shortening velocities between fiber types. Data are from reference 11b.

Type IIb are less efficient than all other fiber types. This low efficiency is due to the high ATPase activity which results in a greater energy expenditure per unit of work performed.

A second type of fast fiber is the **Type IIa fiber** (also called **intermediate fibers** or fast-oxidative glycolytic fibers). These fibers contain biochemical and fatigue characteristics that are between Type IIb and Type I fibers. Therefore, conceptually, Type IIa fibers can be viewed as a mixture of both Type I and Type IIb fiber characteristics. However, note that Type IIa fibers are extremely adaptable. That is, with endurance training, they can increase their oxidative capacity to levels equal with Type I. For more details on muscle fiber characteristics, see references 7, 11, 31, and 50.

Table 8.1 Characteristics of Human Skeletal Muscle Fiber Types

Characteristic	Fast Fibers		Slow Fibers
	Type IIb	Type IIa	Type I
Number of mitochondria	low	high/moderate	high
Resistance to fatigue	low	high/moderate	high
Predominant energy system	anaerobic	combination	aerobic
ATPase activity	highest	high	low
Vmax (speed of shortening)	highest	intermediate	low
Efficiency	low	moderate	high
Specific tension	high	high	moderate

A Closer Look 8.4

How Are Skeletal Muscle Fibers Typed?

The relative percentage of fast or slow fibers contained in a particular muscle can be estimated by removing a small piece of muscle (via a procedure called a biopsy) and performing histochemical or biochemical analysis of the individual muscle cells. An early method used an histochemical procedure that divides muscle fibers into three categories based on the specific "isoform" of myosin ATPase enzyme found in the fiber. This technique applies a chemical stain that darkens muscle cells that contain high concentrations of the type of ATPase found in slow muscles. Using this technique, slow (Type I) fibers become dark, while Type IIa fibers remain light in color. The shade of Type IIb fibers tends to fall somewhere between the Type I and IIa fibers. Hence, this technique provides a means of determining these three fiber types at the same time. Figure 8.12 is an example of a muscle cross section after histochemical staining using an acid preincubation, showing Type I, IIa, and IIb fibers.

Another means of determining the percentage of the various muscle fiber types is by identifying the specific type of myosin found in the muscle using a technique called gel electrophoresis. At present, three different types of myosins (called myosin isoforms) have been reported in adult human skeletal muscle (e.g., Type I, Type IIa, Type IIb). The functional differences between these myosin isoforms explain why fast fibers shorten more rapidly than slow fibers (8, 41). For example, the myosin isoform found in fast fibers has a high ATPase activity; this promotes a rapid breakdown of ATP and provides the needed energy for a high speed of muscle shortening (i.e., high Vmax). In contrast, the myosin isoform found in slow fibers has a low ATPase activity and therefore shortens at a slower rate compared to fast fibers. For details of the different types of myosins found in skeletal muscle see reference 46a and 50.

One of the inherent problems with fiber typing in humans is that a muscle biopsy is usually performed on only one muscle group. Therefore, a single sample from one muscle may not be representative of the entire body. A further complication is that fiber types tend to be layered within muscle, and thus a small sample of muscle taken from a single area of the muscle may not be truly representative of the total fiber population of the muscle biopsied (4, 64). Therefore, it is difficult to make a definitive statement concerning the whole body percentage of a particular fiber type based on the staining of a single muscle biopsy.

Figure 8.12
Histochemical staining of a cross-sectional area of muscle. The darker cells are Type I fibers and the lightest-colored cells are Type IIa fibers. The cells with the brown appearance are Type IIb fibers.

in summary

- Human skeletal muscle fiber types can be divided into three general classes of fibers based on their biochemical and contractile properties. Two categories of fast fibers exist: (1) Type IIb, and (2) Type IIa. One type of slow fiber exists—Type I fibers.
- The biochemical and contractile properties characteristic of all muscle fiber types are summarized in table 8.1.
- Although classifying skeletal muscle fibers into three general groups is a convenient system to study the properties of muscle fibers, it is important to appreciate that human skeletal muscle fibers exhibit a wide range of contractile and biochemical properties. That is, the biochemical and contractile properties of Type IIb, Type IIa, and Type I fibers represent a continuum instead of three neat packages.

Fiber Types and Performance

Descriptive studies have demonstrated several interesting facts concerning the percentages of fast and slow muscle fibers found in humans. First, there are no apparent sex or age differences in fiber distribution (47). Secondly, the average sedentary man or woman possesses approximately 47%–53% slow fibers. Thirdly, it is commonly believed that successful power athletes (e.g., sprinters, fullbacks, etc.) possess a large percentage of fast fibers, whereas endurance athletes generally have a high percentage of slow fibers (17, 21, 68). Table 8.2 presents some examples of the percentage of slow and fast fibers found in successful athletes.

It is clear from table 8.2 that considerable variation in the percentage of various fiber types exists even among successful athletes competing in the same event or sport. In other words, two equally successful 10,000-meter runners might differ in the percentage of slow fibers that each possesses. For example, runner A might be found to possess 70% slow fibers, while runner B might contain 85% slow fibers. This observation demonstrates that an individual's muscle fiber composition is not the only variable that determines success in athletic events. In fact, it is generally believed that success in athletic performance is due to a complex interaction of psychological, biochemical, neurological, cardiopulmonary, and biomechanical factors (12, 13, 43, 70).

Alteration of Muscle Fiber Types by Exercise Training

Can exercise training result in changes in muscle fiber types? In the past, investigators remained divided on the answer. For example, several studies

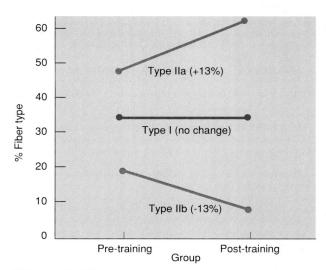

Figure 8.13

Exercise training-induced changes in myosin isoforms (fiber types) in skeletal muscle. Data are from Adams et al. (1a).

Table 8.2	Typical Muscle Fiber Composition in Elite Athletes Representing Different Sports and Nonathletes	
Sport	**% Slow Fibers (Type I)**	**% Fast Fibers (Types IIb and IIa)**
Distance runners	70–80	20–30
Track sprinters	25–30	70–75
Weight lifters	45–55	45–55
Nonathletes	47–53	47–53

Data from references 17, 68, and 70.

have concluded that endurance training does not result in conversion of fast fibers to a slower fiber (6, 7, 23, 27, 34, 40). However, recent investigations using improved techniques to study myosin isoforms have shown that rigorous exercise training results in alterations in muscle fiber types. Interestingly, both endurance training and resistance (weight) training result in a shift from a fast to a slower fiber type (1a,48,57a,65a). Note, however, that the training-induced changes in fiber type are often small and do not result in a complete conversion of Type IIb to Type I fibers (see figure 8.13). For example, resistance training in humans results in a reduction of the percent of Type IIb fibers and an increase in the percent of Type IIa fibers (1a). The transformation of a Type IIb into a Type IIa fiber is considered a fast-to-slow fiber shift because the movement is from the fastest fiber type (i.e., Type IIb) toward a slower fast fiber type (i.e., Type IIa).

Does endurance training result in an increase in the percent of Type I fibers? Current evidence suggests

Skeletal Muscle Is a Plastic Tissue

Skeletal muscle is a highly plastic tissue. Muscle composition (i.e., biochemical and structual makeup) can be altered in response to altered physical activity, changes in the motor neuron, or alterations in blood thyroxine levels. The muscle's response to increased physical activity is specific to the type of exercise training. For example, it is well known that the primary adaptation to strength training (weight lifting) is to increase both muscle size and force production (2, 26, 37, 46, 61, 67). This increase in muscle size is primarily due to muscle fiber enlargement (hypertrophy), although evidence exists that strength training may promote an increase in muscle fiber number (hyperplasia) in both humans and animals (42, 63, 69). In contrast, endurance exercise (e.g., long distance running) results in an elevated muscle oxidative capacity (e.g., mitochondrial number increases) with no increase in muscle size or strength. Details of muscle adaptation to different types of training will be discussed in chapter 13.

It is well known that motor neurons control the characteristic of the muscle fiber that they innervate. When motor nerves innervating Type IIb fibers and Type I fibers are experimentally switched, the two muscle fiber types begin to reverse characteristics (47). That is, the Type II fibers become Type I fibers and the Type I fibers become Type II. Therefore, all of the muscle fibers that are innervated by the same motor neuron (motor unit) are of the same type.

Recent research has shown that thyroxine is a powerful regulator of muscle fiber type (15a,17a). Increases in blood levels of thyroid hormone above normal (hyperthyroidism) result in an increase in the percentage of fast muscle fibers. In contrast, a decrease in blood thyroxine levels (hypothyroidism) promotes an increase in the number of slow fibers in muscle.

---

that 10 weeks of endurance training (30–60 minutes per day) does not increase the number of Type I fibers in trained muscles (57a,65a). However, research shows that chronic electrical stimulation of skeletal muscles can result in large increases in Type I fibers in locomotor muscles of rodents (50a). For example, to gain a better understanding of the effects of chronic exercise on muscle fiber type, investigators have implanted small batteries in animals and electrically stimulated skeletal muscles for up to 12 hours per day. Ninety days of this powerful stimulus results in a large fast-to-slow fiber type shift. That is, this type of training stimulus can completely eliminate Type IIb fibers and results in large increases in Type IIa and Type I fibers (50a). Interestingly, these studies indicate that the training-induced change in fiber type occurs in a stepwise fashion which proceeds in the following order: Type IIb→IIa→I (50a, 61b). That is, a Type IIb fiber cannot be directly converted into a Type I fiber but must be converted to a Type IIa fiber prior to becoming a Type I fiber.

Collectively, the studies discussed above, provide strong evidence that skeletal muscle fibers are "plastic" and can be altered by increased physical activity as well as hormonal factors (see A Closer Look 8.5). The effects of exercise on skeletal muscle is discussed in detail in chapter 13.

in summary

- Successful power athletes (e.g., sprinters) generally possess a high percentage of fast fibers whereas endurance athletes (e.g., distance runners) generally possess a high percentage of slow fibers.
- Both endurance and resistance exercise training have been shown to promote a fast-to-slow shift in skeletal muscle fiber types. However, this shift is often small and generally results in a conversion of Type IIb fibers to Type IIa fibers.

Age-Related Changes in Skeletal Muscle

Aging is associated with a loss of muscle mass. The age-related decline in muscle mass appears to have two phases. A "slow" phase of muscle loss where 10% of muscle mass is lost from age 25 to 50 years. Thereafter, there is a rapid loss in muscle mass. In fact, from age 50 to 80 years, an additional 40% of muscle mass is lost. Thus, by the age of 80 years, one half of the total muscle mass is lost (11a). Also,

(a) Muscle contracts and shortens

Movement

(b) Muscle contracts but does not shorten

No movement

Figure 8.14

(*a*) Isotonic contractions occur when a muscle contracts and shortens. (*b*) Isometric contractions occur when a muscle exerts force but does not shorten.

aging results in a loss of fast fibers (particularly Type IIb) and an increase in slow fibers (65a). See reference 11a for a review.

The loss of muscle size and strength observed in inactive older adults is not isolated to aging populations. A classic example of disuse muscle atrophy in young individuals is the reduction in muscle size observed in a broken limb during the period of immobilization imposed by the plaster "cast" (3). This simple example further illustrates that skeletal muscle is a highly "plastic" tissue that responds to both use and disuse (1, 30, 51, 52, 57).

Does aging impair skeletal muscle's ability to adapt to physical training? The answer to this question is no. Although a loss of muscle mass occurs in aging humans, this decline in muscle size is due not only to the aging process but is often due to atrophy associated with limited physical activity in older individuals. Although regular exercise cannot completely eliminate the age-related loss of muscle, regular exercise can improve muscular endurance and strength in the elderly in a manner similar to that observed in young individuals (9, 11a, 32, 53, 54, 55, 65a).

in summary

- Aging is associated with a loss of muscle mass. This age-related loss of muscle mass is slow from age 25 to 50 years but increases rapidly after 50 years of age.
- Regular exercise training can improve skeletal muscular strength and endurance in the elderly but cannot completely eliminate the age-related loss in muscle mass.

Isometric and Isotonic Contractions

It is possible for skeletal muscle to exert force without a large amount of muscle shortening. This might occur when an individual pulls against a wire attached to the wall of a building (see figure 8.14b). What happens here is that muscle tension increases but the wall does not move and therefore neither does the body part (e.g., arm) that applies the force. Contractions of this type are called **isometric,** or **static.** Isometric contractions are common in the postural muscles of the body, which act to maintain a static body position during periods of standing or sitting.

In contrast, most types of exercise or sports skills involve contractions that result in movement of body parts. In this case, as in an isometric contraction, tension within the muscle increases but the joint angle changes as the body parts move. This type of contraction is termed **isotonic,** or **dynamic.** There are two types of isotonic contractions: (1) concentric and (2) eccentric. A **concentric contraction** occurs when a muscle is activated and shortens (see figure 8.14a). An **eccentric contraction** occurs when a muscle is activated and force is produced but the muscle lengthens.

Speed of Muscle Contraction and Relaxation

If a muscle is given a single stimulus, such as a brief electrical shock applied to the nerve innervating it, the muscle responds with a simple **twitch.** The movement of the muscle can be recorded on a special recording device, and the time periods for contraction and relaxation can be studied. Figure 8.15 demonstrates the time course of a simple twitch in an isolated frog muscle. Notice that the twitch can be divided into three phases. First, immediately after the stimulus, there is a brief latent period (lasting a few milliseconds) prior to the beginning of muscle shortening. The second phase of the twitch is the contraction phase, which lasts approximately 40 milliseconds. Finally, the muscle returns to its original length during the relaxation period, which lasts about 50 milliseconds and thus is the longest of the three phases.

The timing of the phases in a simple twitch varies among muscle fiber types. The variability in speed of contraction arises from differences in the responses of the individual fiber types that make up muscles. Individual muscle fibers behave much like individual neurons in that they exhibit all-or-none responses to stimulation. To contract, an individual muscle fiber must receive an appropriate amount of stimulation. However, fast fibers contract in a shorter time period when stimulated than do slow fibers. The explanation for this observation is as follows. The speed of shortening is greater in fast fibers compared to slow fibers because the sarcoplasmic reticulum in fast fibers releases Ca^{++} at a faster rate and fast fibers possess a higher ATPase activity compared to the slow fiber types (21, 24, 61). The higher ATPase activity results in a more rapid splitting of ATP and a quicker release of the energy required for contraction.

Figure 8.15

A recording of a simple twitch. Note the three time periods (latent period, contraction, and relaxation) following the stimulus.

Force Regulation in Muscle

As stated earlier, the amount of force generated in a single muscle fiber is related to the number of myosin cross-bridges making contact with actin. However, the amount of force exerted during muscular contraction in a group of muscles is complex and dependent on three primary factors: (1) number and types of motor units recruited, (2) the initial length of the muscle, and (3) the nature of the neural stimulation of the motor units (5, 15, 16, 24). A discussion of each of these factors follows.

First, variations in the strength of contraction within an entire muscle depend on both the type and the number of muscle fibers that are stimulated to contract (i.e., recruited). If only a few motor units are recruited, the force is small. If more motor units are stimulated the force is increased. Figure 8.16 illustrates this point. Note that as the stimulus is increased, the force of contraction is increased due to the recruitment of additional motor units. Also, recall that fast fibers exert a greater specific force than slow fibers. Therefore, the types of motor units recruited also influences force production.

A second factor that determines the force exerted by a muscle is the initial length of the muscle at the time of contraction. There exists an "ideal" length of the muscle fiber. The explanation for the existence of an ideal length is related to the overlap between actin and myosin. For instance, when the resting length is longer than optimal, the overlap between actin and myosin is limited and few cross-bridges can attach. This concept is illustrated in figure 8.17. Note that

Figure 8.16

The relationship between increasing stimulus strength and the force of contraction. Weak stimuli do not activate many motor units and do not produce great force. In contrast, increasing the stimulus strength recruits more and more motor units and thus produces more force.

Figure 8.17

Length-tension relationships in skeletal muscle. Note that an optimal length of muscle exists, which will produce maximal force when stimulated. Lengths that are above or below this optimal length result in a reduced amount of force when stimulated.

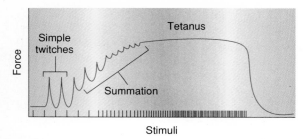

Figure 8.18

Recording showing the change from simple twitches to summation, and finally tetanus. Peaks to the left represent simple twitches, while increasing the frequency of the stimulus results in summation of the twitches, and finally tetanus.

when the muscle is stretched to the point where there is no overlap of actin and myosin, cross-bridges cannot attach and thus tension cannot be developed. At the other extreme, when the muscle is shortened to about 60% of its resting length, the Z lines are very close to the thick myosin filaments, and thus only limited additional shortening can occur.

A final factor that can affect the amount of force a muscle exerts upon contraction is the nature of the neural stimulation. Simple muscle twitches studied under experimental conditions reveal some interesting fundamental properties about how muscles function. However, normal body movements involve sustained contractions that are not simple twitches. The sustained contractions involved in normal body movements can be closely replicated in the laboratory if a series of stimulations are applied to the muscle. The recording pictured in figure 8.18 represents what occurs when successive stimuli are applied to the muscle. The first few contractions represent simple twitches. Note that as the frequency of stimulations is increased, the muscle does not have time to relax between stimuli and the force appears to be additive. This response is called **summation** (addition of successive twitches). If the frequency of stimuli is increased further, individual contractions are blended together in a single sustained contraction called **tetanus.** A tetanic contraction will continue until the stimuli are stopped or the muscle fatigues.

Muscular contractions that occur during normal body movements are tetanic contractions. These sustained contractions result from a series of rapidly repeated neural impulses conducted by the motor neurons that innervate those motor units involved in the movement. It is important to appreciate that in the body neural impulses to various motor units do not arrive at the same time as they do in the laboratory-induced tetanic contraction. Instead, various motor units are stimulated to contract at different times. Thus, some motor units are contracting while some are relaxing. This type of tetanic contraction results

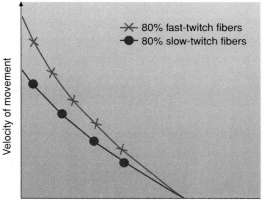

Figure 8.19

Muscle force-velocity relationships. Note that at any given speed of movement, muscle groups with a high percentage of fast-twitch (FT) fibers exert more *force* than those with muscle groups that contain primarily slow-twitch (ST) fibers.

in a smooth contraction and aids in sustaining a coordinated muscle contraction.

Force–Velocity/Power–Velocity Relationships

In most physical activities, muscular force is applied through a range of movement. For instance, an athlete throwing the shot put applies force against the shot over a specified range of movement prior to release. How far the shot travels is a function of both the speed of the shot upon release and the angle of release. Since success in many athletic events is dependent on speed, it is important to appreciate some of the basic concepts underlying the relationship between muscular force and the speed of movement. The relationship between speed of movement and muscular force is shown in figure 8.19. Two important points emerge from an examination of figure 8.19.

1. At any absolute force exerted by the muscle, the velocity or speed of movement is greater in muscles that contain a high percentage of fast fibers when compared to muscles that possess predominantly slow fibers.
2. The maximum velocity of muscle shortening is greatest at the lowest force (i.e., resistance against the muscle). In short, the greatest speed of movement is generated at the lowest work loads (10, 39). This principle holds true for both slow- and fast fibers.

The data contained in figure 8.19 also demonstrate that fast fibers are capable of producing greater muscular force at a faster speed than slow

Figure 8.20

Muscle power-velocity relationships. In general, the power produced by a muscle group increases as a function of velocity of movement. At any given speed of movement, muscles that contain a large percentage of fast-twitch (FT) fibers produce more *power* than those muscles that contain primarily slow-twitch (ST) fibers.

fibers. The biochemical mechanism to explain this observation is related to the fact that fast fibers possess higher ATPase activity than do slow fibers (21, 24). Therefore, ATP is broken down more rapidly in fast fibers when compared to slow fibers. Further, calcium release from the sarcoplasmic reticulum is faster following neural stimulation in fast fibers than in slow fibers (24, 59).

The relationship between force and movement speed has practical importance for the physical therapist, athlete, or physical educator. The message is simply that athletes that possess a high percentage of fast fibers would seem to have an advantage in power-type athletic events. This may explain why successful sprinters and weight lifters typically possess a relatively high percentage of fast fibers.

As might be expected, the fiber-type distribution in muscle influences the power-velocity curve (see figure 8.20). The peak power that can be generated by muscle is greater in muscle that contains a high percentage of fast fibers than in muscle that is largely composed of slow fibers. As with the force-velocity curve, two important points should be retained from examination of the power-velocity curve:

1. At any given velocity of movement, the peak power generated is greater in muscle that contains a high percentage of fast fibers than in muscle with a high percentage of slow fibers. This difference is due to the aforementioned biochemical differences

between fast and slow fibers. Again, athletes who possess a high percentage of fast fibers can generate more power than athletes with predominantly slow fibers.

2. The peak power generated by any muscle increases with increasing velocities of movement up to a movement speed of 200–300 degrees/second. The reason for the plateau of power output with increasing movement speed is that muscular force decreases with increasing speed of movement (see figure 8.19). Therefore, with any given muscle group there is an optimum speed of movement that will elicit the greatest power output.

in summary

- The amount of force generated during muscular contraction is dependent on the following factors: (1) types and number of motor units recruited, (2) the initial muscle length, and (3) the nature of the motor units' neural stimulation.
- The addition of muscle twitches is termed summation. When the frequency of neural stimulation to a motor unit is increased, individual contractions are fused together in a sustained contraction called tetanus.
- The peak force generated by muscle decreases as the speed of movement increases. However, in general, the amount of power generated by a muscle group increases as a function of movement velocity.

Receptors in Muscle

Skeletal muscle contains several types of sensory receptors. These include chemoreceptors, muscle spindles, and Golgi tendon organs (44). Chemoreceptors are specialized free nerve endings that send information to the central nervous system in response to changes in muscle pH, concentrations of extracellular potassium, and changes in O_2 and CO_2 tensions. Chemoreceptors may play a role in cardiopulmonary regulation during exercise and will be discussed in more detail in chapters 9 and 10.

In order for the nervous system to properly control skeletal muscle movements, it must receive continuous sensory feedback from the contracting muscle. This sensory feedback includes (1) information concerning the tension developed by a muscle and (2) an account of the muscle length. **Golgi tendon organs (GTOs)** provide the central nervous system with feedback concerning the tension developed by the muscle, while the **muscle spindle** provides sensory information concerning the relative muscle length (35, 44). A discussion of each sensory organ follows.

Muscle Spindle

As previously stated, the muscle spindle functions as a length detector. Muscle spindles are found in large numbers in most human locomotor muscles (35). Muscles that require the finest degree of control, such as the muscles of the hands, have the highest density of spindles. In contrast, muscles that are responsible for gross movements (e.g., quadriceps) contain relatively few spindles.

The muscle spindle is composed of several thin muscle cells (called *intrafusal fibers*) that are surrounded by a connective tissue sheath. Like normal skeletal muscle fibers (called *extrafusal fibers*), muscle spindles insert into connective tissue within the muscle. Therefore, muscle spindles run parallel with muscle fibers (see figure 8.21).

Muscle spindles contain two types of sensory nerve endings. The primary endings respond to dynamic changes in muscle length. The second type of sensory ending is called the secondary ending and it does not respond to rapid changes in muscle length, but provides the central nervous system with continuous information concerning static muscle length.

In addition to the sensory neurons, muscle spindles are innervated by gamma motor neurons, which stimulate the intrafusal fibers to contract simultaneously along with extrafusal fibers. Gamma motor neuron stimulation causes the central region of the intrafusal fibers to shorten, which serves to tighten the spindle. The need for contraction of the intrafusal fibers can be explained as follows. When skeletal muscles are shortened by motor-neuron stimulation, muscle spindles are passively shortened along with the skeletal muscle fibers. If the intrafusal fibers did not compensate accordingly, this shortening would result in "slack" in the spindle and make them less sensitive. Therefore, their function as length detectors would be compromised.

Muscle spindles are responsible for the observation that rapid stretching of skeletal muscles results in a reflex contraction. This is called the *stretch reflex* and is present in all muscles, but is most dramatic in the extensor muscles of the limbs. The so-called knee-jerk reflex is often evaluated by the physician by tapping the patellar tendon with a rubber mallet. The blow by the mallet stretches the entire muscle and thus "excites" the primary nerve endings located in muscle spindles. The neural impulse from the muscle spindle synapses at the spinal cord level with a motor neuron, which then stimulates the extrafusal fibers of the extensor muscle, resulting in an isotonic contraction.

The function of the muscle spindle is to assist in the regulation of movement and to maintain posture. This is accomplished by the muscle spindle's ability to

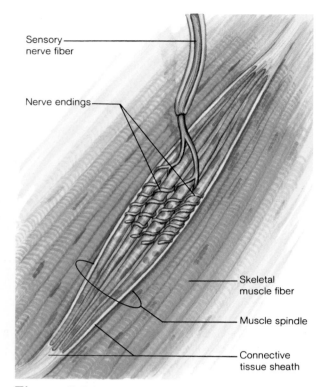

Figure 8.21

The structure of muscle spindles and their location in skeletal muscle.

detect and cause the central nervous system (CNS) to respond to changes in the length of skeletal muscle fibers. The following practical example shows how the muscle spindle assists in the control of movement. Suppose a student is holding a single book in front of him or her with the arm extended. This type of load poses a tonic stretch on the muscle spindle, which sends information to the CNS concerning the final length of the extrafusal muscle fibers. If a second book is suddenly placed upon the first book, the muscles would be suddenly stretched (arm would drop) and a burst of impulses from the muscle spindle would alert the CNS about the change in muscle length (and thus load). The ensuing reflex would recruit additional motor units to raise the arm back to the original position. Generally, this type of reflex action results in an overcompensation. That is, more motor units are recruited than are needed to bring the arm back to the original position. However, immediately following the overcompensation movement, an additional adjustment rapidly occurs and the arm is quickly returned to the original position.

Golgi Tendon Organs

The Golgi tendon organs (GTOs) continuously monitor tension produced by muscle contraction. Golgi tendon

Sensory neuron

Golgi
tendon
organ

Alpha
motoneuron
inhibited

Figure 8.22
The Golgi tendon organ. The Golgi tendon organ is located in series with muscle and serves as a "tension monitor" that acts as a protective device for muscle. See text for details.

organs are located within the tendon and thus are in series with the extrafusal fibers (figure 8.22). In essence, GTOs serve as "safety devices" that help prevent excessive force during muscle contraction. When activated, GTOs send information to the spinal cord via sensory neurons, which in turn excite inhibitory neurons (i.e., send IPSPs). This inhibitory disynaptic reflex (i.e., two synapses are involved) helps prevent excessive muscle contractions and provides a finer control over skeletal movements. This process is pictured in figure 8.22.

It seems likely that GTOs play an important role in the performance of strength activities. For instance, the amount of force that can be produced by a muscle group may be dependent on the ability of the individual to voluntarily oppose the inhibition of the GTO. It seems possible that the inhibitory influences of the GTO could be gradually reduced in response to strength training (70). This would allow an individual to produce a greater amount of muscle force, and in many cases improve sport performance.

in summary

- The muscle spindle functions as a length detector in muscle.
- Golgi tendon organs continuously monitor the tension developed during muscular contraction. In essence, Golgi tendon organs serve as safety devices that help prevent excessive force during muscle contractions.

study questions

1. List the principal functions of skeletal muscles.
2. List the principal proteins contained in skeletal muscle.
3. Outline the contractile process. Use a step-by-step format illustrating the entire process, beginning with the nerve impulse reaching the neuromuscular junction.
4. Outline the mechanical and biochemical properties of human skeletal muscle fiber types.
5. Discuss those factors thought to be responsible for regulating force during muscular contractions.
6. Define the term *summation*.
7. Graph a simple muscle twitch and a contraction that results in tetanus.
8. Discuss the relationship between force and speed of movement during a muscular contraction.
9. Describe the general anatomical design of a muscle spindle and discuss its physiological function.
10. Discuss the function of Golgi tendon organs in monitoring muscle tension.

suggested readings

Conley, K. 1994. Cellular energetics during exercise. *Advances in Veterinary Science and Comparative Medicine.* 38A:1–39.

Hochachka, P. 1994. *Muscles as Molecular and Metabolic Machines.* Boca Raton, FL: CRC Press.

Komi, P., ed. *Strength and Power in Sport.* 1992. Oxford: Blackwell Scientific Publications.

Lieber, R. 1992. *Skeletal Muscle Structure and Function.* Baltimore, MD: Williams and Wilkie.

Moss, R., G. Diffee, and M. Greaser. 1995. Contractile properties of skeletal muscle fibers in relation to myofibrillar protein isoforms. *Review of Physiology, Biochemistry, and Pharmacology.* 126:1–63.

Terjung, T. 1995. Muscle adaptations to aerobic training. *Sports Science Exchange.* 8:54.

references

1. Abernethy, P., R. Thayer, and A. Taylor. 1990. Acute and chronic responses of skeletal muscle to endurance and sprint exercise: A review. *Sports Medicine* 10:365–89.

1a. Adams, G. et al. 1993. Skeletal muscle myosin heavy chain composition and resistance training. *Journal of Applied Physiology.* 74:911–15.

2. Alway, S. et al. 1990. Muscle cross-sectional area and torque in resistance trained subjects. *European Journal of Applied Physiology* 60:86–90.

3. Appell, H. 1990. Muscular atrophy following immobilisation: A review. *Sports Medicine* 10:42–58.

4. Armstrong, R. et al. 1983. Differential inter- and intra-muscular responses to exercise: Considerations in use of the biopsy technique. In *Biochemistry of Exercise,* eds. H. Knuttgen, J. Vogel, and J. Poortmans, 775–80. Champaign, IL: Human Kinetics.

5. Armstrong, R., and H. Laughlin. 1985. Muscle function during locomotion in mammals. In *Circulation, Respiration, and Metabolism,* ed. R. Giles, 56–63. New York: Springer-Verlag.

6. Bagby, G., W. Sembrowich, and P. Gollnick. 1972. Myosin ATPase and fiber type composition from trained and untrained rat skeletal muscle. *Journal of Applied Physiology* 223:1415–17.

7. Baldwin, K. et al. 1972. Respiratory capacity of white, red, and intermediate muscle: Adaptive response to exercise. *Journal of Applied Physiology* 222:373–78.

7a. Bar, A., and D. Pette. 1988. Three fast myosin heavy chains in adult rat skeletal muscle. *FEBS Letters.* 235:153–54.

8. Billeter, R., and H. Hoppeler. 1992. Muscular basis of strength. In *Strength and Power in Sport,* ed. P. Komi, 39–63. Oxford: Blackwell Scientific Publishing.

9. Black, R. 1991. Muscle strength as an indicator of the habitual level of physical activity. *Medicine and Science in Sports and Exercise* 23:1375–81.

10. Bobbert, M., G. Ettema, and P. Huijing. 1990. The force-length relationship of a muscle-tendon complex: Experimental results and model calculations. *European Journal of Applied Physiology* 61:323–29.

11. Booth, F., and D. Thomason. 1991. Molecular and cellular adaptation of muscle in response to exercise: Perspectives of various models. *Physiological Reviews* 71:541–85.

11a. Booth, F. and S. Weeden. 1993. Structural aspects of aging human skeletal muscle. In *Musculoskeletal Soft-tissue Aging: Impact on Mobility.* eds. J. Buckwalter, V. Goldberg, and S. Woo. Rosemont, IL: American Academy of Orthopaedic Surgeons.

11b. Bottinelli, R., M. Canepari, C. Reggiani, and G. Stienen. 1994. Myofibrillar ATPase activity during isometric contractions and isomyosin composition in rat single skinned muscle fibers. *Journal of Physiology* (London). 481:663–75.

12. Brooks, G., and T. Fahey. 1984. *Exercise Physiology: Human Bioenergetics and Its Applications.* New York: John Wiley & Sons.

13. ———. 1987. *Fundamentals of Human Performance.* New York: John Wiley & Sons.

14. Buchthal, F., and H. Schmalbruch. 1970. Contraction times and fiber types in intact human muscle. *Acta Physiologica Scandanavica* 79:435–40.

15. Burke, R. 1986. The control of muscle force: Motor unit recruitment and firing pattern. In *Human Muscle Power,* ed. N. Jones, N. McCartney, and A. McComas, 97–105. Champaign, IL: Human Kinetics.

15a. Caiozzo, V. et al. 1993. Single fiber analyses of Type IIa myosin heavy chain distribution in hyper- and hypothyroid soleus. *American Journal of Physiology.* 265:C842–C849.

16. Carlson, F., and D. Wilkie. 1974. *Muscle Physiology.* Englewood Cliffs, NJ: Prentice-Hall.

16a. Conley, K. 1994. Cellular energetics during exercise. *Advances in Veterinary Science and Comparative Medicine.* 38A:1–39.

17. Costill, D., W. Fink, and M. Pollock. 1976. Muscle fiber composition and enzyme activities of elite distance runners. *Medicine and Science in Sports* 8:96.

17a. Devor, S., and T. White. 1995. Myosin heavy chain phenotype in regenerating skeletal muscle is affected by thyroid hormone. *Medicine and Science in Sports and Exercise* 27:674–81.

18. Ebashi, S. 1976. Excitation-contraction coupling. *Annual Review of Physiology* 38:293–309.

19. ———. 1991. Excitation-contraction coupling. *Annual Review of Physiology* 53:1–16.

20. Edgerton, V. et al. 1983. Muscle fiber activation and recruitment. In *Biochemistry of Exercise,* ed. H. Knuttgen, J. Vogel, and J. Poortmans, 31–49. Champaign, IL: Human Kinetics.

21. Edgerton, V. et al. 1986. Morphological basis of skeletal muscle power output. In *Human Muscle Power,* ed. N. Jones, N. McCartney, and A. McComas, 43–58. Champaign, IL: Human Kinetics.

22. Edman, K. 1992. Contractile performance of skeletal muscle fibres. In *Strength and Power in Sport,* ed. P. Komi, 96–114. Oxford: Blackwell Scientific Publishing.

23. Edstrom, L., and L. Grimby. 1986. Effect of exercise on the motor unit. *Muscle and Nerve* 9:104–26.

24. Faulker, J., D. Claflin, and K. McCully. 1986. Power output of fast and slow fibers from human skeletal muscles. In *Human Muscle Power*, ed. N. Jones, N. McCartney, and A. McComas, 81–90. Champaign, IL: Human Kinetics.

24a. Fauteck, S., and S. Kandarian. 1995. Sensitive detection of myosin heavy chain composition in skeletal muscle under different loading conditions. *American Journal of Physiology* 37:C419–C424.

24b. Fitts, R. 1994. Cellular mechanisms of muscle fatigue. *Physiological Reviews* 74:49–94.

25. Fox, S. 1993. *Human Physiology*. Dubuque, IA: Wm. C. Brown.

26. Goldspink, G. 1992. Cellular and molecular aspects of adaptation in skeletal muscle. In *Strength and Power in Sport*, ed. P. Komi, 211–29. London: Blackwell Scientific Publishing.

27. Gollnick, P. 1985. Metabolism of substrates: Energy substrate metabolism during exercise and as modified by training. *Federation Proceedings* 44:353–56.

28. Gollnick, P., and B. Saltin. 1983. Hypothesis: Significance of skeletal muscle oxidative capacity with endurance training. *Clinical Physiology* 2:1–12.

29. Green, H. 1986. Muscle power: Fiber type recruitment, metabolism, and fatigue. In *Human Muscle Power*, ed. N. Jones, N. McCartney, and A. McComas, 65–79. Champaign, IL: Human Kinetics.

30. Grinton, S. et al. 1992. Exercise training-induced increases in expiratory muscle oxidative capacity. *Medicine and Science in Sports and Exercise* 24:551–55.

31. Gunning, P., and E. Hardeman. 1991. Multiple mechanisms regulate muscle fiber diversity. FASEB *Journal* 5:3064–70.

32. Hammeren, J. et al. 1992. Exercise training-induced alterations in skeletal muscle oxidative and antioxidant enzyme activity in senescent rats. *International Journal of Sports Medicine* 13:412–16.

33. Holloszy, J. 1982. Muscle metabolism during exercise. *Archives of Physical and Rehabilitation Medicine* 63:231–34.

34. Hoppeler, H. 1986. Exercise-induced ultrastructure changes in skeletal muscle. *International Journal of Sports Medicine* 7:187–204.

34a. Hughes, S. et al. 1993. Three slow myosin heavy chains sequentially expressed in developing mammalian skeletal muscle. *Developmental Biology*. 158:183–99.

35. Hunt, C. 1991. Mammalian muscle spindle: Peripheral mechanisms. *Physiological Reviews* 70:643–63.

36. Johnson, L. 1983. *Biology*. Dubuque, IA: Wm. C. Brown.

37. Johnson, T., and K. Klueber. 1991. Skeletal muscle following tonic overload: Functional and structural analysis. *Medicine and Science in Sports and Exercise* 23:49–55.

38. Kodama, T. 1985. Thermodynamic analysis of muscle ATPase mechanisms. *Physiological Reviews* 65:468–540.

39. Kojima, T. 1991. Force-velocity relationship of human elbow flexors in voluntary isotonic contraction under heavy loads. *International Journal of Sports Medicine* 12:208–13.

40. Larsson, L. 1982. Physical training effects on muscle morphology in sedentary males at different ages. *Medicine and Science in Sports and Exercise* 14:203.

41. Lowey, S. 1986. Cardiac and skeletal muscle myosin polymorphism. *Medicine and Science in Sports and Exercise* 18:284–91.

42. MacDougall, J. 1992. Hypertrophy or hyperplasia. In *Strength and Power in Sport*, ed. P. Komi, 230–38. London: Blackwell Scientific Publishing.

43. McArdle, W., F. Katch, and V. Katch. 1991. *Exercise Physiology: Energy, Nutrition, and Human Performance*. Philadelphia: Lea & Febiger.

44. McCloskey, D. et al. 1987. Sensing position and movements of the fingers. *News in Physiological Sciences* 2:226–30.

45. Metzger, J. 1992. Mechanism of chemomechanical coupling in skeletal muscle during work. In *Energy Metabolism in Exercise and Sport*, ed. D. Lamb and C. Gisolfi, 1–43. Dubuque, IA: Brown & Benchmark.

46. Milesky, A. et al. 1991. Changes in muscle fiber size and composition in response to heavy-resistance exercise. *Medicine and Science in Sports and Exercise* 23:1042–49.

46a. Moss, R., G. Diffee, and M. Greaser. 1995. Contractile properties of skeletal muscle fibers in relation to myofibrillar protein isoforms. *Review of Physiology, Biochemistry, and Pharmacology* 126:1–63.

47. Pette, D. 1980. *Plasticity of Muscle*. New York: Walter de Gruyter.

48. ———. 1984. Activity-induced fast-to-slow transitions in mammalian muscle. *Medicine and Science in Sports and Exercise* 16:517–28.

49. Pette, D., and C. Spamer. 1986. Metabolic properties of muscle fibers. *Federation Proceedings* 45:2910–14.

50. Pette, D., and R. Staron. 1990. Cellular and molecular diversities of mammalian skeletal muscle fibers. *Review of Physiology, Biochemistry, and Pharmacology* 116:1–76.

50a. Pette, D., and G. Vrbova. 1992. Adaptation of mammalian muscle fibers to chronic electrical stimulation. *Review of Physiology, Biochemistry, and Pharmacology* 120:115–202.

51. Powers, S. et al. 1990. Endurance-training-induced cellular adaptations in respiratory muscles. *Journal of Applied Physiology* 69:648–50.

52. Powers, S. et al. 1990. Regional metabolic differences in the rat diaphragm. *Journal of Applied Physiology* 68:2114–18.

53. Powers, S. et al. 1991. Age-related changes in enzyme activity in the rat diaphragm. *Respiration Physiology* 83:1–10.

54. Powers, S. et al. 1992. Aging and exercise-induced cellular alterations in the rat diaphragm. *American Journal of Physiology* 32:R1093–R1098.

55. Powers, S. et al. 1992. Aging and respiratory muscle metabolic plasticity: Effects of endurance training. *Journal of Applied Physiology* 72:1068–73.

56. Powers, S. et al. 1992. Diaphragmatic fiber type specific adaptation to endurance training. *Respiration Physiology* 89:195–207.

57. Powers, S. et al. 1992. High intensity exercise training-induced metabolic alterations in respiratory muscles. *Respiration Physiology* 89:169–77.

57a. Powers, S. et al. 1995. Role of beta-adrenergic mechanisms in exercise training-induced metabolic changes in respiratory and locomotor muscle. *International Journal of Sports Medicine* 16:13–18.

57b. Rayment, I. et al. 1993. Structure of the actin myosin complex and its implications for muscle contraction. *Science* 261:58–65.

58. Ruegg, J. 1992. *Calcium in Muscle Activation*. Berlin: Springer-Verlag.

59. Ruegg, J. C. 1987. Excitation-contraction coupling in fast- and slow-twitch muscle fibers. *International Journal of Sports Medicine* 8:360–64.

60. Saltin, B. et al. 1977. Fiber types and metabolic potentials of skeletal muscles in sedentary man and endurance runners. *Annals of New York Academy of Sciences* 301:3–29.

61. Saltin, B., and P. Gollnick. 1983. Skeletal muscle adaptability: Significance for metabolism and performance. In *Handbook of Physiology*, ed. L. Peachy, R. Adrian, and S. Geiger. Section 10: Skeletal Muscle, chapter 19, 555–631. Bethesda, MD: American Physiological Society.

61a. Sant'Ana Pereira, J., S. Ennion, A. Moorman, G. Goldspink, and A. Sargeant. 1994. The predominant fast myHC's in human skeletal muscle corresponds to the rat IIa and IIx and not IIb. *Annual Meeting of Society For Neuroscience*. Abstract. A26.

61b. Schiaffino, S., L. Gorza, L. Saggin, S. Ausoni, M. Vianello, K. Gundersen, and T. Lomo. 1989. Three myosin heavy chain isoforms in type 2 skeletal muscle fibers. *Journal of Muscle Research and Cell Motility* 10:197–205.

61c. Schiaffino, S., and C. Reggiani. 1994. Myosin isoforms in mammalian skeletal muscle. *Journal of Applied Physiology* 77:493–501.

62. Simoneau, J. et al. 1986. Inheritance of human skeletal muscle and anaerobic capacity adaptation to high-intensity intermittent training. *International Journal of Sports Medicine* 7:167–71.

63. Sjostrom, M. et al. 1991. Evidence of fibre hyperplasia in human skeletal muscles from healthy young men? *European Journal of Applied Physiology* 62:301–4.

64. Snow, D., and R. Harris. 1985. Thoroughbreds and greyhounds: Biochemical adaptations in creatures of nature and man. In *Circulation, Respiration, and Metabolism*, ed. R. Giles, 227–39. New York: Springer-Verlag.

65. Staron, R. et al. 1989. Muscle hypertrophy and fast fiber conversions in heavy resistance-trained women. *European Journal of Applied Physiology* 60:71–79.

65a. Sullivan, V. et al. 1995. Myosin heavy chain composition in young and old rat skeletal muscle: Effects of endurance exercise. *Journal of Applied Physiology* 78:2115–20.

66. Tate, C., M. Hyek, and G. Taffet. 1991. The role of calcium in the energetics of contracting skeletal muscle. *Sports Medicine* 12:208–17.

67. Tesch, P. 1992. Short and long-term histochemical and biochemical adaptations in muscle. In *Strength and Power in Sport*, ed. P. Komi, 239–48. Oxford: Blackwell Scientific Publishing.

68. Tesch, P., A. Thorsson, and P. Kaiser. 1984. Muscle capillary supply and fiber type characteristics in weight and power lifters. *Journal of Applied Physiology* 56:35–38.

69. Umnova, M., and T. Seene. 1991. The effect of increased functional load on the activation of satellite cells in the skeletal muscles of adult rats. *International Journal of Sports Medicine* 12:501–4.

69a. Vale, R. 1994. Getting a grip on myosin. *Cell* 78:733–37.

70. Wilmore, J., and Costill, D. 1988. *Training for Sport and Activity*. Dubuque, IA: Wm. C. Brown.

Circulatory Adaptations to Exercise

objectives

By studying this chapter, you should be able to do the following:

1. Give an overview of the design and function of the circulatory system.
2. Describe the cardiac cycle and the associated electrical activity recorded via the electrocardiogram.
3. Discuss the pattern of redistribution of blood flow during exercise.
4. Outline the circulatory responses to various types of exercise.
5. Identify the factors that regulate local blood flow during exercise.
6. List and discuss those factors responsible for regulation of stroke volume during exercise.
7. Discuss the regulation of cardiac output during exercise.

outline

Organization of the Circulatory System 152
  Structure of the Heart 152
  Pulmonary and Systemic Circuits 153
Heart: Myocardium and Cardiac Cycle 153
  Myocardium 153
  Cardiac Cycle 154
  Arterial Blood Pressure 155
  Electrical Activity of the Heart 157
Cardiac Output 160
  Regulation of Heart Rate 160
  Regulation of Stroke Volume 161

Hemodynamics 163
  Physical Characteristics of Blood 163
  Relationships Between Pressure, Resistance, and Flow 163
  Sources of Vascular Resistance 164
Changes in Oxygen Delivery to Muscle During Exercise 165
  Changes in Cardiac Output During Exercise 165
  Changes in Arterial-Mixed Venous O_2 Content During Exercise 166
  Redistribution of Blood Flow During Exercise 167

Regulation of Local Blood Flow During Exercise 167
Circulatory Responses to Exercise 169
  Emotional Influence 169
  Transition from Rest to Exercise 169
  Recovery from Exercise 169
  Incremental Exercise 170
  Arm versus Leg Exercise 170
  Intermittent Exercise 171
  Prolonged Exercise 171
Regulation of Cardiovascular Adjustments to Exercise 172

key terms

arteries
arterioles
atrioventricular node (AV node)
autoregulation
capillaries
cardiac accelerator nerves
cardiac output
cardiovascular control center

central command
diastole
diastolic blood pressure
double product
electrocardiogram (ECG)
intercalated discs
mixed venous blood
myocardium

pulmonary circuit
sinoatrial node (SA node)
stroke volume
systole
systolic blood pressure
vagus nerve
veins
venules

One of the major challenges to homeostasis posed by exercise is the increased muscular demand for oxygen; during heavy exercise the demand may be fifteen to twenty-five times greater than at rest. The primary purpose of the cardiorespiratory system is to deliver adequate amounts of oxygen and remove wastes from body tissues. In addition, the circulatory system transports nutrients and aids in temperature regulation. It is important to note that the respiratory system and the circulatory system function together as a "coupled unit"; the respiratory system adds oxygen and removes carbon dioxide from the blood, while the circulatory system is responsible for delivery of oxygenated blood and nutrients to tissues in accordance with their needs. Stated another way, the "cardiopulmonary system" works to maintain oxygen and carbon dioxide homeostasis in body tissues.

In order to meet the increased oxygen demands of muscle during exercise, two major adjustments of blood flow must be made: (1) an increased **cardiac output** (i.e., increased amount of blood pumped per minute by the heart) and (2) a redistribution of blood flow from inactive organs to the active skeletal muscles. However, while the needs of the muscles are being met, other tissues, such as the brain, cannot be denied blood flow. This is accomplished by maintaining blood pressure, the driving force of the blood. A thorough understanding of the cardiovascular responses to exercise is important for the student of exercise physiology. Therefore, it is the purpose of this chapter to describe the design and function of the circulatory system and how it responds during exercise.

Organization of the Circulatory System

The human circulatory system is a closed loop that circulates blood to all body tissues. Circulation of blood requires the action of a muscular pump, the heart, that creates the "pressure head" needed to move blood through the system. Blood travels away from the heart in **arteries** and returns to the heart by way of **veins.** The system is considered "closed" because arteries and veins are continuous with each other through smaller vessels. Arteries branch extensively to form a "tree" of smaller vessels. As the vessels become microscopic they form **arterioles,** which eventually develop into "beds" of much smaller vessels called **capillaries.** Capillaries are the smallest and most numerous of blood vessels; all exchanges of oxygen, carbon dioxide, and nutrients between tissues and the circulatory system occur across capillary beds. Blood passes from capillary beds to small venous vessels called **venules.** As venules move back toward the heart they increase in size and become veins. Major veins empty directly into the heart. The mixture of venous blood from both the upper and lower body that accumulates in the right side of the heart is termed **mixed venous blood.** Mixed venous blood therefore represents an average of venous blood from the entire body.

Structure of the Heart

The heart is divided into four chambers and is often considered to be two pumps in one. The right atrium and right ventricle form the right pump, while the left atrium and left ventricle combine to make the left pump (see figure 9.1). The right side of the heart is separated from the left side by a muscular wall called the interventricular septum. This septum prevents the mixing of blood from the two sides of the heart.

Blood movement within the heart is from the atria to the ventricles, and from the ventricles blood is pumped into the arteries. To prevent backward movement of blood, the heart contains four one-way valves. The right and left atrioventricular valves connect the atria with the right and left ventricles, respectively (figure 9.1). These valves are also known as the tricuspid valve (right atrioventricular valve) and the bicuspid valve (left atrioventricular valve). Backflow from the arteries into the ventricles is prevented by the pulmonary semilunar valve (right ventricle) and the aortic semilunar valve (left ventricle).

Figure 9.1
An anterior view of the heart.

Labels (clockwise from top left): Superior vena cava, Pulmonary valve, Right pulmonary artery, Right pulmonary veins, Right atrium, Tricuspid valve, Right ventricle, Inferior vena cava, Aorta, Left pulmonary artery, Pulmonary trunk, Left pulmonary veins, Left atrium, Bicuspid valve, Chordae tendineae, Papillary muscle, Left ventricle, Interventricular septum

Pulmonary and Systemic Circuits

As mentioned previously, the heart can be considered as two pumps in one. The right side of the heart pumps blood that is partially depleted of its oxygen content and contains an elevated carbon dioxide content as a result of gas exchange in the various tissues of the body. This blood is delivered from the right heart into the lungs through the **pulmonary circuit.** At the lungs, oxygen is loaded into the blood and carbon dioxide is released. This "oxygenated" blood then travels to the left side of the heart and is pumped to the various tissues of the body via the systemic circuit.

in summary

- The purposes of the cardiovascular system are the following: (1) transport of O_2 to tissues and removal of wastes, (2) transport of nutrients to tissues, and (3) the regulation of body temperature.
- The heart is two pumps in one. The right side of the heart pumps blood through the pulmonary circulation, while the left side of the heart delivers blood to the systemic circulation.

Heart: Myocardium and Cardiac Cycle

In order to better appreciate how the circulatory system adjusts to the stress of exercise, it is important to understand elementary details of heart muscle structure as well as the electrical and mechanical activities of the heart.

Myocardium

The wall of the heart is composed of three layers: (1) an outer layer called the epicardium, (2) a muscular middle layer, the myocardium, and (3) an inner layer known as the endocardium (see figure 9.2). It is the **myocardium,** or heart muscle, that is responsible for contracting and forcing blood out of the heart. The myocardium receives its blood supply via the right and left coronary arteries. These vessels branch off the aorta and encircle the heart. The coronary veins run alongside the arteries and drain all coronary blood into a larger vein called the coronary sinus, which deposits blood into the right atrium.

Heart muscle differs from skeletal muscle in several important ways. First, unlike skeletal muscle cells,

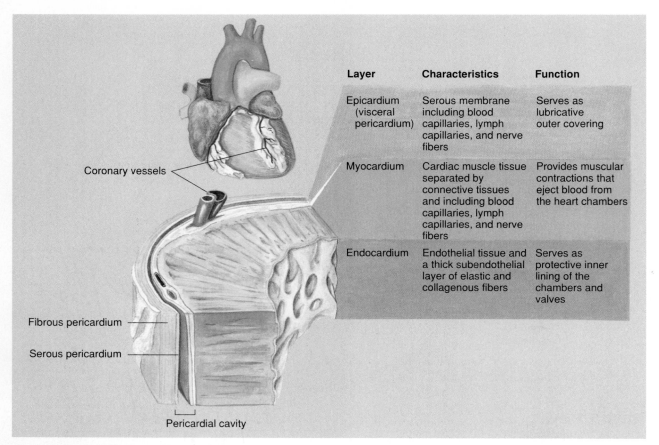

Layer	Characteristics	Function
Epicardium (visceral pericardium)	Serous membrane including blood capillaries, lymph capillaries, and nerve fibers	Serves as lubricative outer covering
Myocardium	Cardiac muscle tissue separated by connective tissues and including blood capillaries, lymph capillaries, and nerve fibers	Provides muscular contractions that eject blood from the heart chambers
Endocardium	Endothelial tissue and a thick subendothelial layer of elastic and collagenous fibers	Serves as protective inner lining of the chambers and valves

Figure 9.2
The heart wall is composed of three distinct layers: (1) epicardium, (2) myocardium, and (3) endocardium.

heart muscle cells are all interconnected via **intercalated discs.** These intercellular connections permit transmission of electrical impulses from one cell to another. Intercalated discs are nothing more than leaky membranes that allow ions to cross from one cell to another. Therefore, when one heart cell is depolarized to contract, all connecting cells also become excited and contract as a unit. This arrangement is referred to as a *functional syncytium*. Heart muscle cells in the atria are separated from ventricular muscle cells by a layer of connective tissue that does not permit transmission of electrical impulses. Hence, the atria contract separately from the ventricles.

A second difference between heart muscle cells and skeletal muscle cells is that human heart muscle cannot be divided into many different fiber types. The ventricular myocardium is thought to be a rather homogenous muscle containing one primary fiber type that is similar in many ways to slow-twitch fibers found in skeletal muscle. That is, heart muscle cells are highly aerobic in nature, contain an extensive capillary supply, and have large numbers of mitochondria (59).

Heart muscle is similar to skeletal muscle in that it is striated (contains actin and myosin protein filaments), requires calcium to activate the myofilaments (4, 5), and contracts via the sliding filament model of muscular contraction (chapter 8). In addition, like skeletal muscle, heart muscle can alter its force of contraction as a function of the degree of overlap between actin-myosin filaments. This length-tension relationship of the heart will be discussed later in the chapter.

Cardiac Cycle

The cardiac cycle refers to the repeating pattern of contraction and relaxation of the heart. The contraction phase is called **systole** and the relaxation period is called **diastole.** Generally, when these terms are used alone, they refer to contraction and relaxation of the ventricles. However, note that the atria also contract and relax; therefore, there is an atrial systole and diastole. Atrial contraction occurs during ventricular diastole and atrial relaxation occurs during ventricular systole. The heart thus has a two-step pumping action. The right and left atria contract together, which empties atrial blood into the ventricles. Approximately 0.1 seconds after the atrial contraction, the ventricles contract and deliver blood into both the systemic and pulmonary circuits.

Systole | Diastole | Rest
Heart rate = 75 beats/min

0.3 seconds | 0.5 seconds

Systole | Diastole | Heavy exercise
Heart rate = 180 beats/min

0.2 seconds | 0.13 seconds

Figure 9.3

Increases in heart rate during exercise are achieved primarily through a decrease in the time spent in diastole; however, at high heart rates, the length of time spent in systole also decreases.

At rest, contraction of the ventricles during systole ejects about two-thirds of the blood in the ventricles, leaving about one-third in the ventricles. The ventricles then fill with blood during the next diastole. A healthy twenty-one-year-old female might have an average resting heart rate of 75 beats per minute. This means that the total cardiac cycle lasts 0.8 seconds, with 0.5 seconds spent in diastole and the remaining 0.3 seconds dedicated to systole (26) (see figure 9.3). If the heart rate increases from 75 beats per minute to 180 beats per minute (e.g., heavy exercise), there is a reduction in the time spent in both systole and diastole (16, 20). This point is illustrated in figure 9.3. Note that a rising heart rate results in a greater time reduction in diastole, while systole is less affected.

Pressure Changes During the Cardiac Cycle

During the cardiac cycle, the pressure within the heart chambers rises and falls. When the atria are relaxed, blood flows into them from the venous circulation. As these chambers fill, the pressure inside gradually increases. Approximately 70% of the blood entering the atria during diastole flows directly into the ventricles through the atrioventricular valves before the atria contract. Upon atrial contraction, atrial pressure rises and forces most of the remaining 30% of the atrial blood into the ventricles.

Pressure in the ventricles is low while they are filling, but when the atria contract, the ventricular pressure increases slightly. Then as the ventricles contract, the pressure rises sharply, which closes the atrioventricular valves and prevents backflow into the atria. As soon as ventricular pressure exceeds the pressure of the pulmonary artery and the aorta, the pulmonary and aortic valves open and blood is forced into both pulmonary and systemic circulations. Figure 9.4 illustrates the changes in ventricular pressure as a function of time during the resting cardiac cycle. Note the occurrence of two heart sounds that are produced by the closing of the atrioventricular valves (first heart sound) and the closing of the aortic and pulmonary valves (second heart sound).

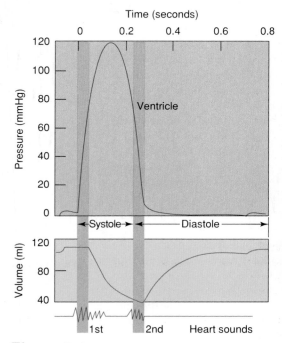

Figure 9.4

Relationship between pressure, volume, and heart sounds during the cardiac cycle. Notice the change in ventricular pressure and volume during the transition from systole to diastole.

Arterial Blood Pressure

Blood exerts pressure throughout the vascular system, but is greatest within the arteries where it is generally measured and used as an indication of health. Blood pressure is the force exerted by blood against the arterial walls and is determined by how much blood is pumped and the resistance to blood flow. The factors that regulate blood pressure will be discussed later in A Closer Look 9.2.

Arterial blood pressure can be estimated by use of a sphygmomanometer (see A Closer Look 9.1). The normal blood pressure of an adult male is 120/80, while that of adult females tends to be lower (110/70). The larger number in the expression of blood pressure is the systolic pressure expressed in millimeters of mercury (mm Hg). The lower number in the blood pressure ratio

A Closer Look 9.1

Measurement of Arterial Blood Pressure

Arterial blood pressure is not usually measured directly but is estimated using an instrument called a sphygmomanometer (see figure 9.5). This device consists of an inflatable arm cuff connected to a column of mercury. The cuff can be inflated by a bulb pump, with the pressure in the cuff measured by the rising column of mercury. For example, a pressure of 100 mm of mercury (mm Hg) would be enough force to raise the column of mercury upward a distance of 100 mm.

Blood pressure is measured in the following way. The rubber cuff is placed around the upper arm so it surrounds the brachial artery. Air is pumped into the cuff so that the pressure around the arm exceeds arterial pressure. Since the pressure applied around the arm is greater than arterial pressure, the brachial artery is squeezed shut and blood flow is stopped. If a stethoscope is placed over the brachial artery (just below the cuff), no sounds are heard since there is no blood flow. However, if the air control valve is slowly opened to release air, the pressure in the cuff begins to decline and soon the pressure around the arm reaches a point that is equal to or just slightly below arterial pressure. At this point blood begins to spurt through the artery and a sharp sound can be heard through the stethoscope. The pressure (i.e.,

height of mercury column) at which the first tapping sound is heard represents systolic blood pressure.

As the cuff pressure continues to decline, a series of increasingly louder sounds can be heard. When the pressure in the cuff is equal to or slightly below diastolic blood pressure, the sounds heard through the stethoscope cease. Therefore, resting diastolic blood pressure represents the height of the mercury column when the sounds disappear.

Figure 9.5
A sphygmomanometer is used to measure arterial blood pressure.

is the diastolic pressure again expressed in mm Hg. **Systolic blood pressure** is the pressure generated as blood is ejected from the heart during ventricular systole. During ventricular relaxation (diastole), the arterial blood pressure decreases and represents **diastolic blood pressure.** The difference between systolic and diastolic blood pressure is called the *pulse pressure*.

The average pressure during a cardiac cycle is called *mean arterial pressure*. Mean arterial blood pressure is important because it determines the rate of blood flow through the systemic circuit.

Determination of mean arterial pressure is not easy. It is not a simple average of systolic and diastolic pressure since diastole generally lasts longer than systole. However, mean arterial pressure can be estimated in the following way:

Mean arterial pressure = DBP + .33 (pulse pressure)

Here DBP is the diastolic blood pressure, and the pulse pressure is the difference between systolic and diastolic pressures. Let's consider a sample calculation of mean arterial pressure at rest.

Factors That Influence Arterial Blood Pressure

Mean arterial blood pressure (MAP) is the product of cardiac output and total vascular resistance. Therefore, an increase in either cardiac output or vascular resistance results in an increase in MAP. In the body, MAP depends on a variety of physiological factors, including cardiac output, blood volume, resistance to flow, and blood viscosity. These relationships are summarized in figure 9.6. An increase in any of the above variables results in an increase in arterial blood pressure. Conversely, a decrease in any of the above variables causes a decrease in blood pressure.

How is blood pressure regulated? Acute (short-term) regulation of blood pressure is achieved by the sympathetic nervous system, while long-term regulation of blood pressure is primarily a function of the kidneys (7). The kidneys regulate blood pressure by their control of blood volume.

Pressure receptors (called baroreceptors) in the carotid artery and the aorta are sensitive to changes in arterial blood pressure.

An increase in arterial pressure triggers these receptors to send impulses to the cardiovascular control center, which responds by decreasing sympathetic activity. A reduction in sympathetic activity may lower cardiac output and/or reduce vascular resistance, which in turn lowers blood pressure. Conversely, a decrease in blood pressure results in a reduction of baroreceptor activity to the brain. This causes the cardiovascular control center to respond by increasing sympathetic outflow, which raises blood pressure back to normal. For a complete discussion of blood-pressure regulation, see Cowley (7) and Rowell (48).

Figure 9.6
Some factors that influence arterial blood pressure.

For example, suppose an individual has a blood pressure of 120/80 mm Hg. The mean arterial pressure would be:

Mean arterial pressure = 80 mm Hg + .33(120−80)
= 80 mm Hg + 13
= 93 mm Hg

Approximately 20% of all adults in the United States have hypertension, which is defined as blood pressure in excess of the normal range for the person's age and sex (16). Blood pressures above 140/90 are considered to be indicators of hypertension (16, 20). Hypertension is generally classified into one or two categories: (1) primary, or essential hypertension, and (2) secondary hypertension. The cause of primary hypertension is unknown. This type of hypertension constitutes 90% of all reported cases of hypertension in the United States. Secondary hypertension is a result of some known disease process and thus the hypertension is "secondary" to another

disease. A Closer Look 9.2 discusses those factors that influence arterial blood pressure.

Electrical Activity of the Heart

Many myocardial cells have the unique potential for spontaneous electrical activity (i.e., each has an intrinsic rhythm). However, in the normal heart, spontaneous electrical activity is limited to a special region located in the right atrium. This region, called the **sinoatrial node (SA node),** serves as the pacemaker for the heart (see figure 9.7). Spontaneous electrical activity in the SA node occurs due to a decay of the resting membrane potential via inward diffusion of sodium during diastole. When the SA node reaches the depolarization threshold and "fires," the wave of depolarization spreads over the atria resulting in atrial contraction. The wave of atrial depolarization cannot directly cross into the ventricles but must be transported by way of specialized conductive tissue. This specialized conductive tissue radiates from a small

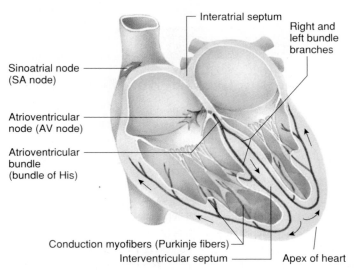

Figure 9.7

Conduction system of the heart.

A Closer Look 9.3

Diagnostic Use of the ECG During Exercise

Cardiologists are physicians who specialize in diseases of the heart and vascular system. One of the diagnostic procedures commonly used to evaluate cardiac function is to make ECG measurements during an incremental exercise test (usually on a treadmill). This allows the physician to observe changes in blood pressure as well as changes in the patient's ECG during periods of stress.

The most common cause of heart disease is the collection of fatty plaque (called atherosclerosis) inside coronary vessels. This collection of plaque reduces blood flow to the myocardium. The adequacy of blood flow to the heart is relative—it depends on the metabolic demand placed on the heart. An obstruction to a coronary artery, for example, may allow sufficient blood flow at rest, but may be inadequate

during exercise due to increased metabolic demand placed on the heart. Therefore, a graded exercise test may serve as a "stress test" to evaluate cardiac function.

An example of an abnormal exercise ECG is illustrated in figure 9.8. Myocardial ischemia (reduced blood flow) may be detected by

changes in the ST segment of the ECG. Notice the depressed ST segment in the picture on the right when compared to the normal ECG on the left. This ST segment depression suggests to the physician that ischemic heart disease may be present and that additional diagnostic procedures may be warranted.

Normal   Ischemia

Figure 9.8

Depression of the S-T segment of the electrocardiogram as a result of myocardial ischemia.

mass of muscle tissue called the **atrioventricular node (AV node).** This node, located in the floor of the right atrium, connects the atria with the ventricles by a pair of conductive pathways called the right and left bundle branches (figure 9.7). Upon reaching the ventricles, these conductive pathways branch into smaller fibers called Purkinje fibers. The Purkinje fibers then spread the wave of depolarization throughout the ventricles.

A recording of the electrical changes that occur in the myocardium during the cardiac cycle is called an **electrocardiogram (ECG).** Analysis of ECG waveforms allows the physician to evaluate the heart's ability to conduct impulses and therefore determine if electrical problems exist. Further, analysis of the ECG during exercise is often used in the diagnosis of coronary artery disease (see A Closer Look 9.3). Figure 9.9 illustrates a

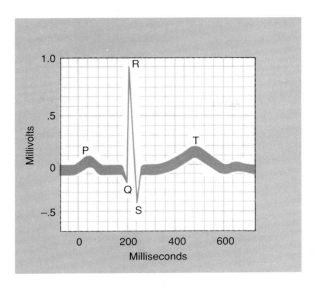

Figure 9.9
The normal electrocardiogram during rest.

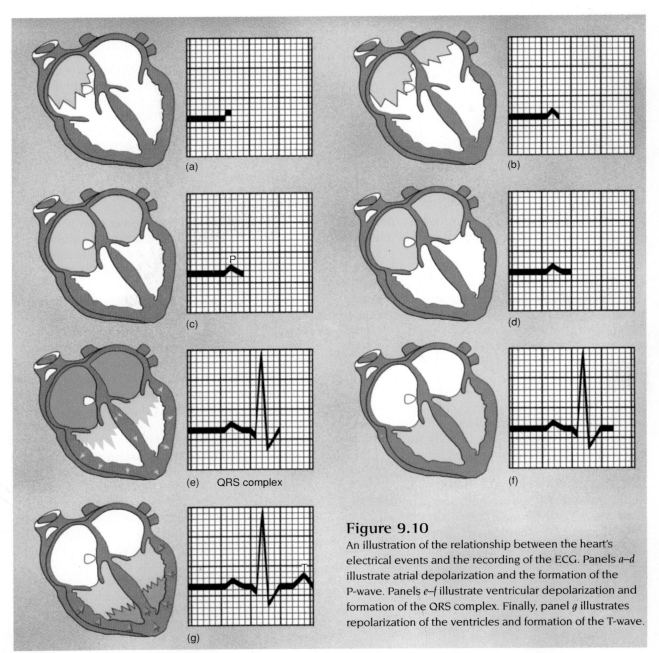

(a)

(b)

(c)

(d)

(e)   QRS complex

(f)

(g)

Figure 9.10
An illustration of the relationship between the heart's electrical events and the recording of the ECG. Panels *a–d* illustrate atrial depolarization and the formation of the P-wave. Panels *e–f* illustrate ventricular depolarization and formation of the QRS complex. Finally, panel *g* illustrates repolarization of the ventricles and formation of the T-wave.

normal ECG pattern. Notice that the ECG pattern contains several different deflections, or waves, during each cardiac cycle. Each of these distinct waveforms is identified by different letters. The P wave results from the depolarization of the atria, the QRS complex results from ventricular depolarization, and the T wave is due to ventricular repolarization. A step-by-step illustration of an ECG recording is given in figure 9.9. Note the formation of each new wave as a result of electrical activity in the heart.

in summary

- The contraction phase of the cardiac cycle is called systole and the relaxation period is called diastole.
- The pacemaker of the heart is the SA node.
- The average blood pressure during a cardiac cycle is called mean arterial blood pressure.
- Blood pressure can be increased by one or all of the following factors:
  a) increase in blood volume,
  b) increase in heart rate,
  c) increased blood viscosity,
  d) increase in stroke volume, and/or
  e) increased peripheral resistance.
- A recording of the electrical activity of the heart during the cardiac cycle is called the electrocardiogram (ECG).

Cardiac Output

Cardiac output ($\dot{Q}$) is the product of the heart rate (HR) and the **stroke volume** (SV) (amount of blood pumped per heartbeat):

$$\dot{Q} = HR \times SV$$

Thus, cardiac output can be increased due to a rise in either heart rate or stroke volume. During exercise in the upright position (e.g., running, cycling, etc.) the increase in cardiac output is due to both an increase in heart rate and stroke volume. Table 9.1 presents typical values at rest and during maximal exercise for heart rate, stroke volume, and cardiac output in both untrained and highly trained endurance athletes. The gender differences in stroke volume and cardiac output are due mainly to differences in body sizes between men and women (3) (see table 9.1).

Regulation of Heart Rate

During exercise the quantity of blood pumped by the heart must change in accordance with the elevated skeletal muscle oxygen demand. Since the SA node controls heart rate, changes in heart rate often involve factors that influence the SA node. The two most prominent factors that influence heart rate are the parasympathetic and sympathetic nervous systems (25, 44, 52, 58a).

The parasympathetic fibers that supply the heart arise from neurons in the **cardiovascular control center** in the medulla oblongata and make up a portion of the **vagus nerve.** Upon reaching the heart, these fibers make contact with both the SA node and the AV node (see figure 9.11). When stimulated, these nerve endings release acetylcholine, which causes a decrease in the activity of both the SA and AV nodes due to hyperpolarization (i.e., moving the resting membrane potential further from threshold). The end result is a reduction of heart rate. Therefore, the parasympathetic nervous system acts as a braking system to slow down heart rate.

Even at rest, the vagus nerves carry impulses to the SA and AV nodes (16, 20, 38). This is often referred to as *parasympathetic tone*. As a consequence, parasympathetic activity can cause heart rate to increase or decrease. For instance, a decrease in parasympathetic tone to the heart can elevate heart rate, while an increase in parasympathetic activity causes a slowing of heart rate.

Studies have shown that the initial increase in heart rate during exercise, up to approximately 100 beats per minute, is due to a withdrawal of parasympathetic tone (48). At higher work rates, stimulation of the SA and AV nodes by the sympathetic nervous system is responsible for increases in heart rate (48). Sympathetic fibers reach the heart by means of the **cardiac accelerator nerves,** which innervate both the SA node and the ventricles (figure 9.11). Endings of these fibers release norepinephrine upon stimulation, which causes an increase in both heart rate and the force of myocardial contraction.

At rest, a normal balance between parasympathetic tone and sympathetic activity to the heart is maintained by the cardiovascular control center in the medulla oblongata. The cardiovascular control center receives impulses from various parts of the circulatory system relative to changes in important parameters (e.g., blood pressure, blood oxygen tension, etc.), and relays motor impulses to the heart in response to a changing cardiovascular need. For example, an increase in resting blood pressure above normal stimulates pressure receptors in the carotid arteries and the arch of the aorta, which in turn send impulses to the cardiovascular control center (figure 9.11). In response, the cardiovascular control center increases parasympathetic activity to the heart to slow the heart rate and reduce cardiac output. This reduction in cardiac output causes blood pressure to decline back toward normal.

Another regulatory reflex involves pressure receptors located in the right atrium. In this case, an increase in right atrial pressure signals the cardiovascular control center that an increase in venous return has occurred; hence, in order to prevent a backup of blood in the systemic venous system, an increase in cardiac output must result. The cardiovascular control center responds by sending sympathetic accelerator nerve impulses to the heart, which increases heart rate and

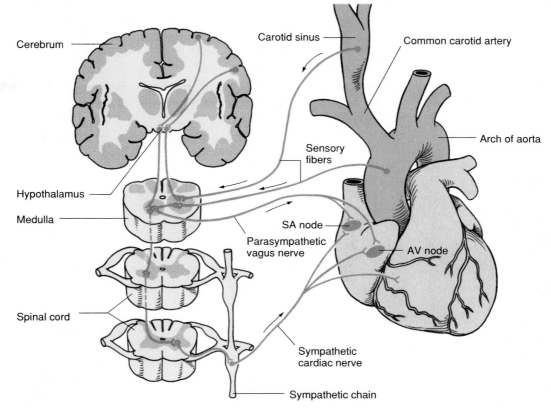

Figure 9.11
The activities of the SA and AV nodes can be altered by both the sympathetic and parasympathetic nervous systems.

Table 9.1	Typical Resting and Maximal Exercise Values for Stroke Volume (SV), Heart Rate (HR), and Cardiac Output ($\dot{Q}$) for College-age Untrained Subjects and Trained Endurance Athletes. (Body Weights for Males are 70 kg and 50 kg for Females.)					
Subject	HR (beat/min)		SV (ml/beat)		$\dot{Q}$ (l/min)	
Rest						
Untrained Male	72	×	70	=	5.00	
Untrained Female	75	×	60	=	4.50	
Trained Male	50	×	100	=	5.00	
Trained Female	55	×	80	=	4.50	
Max Exercise						
Untrained Male	200	×	110	=	22.0	
Untrained Female	200	×	90	=	18.0	
Trained Male	190	×	180	=	34.2	
Trained Female	190	×	125	=	23.9	

Note that values are rounded off. Data from references 3, 16, and 48.

cardiac output. The end result is that the increase in cardiac output lowers right atrial pressure back to normal and venous blood pressure is reduced.

Finally, a change in body temperature can influence heart rate. An increase in body temperature above normal results in an increase in heart rate, while a lowering of body temperature below normal causes a reduction in heart rate (6, 16, 20, 31, 48, 50, 51). This topic will be discussed later in chapter 12.

Regulation of Stroke Volume
Stroke volume, at rest or during exercise, is regulated by three variables: (1) the end-diastolic volume (EDV), which is the volume of blood in the ventricles at the

end of diastole; (2) the average aortic blood pressure; and (3) the strength of ventricular contraction.

EDV is often referred to as "preload" and influences stroke volume in the following way. Two physiologists, Frank and Starling, demonstrated that the strength of ventricular contraction was increased with an enlargement of EDV (i.e., stretch of the ventricles). This relationship has become known as the Frank-Starling law of the heart. The increase in EDV results in a lengthening of cardiac fibers, which improves the force of contraction in a manner similar to that seen in skeletal muscle (chapter 8). A rise in cardiac contractility results in an increase in the amount of blood pumped per beat. The principal variable that influences EDV is the rate of venous return to the heart. An increase in venous return results in a rise in EDV and therefore an increase in stroke volume. Increased venous return and the resulting increase in EDV plays a key role in the increase in stroke volume observed during upright exercise (20).

What factors regulate venous return during exercise? There are three principal mechanisms for increasing venous return during exercise: (1) constriction of the veins (venoconstriction), (2) pumping action of contracting skeletal muscle (muscle pump), and (3) pumping action of the respiratory system (respiratory pump).

1. *Venoconstriction*. Venoconstriction increases venous return by reducing the volume capacity of the veins to store blood. The end result of a reduced volume capacity in veins is to move blood back toward the heart. Venoconstriction occurs via a reflex sympathetic constriction of smooth muscle in veins draining skeletal muscle, which is controlled by the cardiovascular control center (3, 20, 37a, 48).

2. *Muscle pump*. The muscle pump is a result of the mechanical action of rhythmic skeletal muscle contractions. As muscles contract, they compress veins and push blood back toward the heart. Between contractions, blood refills the veins and the process is repeated. Blood is prevented from flowing away from the heart between contractions by one-way valves located in large veins (see figure 9.12). During sustained muscular contractions (isometric exercise), the muscle pump cannot operate and venous return is reduced.

3. *Respiratory pump*. The rhythmic pattern of breathing also provides a mechanical pump by which venous return is promoted. The respiratory pump works in the following way. During inspiration, the pressure within the thorax (chest) decreases and abdominal pressure increases. This creates a flow of venous blood from the abdominal region into the thorax and therefore promotes venous return. Although quiet breathing (rest) aids in

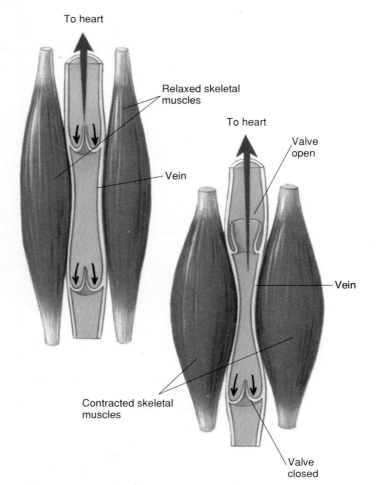

Figure 9.12
The action of the one-way venous valves. Contraction of skeletal muscles helps to pump blood toward the heart, but is prevented from pushing blood away from the heart by closure of the venous valves.

venous return, the role of the respiratory pump is enhanced during exercise due to the greater respiratory rate and depth.

A second variable that affects stroke volume is the aortic pressure (mean arterial pressure). In order to eject blood, the pressure generated by the left ventricle must exceed the pressure in the aorta. Therefore, aortic pressure or mean arterial pressure (called afterload) represents a barrier to the ejection of blood from the ventricles. Stroke volume is thus inversely proportional to the afterload; that is, an increase in aortic pressure produces a decrease in stroke volume. However, it is noteworthy that afterload is minimized during exercise due to arteriole dilation. This arteriole dilation in the working muscles reduces afterload and makes it easier for the heart to pump a large volume of blood.

The final factor that influences stroke volume is the effect of circulating epinephrine/norepinephrine and direct sympathetic stimulation of the heart by

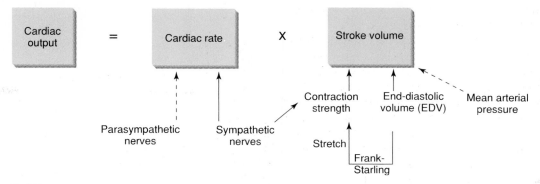

Figure 9.13
Factors that regulate cardiac output. Variables that stimulate cardiac output are shown by solid arrows, while factors that reduce cardiac output are shown by dotted arrows.

cardiac accelerator nerves. Both of these mechanisms increase cardiac contractility by increasing the amount of calcium available to the myocardial cell (16, 20, 48).

in summary

- Cardiac output is the product of heart rate and stroke volume ($\dot{Q} = HR \times SV$). Figure 9.13 summarizes those variables that influence cardiac output during exercise.
- The pacemaker of the heart is the SA node. SA node activity is modified by the parasympathetic nervous system (slows HR) and the sympathetic nervous system (increases HR).
- Heart rate increases at the beginning of exercise due to a withdrawal of parasympathetic tone. At higher work rates the increase in heart rate is achieved via an increased sympathetic outflow to the SA nodes.
- Stroke volume is regulated via: (1) end-diastolic volume, (2) aortic blood pressure, and (3) the strength of ventricular contraction.
- Venous return increases during exercise due to: (1) venoconstriction, (2) the muscle pump, and (3) the respiratory pump.

Hemodynamics

One of the most important features of the circulatory system to remember is that the system is a continuous "closed loop." Blood flow through the circulatory system results from pressure differences between the two ends of the system. In order to understand the physical regulation of blood flow to tissues, it is necessary to appreciate the interrelationships between pressure, flow, and resistance. The study of these factors and the physical principles of blood flow is called *hemodynamics*.

Physical Characteristics of Blood

Blood is composed of two principle components: (1) plasma and (2) cells. Plasma is the "watery" portion of blood that contains numerous ions, proteins, and hormones. The cells that make up blood are red blood cells (RBCs), platelets, and white blood cells. Red blood cells contain hemoglobin used for the transport of oxygen (see chapter 10). Platelets play an important role in blood clotting, and white blood cells are important in preventing infection.

The percent of the blood that is composed of cells is called the *hematocrit*. That is, if 42% of the blood is cells and the remainder is plasma, the hematocrit is 42% (see figure 9.14). On a percentage basis, RBCs constitute the largest fraction of cells found in blood. Therefore, the hematocrit is principally influenced by increases or decreases in RBC numbers. The average hematocrit of a normal college-age male is 42%, while the hematocrit of a normal college-age female averages approximately 38%. These values vary between individuals and are dependent on a number of variables.

Blood is several times more viscous than water, and this viscosity increases the difficulty with which blood flows through the circulatory system. One of the major contributors to viscosity is the concentration of RBCs found in the blood. Therefore, during periods of anemia (decreased RBCs), the viscosity of blood is lowered. Conversely, an increase in hematocrit results in an elevation in blood viscosity. The potential influence of changing blood viscosity on performance will be discussed in chapter 25.

Relationships Between Pressure, Resistance, and Flow

As mentioned earlier, blood flow through the vascular system depends in part on the difference in pressure at the two ends of the system. If the pressure at the two ends of the vessel are equal, there will be no flow. In contrast, if the pressure is higher at one end of the vessel than the other, blood will flow from the region of higher pressure to the region of lower pressure. The

Figure 9.14

Blood cells become packed at the bottom of the test tube when blood is centrifuged; this leaves the plasma at the top of the tube. The percent of whole blood comprised of blood cells is termed the hematocrit.

Figure 9.15

The flow of blood through the systemic circuit is dependent on the pressure difference (ΔP) between the aorta and the right atrium. In this illustration, the mean pressure in the aorta is 100 mm Hg, while the pressure in the right atrium is 0 mm Hg. Therefore, the "driving" pressure across the circuit is 100 mm Hg (100 − 0 = 100).

rate of flow is proportional to the pressure difference ($P_1 - P_2$) between the two ends of the tube. Figure 9.15 illustrates the "pressure head" driving blood flow in the systemic circulatory system under resting conditions. Here the mean arterial pressure is 100 mm Hg (i.e., this is the pressure of blood in the aorta), while the pressure at the opposite end of the circuit (i.e., pressure in the right atrium) is 0 mm Hg. Therefore, the driving pressure across the circulatory system is 100 mm Hg (100 − 0 = 100).

It should be pointed out that the flow rate of blood through the vascular system is proportional to the pressure difference across the system, but is inversely proportional to the resistance. Inverse proportionality is expressed mathematically by the placement of this variable in the denominator of a fraction, since a fraction decreases when the denominator increases.

Therefore, the relationship between blood flow, pressure, and resistance is given by the equation:

$$\text{Blood flow} = \frac{\Delta \text{ Pressure}}{\text{Resistance}}$$

where Δ pressure means the difference in pressure between the two ends of the circulatory system. Notice that blood flow can be increased by either an increase in blood pressure or a decrease in resistance. A five-fold increase in blood flow could be generated by increasing pressure by a factor of five; however, this large increase in blood pressure would be hazardous to health. Fortunately, increases in blood flow during exercise are achieved primarily by a decrease in resistance with a small rise in blood pressure.

What factors contribute to the resistance of blood flow? Resistance to flow is directly proportional to the length of the vessel and the viscosity of blood. However, the most important variable determining vascular resistance is the diameter of the blood vessel, since vascular resistance is inversely proportional to the fourth power of the radius of the vessel:

$$\text{Resistance} = \frac{\text{Length} \times \text{viscosity}}{\text{Radius}^4}$$

In other words, an increase in either vessel length or blood viscosity results in a proportional increase in resistance. However, reducing the radius of a blood vessel by one-half would increase resistance sixteen-fold (i.e., $2^4 = 16$)!

Sources of Vascular Resistance

Under ordinary circumstances, the viscosity of blood and the length of the blood vessels are not manipulated in normal physiology. Therefore, the primary factor regulating blood flow through organs must be the radius of the blood vessel. Since the effect of changes in radius on changes in flow rate are magnified by a

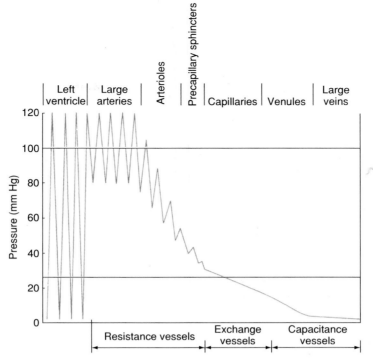

Figure 9.16

Pressure changes across the systemic circulation. Notice the large pressure drop across the arterioles.

power of four, blood can be diverted from one organ system to another by varying degrees of vasoconstriction and vasodilation. This principle is used during heavy exercise to divert blood toward contracting skeletal muscle and away from less-active tissue. This concept will be discussed in detail in the next section.

The greatest vascular resistance in blood flow occurs in arterioles. This point is illustrated in figure 9.16. Note the large drop in arterial pressure that occurs across the arterioles; approximately 70%–80% of the decline in mean arterial pressure occurs across the arterioles.

in summary

- Blood is composed of two principal components: (1) plasma and (2) cells.
- Blood flow through the vascular system is directly proportional to the pressure at the two ends of the system and inversely proportional to resistance:

$$\text{Blood flow} = \frac{\Delta \text{ Pressure}}{\text{Resistance}}$$

- The most important factor determining resistance to blood flow is the radius of the blood vessel. The relationship between vessel radius, vessel length, blood viscosity, and flow is:

$$\text{Resistance} = \frac{\text{Length} \times \text{viscosity}}{\text{Radius}^4}$$

- The greatest vascular resistance to blood flow is offered in the arterioles.

Changes in Oxygen Delivery to Muscle During Exercise

During intense exercise, the metabolic need for oxygen in skeletal muscle increases many times over the resting value (3). In order to meet this rise in oxygen demand, blood flow to the contracting muscle must increase. As mentioned earlier, increased oxygen delivery to exercising skeletal muscle is accomplished via two mechanisms: (1) an increased cardiac output and (2) a redistribution of blood flow from inactive organs to the working skeletal muscle.

Changes in Cardiac Output During Exercise

Cardiac output increases during exercise in direct proportion to the metabolic rate required to perform the exercise task. This is pointed out in figure 9.17. Note that the relationship between cardiac output and percent maximal oxygen uptake is essentially linear. The increase in cardiac output during exercise in the upright position is achieved by both an increase in stroke volume and heart rate. However, note that in untrained or moderately trained subjects, stroke volume does not increase beyond a work load of approximately 40% of $\dot{V}O_2$ max (figure 9.17). Therefore, at work rates greater than 40% $\dot{V}O_2$ max, the rise in cardiac output in these individuals is achieved by increases in heart rate alone (3, 14, 18, 46, 60) (see Research Focus 9.1). The examples presented in

Research Focus 9.1

Stroke Volume Does Not Plateau in Endurance Athletes

It is widely accepted that during incremental exercise, stroke volume in active or untrained subjects reaches a plateau at a submaximal work rate (i.e., approximately 40% $\dot{V}O_2$ max). The physiological explanation for this plateau in stroke volume is that at high heart rates the time available for ventricular filling is decreased.

Therefore, diastole and end-diastolic volume decrease. However, new evidence suggests that during incremental work rates the stroke volume of endurance athletes (e.g., highly-trained distance runners) does not plateau but continues to increase to $\dot{V}O_2$ max (18a). What is the explanation for this observation? It appears

that compared to untrained subjects, endurance athletes have improved ventricular filling during heavy exercise due to increased venous return. This increase in end-diastolic volume results in an increased force of ventricular contraction (Frank-Starling law) and an increase in stroke volume.

Figure 9.17

Changes in blood pressure, stroke volume, cardiac output, heart rate, and the arterial-mixed venous oxygen difference as a function of relative work rates. See text for details.

figure 9.17 for maximal heart rate, stroke volume, and cardiac output are typical values for a 70-kg active (but not highly trained) college-age male. See table 9.1 for examples of maximal stroke volume and cardiac output for trained men and women.

Maximal cardiac output tends to decrease in a linear fashion in both men and women after thirty years of age (18, 21). This is primarily due to a decrease in maximal heart rate with age (18). For example, since cardiac output equals heart rate times stroke volume, any decrease in heart rate would result in a decrease in cardiac output. The decrease in maximal heart rate with age can be estimated by the following formula:

$$\text{Max HR} = 220 - \text{age (years)}$$

According to this formula, a twenty-year-old subject might have a maximal heart rate of 200 beats per minute (220 − 20 = 200), whereas a fifty-year-old would have a maximal heart rate of 170 beats per minute (220 − 50 = 170). However, this is only an estimate and values can be actually 20 beats · min^{-1} higher or lower.

Changes in Arterial–Mixed Venous O_2 Content During Exercise

Note in figure 9.17 the change in the arterial-mixed venous oxygen difference (a − $\bar{v}$ O_2 diff) that occurs during exercise. The a − $\bar{v}$ O_2 difference represents the amount of O_2 that is taken up from 100 ml of blood by the tissues during one trip around the systemic circuit. An increase in the a − $\bar{v}$ O_2 difference during exercise is due to an increase in the amount of O_2 taken up and used for the oxidative production of ATP by skeletal muscle. The relationship between cardiac output ($\dot{Q}$), a − $\bar{v}$ O_2 diff, and oxygen uptake is given by the Fick equation:

$$\dot{V}O_2 = \dot{Q} \times (a - \bar{v}O_2 \text{ diff})$$

Simply stated, the Fick equation says that $\dot{V}O_2$ is equal to the product of cardiac output and the a − $\bar{v}$ O_2 diff. This means that an increase in either cardiac output or a − $\bar{v}$ O_2 diff would elevate $\dot{V}O_2$.

Redistribution of Blood Flow During Exercise

In order to meet the increased oxygen demand of the skeletal muscles during exercise, it is necessary to increase muscle blood flow while at the same time reducing blood flow to less active organs such as the liver, kidneys, and GI tract. Figure 9.18 points out that the change in blood flow to muscle and the splanchnic (pertaining to the viscera) circulation is dictated by the exercise intensity (metabolic rate). That is, the increase in muscle blood flow during exercise and the decrease in splanchnic blood flow change as a linear function of $\% \dot{V}O_2$ max (46, 48).

Figure 9.19 illustrates the change in blood flow to various organ systems between resting conditions and during maximal exercise. Several important points need to be stressed. First, at rest, approximately 15%–20% of total cardiac output is directed toward skeletal muscle (3, 16, 48). However, during maximal exercise 80%–85% of total cardiac output goes to contracting skeletal muscle (34, 48, 56). This is necessary to meet the huge increase in muscle oxygen requirements during intense exercise. Second, notice that during heavy exercise the percent of total cardiac output that goes to the brain is reduced compared to rest. However, the absolute blood flow that reaches the brain is slightly increased above resting values; this is due to the elevated cardiac output during exercise (63). Further, although the percentage of total cardiac output that reaches the myocardium is the same during maximal exercise as it is at rest, the total coronary blood flow is increased due to the increase in cardiac output during heavy exercise. Finally, note the reduction in blood flow to the skin (58) and the abdominal organs that occurs during intense exercise when compared to resting conditions. This reduction in abdominal blood flow during heavy exercise is an important means of shifting blood flow away from "less active" tissues and toward the working skeletal muscles.

Regulation of Local Blood Flow During Exercise

What regulates blood flow to various organs during exercise? Muscle as well as other body tissues have the unique ability to regulate their own blood flow in direct proportion to their metabolic needs. Blood flow to skeletal muscle during exercise is regulated in the following way. First, the arterioles in skeletal muscle have a high vascular resistance at rest. This is due to adrenergic sympathetic stimulation, which causes arteriole smooth muscle to contract (vasoconstriction) (54). This produces a relatively low blood flow to muscle at rest (4–5 ml per minute per 100 grams of muscle), but because muscles have a large mass, this accounts for 20%–25% of total blood flow from the heart.

Figure 9.18

Changes in muscle and splanchnic blood flow as a function of exercise intensity. Notice the large increase in muscle blood flow as the work rate increases.

Data from L. Rowell, *Human Circulation Regulating During Physical Stress*. 1986: Oxford University Press, New York NY

Although controversy exists, it is speculated that at the beginning of exercise, the initial skeletal muscle vasodilation that occurs is due to a withdrawal of sympathetic outflow to arterioles in the working muscles. This initial vasodilation serves to "prime" the skeletal muscle for action. However, as the exercise progresses, vasodilation is maintained and increased by intrinsic metabolic control. This latter type of blood flow regulation is termed **autoregulation,** and is thought to be the most important factor in regulating blood flow to muscle during exercise. The high metabolic rate of skeletal muscle during exercise causes local changes such as decreases in oxygen tension, increases in CO_2 tension, nitric oxide, potassium and adenosine concentrations, and a decrease in pH (increase in acidity) (See Research Focus 9.2). These local changes work together to cause vasodilation of arterioles feeding the contracting skeletal muscle (18, 34, 39a, 56). Vasodilation reduces the vascular resistance and therefore increases blood flow. As a result of these changes, blood delivery to contracting skeletal muscle during heavy exercise may rise fifteen-to-twenty times above rest (3, 6, 16, 53). Further, arteriole vasodilation is combined with "recruitment" of capillaries in skeletal muscle. At rest, only 5%–10% of the capillaries in skeletal muscle are open at any one time; however, during intense exercise almost all of the capillaries in contracting muscle may be open (48).

While the vascular resistance in skeletal muscle decreases during exercise, vascular resistance to flow

Research Focus 9.2

Discovery of a New Vasodilator Substance: Nitric Oxide

Recent research has lead to the discovery of a new and important vasodilator called nitric oxide (see reference 39a for a review). Nitric oxide is produced in the endothelium of arterioles. After production, nitric oxide promotes smooth muscle relaxation in the arteriole which results in vasodilation and therefore causes an increase in blood flow. Current evidence suggests that ni-

tric oxide works in conjunction with other local factors in autoregulation of blood flow.

How important is nitric oxide in the autoregulation of muscle blood flow during exercise? At present, a definitive answer to this question is not available. Nonetheless, it seems likely that nitric oxide is one of several factors involved in regulation of muscle blood flow

during exercise. Current speculation is that muscular contraction results in increased production of nitric oxide which promotes vasodilation in those arterioles leading to the working muscle. Improving our understanding of the role of nitric oxide in the regulation of muscle blood flow is an exciting area for future research.

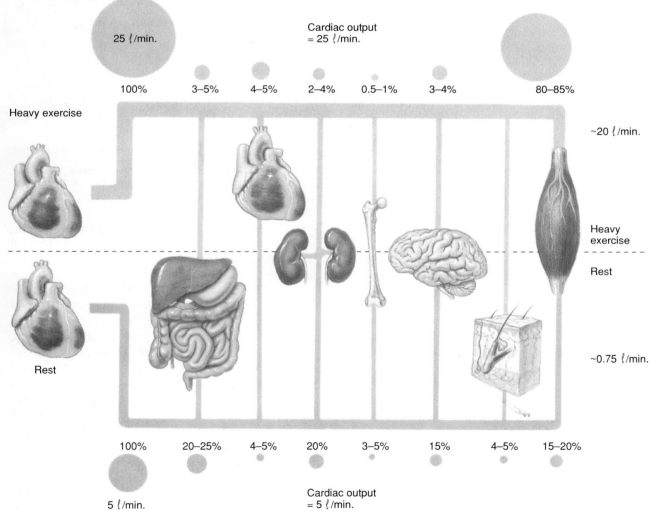

Figure 9.19

Distribution of cardiac output during rest and maximal exercise. At rest, the cardiac output is 5 ℓ/min (bottom of figure); during maximum exercise, the cardiac output increased five-fold to 25 ℓ/min. Note the large increases in blood flow to the skeletal muscle and the reduction in flow to the liver/GI tract.

From P. Astrand and K. Rodahl, *Textbook of Work Physiology*, 3d ed. Copyright © 1986 McGraw-Hill, Inc., New York. Reprinted by permission of the authors.

in the visceral organs increases. This occurs due to an increased adrenergic sympathetic output to these organs, which is regulated by the cardiovascular control center. As a result of the increase in visceral vasoconstriction during exercise (i.e., resistance increases), blood flow to the viscera may decrease to only 20%–30% of resting values (48, 50).

in summary

- Oxygen delivery to exercising skeletal muscle increases due to: (1) an increased cardiac output and (2) a redistribution of blood flow from inactive organs to the contracting skeletal muscles.
- Cardiac output increases as a linear function of oxygen uptake during exercise. During exercise in the upright position, stroke volume reaches a plateau at approximately 40% of $\dot{V}O_2$ max; therefore, at work rates above 40% $\dot{V}O_2$ max the rise in cardiac output is due to increases in heart rate alone.
- During exercise, blood flow to contracting muscle is increased and blood flow to less active tissues is reduced.
- Regulation of muscle blood flow during exercise is regulated by: (1) withdrawal of the sympathetic outflow and (2) autoregulation. Autoregulation refers to intrinsic control of blood flow by change in local metabolites (e.g., oxygen tension, pH, potassium, adenosine, and nitric oxide) around arterioles.

Circulatory Responses to Exercise

The changes in heart rate and blood pressure that occur during exercise reflect the type and intensity of exercise performed, the duration of exercise, and the environmental conditions under which the work was performed. For example, heart rate and blood pressure, at any given oxygen uptake, are higher during arm work when compared to leg work. Further, exercise in a hot/humid condition results in higher heart rates when compared to the same exercise in a cool environment. The next several sections discuss the cardiovascular responses to exercise under varying conditions.

Emotional Influence

Submaximal exercise in an emotionally charged atmosphere results in higher heart rates and blood pressures when compared to the same work in a psychologically "neutral" environment (3, 24, 55). This emotional elevation in heart rate and blood pressure response to exercise is mediated by an increase in sympathetic nervous system activity. If the exercise is maximal (e.g., 400-meter dash), high emotion elevates

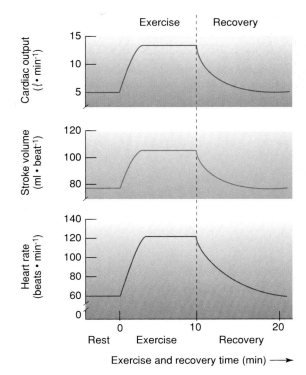

Figure 9.20

Changes in cardiac output, stroke volume, and heart rate during the transition from rest to submaximal constant intensity exercise and during recovery. See text for discussion.

Data from L. Rowell, 1974, "Human Cardiovascular Adjustments to Exercise and Thermal Stress" American Physiological Society, Bethesda MD: *Physiological Reviews*, 54:75–159; and L. Rowell, *Human Circulation Regulating During Physical Stress.* 1986: Oxford University Press, New York NY

the pre-exercise heart rate and blood pressure but does not generally alter the peak heart rate or blood pressure observed during the exercise itself.

Transition from Rest to Exercise

At the beginning of exercise there is a rapid increase in heart rate, stroke volume, and cardiac output. It has been demonstrated that heart rate and cardiac output begin to increase within the first second after muscular contraction begins (55) (see figure 9.20). If the work rate is constant and below the lactate threshold, a steady state plateau in heart rate, stroke volume, and cardiac output is reached within two to three minutes. This response is similar to that observed in oxygen uptake at the beginning of exercise (chapter 4).

Recovery from Exercise

Recovery from short-term, low-intensity exercise is generally rapid. This is illustrated in figure 9.20. Notice that heart rate, stroke volume, and cardiac output all decrease rapidly back toward resting levels following this type of exercise. Recovery speed varies from individual to individual, with well-conditioned subjects demonstrating better recuperative powers than untrained subjects. In

Table 9.2 — Changes in the Double Product (i.e., Heart Rate × Systolic Blood Pressure) During an Incremental Exercise Test in a Healthy 21-year Old Female Subject

Note that the double product is a dementionless term which reflects the relative changes in the work load placed on the heart during exercise and other forms of stress.

Condition	Heart Rate (beats · min⁻¹)	Systolic Blood Pressure (mm Hg)	Double Product
Rest	75	110	8,250
Exercise			
25% $\dot{V}O_2$ max	100	130	13,000
50% $\dot{V}O_2$ max	140	160	22,400
75% $\dot{V}O_2$ max	170	180	30,600
100% $\dot{V}O_2$ max	200	210	42,000

regard to recovery heart rates, the slopes of heart-rate decay following exercise are generally the same for trained and untrained subjects. However, trained subjects recover faster following exercise since they don't achieve as high a heart rate as untrained subjects during a particular exercise.

Recovery from long-term exercise is much slower than the response depicted in figure 9.20. This is particularly true when the exercise is performed in hot/humid conditions, since an elevated body temperature delays the fall in heart rate during recovery from exercise (51).

Incremental Exercise

The cardiovascular responses to dynamic incremental exercise are illustrated in figure 9.17. Heart rate and cardiac output increase in direct proportion to oxygen uptake. Further, blood flow to muscle increases as a function of oxygen uptake (figure 9.18). This ensures that as the need to synthesize ATP to supply the energy for muscular contraction increases, the supply of O_2 reaching the muscle rises. However, both cardiac output and heart rate reach a plateau at 100% $\dot{V}O_2$ max (figure 9.17). This point represents a maximal ceiling for oxygen transport to exercising skeletal muscles, and is thought to occur simultaneously with the attainment of maximal oxygen uptake.

The increase in cardiac output during incremental exercise is achieved via a decrease in vascular resistance to flow and an increase in mean arterial blood pressure. The elevation in mean arterial blood pressure during exercise is due to an increase in systolic pressure, since diastolic pressure remains fairly constant during incremental work (figure 9.17).

As mentioned earlier, the increase in heart and systolic blood pressure that occurs during exercise results in an increased work load on the heart. The increased metabolic demand placed on the heart during exercise can be estimated by examining the double product. The **double product** is computed by multiplying heart rate times systolic blood pressure:

Double product =
heart rate × systolic blood pressure

Table 9.2 contains an illustration of changes in the double product during an incremental exercise test. The take-home message in table 9.2 is simply that increases in exercise intensity result in an elevation in both heart rate and systolic blood pressure; each of these factors increases the work load placed on the heart.

Careful examination of table 9.2 reveals that the double product during exercise at $\dot{V}O_2$ max is five-times greater than the double product at rest. This implies that maximal exercise increases the work load on the heart by 500% over rest.

The practical application of the double product is that this measure can be used as a guideline to prescribe exercise for patients with coronary artery blockage. For example, suppose a patient develops chest pain (called angina pectoris) at a certain intensity of exercise due to myocardial ischemia at a double product of >30,000. Because chest pain appears at a double product of >30,000, the cardiologist or exercise physiologist would recommend that this patient perform types of exercise that result in a double product of < 30,000. This would reduce the risk of the patient developing chest pain due to a high metabolic demand on the heart.

Arm versus Leg Exercise

As mentioned earlier, at any given level of oxygen consumption, both heart rate and blood pressure are higher during arm work when compared to leg work (1, 2, 13, 32, 37, 45) (see figure 9.21). The explanation for the higher heart rate seems to be linked to a greater sympathetic outflow to the heart during arm work when compared to leg exercise (3). Additionally, isometric exercise also increases the heart rate above the expected value based on relative oxygen consumption (1, 2, 6, 28, 30, 32).

The relatively large increase in blood pressure for arm work is due to a vasoconstriction in the inactive muscle groups (3). For example, the larger the muscle group (e.g., legs) involved in performing the exercise, the more resistance vessels (arterioles) that are dilated. Therefore, this lower peripheral resistance is reflected in lower blood pressure (since cardiac output × resistance = pressure).

Figure 9.21

Comparison of mean arterial blood pressures and heart rate during submaximal rhythmic arm and leg exercise.

Intermittent Exercise

If exercise is discontinuous (e.g., interval training), the extent of the recovery of heart rate and blood pressure between bouts depends on the level of subject fitness, environmental conditions (temperature, humidity), and the duration and intensity of the exercise. With a relatively light effort in a cool environment, there is generally complete recovery between exercise bouts within several minutes. However, if the exercise is intense or the work is performed in a hot/humid environment, there is a cumulative increase in heart rate between efforts and thus recovery is not complete (53). The practical consequence of performing repeated bouts of light exercise is that many repetitions can be performed. In contrast, the nature of high-intensity exercise dictates that a limited number of efforts can be tolerated.

Prolonged Exercise

Figure 9.22 illustrates the change in heart rate, stroke volume, and cardiac output that occurs during prolonged exercise at a constant work rate. Note that cardiac output is maintained at a constant level throughout the duration of the exercise. However, stroke volume declines while heart rate increases (6, 10, 23, 31, 41, 50, 51, 53). Figure 9.22 demonstrates that the ability to maintain a constant cardiac output in the face of declining stroke volume is due to the increase in heart rate being equal in magnitude to the decline in stroke volume.

The increase in heart rate and decrease in stroke volume observed during prolonged exercise is often referred to as *cardiovascular drift* and is due to the influence of rising body temperature on cutaneous vasodilation and dehydration (reduction in plasma volume) (42, 48);

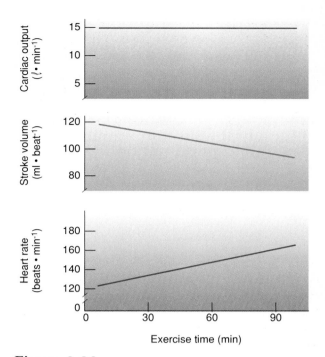

Figure 9.22

Changes in cardiac output, stroke volume, and heart rate during prolonged exercise at a constant intensity. Notice that cardiac output is maintained by an increase in heart rate to offset the fall in stroke volume that occurs during this type of work.

an increase in skin blood flow and a reduction in plasma volume act in concert to reduce venous return to the heart and therefore reduce stroke volume (see chapters 12 and 24). If prolonged exercise is performed in a hot/humid environment, the increase in heart rate and decrease in stroke volume is exaggerated even more than depicted in figure 9.22 (40, 43). In fact, it is not surprising to find near-maximal heart rates during submaximal exercise in the heat. For example, it has been demonstrated that during a 2.5-hour marathon race at a work rate of 70%–75% $\dot{V}O_2$ max, maximal heart rates may be maintained during the last hour of the race (15).

in summary

- The changes in heart rate and blood pressure that occur during exercise are a function of the type and intensity of exercise performed, the duration of exercise, and the environmental conditions.
- The increased metabolic demand placed on the heart during exercise can be estimated by examining the double product.
- At the same level of oxygen consumption, heart rate and blood pressure is greater during arm exercise compared to leg exercise.
- The increase in heart rate that occurs during prolonged exercise is called "cardiovascular drift."

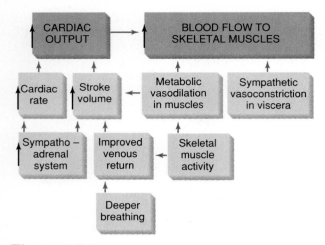

Figure 9.23
A summary of cardiovascular responses to exercise.

Figure 9.24
A summary of cardiovascular control during exercise. See text for discussion.

Regulation of Cardiovascular Adjustments to Exercise

The cardiovascular adjustments at the beginning of exercise are rapid. Within one second after the commencement of muscular contraction there is a withdrawal of vagal outflow to the heart, which is followed by an increase in sympathetic stimulation of the heart (48). At the same time there is a vasodilation of arterioles in active skeletal muscles and a reflex increase in the resistance of vessels in less active areas. The end result is an increase in cardiac output to ensure that blood flow to muscle matches the metabolic needs (see figure 9.23). What is the signal to "turn on" the cardiovascular system at the onset of exercise? This question has puzzled physiologists for nearly one hundred years (19). At present, a complete answer is not available. However, recent advances in understanding cardiovascular control has led to the development of the *central command theory* (8, 11, 12, 37, 57, 61a).

The term **central command** refers to a motor signal developed within the brain. The central command theory of cardiovascular control argues that the initial cardiovascular changes at the beginning of dynamic exercise (e.g., cycle ergometer exercise) are due to centrally generated cardiovascular motor signals, which set the general pattern of the cardiovascular response. However, it is believed that cardiovascular activity can be and is modified by heart mechanoreceptors, muscle chemoreceptors, muscle mechanoreceptors, and pressure-sensitive receptors (baroreceptors) located

within the carotid arteries and the aortic arch (22, 32a, 34a, 36, 49, 50a, 58a). Muscle chemoreceptors are sensitive to increases in muscle metabolites (e.g., potassium, lactic acid, etc.) and send messages to higher brain centers to "fine-tune" the cardiovascular responses to exercise (6, 17, 27–35, 39). This type of peripheral feedback to the cardiovascular control center (medulla oblongata) has been termed the *exercise pressor reflex* (9, 36).

Muscle mechanoreceptors (e.g., muscle spindles, Golgi tendon organs) are sensitive to the force and speed of muscular movement. These receptors, like muscle chemoreceptors, send information to higher brain centers to aid in modification of the cardiovascular responses to a given exercise task (47, 48, 61, 62).

Finally, baroreceptors, which are sensitive to changes in arterial blood pressure, may also send afferent information back to the cardiovascular control center to add precision to the cardiovascular activity during exercise. These pressure receptors are important since they regulate arterial blood pressure around an elevated systemic pressure during exercise (47, 48).

In review, the central command theory proposes that the initial signal to the cardiovascular system at the beginning of exercise comes from higher brain centers. However, fine-tuning of the cardiovascular response to a given exercise test is accomplished via a series of feedback loops from muscle chemoreceptors, muscle mechanoreceptors, and arterial baroreceptors (see figure 9.24). The fact that there appears to be some overlap between these three feedback systems during submaximal exercise suggests that redundancy in cardiovascular control exists (47, 48). This is not surprising considering the importance of matching blood flow to the metabolic needs of exercising skeletal muscle. Whether or not one or many of these feedback loops becomes more important during heavy exercise is not presently known and poses an interesting question for future research.

in summary

- The central command theory of cardiovascular control during exercise proposes that the initial signal to "drive" the cardiovascular system at the beginning of exercise comes from higher brain centers.
- Although central command is the primary drive to increase heart rate during exercise, the cardiovascular response to exercise is fine-tuned by feedback from muscle chemoreceptors, muscle mechanoreceptors, and arterial baroreceptors to the cardiovascular control center.

study questions

1. What are the major purposes of the cardiovascular system?
2. Briefly, outline the design of the heart. Why is the heart often called "two pumps in one?"
3. Outline the cardiac cycle and the associated electrical activity recorded via the electrocardiogram.
4. Graph the heart rate, stroke volume, and cardiac output response to incremental exercise.
5. What factors regulate heart rate during exercise? Stroke volume?
6. How does exercise influence venous return?
7. What factors determine local blood flow during exercise?
8. Graph the changes that occur in heart rate, stroke volume, and cardiac output during prolonged exercise. What happens to these variables if the exercise is performed in a hot/humid environment?
9. Compare heart rate and blood pressure responses to arm and leg work at the same oxygen uptake. What factors might explain the observed differences?
10. Explain the central command theory of cardiovascular regulation during exercise.

suggested readings

Gledhill, N. et al. 1994. Endurance athletes' stroke volume does not plateau: Major advantage is diastolic function. *Medicine and Science in Sports and Exercise* 26:1116–21.

Kjaer, M., and N. Secher. 1992. Neural influence on cardiovascular and endocrine responses to static exercise in humans. *Sports Medicine* 13:303–9.

Opie, L. 1991. *The Heart: Physiology and Metabolism*. New York: Raven Press.

Rowell, L. 1986. *Human Circulation Regulation during Physical Stress*. New York: Oxford University Press.

Rowell, L. 1992. Reflex control of the circulation during exercise. *International Journal of Sports Medicine* 13:(Suppl. 1) S25–S27.

Spyer, K. 1994. Central nervous mechanisms contributing to cardiovascular control. *Journal of Physiology* (London). 474:1–19.

references

1. Asmussen, E. 1981. Similarities and dissimilarities between static and dynamic exercise. *Circulation Research* 48 (Suppl. 1):3–10.
2. Åstrand, P. et al. 1965. Intra-arterial blood pressure during exercise with different muscle groups. *Journal of Applied Physiology* 20:253–57.
3. Åstrand, P., and K. Rodahl. 1986. *Textbook of Work Physiology*. New York: McGraw-Hill.
4. Bers, D. 1991. Calcium regulation in cardiac muscle. *Medicine and Science in Sports and Exercise* 23:1157–62.
5. Brady, A. 1991. Mechanical properties of isolated cardiac myocytes. *Physiological Reviews* 71:413–28.
6. Brengelmann, G. 1983. Circulatory adjustments to exercise and heat stress. *Annual Review of Physiology* 45:191–212.
7. Cowley, A. 1992. Long-term control of arterial blood pressure. *Physiological Reviews* 72:231–300.
8. Dormer, J., and H. L. Stone. 1982. Fastigial nucleus and its possible role in the cardiovascular response to exercise. In *Circulation, Neurobiology and Behavior*, ed. O. Smith, R. Galosy, and S. Weiss. New York: Elsevier.
9. Duncan, G., R. Johnson, and D. Lambie. 1981. Role of sensory nerves in the cardiovascular and respiratory changes with isometric forearm exercise in man. *Clinical Science* 60:145–55.
10. Ekelund, L., and A. Holmgren. 1964. Circulatory and respiratory adaptation during long-term, non-steady state exercise, in the sitting position. *Acta Physiologica Scandanavica* 62:240–55.

11. Eldridge, F., D. Milhorn, and T. Waldrop. 1981. Exercise hyperpnea and locomotion: Parallel activation from the hypothalamus. *Science* 211:844–46.

12. Eldridge, F. et al. 1985. Stimulation by central command of locomotion, respiration, and circulation during exercise. *Respiratory Physiology* 59:313–37.

13. Eston, R., and D. Brodie. 1986. Responses to arm and leg ergometry. *British Journal of Sports Medicine* 20:4–6.

14. Fox, E., R. Bowers, and M. Foss. 1993. *Physiological Basis of Physical Education and Athletics*. Dubuque, IA: Brown & Benchmark.

15. Fox, E., and D. Costill. 1972. Estimated cardiorespiratory responses during marathon running. *Archives of Environmental Health* 24:315–24.

16. Fox, S. 1993. *Human Physiology*. Dubuque, IA: Wm. C. Brown.

17. Freund, P., S. Hobbs, and L. Rowell. 1978. Cardiovascular responses to muscle ischemia in man—dependency on muscle mass. *Journal of Applied Physiology* 45:762–67.

18. Gerstenblith, G., D. Renlund, and E. Lakatta. 1987. Cardiovascular response to exercise in younger and older men. *Federation Proceedings* 46:1834–39.

18a. Gledhill, N. et al. 1994. Endurance athletes' stroke volume does not plateau: Major advantage is diastolic function. *Medicine and Science in Sports and Exercise* 26:1116–21.

19. Gorman, M., and H. Sparks. 1991. The unanswered question. *News in Physiological Sciences* 6:191–93.

20. Guyton, A. 1991. *Textbook of Medical Physiology*. Philadelphia: W. B. Saunders.

21. Hagberg, J. 1987. Effect of training on the decline of O_2 max with aging. *Federation Proceedings* 46:1830–33.

22. Hainsworth, R. 1991. Reflexes from the heart. *Physiological Reviews* 71:617–58.

23. Hartley, L. 1977. Central circulatory function during prolonged exercise. *Annals of New York Academy of Sciences* 301:189–94.

24. Herd, J. 1991. Cardiovascular response to stress. *Physiological Reviews* 71:305–30.

25. Hirst, G., F. Edwards, N. Bramich, and M. Klemm. 1991. Neural control of cardiac pacemaker potentials. *News in Physiological Sciences* 6:185–90.

26. Hole, J. 1993. *Human Anatomy and Physiology*. Dubuque, IA: Wm. C. Brown.

27. Johansson, B. 1962. Circulatory responses to stimulation of somatic afferents. *Acta Physiologica Scandanavica* (Suppl. 198):1–91.

28. Kaufman, M. et al. 1983. Effects of static muscular contraction on impulse activity of groups III and IV afferents in cats. *Journal of Applied Physiology* 55:105–12.

29. Kaufman, M. et al. 1984. Effect of ischemia on responses of group III and IV afferents to contraction. *Journal of Applied Physiology* 57:644–50.

30. Kaufman, M. et al. 1984. Effects of static and rhythmic twitch contractions on the discharge of group III and IV muscle afferents. *Cardiovascular Research* 18:663–68.

31. Kenny, W. L. 1988. Control of heat-induced cutaneous vasodilation in relation to age. *European Journal of Applied Physiology* 57:120–25.

32. Kilbom, A., and T. Brunkin. 1976. Circulatory effects of isometric muscle contractions, performed separately and in combination with dynamic exercise. *European Journal of Applied Physiology* 36:7–27.

32a. Kjaer, M., and N. Secher. 1992. Neural influence on cardiovascular and endocrine responses to static exercise in humans. *Sports Medicine* 13:303–9.

33. Kniffki, K., S. Mense, and R. Schmidt. 1981. Muscle receptors with fine afferent fibers which may evoke circulatory reflexes. *Circulation Research* 48 (Suppl. 1):25–31.

34. Laughlin, M. H., and R. Korthius. 1987. Control of muscle blood flow during sustained physiological exercise. *Canadian Journal of Applied Sports Sciences* 12 (Suppl.):775–835.

34a. Marshall, J. 1994. Peripheral chemoreceptors and cardiovacular regulation. *Physiological Reviews* 74:543–79.

35. McCloskey, D., and J. Mitchell. 1972. Reflex cardiovascular and respiratory responses originating in exercising muscle. *Journal of Physiology* (London) 224:173–86.

36. Mitchell, J. 1990. Neural control of the circulation during exercise. *Medicine and Science in Sports and Exercise* 22:141–54.

37. Mitchell, J. et al. 1980. The role of muscle mass in the cardiovascular response to static contraction. *Journal of Physiology* (London) 309:45–54.

37a. Monos, E., V. Berczi, and G. Nadasy. 1995. Local control of veins: Biomechanical, metabolic, and humoral aspects. *Physiological Reviews* 75:611–53.

38. Opie, L. 1991. *The Heart: Physiology and Metabolism*. New York: Raven Press.

39. Paterson, D., and A. Morton. 1986. Maximal aerobic power, ventilatory and respiratory compensation thresholds during arm cranking and bicycle ergometry. *Australian Journal of Science and Medicine in Sport* 18:11–15.

39a. Pearson, P., and P. Vanhoutte. 1993. Vasodilator and vascoconstrictor substances produced by the endothelium. *Review of Physiology, Biochemistry, and Pharmacology*. 122:2–37.

40. Powers, S., E. Howley, and R. Cox. 1982. A differential catecholamine response to prolonged exercise and passive heating. *Medicine and Science in Sports* 14:435–39.

41. ———. 1982. Ventilatory and metabolic responses to heat stress during prolonged exercise. *Journal of Sports Medicine and Physical Fitness* 22:32–36.

42. Raven, P., and G. Stevens. 1988. Cardiovascular function during prolonged exercise. In *Perspectives in Exercise Science and Sports Medicine: Prolonged Exercise*, ed. D. Lamb and R. Murray, 43–71. Indianapolis: Benchmark Press.

43. Ridge, B., and F. Pyke. 1986. Physiological responses to combinations of exercise and sauna. *Australian Journal of Science and Medicine in Sports* 18:25–28.

44. Rosen, M., E. Anyukhovsky, and S. Steinberg. 1991. Alpha-adrenergic modulation of cardiac rhythm. *News in Physiological Sciences* 6:135–38.

45. Rosiello, R., D. Mahler, and J. Ward. 1987. Cardiovascular responses to rowing. *Medicine and Science in Sports and Exercise* 19:239–45.

46. Rowell, L. 1974. Human cardiovascular adjustments to exercise and thermal stress. *Physiological Reviews* 54:75–159.

47. ———. 1980. What signals govern the cardiovascular response to exercise? *Medicine and Science in Sports and Exercise* 12:307–15.

48. ———. 1986. *Human Circulation Regulation during Physical Stress.* New York: Oxford University Press.

49. ———. 1992. Reflex control of the circulation during exercise. *International Journal of Sports Medicine* 13:(Suppl. 1) S25–S27.

50. Rowell, L., L. Hermansen, and J. Blackmon. 1976. Human cardiovascular and respiratory responses to graded muscle ischemia. *Journal of Applied Physiology* 41:693–701.

50a. Rowell, L., and D. O'Leary. 1990. Reflex control of the circulation during exercise: Chemoreflexes and mechanoreflexes. *Journal of Applied Physiology* 69:407–18.

51. Rubin, S. 1987. Core temperature regulation of heart rate during exercise in humans. *Journal of Applied Physiology* 62:1997–2002.

52. Saul, J. 1990. Beat-to-beat variations of heart rate reflect modulation of cardiac autonomic outflow. *News in Physiological Sciences* 5:32–37.

53. Sawka, M., R. Knowlton, and J. Critz. 1979. Thermal and circulatory responses to repeated bouts of prolonged running. *Medicine and Science in Sports* 11:177–80.

54. Seals, D., and R. Victor. 1991. Regulation of muscle sympathetic nerve activity during exercise in humans. In *Exercise and Sport Science Reviews*, ed. J. Holloszy, 313–50. Baltimore: Williams & Wilkins.

55. Shephard, R. 1981. *Physiology and Biochemistry of Exercise.* New York: Praeger.

56. Sjogaard, G., G. Sauard, and C. Juel. 1988. Muscle blood flow during isometric activity and its relation to muscle fatigue. *European Journal of Applied Physiology* 57:327–35.

57. Smith, O., R. Rushmer, and E. Lasher. 1960. Similarity of cardiovascular responses to exercise and to diencephalic stimulation. *American Journal of Physiology* 198:1139–42.

58. Smolander, J., J. Saalo, and O. Korhonen. 1991. Effect of work load on cutaneous vascular response to exercise. *Journal of Applied Physiology* 71:1614–19.

58a. Spyer, K. 1994. Central nervous mechanisms contributing to cardiovascular control. *Journal of Physiology* (London). 474:1–19.

59. Suga, H. 1990. Ventricular energetics. *Physiological Reviews* 70:247–77.

60. Sullivan, M., F. Cobb, and M. Higginbotham. 1991. Stroke volume increases by similar mechanisms during upright exercise in normal men and women. *American Journal of Cardiology* 67:1405–12.

61. Tibes, V. 1977. Reflex inputs to the cardiovascular and respiratory centers from dynamically working canine muscles. *Circulation Research* 41:332–41.

61a. Williamson, J. 1995. Instantaneous heart rate increase with dynamic exercise: Central command and muscle-heart reflex contributions. *Journal of Applied Physiology* 78:1273–79.

62. Wyss, C. et al. 1983. Cardiovascular responses to graded reductions in hindlimb perfusion in exercising dogs. *American Journal of Physiology* 245:H481–H486.

63. Zobl, E. et al. 1965. Effect of exercise on the cerebral circulation and metabolism. *Journal of Applied Physiology* 20:1289–93.

Respiration During Exercise

objectives

By studying this chapter, you should be able to do the following:

1. Explain the principal physiological function of the pulmonary system.
2. Outline the major anatomical components of the respiratory system.
3. List the major muscles involved in inspiration and expiration at rest and during exercise.
4. Discuss the importance of matching blood flow to alveolar ventilation in the lung.
5. Explain how gases are transported across the blood-gas interface in the lung.
6. Discuss the major transportation modes of O_2 and CO_2 in the blood.
7. Discuss the effects of increasing temperature, decreasing pH, and increasing levels of 2-3 DPG on the oxygen-hemoglobin dissociation curve.
8. Describe the ventilatory response to constant load steady state exercise. What happens to ventilation if exercise is prolonged and performed in a high-temperature/humid environment?
9. Describe the ventilatory response to incremental exercise. What factors are thought to contribute to the alinear rise in ventilation at work rates above 50%–70% of $\dot{V}O_2$ max?
10. Identify the location and function of chemoreceptors and mechanoreceptors that are thought to play a role in the regulation of breathing.
11. Discuss the neural-humoral theory of respiratory control during exercise.

outline

Function of the Lung 178
Structure of the Respiratory System 178
  Conducting Zone 179
  Respiratory Zone 180
Mechanics of Breathing 181
  Inspiration 182
  Expiration 182
  Airway Resistance 182
Pulmonary Ventilation 184
Pulmonary Volumes and Capacities 184
Diffusion of Gases 185

Blood Flow to the Lung 187
Ventilation-Perfusion Relationships 188
O_2 and CO_2 Transport in Blood 188
  Hemoglobin and O_2 Transport 188
  Oxyhemoglobin Dissociation Curve 189
  O_2 Transport in Muscle 191
  CO_2 Transport in Blood 191
Ventilation and Acid–Base Balance 192
Ventilatory and Blood-Gas Responses to Exercise 193

Rest-to-Work Transitions 193
Prolonged Exercise in a Hot Environment 194
Incremental Exercise 194
Control of Ventilation 195
  Ventilatory Regulation at Rest 195
  Ventilatory Control During Submaximal Exercise 198
  Ventilatory Control During Heavy Exercise 198
Do the Lungs Limit Maximal Exercise Performance? 200

key terms

alveolar ventilation ($\dot{V}_A$)
alveoli
anatomical dead space
aortic bodies
Bohr effect
bulk flow
carotid bodies
cellular respiration
deoxyhemoglobin

diaphragm
diffusion
hemoglobin
myoglobin
oxyhemoglobin
partial pressure
pleura
pulmonary respiration
residual volume (RV)

respiration
spirometry
tidal volume
total lung capacity (TLC)
ventilation
ventilatory threshold (Tvent)
vital capacity (VC)

he word **respiration** can have two definitions in physiology. These definitions can be divided into two separate but related subdivisions: (1) **pulmonary respiration** and (2) **cellular respiration.** Pulmonary respiration refers to ventilation (breathing) and the exchange of gases (O_2 and CO_2) in the lungs. Cellular respiration relates to O_2 utilization and CO_2 production by the tissues (chapter 3). This chapter will be concerned with pulmonary respiration, and the term *respiration* will be used in the text as a synonym for pulmonary respiration. Since the respiratory, or pulmonary, system plays a key role in maintaining blood-gas homeostasis (i.e., O_2 and CO_2 tensions) during exercise, an understanding of lung function during work is important for the student of exercise physiology. It is the purpose of this chapter to discuss the design and function of the respiratory system during exercise.

Function of the Lung

The primary purpose of the respiratory system is to provide a means of gas exchange between the external environment and the body. That is, the respiratory system provides the individual with a means of replacing O_2 and removing CO_2 from the blood. The exchange of O_2 and CO_2 between the lung and blood occurs as a result of ventilation and diffusion. The term **ventilation** refers to the mechanical process of moving air into and out of the lungs. **Diffusion** is the random movement of molecules from an area of high concentration to an area of lower concentration. Since O_2 tension in the lung is greater than in the blood, O_2 moves from the lungs into the blood. Similarly, the tension of CO_2 in the blood is greater than the tension of CO_2 in the lungs, and thus CO_2 moves from the blood into the lung and is expired. Diffusion in the respiratory system occurs rapidly because there is a large surface area within the lungs and a very short diffusion distance between blood and gas in the lungs. The fact that the O_2 and CO_2 tensions in the blood leaving the lung is almost in complete equilibrium with the O_2 and CO_2 tension found within the lung is testimony to the high efficiency of normal lung function.

The respiratory system also plays an important role in regulation of the acid-base balance during heavy exercise. This important topic will be discussed later in this chapter and again in chapter 11.

in summary

- The primary function of the pulmonary system is to provide a means of gas exchange between the environment and the body. Further, the respiratory system plays an important role in the regulation of the acid-base balance during exercise.

Structure of the Respiratory System

The human respiratory system consists of a group of passages that filter air and transport it into the lungs where gas exchange occurs within microscopic air sacs called **alveoli.** The major components of the respiratory system are pictured in figure 10.1. The organs of the respiratory system include the nose, nasal cavity, pharynx, larynx, trachea, bronchial tree, and the lungs themselves. The anatomical position of the lungs relative to the major muscle of inspiration, the diaphragm, is pictured in figure 10.2. Note that both the right and left lungs are enclosed by a set of membranes called **pleura.** The visceral pleura adheres to the outer surface of the lung, whereas the parietal pleura lines the thoracic walls and the diaphragm. These two pleura are separated by a thin layer of fluid that acts as a lubricant, allowing a gliding action of one pleura on the other. The pressure in the pleural cavity (intrapleural pressure) is less than atmospheric and becomes even lower during inspiration, causing air to inflate the lungs. The fact that intrapleural pressure is less than atmospheric is important since it prevents the collapse of the fragile air sacs within the lungs. More will be said about this later.

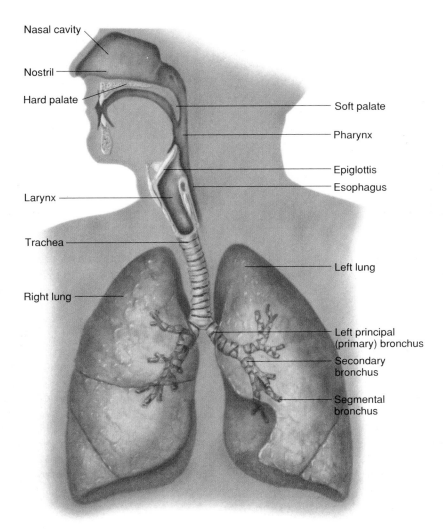

Figure 10.1
Major organs of the respiratory system.

Nasal cavity
Nostril
Hard palate
Soft palate
Pharynx
Epiglottis
Esophagus
Larynx
Trachea
Left lung
Right lung
Left principal (primary) bronchus
Secondary bronchus
Segmental bronchus

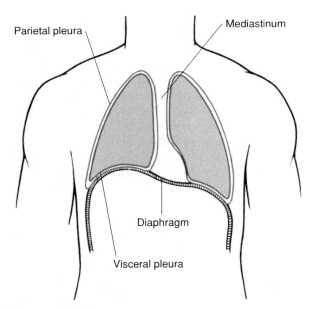

Figure 10.2
Position of the lungs, diaphragm, and pleura.

Parietal pleura
Mediastinum
Diaphragm
Visceral pleura

Conducting Zone

The air passages of the respiratory system are divided into two functional zones: (1) the conducting zone and (2) the respiratory zone (see figure 10.3). The conducting zone includes all those anatomical structures (e.g., trachea, bronchial tree, bronchioles) that air passes through to reach the respiratory zone. The region of the lung where gas exchange occurs is labeled the respiratory zone and includes the respiratory bronchioles and alveolar sacs. Respiratory bronchioles are included in this region since they contain small clusters of alveoli.

Air enters the trachea from the pharynx (throat), which receives air from both the nasal and oral cavities. In general, humans breathe through the nose until ventilation is increased to approximately 20–30 liters per minute, at which time the mouth becomes the primary passageway for air (26). In order for gas to enter or leave the trachea, it must pass through a valvelike opening called the *epiglottis*, which is located between the vocal cords.

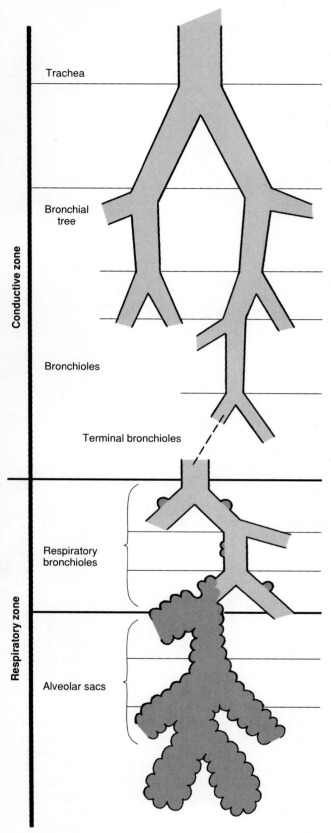

Conductive zone

Trachea

Bronchial tree

Bronchioles

Terminal bronchioles

Respiratory zone

Respiratory bronchioles

Alveolar sacs

Figure 10.3

The conducting zones and respiratory zones of the pulmonary system.

The trachea branches into two primary bronchi (right and left) that enter each lung. The bronchial tree then branches several more times before forming bronchioles (bronchioles are small branches of the segmental bronchi). The bronchioles then branch several times before they become the alveolar ducts leading to the alveolar sacs and respiratory zone of the lung (see figure 10.4).

The conducting zone of the respiratory system serves not only as a passageway for air, but also functions to humidify and filter the air as it moves toward the respiratory zone of the lung. Regardless of the temperature or humidity of the environment, the air that reaches the lung is warmed and is saturated with water vapor (47). This warming and humidification of air serves to protect body temperature and prevents the delicate lung tissue from desiccation (drying out).

The role of the conducting zone and the respiratory zone in filtration of the inspired gas is critical in order to prevent lung damage due to the collection of inhaled particles in the respiratory zone. These filtration and cleaning processes are achieved via two principal means. First, mucus, secreted by the cells of the conducting zone, serves to trap small inhaled particles. This mucus is moved toward the oral cavity via tiny fingerlike projections called *cilia*. These cilia move in a wavelike fashion, which propels the mucus at a rate of 1–2 centimeters/minute. When a particle becomes trapped in the mucus, it is moved toward the pharynx via ciliary action, where it can be either swallowed or expectorated.

A second means of protecting the lung from foreign particles is by the action of cells called *macrophages* that reside primarily in the alveoli (72). These macrophages literally engulf particles that reach the alveoli. The cleansing action of both the cilia and macrophages has been shown to be hindered by cigarette smoke and certain types of air pollution (47).

Respiratory Zone

Gas exchange in the lungs occurs across about 300 million tiny (0.25–0.50 mm diameter) alveoli. The enormous number of these structures provides the lung with a large surface area for diffusion. It is estimated that the total surface area available for diffusion in the human lung is 60–80 square meters, or about the size of a tennis court. The rate of diffusion is further assisted by the fact that each alveolus is only one cell layer thick, so that the total *blood-gas barrier* is only two cell layers thick (alveolar cell and capillary cell) (see figure 10.5).

Although the 300 million alveoli provide the ideal structure for gas exchange, the fragility of these tiny "bubbles" presents some problems for the lung. For example, because of the surface tension (pressure exerted due to the properties of water) of the liquid lining the alveoli, relatively large forces develop, which tend to collapse alveoli. Fortunately, some of the alveolar cells

Section One Physiology of Exercise

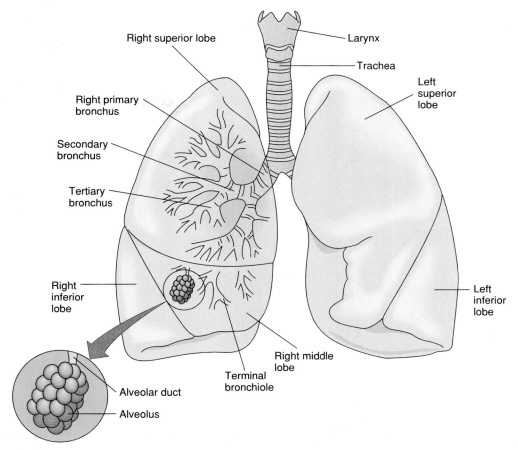

Figure 10.4

The bronchial tree consists of the passageways that connect the trachea and the alveoli.

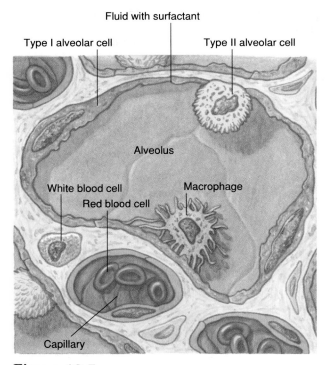

Figure 10.5

Relationship between Type II alveolar cells and the alveolus.

(called Type II, see figure 10.5) synthesize and release a material called *surfactant*, which lowers the surface tension of the alveoli and thus prevents their collapse (44).

in summary

- Anatomically, the pulmonary system consists of a group of passages that filter air and transport it into the lungs where gas exchange occurs within tiny air sacs called alveoli.

Mechanics of Breathing

As previously mentioned, movement of air from the environment to the lungs is called pulmonary ventilation and occurs via a process known as **bulk flow.** Bulk flow refers to the movement of molecules along a passageway due to a pressure difference between the two ends of the passageway. Thus inspiration occurs due to the pressure in the lungs (intrapulmonary) being reduced below atmospheric pressure. Conversely, expiration occurs when the pressure within the lungs

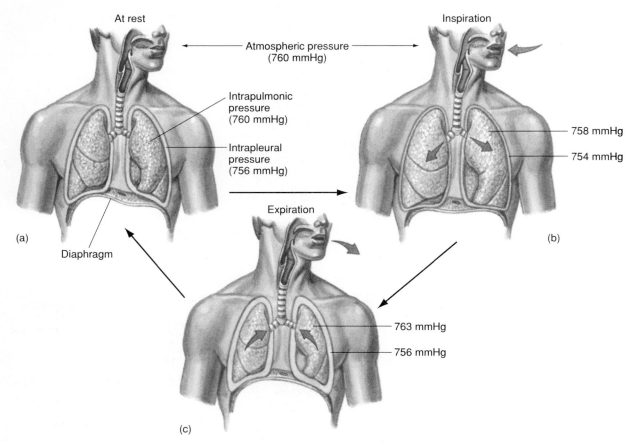

At rest

Atmospheric pressure
(760 mmHg)

Intrapulmonic
pressure
(760 mmHg)

Intrapleural
pressure
(756 mmHg)

(a)

Diaphragm

Inspiration

758 mmHg

754 mmHg

(b)

Expiration

763 mmHg

756 mmHg

(c)

Figure 10.6
Illustration of the mechanics of inspiration and expiration.

exceeds atmospheric pressure. The means by which this pressure change within the lungs is achieved will be discussed within the next several paragraphs.

Inspiration

Any muscle capable of increasing the volume of the chest is considered to be an inspiratory muscle. The **diaphragm** is the most important muscle of inspiration and is the only skeletal muscle considered essential for life (22, 26, 47, 66, 67, 69). This thin, dome-shaped muscle inserts into the lower ribs and is innervated by the phrenic nerves. When the diaphragm contracts, it forces the abdominal contents downward and forward. Further, the ribs are lifted outward (see figure 10.6). The outcome of these two actions is to reduce intrapleural pressure, which in turn causes the lungs to expand. This expansion of the lungs results in a reduction in intrapulmonary pressure below atmospheric, which allows airflow into the lungs.

During normal quiet breathing the diaphragm performs most of the work of inspiration. However, during exercise, accessory muscles of inspiration are called into play (50, 51, 71). These include the external intercostal muscles, pectoralis minor, the scalene muscles, and the sternomastoids (see figure 10.7). Collectively, these muscles assist the diaphragm in increasing the volume of the thorax, which aids in inspiration.

Expiration

Expiration is passive during normal quiet breathing. That is, no muscular effort is necessary for expiration to occur at rest. This is true because the lungs and chest walls are elastic and tend to return to equilibrium position after expanding during inspiration (76). During exercise and voluntary hyperventilation, expiration becomes active. The most important muscles involved in expiration are those found in the abdominal wall, which include the rectus abdominus and the internal oblique (50, 71, 78). When these muscles contract, the diaphragm is pushed upward and the ribs are pulled downward and inward. This results in an increase in intrapulmonary pressure and expiration occurs.

Airway Resistance

At any given rate of airflow into the lungs, the pressure difference that must be developed depends on the resistance of the airways. Airflow through the airways of the respiratory system can be mathematically defined by the following relationships:

$$\text{Airflow} = \frac{P_1 - P_2}{\text{Resistance}}$$

where $P_1 - P_2$ is the pressure difference at the two ends of the airway, and resistance is the resistance to flow offered by the airway. Airflow is increased any time

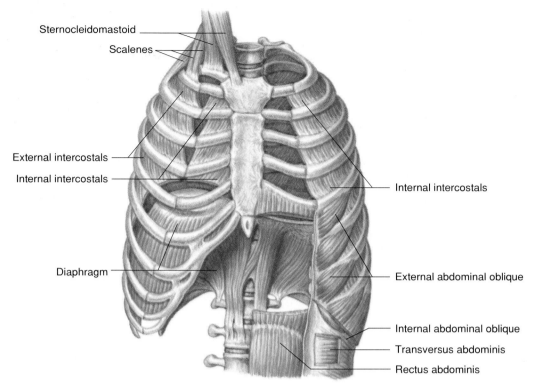

Sternocleidomastoid

Scalenes

External intercostals

Internal intercostals

Internal intercostals

Diaphragm

External abdominal oblique

Internal abdominal oblique

Transversus abdominis

Rectus abdominis

Figure 10.7

The muscles of respiration. The principal muscles of inspiration are shown on the left side of the trunk; the principal muscles of expiration are shown on the right side.

A Closer Look 10.1

Exercise-induced Asthma

Asthma is a disease that promotes a reversible narrowing of the airways (called a bronchospasm). This reduction in airway diameter results in an increased work of breathing and individuals suffering from asthma generally report being short of breath (called dyspnea).

Although there are many potential causes of asthma (20c),

some asthmatic patients develop a bronchospasm during or immediately after exercise. This type of asthma is called "exercise-induced asthma." When an individual experiences an asthma attack during exercise, breathing becomes labored and a wheezing sound is often heard during expiration. If the asthmatic attack is severe, it becomes

impossible for the individual to exercise at even low intensities because of the dsypnea associated with the increased work of breathing. Asthma is an excellent example of how even a small decrease in airway diameter can result in a large increase in breathing resistance. See chapter 17 for more details.

there is an increase in the pressure gradient across the pulmonary system, or if there is a decrease in airway resistance. This same relationship for blood flow was discussed in chapter 9.

What factors contribute to airway resistance? By far the most important variable contributing to airway resistance is the diameter of the airway. Airways that are reduced in size due to disease (chronic obstructive lung disease, asthma, etc.) offer more resistance to

flow than healthy, open airways. Recall from chapter 9 that if the radius of a blood vessel (or airway) is reduced by one-half, the resistance to flow is increased sixteen times! Therefore, one can easily understand the effect of obstructive lung diseases (e.g., exercise-induced asthma) on increasing the work of breathing, especially during exercise when pulmonary ventilation is ten to twenty times greater than at rest (see A Closer Look 10.1).

in summary

- The major muscle of inspiration is the diaphragm. Air enters the pulmonary system due to intrapulmonary pressure being reduced below atmospheric pressure (bulk flow). At rest, expiration is passive. However, during exercise expiration becomes active using muscles located in the abdominal wall (e.g., rectus abdominus and internal oblique).
- The primary factor that contributes to airflow resistance in the pulmonary system is the diameter of the airway.

Pulmonary Ventilation

Prior to beginning a discussion of ventilation, it is helpful to define some commonly used pulmonary physiology symbols:

1. V is used to denote volume
2. $\dot{V}$ means volume per unit of time (generally one minute)
3. the subscripts $_{T, D, A, I, E}$ are used to denote tidal, dead space, alveolar, inspired, and expired, respectively.

Pulmonary ventilation refers to the movement of gas into and out of the lungs. The amount of gas ventilated per minute is the product of the frequency of breathing (f) and the amount of gas moved per breath **(tidal volume):**

$$\dot{V} = V_T \times f$$

In a 70-kg man the $\dot{V}$ at rest is generally around 7.5 liters/minute, with a tidal volume of 0.5 liters and a frequency of 15. During maximal exercise, ventilation may reach 120–175 liters per minute, with a frequency of 40–50 and a tidal volume of approximately 3–3.5 liters.

It is important to understand that not all of the air that passes the lips reaches the alveolar gas compartment, where gas exchange occurs. Part of each breath remains in conducting airways (trachea, bronchi, etc.) and thus does not participate in gas exchange. This "unused" ventilation is called dead-space ventilation (V_D), and the space it occupies is known as **anatomical dead space.** The volume of inspired gas that reaches the respiratory zone is referred to as **alveolar ventilation ($\dot{V}_A$).** Thus total minute ventilation can be subdivided into dead space ventilation and alveolar ventilation:

$$\dot{V} = \dot{V}_A + \dot{V}_D$$

Note that pulmonary ventilation is not equally distributed throughout the lung. The basal (bottom) region of the lung receives more ventilation than the apex (top region), particularly during quiet breathing (47). This changes to some degree during exercise, with the apical (top) regions of the lung receiving an increased percentage of the total ventilation (43).

in summary

- Pulmonary ventilation refers to the amount of gas moved in and out of the lungs.
- The amount of gas moved per minute is the product of tidal volume times breathing frequency.

Pulmonary Volumes and Capacities

Pulmonary volumes can be measured via a technique known as **spirometry.** Using this procedure, the subject breathes into a device that is capable of measuring inspired and expired gas volumes. Modern spirometers use computer technology to measure pulmonary volumes and the rate of expired airflow (see figure 10.8). Figure 10.9 is a spirogram showing the measurement of tidal volumes during quiet breathing and the various lung volumes and capacities that are defined in table 10.1. Several of these terms require special mention. First, **vital capacity (VC)** is defined as the maximum amount of gas that can be expired after a maximum inspiration. Secondly, the **residual volume (RV)** is the volume of gas remaining in the lungs after a maximum expiration. Finally, **total lung capacity (TLC)** is defined as the amount of gas in the lungs after a maximum inspiration, and is the sum of the two lung volumes (VC + RV) just mentioned.

Figure 10.8

Photograph of a computerized spirometer used to measure lung volumes. Courtesy of Sensor-medics Corp.

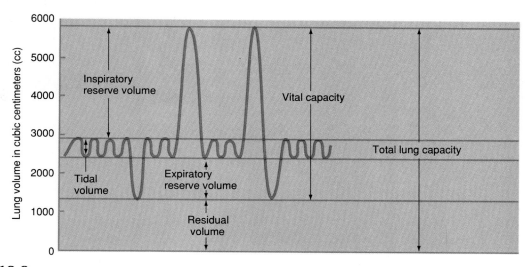

Figure 10.9
A spirogram showing lung volumes and capacities at rest.

Table 10.1	Definitions of Terms Used to Describe Lung Volumes and Capacities
Term	Definitions
Lung Volumes	
Tidal volume	Volume of gas inspired or expired during unforced respiratory cycle
Inspiratory reserve	The volume of gas that can be inspired at the end of a tidal inspiration
Expiratory reserve	The volume of gas that can be expired at the end of a tidal expiration
Residual volume	The volume of gas left in the lungs after a maximal expiration
Lung Capacities	
Total lung capacity	The total amount of gas in the lungs at the end of a maximal inspiration
Vital capacity	The maximum amount of gas that can be expired after a maximum inspiration
Inspiratory capacity	The maximum amount of gas that can be inspired at the end of a tidal expiration
Functional residual capacity	The amount of gas remaining in the lungs after a normal quiet tidal expiration

Lung volumes are the four nonoverlapping components of the total lung capacity. Lung capacities are the sum of two or more lung volumes.

in summary
- Pulmonary volumes can be measured using spirometry.
- Vital capacity is the maximum amount of gas that can be expired after a maximal inspiration.
- Residual volume is the amount of gas left in the lungs after a maximal expiration.

Diffusion of Gases
Prior to discussing diffusion of gases across the alveolar membrane into the blood, it is necessary to introduce the concept of **partial pressure.** According to Dalton's law, the total pressure of a gas mixture is equal to the sum of the pressures that each gas would exert independently. Thus, the pressure that each gas exerts independently can be calculated by multiplying the fractional composition of the gas by the absolute pressure (barometric pressure). Let's consider an example calculating the partial pressure of oxygen in air at sea level. The barometric pressure at sea level is 760 mm Hg (barometric pressure is the force exerted by the weight of the gas contained within the atmosphere). The composition of air is generally considered to be:

Gas	Percentage	Fraction
Oxygen	20.93	.2093
Nitrogen	79.04	.7904
Carbon dioxide	0.03	.0003
Total	100.0	

Therefore the partial pressure of oxygen (PO_2) at sea level can be computed as:

$$PO_2 = 760 \times .2093$$
$$PO_2 = 159 \text{ mm Hg}$$

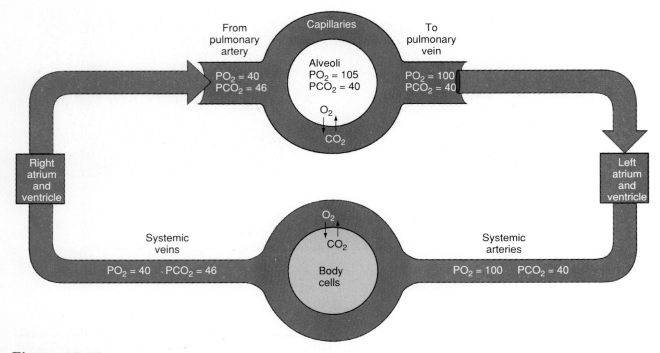

Figure 10.10
Partial pressures of O_2 (PO_2) and CO_2 (PCO_2) in blood as a result of gas exchange in the lung and gas exchange between capillaries and tissues.

In a similar manner, the partial pressure of nitrogen can be calculated to be:

$$PN_2 = 760 \times .7904$$
$$PN_2 = 600.7 \text{ mm Hg}$$

Since O_2, CO_2, and N_2 make up almost 100% of the atmosphere, the total barometric pressure (P) can be computed as:

$$P \text{ (dry atmosphere)} = PO_2 + PN_2 + PCO_2$$

Diffusion of a gas across tissues is described by Fick's law of diffusion, which states that the rate of gas transfer (V gas) is proportional to the tissue area, the diffusion coefficient of the gas, and the difference in the partial pressure of the gas on the two sides of the tissue, and is inversely proportional to the thickness:

$$V \text{ gas} = \frac{A}{T} \times D \times (P_1 - P_2)$$

where A is the area, T is the thickness of the tissue, D is the diffusion coefficient of the gas, and $P_1 - P_2$ is the difference in the partial pressure between the two sides of the tissue. In simple terms, the rate of diffusion for any single gas is greater when the surface area for diffusion is large and the "driving pressure" between the two sides of the tissue is high. In contrast, an increase in tissue thickness impedes diffusion. The lung is well designed for the diffusion of gases across the alveolar membrane into and out of the blood. First, the total surface area available for diffusion is large. Secondly, the alveolar membrane is extremely thin. The fact that the lung is an ideal organ for gas exchange is important since during maximal exercise the rate of O_2 uptake and CO_2 output may increase twenty to thirty times above resting condition.

The amount of O_2 or CO_2 dissolved in blood obeys Henry's law and is dependent on the temperature of blood, the partial pressure of the gas, and the solubility of the gas. Since the temperature of the blood does not change a great deal during exercise (i.e., 1–3° C), and the solubility of the gas remains constant, the major factor that determines the amount of dissolved gas is the partial pressure.

Figure 10.10 illustrates gas exchange via diffusion across the alveolar-capillary membranes and at the tissue level. Note that the PCO_2 and PO_2 of blood entering the lung are approximately 46 and 40 mm Hg, respectively. In contrast, the PCO_2 and PO_2 in alveolar gas are around 40 and 105 mm Hg, respectively. As a consequence of the difference in partial pressure across the blood-gas interface, CO_2 leaves the blood and diffuses into the alveolus, and O_2 diffuses from the alveolus into the blood. Blood leaving the lung has a PO_2 of approximately 100 mm Hg and a PCO_2 of 40 mm Hg.

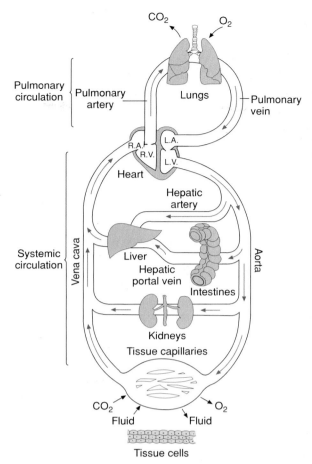

Figure 10.11
The pulmonary circulation is a low-pressure system that pumps mixed venous blood through the pulmonary capillaries for gas exchange. After completion of gas exchange, this oxygenated blood is returned to the left heart to be circulated throughout the body.

in summary

- Gas moves across the blood-gas interface in the lung due to simple diffusion.
- The rate of diffusion is described by Fick's law which states: the volume of gas that moves across a tissue is proportional to the area for diffusion and the difference in partial pressure across the membrane, and is inversely proportional to membrane thickness.

Blood Flow to the Lung

The pulmonary circulation begins at the pulmonary artery, which receives venous blood from the right ventricle (recall that this is mixed venous blood). Mixed venous blood is then circulated through the pulmonary

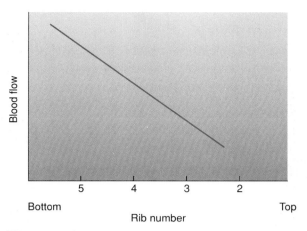

Figure 10.12
Regional blood flow within the lung. Note that there is a linear decrease in blood flow from the lower regions of the lung toward the upper regions.

capillaries where gas exchange occurs, and this oxygenated blood is returned to the left atrium via the pulmonary vein to be circulated throughout the body (see figure 10.11).

In the adult, the right ventricle of the heart (like the left) has an output of approximately 5 liters/minute. Therefore, the rate of blood flow throughout the pulmonary circulation is equal to that of the systemic circulation. The pressures in the pulmonary circulation are relatively low when compared to those in the systemic circulation (chapter 9). This low-pressure system is due to low vascular resistance in the pulmonary circulation (47). An interesting feature of pulmonary circulation is that during periods of increased pulmonary blood flow during exercise, the resistance in the pulmonary vascular system falls due to distension of vessels and the recruitment of previously unused capillaries. This decrease in pulmonary vascular resistance allows lung blood flow to increase during exercise with relatively small increases in pulmonary arterial pressure.

When standing, considerable inequality of blood flow exists within the human lung due to gravity. For example, in the upright position, blood flow decreases almost linearly from bottom to top, reaching very low values at the top (apex) of the lung (see figure 10.12). This distribution may be altered during exercise and with a change in posture. During light exercise, blood flow to the apex of the lung is increased (18). This is advantageous for improved gas exchange and will be discussed in the next section. When an individual is supine, blood flow becomes uniform within the lung. In contrast, measurements of blood flow in humans who are suspended upside down show that blood flow to the apex of the lung greatly exceeds that found in the base.

in summary

- The pulmonary circulation is a low-pressure system with a rate of blood flow equal to that in the systemic circuit.
- In a standing position, most of the blood flow to the lung is distributed to the base of the lung due to gravitational force.

Ventilation–Perfusion Relationships

Thus far we have discussed pulmonary ventilation, blood flow to the lungs, and diffusion of gases across the blood-gas barrier in the lung. It seems reasonable to assume that if all these processes were adequate, normal gas exchange would occur in the lung. However, normal gas exchange requires a matching of ventilation to blood flow (perfusion, Q). In other words, an alveolus can be well ventilated, but if blood flow to the alveolus does not adequately match ventilation, normal gas exchange does not occur. Indeed, mismatching of ventilation and perfusion is responsible for most of the problems of gas exchange that occur due to lung diseases.

The ideal ventilation-to-perfusion ratio (V/Q) is 1.0 or slightly greater. That is, there is a one-to-one matching of ventilation to blood flow, which results in optimum gas exchange. Unfortunately, the V/Q ratio is generally not equal to 1.0 throughout the lung, but varies depending on the section of the lung being considered (22, 31, 47, 86). This concept is illustrated in figure 10.13, where the V/Q ratio at the apex and the base of the lung is calculated for resting conditions.

Let's discuss the (V/Q) ratio in the apex of the lung first. Here the ventilation (at rest) in the upper region of the lung is estimated to be 0.24 liters/minute, while the blood flow is considered to be 0.07 liters/minute. Thus, the V/Q ratio is 3.3 (i.e., 0.24/0.07 = 3.3). A large V/Q ratio represents a disproportionately high ventilation relative to blood flow, which results in poor gas exchange. In contrast, the ventilation at the base of the lung (figure 10.13) is 0.82 liters/minute, with a blood flow of 1.29 liters/minute (V/Q ratio = 0.82/1.29 = 0.63). A V/Q ratio less than 1.0 represents a greater blood flow than ventilation to the region in question. Although V/Q ratios less than 1.0 are not indicative of ideal conditions for gas exchange, in most cases V/Q ratios greater than 0.50 are adequate to meet the gas exchange demands at rest (86).

What effect does exercise have on the V/Q ratio? The complete answer to this question is not currently available. However, it appears that light exercise may improve the V/Q relationship, while heavy exercise may result in a small V/Q inequality, and thus a minor impairment in gas exchange (43). Whether the increase in V/Q inequality is due to low ventilation or low perfusion is not clear. The possible effects of this V/Q mismatch on blood gases will be discussed later in the chapter.

Figure 10.13
The relationship between ventilation and blood flow (ventilation/perfusion ratios) at the top (apex) and the base of the lung. The ratios indicate that the base of the lung is overperfused relative to ventilation and that the apex is underperfused relative to ventilation. This uneven matching of blood flow to ventilation results in less than perfect gas exchange.

in summary

- Efficient gas exchange between the blood and the lung requires proper matching of blood flow to ventilation (called ventilation-perfusion relationships).
- The ideal ratio of ventilation to perfusion is 1.0 or slightly greater, since this ratio implies a perfect matching of blood flow to ventilation.

O_2 and CO_2 Transport in Blood

Although some O_2 and CO_2 are transported as dissolved gases in the blood, the major portion of O_2 and CO_2 transported via blood is done by O_2 combining with hemoglobin and CO_2 being transformed into bicarbonate (HCO_3^-). A complete discussion of how O_2 and CO_2 are transported in blood follows.

Hemoglobin and O_2 Transport

Approximately 99% of the O_2 transported in the blood is chemically bound to **hemoglobin,** which is a protein contained in the red blood cells (erythrocytes). Each molecule of hemoglobin can transport four O_2 molecules. The binding of O_2 to hemoglobin forms **oxyhemoglobin;** hemoglobin that is not bound to O_2 is referred to as **deoxyhemoglobin.**

The amount of O_2 that can be transported per unit volume of blood is dependent on the concentration of hemoglobin. Normal hemoglobin concentration for a healthy male and female is approximately 150 grams and 130 grams, respectively, per liter of blood. When completely saturated with O_2, each gram

Figure 10.14
The relationship between the partial pressure of O_2 in blood and the relative saturation of hemoglobin with O_2 is pictured here in the oxygen-hemoglobin dissociation curve. Notice the relatively steep portion of the curve up to PO_2 values of 40 mm Hg, after which there is a gradual rise to reach a plateau.

of hemoglobin can transport 1.34 ml of O_2 (47). Therefore, if hemoglobin is 100% saturated with O_2, the healthy male and female can transport approximately 200 ml and 174 ml of O_2, respectively, per liter of blood at sea level.

Oxyhemoglobin Dissociation Curve
The combination of O_2 with hemoglobin in the lung (alveolar capillaries) is sometimes referred to as *loading*, and the release of O_2 from hemoglobin at the tissues is called *unloading*. Loading and unloading is thus a reversible reaction:

$$Deoxyhemoglobin + O_2 \longleftrightarrow Oxyhemoglobin$$

The factors that determine the direction of this reaction are (1) the PO_2 of the blood and (2) the affinity or bond strength between hemoglobin and O_2. A high PO_2 drives the reaction to the right, while low PO_2 and a reduced affinity of hemoglobin for O_2 moves the reaction to the left. For example, a high PO_2 in the lungs results in an increase in arterial PO_2 and the formation of oxyhemoglobin (i.e., reaction moves right). In contrast, a low PO_2 in the tissue results in a decrease of PO_2 in the systemic capillaries, and thus unloads O_2 to be used by the tissues (reaction moves left).

The effect of PO_2 on the combination of O_2 with hemoglobin can be best illustrated by the oxyhemoglobin dissociation curve, which is presented in figure 10.14. This sigmoidal (S shaped) curve has several interesting features. First, the percent hemoglobin saturated with O_2 (% HbO_2) increases sharply up to an arterial PO_2 of 40 mm Hg. At PO_2 values above 40 mm Hg, the increase in % HbO_2 rises slowly to a plateau around 90–100 mm Hg, at which the % HbO_2 is approximately 97%. At rest, the body's O_2 requirements are relatively low and only about 25% of the O_2 transported

in the blood is unloaded to the tissues. In contrast, during intense exercise the mixed venous PO_2 may reach a value of 18–20 mm Hg, and the tissues may extract up to 90% of the O_2 carried by hemoglobin.

The shape of the oxyhemoglobin dissociation curve is well designed to meet human O_2 transport needs. The relatively flat portion of the curve (above a PO_2 of approximately 90 mm Hg) allows arterial PO_2 to oscillate from 90–100 mm Hg without a large drop in % HbO_2. This is important since there is a decline in arterial PO_2 with aging and upon ascent to altitude. At the other end of the curve (steep portion, 0–40 mm Hg), small changes in PO_2 result in a release of large amounts of O_2 from hemoglobin. This is critical during exercise when tissue O_2 consumption is high.

Effect of pH on O_2-Hb Dissociation Curve
In addition to the effect of blood PO_2 on O_2 binding to hemoglobin, a change in acidity, temperature, or red blood cell (RBC) levels of 2,3-diphosphoglyceric acid (2–3 DPG) can affect the loading/unloading reaction. First, let's consider the effect of changing blood acid-base status on hemoglobin's affinity for O_2. The strength of the bond between O_2 and hemoglobin is weakened by a decrease in blood pH (increased acidity), which results in increased unloading of O_2 to the tissues. This is represented by a "right" shift in the oxyhemoglobin curve and is called the **Bohr effect** (see figure 10.15). A right shift in the oxyhemoglobin dissociation curve might be expected during heavy exercise due to the rise in blood lactic acid levels observed in this type of work. After being produced in the muscle cell, lactic acid gives up a proton (H^+), which results in the decrease in pH. The mechanism to explain the Bohr effect is the fact that protons bind to hemoglobin, which reduces its O_2 transport capacity. Therefore,

Figure 10.15
The effect of changing blood pH on the shape of the oxygen-hemoglobin dissociation curve. A decrease in pH results in a rightward shift of the curve (Bohr effect), while an increase in pH results in a leftward shift of the curve.

when there is a higher than normal concentration of H^+ in the blood (a condition called *acidosis*), there is a reduction in hemoglobin affinity for O_2. This facilitates the unloading of O_2 to the tissues during exercise since the acidity level is higher in muscles.

Temperature Effect on O_2-Hb Dissociation Curve

Another factor that affects hemoglobin affinity for O_2 is temperature. At a constant pH, the affinity of hemoglobin for O_2 is inversely related to blood temperature. That is, a decrease in temperature results in a left shift in the oxyhemoglobin curve, while an increase in temperature causes a right shift of the curve. This means that an increase in blood temperature weakens the bond between O_2 and hemoglobin, which assists in the unloading of O_2 to muscle. Conversely, a decrease in blood temperature results in a stronger bond between O_2 and hemoglobin, which hinders O_2 release. The effect of increasing blood temperature on the oxyhemoglobin dissociation curve is presented in figure 10.16. During exercise, increased heat production in the contracting muscle would promote a right shift in the oxyhemoglobin dissociation curve and facilitate unloading of O_2 to the tissue.

2–3 DPG and the O_2-Hb Dissociation Curve

A final factor that potentially can affect the shape of the oxyhemoglobin dissociation curve is the concentration of 2–3 DPG in red blood cells (RBCs). Red blood cells are unique in that they do not contain a nucleus or mitochondria. Therefore, they must rely on anaerobic glycolysis to meet the cell's energy needs. A by-

Figure 10.16
The effect of changing blood temperature on the shape of the oxygen-hemoglobin dissociation curve. An increase in temperature results in a rightward shift in the curve, while a decrease in blood temperature results in a leftward shift in the curve.

product of RBC glycolysis is the compound 2–3 DPG, which can combine with hemoglobin and reduce hemoglobin's affinity for O_2 (i.e., right shift in oxyhemoglobin dissociation curve).

Red blood cell concentrations of 2–3 DPG are known to increase during exposure to altitude and in

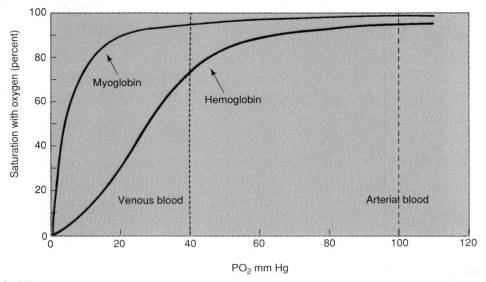

Figure 10.17

Comparison of the dissociation curve for myoglobin and hemoglobin. The steep myoglobin dissociation demonstrates a higher affinity for O_2 than hemoglobin.

anemia (low blood hemoglobin) (47). However, reports in the literature about the acute effects of exercise on blood 2–3 DPG levels remain controversial. In an effort to resolve this issue, a group of Austrian researchers (49) performed a series of well-designed experiments that demonstrated that moderate exercise resulted in no change in blood levels of 2–3 DPG, and that severe exercise resulted in a small decrease in blood 2–3 DPG. Therefore, although an increase in blood 2–3 DPG can alter Hb-O_2 affinity, it appears that exercise at sea level does not increase 2–3 DPG in the red blood cell. Therefore, the right shift in the oxyhemoglobin curve during heavy exercise is not due to changes in 2–3 DPG but to the degree of acidosis and blood temperature elevation.

O_2 Transport in Muscle

Myoglobin is an oxygen-binding protein found in skeletal muscle fibers and cardiac muscle (not in blood) and acts as a "shuttle" to move O_2 from the muscle cell membrane to the mitochondria. Myoglobin is found in large quantities in slow-twitch fibers (i.e., high aerobic capacity), in smaller amounts in intermediate fibers, and in only limited amounts in fast-twitch fibers. Myoglobin is similar in structure to hemoglobin, but is about one-fourth the weight. The difference in structure between myoglobin and hemoglobin results in a difference in O_2 affinity between the two molecules. This point is illustrated in figure 10.17. Myoglobin has a greater affinity for O_2 than hemoglobin and therefore the myoglobin-O_2 dissociation curve is much steeper than that of hemoglobin's for PO_2 values below 20 mm Hg. The practical implication of the shape of the myoglobin-O_2 dissociation curve is that myoglobin discharges its O_2 at very low

PO_2 values. This is important since the PO_2 in the mitochondria of contracting skeletal muscle may be as low as 1–2 mm Hg.

Myoglobin O_2 stores may serve as an "O_2 reserve" during transition periods from rest to exercise. At the beginning of exercise, there is a time lag between the onset of muscular contraction and an increased O_2 delivery to the muscle. Therefore, O_2 bound to myoglobin prior to the initiation of exercise serves to buffer the O_2 needs of the muscle until the cardiopulmonary system can meet the new O_2 requirement. At the conclusion of exercise, myoglobin O_2 stores must be replenished and this O_2 consumption above rest contributes to the O_2 debt (chapter 4).

CO_2 Transport in Blood

Carbon dioxide is transported in the blood in three forms: (1) dissolved CO_2 (about 10% of blood CO_2 is transported this way), (2) CO_2 bound to hemoglobin (called carbaminohemoglobin; about 20% of blood CO_2 is transported via this form), and (3) bicarbonate (70% of CO_2 found in blood is transported as bicarbonate: HCO_3^-. The three forms of CO_2 transport in the blood are illustrated in figure 10.18.

Since most of the CO_2 that is transported in blood is transported as bicarbonate, this mechanism deserves special attention. Carbon dioxide can be converted to bicarbonate (within RBCs) in the following way:

$$CO_2 + H_2O \underset{\text{Carbonic anhydrase}}{\longleftrightarrow} H_2CO_3 \underset{\text{Carbonic acid}}{\longleftrightarrow} H^+ + HCO_3^-$$

Figure 10.18
The three forms of CO_2 transport in blood. See text for discussion.

A high PCO_2 causes CO_2 to combine with water to form carbonic acid. This reaction is catalyzed by the enzyme carbonic anhydrase, which is found in RBCs. After formation, carbonic acid dissociates into a hydrogen ion and a bicarbonate ion. The hydrogen ion then binds to hemoglobin, and the bicarbonate ion diffuses out of the RBC into the plasma (figure 10.18). Since bicarbonate carries a negative charge (anion), the removal of a negatively charged molecule from a cell without replacement would result in an electrochemical imbalance across the cell membrane. This problem is avoided by the replacement of bicarbonate by chloride (Cl^-), which diffuses from the plasma into the RBC. This exchange of anions occurs in the RBC as blood moves through the tissue capillaries, and is called the *chloride shift* (figure 10.18).

When blood reaches the pulmonary capillaries, the PCO_2 of the blood is greater than that of the alveolus, and thus CO_2 diffuses out of the blood across the blood-gas interface. At the lung, the binding of O_2 to Hb results in a release of the hydrogen ions bound to hemoglobin and promotes the formation of carbonic acid:

$$H^+ + HCO_3^- \longrightarrow H_2CO_3$$

Under conditions of low PCO_2 that exist at the alveolus, carbonic acid then dissociates into CO_2 and H_2O:

$$H_2CO_3 \longrightarrow CO_2 + H_2O$$

The release of CO_2 from the blood is summarized in figure 10.19.

in summary

- Over 99% of the O_2 transported in blood is chemically bonded with hemoglobin. The effect of the partial pressure of O_2 on the combination of O_2 with hemoglobin is illustrated by the S-shaped O_2-hemoglobin dissociation curve.
- An increase in body temperature and a reduction in blood pH results in a right shift in the O_2-hemoglobin dissociation curve and a reduced affinity of hemoglobin for O_2.
- Carbon dioxide is transported in blood in three forms: (1) dissolved CO_2 (10% is transported in this way), (2) CO_2 bound to hemoglobin (called carbaminohemoglobin; about 20% of blood CO_2 is transported via this form), and (3) bicarbonate (70% of CO_2 found in blood is transported as bicarbonate (HCO_3^-).

Ventilation and Acid–Base Balance

Pulmonary ventilation can play an important role in removing H^+ from the blood by the HCO_3^- reaction discussed above (77). For example, an increase in CO_2 in blood or body fluids results in an increase in hydrogen

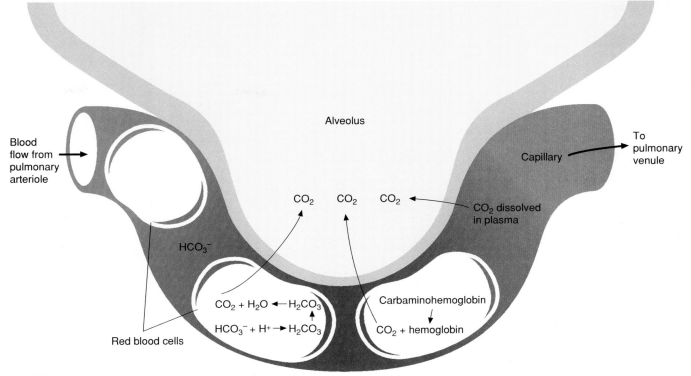

Figure 10.19
Carbon dioxide is released from the blood in the pulmonary capillaries. At the time of CO_2 release in the lung, there is a "reverse chloride shift" and carbonic acid dissociates into CO_2 and H_2O.

ion accumulation and thus a decrease in pH. In contrast, removal of CO_2 from blood or body fluids may decrease hydrogen ion concentration and thus increase pH. Recall that the CO_2-carbonic anhydrase reaction occurs as follows:

$$CO_2 + H_2O \longleftrightarrow H_2CO_3 \longleftrightarrow H^+ + HCO_3^-$$

Therefore, an increase in pulmonary ventilation causes exhalation of additional CO_2 and results in a reduction of blood PCO_2 and a lowering of hydrogen ion concentration. On the other side, a reduction in pulmonary ventilation would result in a buildup of CO_2 and an increase in hydrogen ion concentration (pH would decrease). The role of the pulmonary system in acid-base balance will be discussed in detail in chapter 11.

in summary
- An increase in pulmonary ventilation causes exhalation of additional CO_2 which results in a reduction of blood PCO_2 and a lowering of hydrogen ion concentration (i.e., pH increases).

Ventilatory and Blood-Gas Responses to Exercise

Prior to discussing ventilatory control during exercise, it is useful to examine the ventilatory response to several different types of exercise.

Rest-to-Work Transitions

The change in pulmonary ventilation observed in the transition from rest to constant-load submaximal exercise (i.e., below the lactate threshold) is pictured in figure 10.20. Note that expired ventilation ($\dot{V}_E$) increases abruptly at the beginning of exercise, followed by a slower rise toward a steady state value (7, 19, 20, 29, 41, 60, 61, 87).

Figure 10.20 also points out that arterial tensions of PCO_2 and PO_2 are relatively unchanged during this type of exercise (27, 28a, 84). However, note that arterial PO_2 decreases and arterial PCO_2 tends to increase slightly in the transition from rest to steady state exercise (28a). This observation suggests that the increase in alveolar ventilation at the beginning of exercise is not as rapid as the increase in metabolism.

Figure 10.20

The changes in ventilation and partial pressures of O_2 and CO_2 in the transition from rest to steady state submaximal exercise.

Figure 10.21

Changes in ventilation and blood gas tensions during prolonged submaximal exercise in a hot/humid environment.

Prolonged Exercise in a Hot Environment

Figure 10.21 illustrates the change in pulmonary ventilation during prolonged constant-load submaximal exercise (below the lactate threshold) in two different environmental conditions. The neutral environment represents exercise in a cool, low-relative-humidity environment (19° C, 45% relative humidity). The second condition represented in figure 10.21 is a hot/high-humidity environment, which hampers heat loss from the body. The major point to appreciate from figure 10.21 is that ventilation tends to "drift" upward during prolonged work. The mechanism to explain this increase in $\dot{V}_E$ during work in the heat is an increase in blood temperature, which directly affects the respiratory control center (56).

Another interesting point to gain from figure 10.21 is that although ventilation is greater during exercise in a hot/humid environment when compared to work in a cool environment, there is little difference in arterial PCO_2 between the two types of exercise. This finding suggests that the increase in ventilation seen during work in the heat is due to an increase in breathing frequency and dead-space ventilation (22). This type of breathing in humans in hot weather is similar to the panting observed in dogs and cats during warm conditions (22).

Incremental Exercise

The ventilatory response for an elite male distance runner and an untrained college student during an incremental exercise test is illustrated in figure 10.22. In both subjects, ventilation increases as a linear function of oxygen uptake up to 50%–75% of O_2 max, where

ventilation begins to rise exponentially. This $\dot{V}_E$ "inflection point" has been called the **ventilatory threshold (Tvent)** (42, 55, 58).

An interesting point that emerges from figure 10.22 is the startling difference between the highly trained elite athlete and the untrained subject in arterial PO_2 during heavy exercise. The untrained subject is able to maintain arterial PO_2 within 10–12 mm Hg of the normal resting value, while the highly trained distance runner shows a decrease of 30–40 mm Hg at near-maximal work (22, 23, 26). This drop in arterial PO_2, often observed in the healthy, trained athlete, is similar to that observed in exercising patients who possess severe lung disease. However, not all healthy, elite endurance athletes develop low-arterial PO_2 values (low PO_2 is called *hypoxemia*) during heavy exercise. It appears that only about 40%–50% of highly trained endurance athletes ($\dot{V}O_2$ max 4.5 ℓ/min or > 68 ml · kg · min^{-1}) show this marked hypoxemia (62, 70). In addition, the degree of hypoxemia observed in these athletes during heavy work varies considerably among individuals (23, 59, 70, 81). The reason for the subject differences is unclear.

Perhaps the most important question concerning this exercise-induced hypoxemia is what factor(s) accounts for this failure of the pulmonary system? Unfortunately, a complete answer to this question cannot be provided. Although direct evidence is lacking, it seems possible that much of the decline in arterial PO_2 during heavy exercise in the elite athlete is due to diffusion limitations caused by a reduced amount of time that the RBC spends in the pulmonary capillaries (22, 28). This short transit time for RBCs in the pulmonary capillary is probably due to high cardiac output achieved by these athletes during maximal exercise. This short RBC transit time may be less than the required time for gas equilibrium to be achieved between the lung and blood (23, 64, 88).

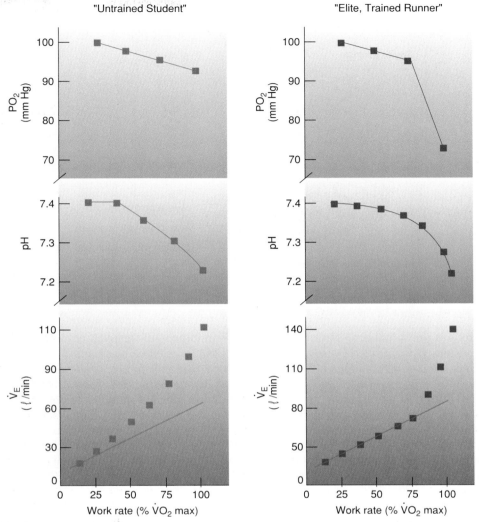

Figure 10.22
Changes in ventilation, blood gas tensions, and pH during incremental exercise in a highly trained male distance runner and an untrained male college student.

in summary

- At the onset of constant-load submaximal exercise, ventilation increases rapidly, followed by a slower rise toward a steady state value. Arterial PO_2 and PCO_2 are maintained relatively constant during this type of exercise.
- During prolonged exercise in a hot/humid environment, ventilation "drifts" upward due to the influence of rising body temperature on the respiratory control center.
- Incremental exercise results in a linear increase in $\dot{V}_E$ up to approximately 50%–70% of O_2 max; at higher work rates, ventilation begins to rise exponentially. This ventilatory inflection point has been called the ventilatory threshold.

Control of Ventilation

Obviously, precise regulation of pulmonary gas exchange during rest and exercise is important in maintaining homeostasis by providing normal arterial O_2 content and maintenance of the acid-base balance within the body. Although the control of breathing has been actively studied by physiologists for many years, many unanswered questions remain. Let's begin our discussion of ventilatory control during exercise with a review of ventilatory regulation at rest.

Ventilatory Regulation at Rest

As mentioned earlier, inspiration and expiration are produced by contraction and relaxation of the diaphragm during quiet breathing, and by accessory muscles during exercise. Contraction and relaxation of these respiratory muscles are directly controlled by

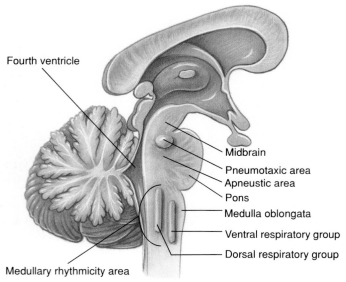

Fourth ventricle

Midbrain
Pneumotaxic area
Apneustic area
Pons
Medulla oblongata
Ventral respiratory group
Dorsal respiratory group

Medullary rhythmicity area

Figure 10.23
Locations of the brain stem respiratory control centers.

somatic motor neurons in the spinal cord. Motor neuron activity, in turn, is directly controlled by the respiratory control center in the medulla oblongata.

Respiratory Control Center
The initial drive to inspire or expire comes from neurons located in the medulla oblongata (labeled as the "rhythmicity area" in figure 10.23). Discharges from some of these neurons produce inspiration, while discharges from other neurons produce expiration. These respiratory neurons act in a reciprocal way to produce a rhythmic pattern of breathing (9a,31b,73, 74). At rest, the cycle of inspiration and a passive expiration is built in, or intrinsic to, the neural activity of the medulla. However, neural activity in the medulla can be modified by neurons located outside the respiratory rhythmicity center.

Two additional areas located in the region of the brainstem called the *pons* contribute to respiratory control; these are the *apneustic area* and the *pneumotaxic area*. The apneustic area directly communicates with inspiratory neurons located in the rhythmicity area to stop inspiratory neuronal activity. Therefore, it is believed that the apneustic area functions as an "inspiratory cutoff switch" that terminates inspiration. Another group of respiratory neurons, the pneumotaxic area, functions to fine tune the activity of the apneustic area (figure 10.23). The practical function of the apneustic/pneumotaxic areas is that they work in concert to regulate the depth of breathing (47).

Input to the Respiratory Control Center
Several types of receptors are capable of modifying the actions of neurons contained in the respiratory control center. In general, input to the respiratory control center can be classified into two types: (1) neural and (2) humoral (blood-borne). Neural input refers to afferent or efferent input to the respiratory control center from neurons that are excited by means other than blood-borne stimuli. Humoral input to the respiratory control center refers to the influence of some blood-borne stimuli reaching a specialized chemoreceptor. This receptor reacts to the strength of the stimuli and sends the appropriate message to the medulla. A brief overview of each of these receptors will be presented prior to a discussion of ventilatory control during exercise.

Humoral Chemoreceptors
Chemoreceptors are specialized neurons that are capable of responding to changes in the internal environment. Traditionally, respiratory chemoreceptors are classified according to their location as being either *central chemoreceptors* or *peripheral chemoreceptors*.

Central Chemoreceptors The central chemoreceptors are located in the medulla (anatomically separate from the respiratory center) and are affected by changes in PCO_2 and H^+ of the cerebral spinal fluid (CSF). An increase in either PCO_2 or H^+ of the CSF results in the central chemoreceptors sending afferent input into the respiratory center to increase ventilation (27).

Peripheral Chemoreceptors The primary peripheral chemoreceptors are located in the aortic arch and at the bifurcation of the common carotid artery. The receptors located in the aorta are called **aortic bodies** and those found in the carotid artery are **carotid bodies.** These peripheral chemoreceptors respond to increases in arterial H^+ concentrations and PCO_2 (1, 3, 10, 89). Additionally, the carotid bodies are sensitive to increases in blood potassium levels (16, 52) and decreases in arterial PO_2 (16, 52). When comparing these two sets of peripheral chemoreceptors, it appears that the carotid bodies are more important (27, 47).

Figure 10.24

Changes in ventilation as a function of increasing arterial PCO_2. Notice that ventilation increases as a linear function of increasing PCO_2.

Figure 10.25

Changes in ventilation as a function of decreasing arterial PO_2. Note the existence of a "hypoxic threshold" for ventilation as arterial PO_2 declines.

There is evidence that specialized (peripheral) chemoreceptors in the lungs of dogs and rabbits are sensitive to CO_2 and act to match ventilation with CO_2 return to the lungs (4, 9, 14, 38–40, 78, 80, 84, 85). In other words, an increase in CO_2 return to the lung stimulates lung receptors, which send a message to the respiratory control center to increase $\dot{V}_E$. This increase in $\dot{V}_E$ is hypothesized to be precisely matched to the amount of the CO_2 returned to the lung, and thus arterial PCO_2 remains constant. Do these lung CO_2 receptors exist in humans? At present, a definitive answer to this question is not available; exciting research in this area continues.

Effect of Blood PCO_2, PO_2, *and Potassium on Ventilation* How do the central and peripheral chemoreceptors respond to changes in chemical stimuli? The effects of increases in arterial PCO_2 on minute ventilation can be seen in figure 10.24. Note that $\dot{V}_E$ increases as a linear function of arterial PCO_2. In general, a 1 mm Hg rise in PCO_2 results in a 2 liter/minute increase in $\dot{V}_E$ (27). The increase in $\dot{V}_E$ that results from a rise in arterial PCO_2 is likely due to CO_2 stimulation of both the carotid bodies and the central chemoreceptors (27, 53).

In healthy individuals breathing at sea level, changes in arterial PO_2 have little effect on the control of ventilation (47). However, exposure to an environment with a barometric pressure much lower than sea level (i.e., high altitude), can alter arterial PO_2 and stimulate the carotid bodies, which in turn signal the respiratory center to increase ventilation. The relationship between arterial PO_2 and $\dot{V}_E$ is illustrated in figure 10.25. The point on the $PO_2/\dot{V}_E$ curve where $\dot{V}_E$ begins to rise rapidly is often referred to as the *hypoxic threshold* ("hypoxic" means low PO_2) (2). This hypoxic threshold usually occurs around an arterial PO_2 of 60–75 mm Hg. The chemoreceptors responsible for the increase in $\dot{V}_E$ following exposure to low PO_2 are the carotid bodies, since the aortic and central chemoreceptors in humans do not respond to changes in PO_2 (27, 47).

Recent evidence demonstrates that increases in blood levels of potassium stimulate the carotid bodies and promote an increase in ventilation (16, 52). Since blood potassium levels rise during exercise due to a net potassium efflux from the contracting muscle, some investigators have suggested that potassium may play a role in regulating ventilation during exercise (16, 52). More will be said about this later.

Neural Input to the Respiratory Control Center

Evidence obtained from animal experiments shows that neural input to the respiratory control center can come from both efferent and afferent pathways. For example, it has been demonstrated in cats that impulses from the motor cortex (i.e., central command) can control both skeletal muscle and drive ventilation in proportion to the amount of work being performed (32, 33). In short, neural impulses originating in the motor cortex may pass through the medulla and "spill over," causing an increase in $\dot{V}_E$ that reflects the number of muscle motor units being recruited.

Afferent input to the respiratory control center during exercise may come from one of several peripheral receptors such as the muscle spindles, Golgi tendon organs, or joint pressure receptors (6, 46, 79). In addition, it is possible that special chemoreceptors located in muscle may respond to changes in potassium and H^+ concentrations and send afferent information to the respiratory control center. This type of input to the medulla is considered afferent neural information, since the stimuli is not humorally mediated. Finally, recent evidence suggests that the right ventricle of the heart contains mechanoreceptors that send afferent information back to the respiratory control center relative to increases in cardiac output (e.g., during exercise) (85). These mechanoreceptors might play important roles in providing afferent input to the respiratory control center at the onset of exercise.

Ventilatory Control During Submaximal Exercise

In the previous sections, we have discussed several possible sources of input to the respiratory control center. Unfortunately, at present, which of these factors is most responsible for ventilatory control during exercise remains controversial (6, 8, 15, 17, 21, 28b, 31a, 32, 36, 46, 54, 63, 84, 89). Nonetheless, it appears that ventilatory control during exercise has similarities to the control of the cardiovascular system. Indeed, there is growing evidence that the "primary" drive to increase ventilation during exercise is due to neural input from higher brain centers (central command) to the respiratory control center (25). However, the fact that arterial PCO_2 is tightly regulated during most types of submaximal exercise suggests that humoral chemoreceptors and afferent neural feedback from working muscles act to fine-tune breathing to match the metabolic rate and thus maintain a rather constant arterial PCO_2 (12, 13, 51a, 84). Therefore, ventilation during exercise is regulated by several overlapping factors which provides redundancy to the control system.

During prolonged exercise in a hot environment, ventilation can be influenced by factors other than those discussed above. For example, the drift upward in $\dot{V}_E$ seen in figure 10.21 may be due to a direct influence of rising blood temperature on the respiratory control center, and rising blood catecholamines (epinephrine and norepinephrine) stimulating the carotid bodies to increase $\dot{V}_E$ (56).

To summarize, the increase in ventilation during submaximal exercise is due to an interaction of both neural and humoral input to the respiratory control center. It seems likely that efferent neural mechanisms from higher brain centers (central command) provide the primary drive to breathe during exercise, with humoral chemoreceptors and neural feedback from working muscles providing a means of precisely matching ventilation with the amount of CO_2 produced via metabolism. This apparent redundancy in mechanisms is not surprising when one considers the important role that respiration plays in sustaining life and maintaining a steady state during exercise (37, 40). A summary of respiratory control during submaximal exercise appears in figure 10.26.

Ventilatory Control During Heavy Exercise

Controversy exists concerning the mechanism to explain the alinear rise in ventilation (ventilatory threshold) that occurs during an incremental exercise test. However, several factors may contribute to this rise. First, examination of figure 10.22 suggests that the alinear rise in $\dot{V}_E$ and the decrease in pH often occur simultaneously. Since rising H^+ levels in blood have been shown to stimulate the carotid bodies and increase $\dot{V}_E$, it has been proposed that the rise in blood lactate, which occurs during incremental exercise, is the stimulus causing the

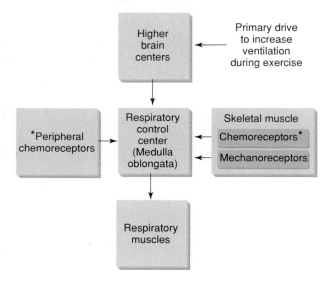

*Act to fine tune ventilation during exercise

Figure 10.26

A summary of respiratory control during submaximal exercise. See text for details.

alinear rise in $\dot{V}_E$ (i.e., ventilatory threshold). Based on this belief, it is common for researchers to estimate the lactate threshold noninvasively by measurement of the ventilatory threshold (5, 17, 82). However, several studies have shown that this technique is not perfect and that the ventilatory threshold and the lactate threshold do not always occur at the same work rate (34, 55).

What additional factors, other than rising blood lactate, might cause the alinear rise in $\dot{V}_E$ observed during incremental exercise? The close relationship between blood potassium levels and ventilation during heavy exercise has led several investigators to speculate that potassium is an important factor in controlling ventilation during heavy exercise (16, 48, 52). Certainly other secondary factors, such as rising body temperature and blood catecholamines, might play a small contributory role to the increasing $\dot{V}_E$ during heavy exercise. Further, it is likely that neural input to the respiratory control center influences the ventilatory pattern during incremental exercise. For example, as exercise intensity increases, motor unit recruitment may occur in a nonlinear fashion and the associated efferent and afferent neural signals to the respiratory control center may promote the alinear rise in $\dot{V}_E$ seen at the ventilatory threshold (55).

To review, it is logical that the rise in blood lactate and reduction in blood pH observed at the lactate threshold can stimulate ventilation and thus may be a primary mechanism to explain the ventilatory threshold. However, secondary factors such as an increase in blood potassium levels, rising body temperature, elevated blood catecholamines, and possible neural influences might also contribute to ventilatory control during heavy exercise.

Training Reduces the Ventilatory Response to Exercise

Although exercise training does not alter the structure of the lung, endurance training does promote a decrease in ventilation during submaximal exercise at moderate-to-high intensity work rates. For example, when comparisons are made at a fixed submaximal work rate, a training program can reduce exercise ventilation by 20%–30% below pretraining levels (20a, 20b)(see figure 10.27).

What is the mechanism to explain this training-induced reduction in exercise ventilation? A definitive answer is not known. However, it seems likely that this training effect is due to changes in the aerobic capacity of the locomotor skeletal muscles. These training-induced changes result in less production of lactic acid and probably less afferent feedback from the working muscles to stimulate breathing (20a).

Figure 10.27

Illustration of the effects of endurance training on ventilation during exercise.

in summary

- The respiratory control center is contained in the medulla oblongata. At rest, the normal breathing pattern is determined by intrinsic firing of inspiratory neurons. This can be modified by neurons outside the medulla oblongata. The apneustic center and the pneumotaxic center (both located in the pons) work together to regulate the depth of breathing by acting as a cutoff switch for inspiratory neurons.

- Input into the respiratory control center to increase ventilation can come from both neural and humoral sources. Neural input may come from higher brain centers, or it may arise from receptors in the exercising muscle. Humoral input may arise from central chemoreceptors, peripheral chemoreceptors, and/or lung CO_2 receptors. The central chemoreceptors are sensitive to increases in PCO_2 and decreases in pH. The peripheral chemoreceptors (carotid bodies are the most important) are sensitive to increases in PCO_2 and decreases in PO_2 or pH. Receptors in the lung that are sensitive to an increase in PCO_2 are hypothesized to exist.

- The primary drive to increase ventilation during exercise probably comes from higher brain centers (central command). Also, humoral chemoreceptors and neural feedback from working muscles act to fine-tune ventilation.

- Controversy exists concerning the mechanism to explain the alinear rise in ventilation (ventilatory threshold) that occurs during an incremental exercise test. However, it appears that the rise in blood H^+ concentration that occurs during this type of exercise provides the principal stimulus to increase ventilation via stimulation of the carotid bodies.

Do the Lungs Limit Maximal Exercise Performance?

Though some controversy exists (11), the pulmonary system is not generally considered to be the limiting factor during prolonged submaximal exercise (18, 22, 24, 30, 35). Although respiratory muscle failure can occur during certain disease states (e.g., obstructive lung disease), respiratory muscle fatigue is not thought to limit exercise in healthy humans exercising at sea level (24, 30). Indeed, the major muscle of inspiration, the diaphragm, is a highly oxidative muscle that resists fatigue (66, 69, 70a). The best evidence that the lungs and respiratory muscles are performing well during prolonged submaximal exercise is the observation that arterial oxygen content does not decrease during this type of work (68).

As in prolonged submaximal exercise, the lungs are not thought to limit performance in young healthy subjects during high-intensity (e.g., 90%–100% $\dot{V}O_2$ max) exercise at sea level (30, 35, 45). However, there is one possible exception to this rule—the elite endurance athlete. That is, the elite endurance athlete who demonstrates exercise-induced hypoxemia is a paradoxical example of a healthy individual in which the pulmonary system may not keep pace with the body's need for oxygen (the mechanism to explain this pulmonary failure was discussed earlier in this chapter). Recall that in approximately 40%–50% of elite endurance athletes, arterial PO_2 declines during heavy exercise to a level that may negatively impact their ability to transport oxygen to the working muscle (22, 28, 62, 65) (figure 10.22). Evidence from the University of Florida suggests that the pulmonary system may limit $\dot{V}O_2$ max in this unique group of athletes (23, 65, 70). In healthy people, this is the only example of a pulmonary limitation to exercise performance.

in summary

- The pulmonary system is not generally considered to be the limiting factor during prolonged submaximal exercise.
- The lungs are not thought to limit performance in young healthy subjects during high-intensity exercise at sea level. However, the elite endurance athlete who demonstrates exercise-induced hypoxemia is an example of where the pulmonary system may not keep pace with the body's need for oxygen. Indeed, evidence demonstrates that the pulmonary system may limit $\dot{V}O_2$ max in this unique group of athletes.

study questions

1. What is the primary function of the pulmonary system? What secondary functions does it serve?
2. List and discuss the major anatomical components of the respiratory system.
3. What muscle groups are involved in ventilation during rest? During exercise?
4. What is the functional significance of the ventilation-perfusion ratio? How would a high V/Q ratio affect gas exchange in the lung?
5. Discuss those factors that influence the rate of diffusion across the blood-gas interface in the lung.
6. Graph the relationship between hemoglobin-O_2 saturation and the partial pressure of O_2 in the blood. What is the functional significance of the shape of the O_2-hemoglobin dissociation curve? What factors affect the shape of the curve?
7. Discuss the modes of transportation for CO_2 in the blood.
8. Graph the ventilatory response in the transition from rest to constant-load submaximal exercise. What happens to ventilation if the exercise is prolonged and performed in a hot/humid environment? Why?
9. Graph the ventilatory response to incremental exercise. Label the ventilatory threshold. What factor(s) might explain the ventilatory threshold?
10. List and identify the functions of the chemoreceptors that contribute to the control of breathing.
11. What neural afferents might also contribute to the regulation of ventilation during exercise?
12. Discuss the control of ventilation during exercise.

suggested readings

Dempsey, J., H. Forster, and D. Ainsworth. 1994. Regulation of hyperpnea, hyperventilation, and respiratory muscle recruitment during exercise. In *Regulation of Breathing*, eds. A. Pack and J. Dempsey, 1065–1134. New York: Marcel Dekker.

Dempsey, J. et al. 1996. *Handbook of Physiology: Exercise*. Section 12: Integration of motor, circulatory, respiratory, and metabolic control. (L. Rawl and J. Sheppard) New York: Oxford University Press.

Dempsey, J., S. Powers, and N. Gledhill. 1990. Cardiovascular and pulmonary adaptation to physical activity. In *Exercise, Fitness, and Health: A Consensus of Current Knowledge*, ed. C. Bouchard et al., 205–16. Champaign, IL: Human Kinetics.

Duffin, J., K. Enzure, and J. Lipski. 1995. Breathing rhythm generation: Focus on the rostal ventrolateral medulla. *News in Physiological Sciences* 10:133–40.

references

1. Allen, C., and N. Jones. 1984. Rate of change of alveolar carbon dioxide and the control of ventilation during exercise. *Journal of Physiology* (London) 355:1–9.

2. Asmussen, E. 1983. Control of ventilation in exercise. In *Exercise and Sport Science Reviews*, vol. 2., ed. R. Terjung. Philadelphia: Franklin Press.

3. Band, D. et al. 1980. Respiratory oscillations in arterial carbon dioxide tension as a signal in exercise. *Nature* 283:84–85.

4. Banzett, R., H. Coleridge, and J. Coleridge. 1978. Pulmonary CO_2 ventilatory reflex in dogs: Effective range of CO_2 and vagal cooling. *Respiration Physiology* 34:121–34.

5. Beaver, W., K. Wasserman, and B. Whipp. 1986. A new method for detecting anaerobic threshold by gas exchange. *Journal of Applied Physiology* 60:2020–27.

6. Bennett, F. 1984. A role for neural pathways in exercise hyperpnea. *Journal of Applied Physiology* 56:1559–64.

7. Bennett, F., and W. Fordyce. 1985. Characteristics of the ventilatory exercise stimulus. *Respiration Physiology* 59:55–63.

8. Bennett, F., R. Tallman, and G. Grodins. 1984. Role of $\dot{V}CO_2$ in control of breathing in awake exercising dogs. *Journal of Applied Physiology* 56:1335–37.

9. Beon, J., W. Kuhlmann, and M. Fedde. 1980. Control of respiration in the chicken: Effects of venous CO_2 loading. *Respiration Physiology* 39:169–81.

9a. Bianchi, A., M. Denavit-Saubie, and J. Champagnat. 1995. Central control of breathing in mammals: Neuronal circuitry, membrane properties, and neurotransmitters. *Physiological Reviews* 75:1–45.

10. Bisgard, G. et al. 1982. Role of the carotid body in hyperpnea of moderate exercise in goats. *Journal of Applied Physiology* 52:1216–22.

11. Boutellier, U., and P. Piwko. 1992. The respiratory system as an exercise limiting factor in normal sedentary subjects. *European Journal of Applied Physiology* 64:145–52.

12. Brice, A. et al. 1988. Is the hyperpnea of muscular contractions critically dependent upon spinal afferents? *Journal of Applied Physiology* 64:226–33.

13. Brice, A. et al. 1988. Ventilatory and $PaCO_2$ responses to voluntary and electrically induced leg exercise. *Journal of Applied Physiology* 64:218–25.

14. Brown, H., K. Wasserman, and B. Whipp. 1976. Effect of beta-adrenergic blockade during exercise on ventilation and gas exchange. *Journal of Applied Physiology* 41:886–92.

15. Brown, D. et al. 1990. Ventilatory response of spinal cord-lesioned subjects to electrically induced exercise. *Journal of Applied Physiology* 68:2312–21.

16. Busse, M., N. Maassen, and H. Konrad. 1991. Relation between plasma K^+ and ventilation during incremental exercise after glycogen depletion and repletion in man. *Journal of Physiology* (London) 443:469–76.

17. Caiozzo, V. et al. 1982. A comparison of gas exchange indices used to detect the anaerobic threshold. *Journal of Applied Physiology* 53:1184–89.

18. Capen, R. et al. 1990. Distribution of pulmonary capillary transit times in recruited networks. *Journal of Applied Physiology* 69:473–78.

19. Casaburi, R. et al. 1977. Ventilatory and gas exchange dynamics in response to sinusoidal work. *Journal of Applied Physiology* 42:300–11.

20. Casaburi, R. et al. 1978. Ventilatory control characteristics of the exercise hyperpnea discerned from dynamic forcing techniques. *Chest* 73:280–83.

20a. Casaburi, R. et al. 1987. Mediation of reduced ventilatory response to exercise after endurance training. *Journal of Applied Physiology* 63:1533–38.

20b. Clanton, T. et al. 1987. Effects of swim training on lung volumes and inspiratory muscle conditioning. *Journal of Applied Physiology* 62:39–46.

20c. Coleridge, H., and J. Coleridge. 1995. Airway axon reflexes-where now? *News in Physiological Sciences* 10:91–96.

21. Dejours, P. 1964. Control of respiration in muscular exercise. In *Handbook of Physiology*, section 3, ed. W. Fenn. Washington: American Physiological Society.

22. Dempsey, J. 1986. Is the lung built for exercise? *Medicine and Science in Sports and Exercise* 18:143–55.

23. Dempsey, J. et al. 1982. Limitation to exercise capacity and endurance: Pulmonary system. *Canadian Journal of Applied Sports Sciences* 7:4–13.

24. Dempsey, J., E. Aaron, and B. Martin. 1988. Pulmonary function during prolonged exercise. In *Perspectives in Exercise and Sports Medicine: Prolonged Exercise*, ed. D. Lamb and R. Murray, 75–119. Indianapolis: Benchmark Press.

25. Dempsey, J., H. Forster, and D. Ainsworth. 1994. Regulation of hyperpnea, hyperventilation, and respiratory muscle recruitment during exercise. In *Regulation of Breathing*. eds. A Pack and J. Dempsey, 1065–1134. New York: Marcel Dekker.

26. Dempsey, J., and R. Fregosi. 1985. Adaptability of the pulmonary system to changing metabolic requirements. *American Journal of Cardiology* 55:59D–67D.

27. Dempsey, J., G. Mitchell, and C. Smith. 1984. Exercise and chemoreception. *American Review of Respiratory Disease* 129:31–34.

28. Dempsey, J., S. Powers, and N. Gledhill. 1990. Cardiovascular and pulmonary adaptation to physical activity. In *Exercise, Fitness, and Health: A Consensus of Current Knowledge*, ed. C. Bouchard et al., 205–16. Champaign, IL: Human Kinetics.

28a. Dempsey, J., E. Vidruk, and G. Mitchell. 1985. Pulmonary control systems in exercise: Update. *Federation Proceedings* 44:2260–70.

28b. Dempsey, J. et al. 1996. *Handbook of Physiology: Exercise*. Section 12: Integration of motor, circulatory, respiratory, and metabolic control. L. Rawl and J. Sheppard. New York: Oxford University Press.

29. Dodd, S. et al. 1988. Effects of acute beta-adrenergic blockade on ventilation and gas exchange during the rest-to-work transition. *Aviation, Space, and Environmental Medicine* 59:255–58.

30. Dodd, S. et al. 1989. Exercise performance following intense, short-term ventilatory work. *International Journal of Sports Medicine* 10:48–52.

31. Domino, K. et al. 1991. Pulmonary blood flow and ventilation-perfusion heterogeneity. *Journal of Applied Physiology* 71:252–58.

31a. Duffin, J. 1994. Neural drives to breathing during exercise. Canadian *Journal of Applied Physiology* 19:289–304.

31b. Duffin, J., K. Enzure, and J. Lipski. 1995. Breathing rhythm generation: Focus on the rostal ventrolateral medulla. *News in Physiological Sciences* 10:133–40.

~~...and T. Waldron. 1981.~~

50. McParland, C., J. Mink, and C. Gallagher. 1991. Respiratory adaptations to dead space loading during maximal incremental exercise. *Journal of Applied Physiology* 70:55–62.

51. Mercier, J., M. Ramonatxo, and C. Prefaut. 1992. Breathing pattern and ventilatory response to CO_2 during exercise. *International Journal of Sports Medicine*

Acid-Base Balance During Exercise

objectives

By studying this chapter, you should be able to do the following:

1. Define the terms *acid*, *base*, and *pH*.
2. Discuss the importance of acid-base regulation to exercise performance.
3. List the principal intracellular and extracellular buffers.
4. Explain the role of respiration in the regulation of acid-base status during exercise.
5. Outline acid-base regulation during exercise.
6. Discuss the principal ways that hydrogen ions are produced during exercise.

outline

Acids, Bases, and pH   206
Hydrogen Ion Production During Exercise   207
Importance of Acid-Base Regulation During Exercise   207

Acid-Base Buffer Systems   208
  Intracellular Buffers   208
  Extracellular Buffers   208
Respiratory Influence on Acid-Base Balance   209

Regulation of Acid-Base Balance via the Kidneys   210
Regulation of Acid-Base Balance During Exercise   210

key terms

acidosis
acid
alkalosis
base

buffer
hydrogen ions
ion
pH

respiratory compensation
strong acids
strong bases

lectrolytes that release **hydrogen ions** are called acids (an **ion** is any atom that is missing electrons or has gained electrons). Substances that readily combine with hydrogen ions are termed *bases*. In physiology, the concentration of hydrogen ions is expressed in pH units. The pH of body fluids must be regulated (i.e., normal arterial blood pH = 7.40 ± .02) in order to maintain homeostasis. Regulation of the pH of body fluids is extremely important since changes in hydrogen ion concentrations can alter the rates of enzyme-controlled metabolic reactions and modify numerous other normal body functions. Therefore, acid-base balance is primarily concerned with the regulation of hydrogen ion concentrations. Heavy exercise can present a serious challenge to hydrogen ion control systems due to lactic acid production, and hydrogen ions may limit performance in some types of intense activities (2, 3, 9, 13, 15, 16, 20, 23, 24, 26, 27). Given the potential detrimental influence of hydrogen ion accumulation on exercise performance, it is important that the student of exercise physiology have an understanding of acid-base regulation.

Acids, Bases, and pH

In biological systems, one of the simplest, but most important ions is the hydrogen ion. The concentration of the hydrogen ion influences the rates of chemical reaction, the shape and function of enzymes as well as other cellular proteins, and the integrity of the cell itself (5, 7, 11, 29, 32).

An **acid** is defined as a molecule that can liberate hydrogen ions and thus can raise the hydrogen ion concentration of an aqueous solution above that of pure water. In contrast, a **base** is a molecule that is capable of combining with hydrogen ions and therefore lowers the hydrogen ion concentration of the solution.

Acids that tend to give up hydrogen ions (ionize) more completely are termed **strong acids.** For example, lactic acid produced during heavy exercise as a result of glycolysis is a relatively strong acid. At normal body pH, lactic acid tends to liberate almost all of its hydrogen ions and therefore elevates the hydrogen ion concentration of the body.

Bases that ionize completely are defined as **strong bases.** The bicarbonate ion (HCO_3^-) is an example of a biologically important strong base. Bicarbonate ions are found in relatively large concentrations in blood and are capable of combining with hydrogen ions to form a weak acid called carbonic acid. The role of HCO_3^- in the regulation of acid-base balance during exercise will be discussed later in the chapter.

As stated earlier, the concentration of hydrogen ions is expressed in pH units. The **pH** of a solution is defined as the negative logarithm of the hydrogen ion concentration (H^+). Recall that a logarithm is the exponent that indicates the power to which one number must be raised to obtain another number. For instance,

the logarithm of 100 to the base 10 is 2. Thus, the definition of pH can be written mathematically as:

$$pH = -\log_{10} [H^+]$$

As an example, if the $[H^+]$ = 40nM (0.000000040 M), then the pH would be 7.40.

A solution is considered neutral (in terms of acid-base status) if the concentration of H^+ and hydroxyl ions (OH^-) are equal. This is the case for pure water, in which the concentrations are both 0.00000010 M. Thus, the pH of pure water is:

$$pH \text{ (pure water)} = -\log_{10} [H^+]$$
$$= 7.0$$

Figure 11.1 shows the continuum of the pH scale. Note that as the hydrogen ion concentration increases, pH declines and the acidity of the blood increases, resulting in a condition termed **acidosis.** Conversely, as the hydrogen ion concentration decreases, pH increases and the solution becomes more basic (alkalotic). This condition is termed **alkalosis.** Conditions leading to acidosis or alkalosis are summarized in figure 11.2.

Figure 11.1

The pH scale. If the pH of arterial blood drops below the normal value of 7.4, the resulting condition is termed acidosis. In contrast, if the pH increases above 7.4, blood alkalosis occurs.

Figure 11.2

Acidosis results from an accumulation of acids or a loss of bases. Alkalosis results from a loss of acids or an accumulation of bases.

- Acids are defined as molecules that can liberate hydrogen ions, which increases the hydrogen ion concentration of an aqueous solution.
- Bases are molecules that are capable of combining with hydrogen ions.
- The concentration of hydrogen ions in a solution is quantified by pH units. The pH of a solution is defined as the negative logarithm of the hydrogen ion concentration:

$$pH = -\log_{10} [H^+]$$

Hydrogen Ion Production During Exercise

Although small quantities of acids or bases are present in foods, the major threat to the pH of body fluids is acids formed in metabolic processes. These metabolic acids can be divided into three major groups (6, 16):

1. Volatile acids (e.g., carbon dioxide). Carbon dioxide, an end product in the oxidation of carbohydrates, fats, and proteins, can be regarded as an acid by virtue of its ability to react with water to form carbonic acid (H_2CO_3), which in turn dissociates to form H^+ and HCO_3^-:

$$CO_2 + H_2O \longleftrightarrow H_2CO_3 \longleftrightarrow H^+ + HCO_3^-$$

Because CO_2 is a gas and can be eliminated by the lungs, it is often referred to as a volatile acid. During the course of a day, the body produces large amounts of CO_2 due to normal metabolism. During exercise, metabolic production of CO_2 increases and therefore adds an additional "volatile acid" load on the body.

2. Fixed acids (e.g., sulfuric acid and phosphoric acid). Sulfuric acid is a product of the oxidation of certain amino acids, while phosphoric acid is formed in the metabolism of various phospholipids and nucleic acids. In contrast to CO_2, both sulfuric acid and phosphoric acid are nonvolatile and therefore are referred to as fixed acids. The production of fixed acids varies with the diet and is not greatly influenced by acute exercise. Hence, fixed acids are not a major contributor of hydrogen ions during heavy exercise.

3. Organic acids (e.g., lactic acid). Organic acids, such as lactic acid and acetoacetic acid, are formed in the metabolism of carbohydrates and fats, respectively (chapters 3 and 4). Under normal resting conditions, both of these acids

Figure 11.3
Sources of hydrogen ions due to metabolic processes.

are further metabolized to CO_2 and therefore do not greatly influence the pH of body fluids. However, an exception to this rule is during heavy exercise (i.e., work above the lactate threshold). During periods of intense physical efforts, contracting skeletal muscles can produce large amounts of lactic acid, resulting in acidosis. In general, it appears that production of lactic acid during heavy exercise presents the greatest challenge to maintaining pH homeostasis during exercise. Some metabolic processes that serve as sources of hydrogen ions are illustrated in figure 11.3.

in summary

- Metabolic acids can be subdivided into three major groups: (1) volatile acids (e.g., carbon dioxide), (2) fixed acids (e.g., sulfuric acid, phosphoric acid), and (3) organic acids (e.g., lactic acid).

Importance of Acid-Base Regulation During Exercise

As discussed earlier, heavy exercise results in the production of large amounts of lactic acid by the contracting skeletal muscle. Lactic acid, a strong acid, ionizes and releases hydrogen ions. These hydrogen ions can exert a powerful effect on other molecules due to their small size and positive charge. Hydrogen ions exert their influence by attaching to molecules and thus altering their original size and shape (3, 9, 12, 22, 28). This change in size and shape may alter the normal function of the molecule (enzyme) and therefore influence metabolism in an important way.

An increase in the intramuscular hydrogen ion concentration can impair exercise performance in at least two ways. First, an increase in the hydrogen ion concentration reduces the muscle cell's ability to produce ATP by inhibiting key enzymes involved in both anaerobic and aerobic production of ATP (3, 9, 14). Second, hydrogen ions compete with calcium ions for binding sites on troponin, thereby hindering the contractile process (3, 9, 31). This will be discussed again in chapter 19.

in summary

- Failure to maintain acid-base homeostasis during exercise can impair performance by inhibition of metabolic pathways responsible for production of ATP or by interference with the contractile process in the working muscle.

Acid–Base Buffer Systems

From the preceding discussion, it is clear that a rapid accumulation of hydrogen ions during heavy exercise can negatively influence muscular performance. Therefore, it is important that the body have control systems capable of regulating acid-base status to prevent drastic decreases or increases in pH. How does the body regulate pH? One of the most important means of regulating hydrogen ion concentrations in body fluids is by the aid of buffers. A **buffer** resists pH change by removing hydrogen ions when the hydrogen ion concentration increases, and releasing hydrogen ions when the hydrogen ion concentration falls.

Buffers often consist of a weak acid and its associated base (called a conjugate base). The ability of individual buffers to resist pH change is dependent upon two factors. First, individual buffers differ in their intrinsic physiochemical ability to act as buffers. Simply stated, some buffers are better than others. A second factor influencing buffering capacity is the concentration of the buffer present. The greater the concentration of a particular buffer, the more effective the buffer can be in preventing pH change.

Intracellular Buffers

The first line of defense in protecting against pH change during exercise is in the cell itself. The most common intracellular buffers are proteins and phosphate groups

Table 11.1	Chemical Acid-Base Buffer Systems	
Buffer System	**Constituents**	**Actions**
Bicarbonate system	Sodium bicarbonate ($NaHCO_3$)	Converts strong acid into weak acid
	Carbonic acid (H_2CO_3)	Converts strong base into weak base
Phosphate system	Sodium phosphate ($Na_2HPO_4^-$)	Converts strong acid into weak acid
Protein system	COO^- group of a molecule	Accepts hydrogens in the presence of excess acid
	NH_3 group of a molecule	Accepts hydrogens in the presence of excess acid

(16). Many intracellular proteins contain ionizable groups that are weak acids capable of accepting hydrogen ions. Intracellular phosphocreatine (chapter 3) has been shown to be a useful buffer at the onset of exercise (1). Further, weak phosphoric acids are found in relatively large concentrations in cells and also serve as an intracellular buffer system. In addition, bicarbonate in muscle has been demonstrated to be a useful buffer during exercise (12). A summary of the chemical action of intracellular buffer systems is presented in table 11.1.

Extracellular Buffers

The blood contains three principal buffer systems (12, 16): (1) proteins, (2) hemoglobin, and (3) bicarbonate. Blood proteins act as buffers in the extracellular compartment. Like intracellular proteins, these blood proteins contain ionizable groups that are weak acids and therefore act as buffers. However, because blood proteins are found in small quantities, their usefulness as buffers during heavy exercise is limited.

In contrast, hemoglobin is a particularly important protein buffer and is a major blood buffer during resting conditions. In fact, hemoglobin has approximately six times the buffering capacity of plasma proteins due to its high concentration (16). Also contributing to the effectiveness of hemoglobin as a buffer is the fact that deoxygenated hemoglobin is a better buffer than oxygenated hemoglobin. As a result, once hemoglobin becomes deoxygenated in the capillaries, it is better able to bind hydrogen ions formed when CO_2 enters the blood from the tissues. Thus, hemoglobin helps to minimize pH changes caused by loading of CO_2 into the blood.

Ingestion of Sodium Buffers and Performance

Recent evidence suggests that performance during high-intensity exercise is improved when athletes ingest a sodium buffer prior to exercise as a means of increasing blood buffering capacity (1a, 2, 18, 24). Two buffers that have been studied extensively are sodium bicarbonate and sodium citrate. In general, these data suggest that boosting the blood buffering capacity by ingestion of these buffers increases time to exhaustion during high intensity exercise (e.g., 80%–120% $\dot{V}O_2$ max). It seems likely that if ingestion of a buffer improves physical performance it does so by increasing the extracellular buffering capacity which in turn, increases the transport of lactate and hydrogen ions out of the muscle fiber (25a). This would reduce the interference of hydrogen ions on bioenergetic ATP production and/or the contractile process itself.

In deciding to use sodium bicarbonate or sodium citrate prior to an exercise event, one should understand risks associated with the procedure. Ingestion of sodium bicarbonate in the doses that are required to improve blood buffering capacity can cause gastrointestinal problems including diarrhea and vomiting (2, 24). Extremely large doses of this buffer could be fatal. In contrast, ingestion of sodium citrate has been shown to improve performance without the same gastrointestinal side effects associated with sodium bicarbonate (15a, 20a). Another important consideration for the use of any ergogenic aid is legality. The International Olympic Committee has ruled that the use of any sodium buffers during Olympic competition is illegal.

The bicarbonate buffer system is probably the most important buffer system in the body (16). This fact has been exploited by some investigators who have demonstrated that an increase in blood bicarbonate concentration (ingestion of bicarbonate) results in an improvement in performance in some types of exercise (2, 15, 18) (see A Closer Look 11.1).

The bicarbonate buffer system involves the weak acid H_2CO_3, which undergoes the following dissociation reaction:

$$CO_2 + H_2O \longleftrightarrow H_2CO_3 \longleftrightarrow H^+ + HCO_3^-$$

The ability of carbonic acid (H_2CO_3) to act as a buffer is described mathematically by a relationship known as the Henderson-Hasselbalch equation:

$$pH = pKa + \log_{10}\left(\frac{HCO_3^-}{H_2CO_3}\right)$$

where pKa is the dissociation constant for H_2CO_3 and has a constant value of 6.1. In short, the Henderson-Hasselbalch equation states that the pH of a weak acid solution is determined by the ratio of the concentration of base (i.e., bicarbonate) in solution to the concentration of acid (i.e., carbonic acid). The normal pH of arterial blood is 7.4, and the ratio of bicarbonate to carbonic acid is 20 to 1. Let's consider an example using the Henderson-Hasselbalch equation to calculate arterial blood pH. Normally the concentration of blood bicarbonate is 24 m Eq/l and the concentration of carbonic acid is 1.2 m Eq/l. Therefore, the blood pH can be calculated as follows:

$$pH = pKa + \log_{10} 24/1.2$$
$$= 6.1 + \log_{10} 20$$
$$= 6.1 + 1.3$$
$$pH = 7.4$$

in summary

- The body maintains acid-base homeostasis by buffer-control systems. A buffer resists pH change by removing hydrogen ions when the pH declines and by releasing hydrogen ions when the pH increases.
- The principal intracellular buffers are proteins, phosphate groups, and bicarbonate. Primary extracellular buffers are bicarbonate, hemoglobin, and blood proteins.

Respiratory Influence on Acid–Base Balance

Recall that CO_2 is considered a volatile acid because it can be readily changed from CO_2 to carbonic acid. Also, recall that it is the partial pressure of CO_2 in the blood that determines the concentration of carbonic acid. For example, according to Henry's law, the concentration of a gas in solution is directly proportional to its partial pressure. That is, as the partial pressure increases, the concentration of the gas in solution increases and vice versa.

Because CO_2 is a gas, it can be eliminated by the lungs. Therefore the respiratory system is an important regulator of blood carbonic acid and pH. To better understand the role of the lungs in acid-base balance, let's reexamine the carbonic acid dissociation equation:

$$CO_2 + H_2O \longleftrightarrow H_2CO_3 \longleftrightarrow H^+ + HCO_3^-$$

This relationship demonstrates that when the amount of CO_2 in the blood increases, the amount of H_2CO_3 increases, which lowers pH by elevating the acid concentration of the blood (i.e., the reaction moves to the right). In contrast, when the CO_2 content of the blood is lowered (i.e., CO_2 is "blown off" by the lungs), the pH of the blood increases because less acid is present (reaction moves to the left). Therefore, the respiratory system provides the body with a rapid means of regulating blood pH by controlling the amount of CO_2 present in the blood.

in summary

- Respiratory control of acid-base balance involves the regulation of blood PCO_2. An increase in blood PCO_2 lowers pH, whereas, a decrease in blood PCO_2 increases pH.

Regulation of Acid–Base Balance via the Kidneys

Since the kidneys do not play an important part in acid-base regulation during short-term exercise, only a brief overview of the kidney's role in acid-base balance will be presented here. The principal means by which the kidneys regulate hydrogen ion concentration is by increasing or decreasing the bicarbonate concentration (4–6). When the hydrogen ion concentration increases in body fluids, the kidney responds by a reduction in the rate of bicarbonate excretion. This results in an increase in the blood bicarbonate concentration and therefore assists in buffering the increase in hydrogen ions. Conversely, when the pH of body fluids rises (hydrogen ion concentration decreases), the kidneys increase the rate of bicarbonate excretion. Therefore, by changing the amount of buffer present in body fluids, the kidneys aid in the regulation of the hydrogen ion concentration. The kidney mechanism involved in regulating the bicarbonate concentration is located in a portion of the kidney called the *tubule*, and acts through a series of complicated reactions and active transport across the tubular wall. For additional information on this topic, the student is referred to Fox (1996) in the suggested reading list.

Why is the kidney not an important regulator of acid-base balance during exercise? The answer lies in the amount of time required for the kidney to respond to an acid-base disturbance. It takes several hours for the kidneys to react effectively in response to an increase in blood hydrogen ions (4–6). Therefore, the kidneys respond too slowly to be of major benefit in the regulation of hydrogen ion concentration during exercise.

in summary

- Although the kidneys play an important role in the long-term regulation of acid-base balance, the kidneys are not important in the regulation of acid-base balance during exercise.

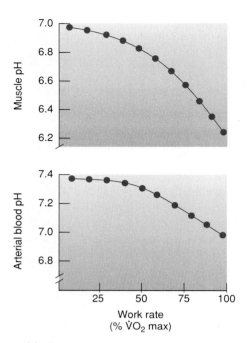

Figure 11.4
Changes in arterial blood pH and muscle pH during incremental exercise. Notice that arterial and muscle pH begin to fall together at work rates above 50% $\dot{V}O_2$ max.

Regulation of Acid–Base Balance During Exercise

During the final stages of an incremental exercise test or during near-maximal exercise of short duration, there is a decrease in both muscle and blood pH primarily due to the increase in the production of lactic acid by the muscle (8, 10, 19). This point is illustrated in figure 11.4, where the changes in blood and muscle pH during an incremental exercise test are graphed as a function of % $\dot{V}O_2$ max. Note that muscle and blood pH follow similar trends during this type of exercise, but that muscle pH is always 0.4 to 0.6 pH units lower than blood pH (17, 21). This is because muscle lactic acid concentration is higher than that of blood, and muscle buffering capacity is lower than that of blood.

The amount of lactic acid produced during exercise is dependent on: (1) the exercise intensity, (2) the amount of muscle mass involved, and (3) the duration of the work (8, 10). Exercise involving high-intensity leg work (e.g., running) may reduce arterial pH from 7.4 to a value of 7.0 within a few minutes (8, 13, 17, 25). Further, repeated bouts of this type of exercise may cause blood pH to decline even further to a value of 6.8 (8). This blood pH value is the lowest ever recorded and would present a life-threatening situation if it were not corrected within a few minutes.

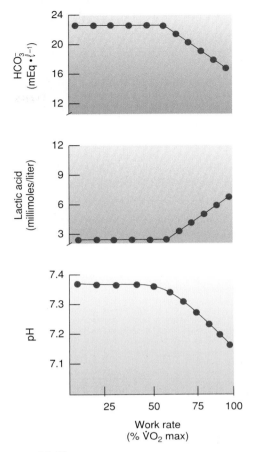

Figure 11.5
Changes in blood concentrations of lactic acid, bicarbonate, and pH as a function of work rate.

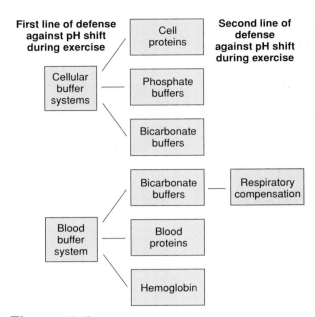

Figure 11.6
Lines of defense against pH change during intense exercise.

How does the body act to regulate acid-base balance during exercise? Since the primary source of hydrogen ions released during exercise is lactic acid produced within the working muscles, it is reasonable that the first line of defense against a rise in acid production would reside in the muscle itself. This is indeed the case. It is estimated that intracellular proteins contribute as much as 60% of the cell's buffering capacity, with an additional 20%–30% of the total buffering capacity coming from muscle bicarbonate (16). The final 10%–20% of muscle buffering capacity comes from intracellular phosphate groups.

Since the muscle's buffering capacity is limited, extracellular fluid (principally the blood) must possess a means of buffering hydrogen ions as well. The principal extracellular buffer and probably the most important buffer in the body is blood bicarbonate (16). Hemoglobin and blood proteins assist in this buffer process, but play only a minor role in blood buffering of lactic acid during exercise (16). Figure 11.5 illustrates the role of blood bicarbonate as a buffer during incremental exercise. Note that as blood lactic acid concentration increases, blood bicarbonate concentration decreases proportionally (30). Also

note that at approximately 50%–60% of $\dot{V}O_2$ max, blood pH begins to decline due to the rise in lactic acid production. This increase in blood hydrogen ion concentration stimulates the carotid bodies, which then signal the respiratory control center to increase alveolar ventilation (i.e., ventilatory threshold, chapter 10). An increase in alveolar ventilation results in the reduction of blood PCO_2 and therefore acts to reduce the acid load produced by exercise. The overall process of respiratory assistance in buffering lactic acid during exercise is referred to as **respiratory compensation** for metabolic acidosis.

in summary

- Figure 11.6 outlines the process of buffering exercise-induced acidosis.
- The first line of defense against exercise-produced hydrogen ions is the chemical buffer systems of the intracellular compartment and the blood. These buffer systems act rapidly to convert strong acids into weak acids.
- Intracellular buffering occurs with the aid of cellular proteins, bicarbonate, and phosphate groups.
- Blood buffering of hydrogen ions occurs through bicarbonate, hemoglobin, and blood proteins, with bicarbonate playing the most important role.
- The second line of defense against pH shift during exercise is respiratory compensation for metabolic acidosis.

study questions

1. Define the terms *acid, base, buffer, acidosis, alkalosis,* and *pH.*
2. Graph the pH scale. Label the pH values that represent normal arterial and intracellular pH.
3. List and briefly discuss the three major groups of acids formed by the body.
4. Why is the maintenance of acid-base homeostasis important to physical performance?
5. What are the principal intracellular and extracellular buffers?
6. Discuss respiratory compensation for metabolic acidosis. What would happen to blood pH if an individual began to hyperventilate at rest? Why?
7. Briefly, outline how the body resists pH change during exercise.

suggested readings

Edwards, R. H. T. 1983. Biochemical bases of fatigue in exercise performance: Catastrophe theory of muscular fatigue. In *Biochemistry of Exercise.* Champaign, IL: Human Kinetics.

Fox, E., R. Bowers, and M. Foss. 1993. *The Physiological Basis of Physical Education and Athletics.* Dubuque, IA: Brown & Benchmark.

Fox, S. I. 1996. *Human Physiology.* Dubuque, IA: Wm. C. Brown.

Linderman, J., and T. Fahey. 1991. Sodium bicarbonate ingestion and exercise performance: An update. *Sports Medicine* 11:71–77.

Vollestad, N., and O. M. Sejersted. 1988. Biochemical correlates of fatigue. *European Journal of Applied Physiology* 57:336–47.

references

1. Adams, G., J. Foley, and R. Meyer. 1990. Muscle buffer capacity estimated from pH changes during rest-to-work transitions. *Journal of Applied Physiology* 69:968–72.

1a. Coombes, J. S., and L. McNaughton. 1993. The effects of bicarbonate ingestion on leg strength and power during isokinetic knee flexion and extension. *Journal of Strength and Conditioning Research* 7(4):241–49.

2. Costill, D. et al. 1984. Acid-base balance during repeated bouts of exercise: Influence of bicarbonate. *International Journal of Sports Medicine* 5:228–31.

3. Edwards, R. H. T. 1983. Biochemical bases of fatigue in exercise performance: Catastrophe theory of muscular fatigue. In *Biochemistry of Exercise.* Champaign, IL: Human Kinetics.

4. Fox, E., R. Bowers, and M. Foss. 1993. *The Physiological Basis of Physical Education and Athletics.* Dubuque, IA: Brown & Benchmark.

5. Fox, S. I. 1993. *Human Physiology.* Dubuque, IA: Wm. C. Brown.

6. Guyton, Arthur. 1991. *Textbook of Medical Physiology.* Philadelphia: W. B. Saunders.

7. Hole, J. 1991. *Human Anatomy and Physiology.* Dubuque, IA: Wm. C. Brown.

8. Hultman, E., and K. Sahlin. 1980. Acid-base balance during exercise. In *Exercise and Sport Science Reviews,* vol. 8, eds. R. Hutton and D. Miller, 41–128. Philadelphia: Franklin Institute Press.

9. Hultman, E., and J. Sjoholm. 1986. Biochemical causes of fatigue. In *Human Muscle Power,* eds. N. Jones, N. McCartney, and A. McComas. Champaign, IL: Human Kinetics.

10. Itoh, H., and T. Ohkuwa. 1991. Ammonia and lactate in the blood after short-term sprint exercise. *European Journal of Applied Physiology* 62:22–25.

11. Johnson, L. 1983. *Biology.* Dubuque, IA: Wm. C. Brown.

12. Jones, N. L. 1980. Hydrogen ion balance during exercise. *Clinical Science* 59:85–91.

13. Jones, N. et al. 1977. Effect of pH on cardiorespiratory and metabolic responses to exercise. *Journal of Applied Physiology* 43:959–64.

14. Karlsson, J. 1979. Localized muscular fatigue: Role of metabolism and substrate depletion. In *Exercise and Sport Science Reviews,* vol. 7, eds. R. Hutton and D. Miller, 1–42. Philadelphia: Franklin Institute Press.

15. Katz, A. et al. 1984. Maximal exercise tolerance after induced alkalosis. *International Journal of Sports Medicine* 5:107–10.

15a. Kowalchuk, J. et al. 1989. The effect of citrate loading on exercise performance, acid-base balance and metabolism. *European Journal of Applied Physiology* 58:858–64.

16. Laiken, N., and D. Fanestil. 1985. Acid-base balance and regulation of hydrogen ion excretion. In *Physiological Basis of Medical Practice,* ed. J. West. Baltimore: Williams & Wilkins.

17. Linderman, J. et al. 1990. A comparison of blood gases and acid-base measurements in arterial, arterialized venous, and venous blood during short-term maximal exercise. *European Journal of Applied Physiology* 61:294–301.

18. Linderman, J., and T. Fahey. 1991. Sodium bicarbonate ingestion and exercise performance: An update. *Sports Medicine* 11:71–77.

19. Marsh, G. et al. 1991. Coincident thresholds in intracellular phosphorylation potential and pH during progressive exercise. *Journal of Applied Physiology* 71:1076–81.

20. McCartney, N., G. Heigenhauser, and N. Jones. 1983. Effects of pH on maximal power output and fatigue during short-term dynamic exercise. *Journal of Applied Physiology* 55:225–29.

20a. McNaughton, L. R. 1990. Sodium citrate and anaerobic performance: Implications of dosage. *European Journal of Applied Physiology* 61:392–97.

descriptive terms such as *core temperature* or *skin temperature*, depending on which temperature is being discussed (2).

in summary

- Homeotherms are animals that maintain a rather constant body core temperature. In order to maintain a constant core temperature, heat loss must match heat gain.
- Temperature varies a great deal within the body. In general, there is a thermal gradient from deep body temperature (core temperature) to the shell (skin) temperature.

Temperature Measurement During Exercise

Measurements of deep-body temperatures may be accomplished via mercury thermometers, or devices known as *thermocouples* or *thermistors*. One of the most common sites of core temperature measurement is the rectum. Although rectal temperature is not the same as the temperature in the brain where temperature is regulated, it can be used to estimate changes in deep-body temperature during exercise. In addition, temperature measurements near the eardrum (called tympanic temperature) have been found to be a good estimate of the actual brain temperature. Another alternative is to measure the temperature of the esophagus as an indication of core temperature. Like rectal temperature, esophageal temperature is not identical to brain temperature, but offers a measure of deep-body temperature.

Skin temperature can be measured by placing temperature sensors (thermistors) on the skin at various locations. The mean skin temperature can be calculated by assigning certain factors to each individual skin measurement in proportion to the fraction of the body's total surface area that each measurement represents. For example, mean skin temperature (T_s) can be estimated by the following formula (21):

$$T_s = (T_{forehead} + T_{chest} + T_{forearm} + T_{thigh} + T_{calf} + T_{abdomen} + T_{back}) \div 7$$

where $T_{forehead}$, T_{chest}, $T_{forearm}$, T_{thigh}, T_{calf}, $T_{abdomen}$, and T_{back} represent skin temperatures measured on the forehead, chest, forearm, thigh, calf, abdomen, and back, respectively.

in summary

- Measurements of deep-body temperatures may be accomplished via mercury thermometers, or devices known as thermocouples or thermistors. Common sites of measurement include the rectum, ear (tympanic temperature), and the esophagus.
- Skin temperature can be measured by placing temperature sensors (thermistors) on the skin at various locations.

Overview of Heat Production/Heat Loss

As previously stated, the goal of temperature regulation is to maintain a constant core temperature. This regulation is achieved by controlling the rate of heat production and heat loss. When out of balance, the body either gains or loses heat. The temperature control center is an area in the brain called the hypothalamus. The hypothalamus works like a thermostat by initiating an increase in heat production when body temperature falls, and an increase in the rate of heat loss when body temperature rises. Temperature regulation is controlled by both physical and chemical processes. Let's begin our discussion of temperature regulation by introducing those factors that govern heat production and heat loss.

Heat Production

The body produces internal heat due to normal metabolic processes. At rest or during sleep, metabolic heat production is small; however, during intense exercise, heat production is large. Heat production can be classified as (1) voluntary (exercise) or (2) involuntary (shivering or biochemical heat production caused by the secretion of hormones such as thyroxine and catecholamines) (see figure 12.2).

Since the body is at most 20%–30% efficient, 70%–80% of the energy expended during exercise appears as heat. During heavy exercise, this can result in a large heat load. Indeed, work in a hot/humid environment serves as a serious test of the body's ability to lose heat.

Involuntary heat production by shivering is the primary means of increasing heat production during exposure to cold. Maximal shivering can increase the body's heat production by approximately five times the resting value (4, 10). In addition, release of thyroxine from the thyroid gland can also increase metabolic rate. Thyroxine acts by increasing the metabolic rate of all cells in the body (6, 10, 16). Finally, an increase in

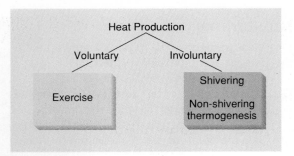

Figure 12.2

The body produces heat due to normal metabolic processes. Heat production can be classified as being either (1) voluntary or (2) involuntary.

blood levels of catecholamines (epinephrine and norepinephrine) can cause an increase in the rate of cellular metabolism (13). The increase in heat production due to the combined influences of thyroxine and catecholamines is called *nonshivering thermogenesis.*

Heat Loss

Heat loss from the body may occur by four processes: (1) radiation, (2) conduction, (3) convection, and/or (4) evaporation. The first three of these heat loss mechanisms require a temperature gradient to exist between the skin and the environment. **Radiation** is heat loss in the form of infrared rays. This involves the transfer of heat from the surface of one object to the surface of another, with no physical contact being involved (i.e., sun transferring heat to the earth via radiation). At rest in a comfortable environment (e.g., room temperature = 21° C), 60% of the heat loss occurs via radiation. This is possible because skin temperature is greater than the temperature of surrounding objects (walls, floor, etc.), and a net loss of body heat occurs due to the thermal gradient. Note that on a hot, sunny day when surface temperatures are greater than skin temperature, the body can also gain heat via radiation (28). Therefore, it is important to remember that radiation is heat transfer by infrared rays and can result in either heat loss or heat gain depending on the environmental conditions.

Conduction is defined as the transfer of heat from the body into the molecules of cooler objects in contact with its surface. In general, the body loses only small amounts of heat due to this process. An example of heat loss due to conduction is the transfer of heat from the body to a metal chair while a person is sitting on it. The heat loss occurs as long as the chair is cooler than the body surface in contact with it.

Convection is a form of conductive heat loss in which heat is transmitted to either air or water molecules in contact with the body. In convective heat loss, air or water molecules are warmed and move away from the source of the heat and are replaced by cooler

molecules. An example of *forced convection* is a fan moving large quantities of air past the skin; this would increase the number of air molecules coming in contact with the skin and thus promote heat loss. Practically speaking, the amount of heat loss due to convection is dependent on the air flow over the skin. Therefore, under the same wind conditions, cycling at high speeds would improve convective cooling when compared to cycling at slow speeds or running. Swimming in cool water (water temperature less than skin temperature) also results in convective heat loss. In fact, water's effectiveness in cooling is about 25 times greater than that of air at the same temperature.

The final means of heat loss is **evaporation.** Evaporation accounts for approximately 25% of the heat loss at rest, but under most environmental conditions it is the most important means of heat loss during exercise (26). In evaporation, heat is transferred from the body to water on the surface of the skin. When this water gains sufficient heat (energy), it is converted to a gas (water vapor), taking the heat away from the body. Note that evaporation occurs due to a vapor pressure gradient between the skin and the air. Vapor pressure is the pressure exerted by water molecules that have been converted to gas (water vapor). Evaporative cooling during exercise occurs in the following way. When body temperature rises above normal, the nervous system stimulates sweat glands to secrete sweat onto the surface of the skin. As sweat evaporates, heat is lost to the environment, which in turn lowers skin temperature.

Evaporation of sweat from the skin is dependent on three factors: (1) the temperature and relative humidity, (2) the convective currents around the body, and (3) the amount of skin surface exposed to the environment (2, 25). At high environmental temperatures, relative humidity is the most important factor by far in determining the rate of evaporative heat loss. High relative humidity reduces the rate of evaporation. In fact, when the relative humidity is near 100%, evaporation is limited. Therefore, cooling by way of evaporation is most effective under conditions of low humidity.

Why does high relative humidity reduce the rate of evaporation? The answer is linked to the fact that high relative humidity (RH) reduces the vapor pressure gradient between the skin and the environment. On a hot/humid day (e.g., RH = 80%–90%) the vapor pressure in the air is close to the vapor pressure on moist skin. Therefore, the rate of evaporation is greatly reduced. High sweat rates during exercise in a hot/high humidity environment result in useless water loss. That is, sweating per se does not cool the skin; it is evaporation that cools the skin (24).

Let's explore in more detail those factors that regulate the rate of evaporation. The major point to keep in mind is that evaporation occurs due to a vapor pressure gradient. That is, in order for evaporative cooling to occur

A Closer Look 12.1

Calculation of Heat Loss via Evaporation

Knowing that evaporation of 1,000 ml of sweat results in 580 kcal of heat loss permits one to calculate the sweat and evaporation rate necessary to maintain a specified body temperature during exercise. Consider the following example: John Hothead is working on a cycle ergometer at a $\dot{V}O_2$ of 2.0 liters · min^{-1}, (energy expenditure of 10.0 kcal · min^{-1}). If John exercises for twenty minutes at this metabolic rate and is 20% efficient, how much

evaporation would be necessary to prevent an increase in core temperature?[1] The total heat produced can be calculated as:

Total energy expenditure
= 20 min × 10 kcal/min
= 200 kcal

Total heat produced
= 200 kcal × .80
= 160 kcal

The total evaporation necessary to prevent any heat gain would be computed as:

$$\frac{160 \text{ kcal}}{580 \text{ kcal} / \text{liter}} = .276 \text{ liters}$$
(evaporation necessary to prevent heat gain)

[1]Assumes no other heat-loss mechanism is active.

[2]If efficiency is 20%, then 80%, or .80 of the total energy expenditure, must be released as heat.

during exercise, the vapor pressure on the skin must be greater than the vapor pressure in the air. Vapor pressure is influenced by both temperature and relative humidity. This relationship is illustrated in table 12.1, which states that at any given temperature, a rise in relative humidity results in increased vapor pressure. Practically speaking, this means that less evaporative cooling occurs during exercise on a hot/humid day when compared to a cool/low humidity day. For example, an athlete running on a hot/humid day (e.g., air temperature = 30° C; RH = 100%) might have a mean skin temperature in the range of 33°–34° C. The vapor pressure on the skin would be approximately 35 mm Hg and the air vapor pressure would be around 32 mm Hg (table 12.1). This small vapor pressure gradient between the skin and air (3 mm Hg) would permit only limited evaporation, and therefore little cooling would occur. In contrast, the same athlete running on a cool/low humidity day (e.g., air temperature = 10° C; RH = 50%) might have a mean skin temperature of 30° C. The vapor pressure gradient between the skin and air under these conditions would be approximately 28 mm Hg (32 − 4 = 28) (table 12.1). This relatively large skin-to-air vapor pressure gradient would permit a reasonably large evaporative rate, and therefore adequate body cooling would occur under these conditions.

How much heat can be lost via evaporation during exercise? Heat loss due to evaporation can be calculated in the following manner. The body loses 0.58 kcal of heat for each ml of water that evaporates (43). Therefore, evaporation of 1 liter of sweat would result in a heat loss of 580 kcal (1,000 ml × 0.58 kcal/ml = 580 kcal). See A Closer Look 12.1 for additional examples of body heat loss calculations.

In summary, heat loss during exercise (other than swimming) in a cool/moderate environment occurs

primarily due to evaporation. In fact, when exercise is performed in a hot environment (where air temperature is greater than skin temperature), evaporation is the only means of losing body heat. The means by which the body gains and loses heat during exercise are summarized in figure 12.3.

Table 12.1	The Relationship Between Temperature and Relative Humidity (RH) on Vapor Pressure

50% RH Temperature °C	Vapor Pressure (mm Hg)
0	2.3
10	4.6
20	8.8
30	15.9

75% RH Temperature °C	Vapor Pressure (mm Hg)
0	3.4
10	6.9
20	13.2
30	23.9

100% RH Temperature °C	Vapor Pressure (mm Hg)
0	4.6
10	9.2
20	17.6
30	31.9

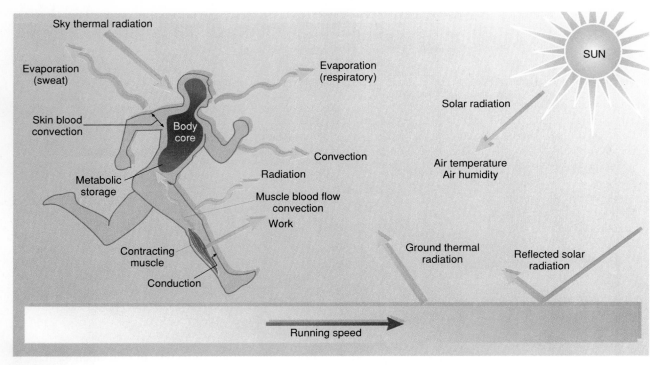

Figure 12.3

A summary of heat exchange mechanisms during exercise.

in summary

- Muscular exercise can result in large amounts of heat production. Since the body is at most 20%–30% efficient, 70%–80% of the energy expended during exercise is released as heat.
- Body heat can be lost by evaporation, convection, conduction, and radiation. During exercise in a cool environment, evaporation is the primary avenue for heat loss.
- The rate of evaporation from the skin is dependent upon three factors: (1) temperature and relative humidity, (2) convective currents around the body, and (3) the amount of skin exposed to the environment.

Body's Thermostat— Hypothalamus

Again, the body's temperature regulatory center is located in the hypothalamus. The **anterior hypothalamus** is primarily responsible for dealing with increases in body heat, while the **posterior hypothalamus** is responsible for reacting to a decrease in body temperature. In general, the hypothalamus operates much like a thermostat in your home—that is, it attempts to maintain a relatively constant core temperature around some "set point." The set-point temperature in humans is approximately 37° C.

The input to the temperature-regulating centers in the hypothalamus comes from receptors in both the skin and the core. Changes in environmental temperature are first detected by thermal receptors (both heat and cold) located in the skin. These skin temperature receptors transmit nerve impulses to the hypothalamus, which then initiates the appropriate response in an effort to maintain the body's set-point temperature. Further, heat-/cold-sensitive neurons are located in both the spinal cord and the hypothalamus itself, sensing changes in the core temperature.

An increase in core temperature above the set point results in the hypothalamus initiating a series of physiological actions aimed at increasing the amount of heat loss. First, the hypothalamus stimulates the sweat glands, which results in an increase in evaporative heat loss (19, 22). In addition, the vasomotor control center withdraws the normal vasoconstrictor tone to the skin, promoting increased skin blood flow and therefore allowing increased heat loss. Figure 12.4 illustrates the physiological responses associated with an increase in core temperature. When core temperature returns to normal, the stimulus to promote both sweating and vasodilation is removed. This is an example of a control system using negative feedback (chapter 2).

Physiological response to a "Heat Load"

Figure 12.4

A summary illustration of the physiological responses to an increase in "heat load."

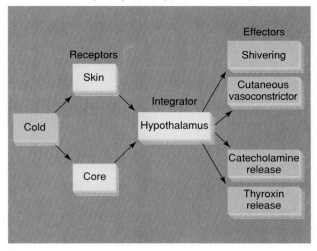

Physiological Responses to Cold

Figure 12.5

An illustration of the physiological responses to cold stress.

When cold receptors are stimulated in the skin or the hypothalamus, the thermoregulatory control center sets forth a plan of action to minimize heat loss and increase heat production. First, the vasomotor center directs peripheral blood vessels to vasoconstrict, which reduces heat loss (16). Second, if core temperature drops significantly, involuntary shivering begins (42). Additional responses include stimulation of the pilomotor center, which promotes piloerection (goosebumps). This piloerection reflex is an effective means of increasing the insulation space over the skin in fur-bearing animals, but is not an effective means of preventing heat loss in humans. Further, the hypothalamus indirectly increases thyroxine production and release, which increases cellular heat production (5). Finally, the posterior hypothalamus initiates the release of norepinephrine, which increases the rate of cellular metabolism (nonshivering thermogenesis). The physiological responses to a drop in core temperature are summarized in figure 12.5.

Shift in the Hypothalamic Thermostat Set Point Due to Fever

A fever is an increase in body temperature above the normal range, and may be caused by a number of bacterial diseases or brain disorders. During a fever, certain proteins and other toxins secreted by bacteria can cause the set point of the hypothalamic thermostat to rise above the normal level. Substances that cause this effect are called *pyrogens*. When the set point of the hypothalamic thermostat is raised to a higher level than normal, all the mechanisms for raising body temperature are called into play (13). Within a few hours after the thermostat has been set to a higher level, the body core temperature reaches this new level due to heat conservation.

in summary

- The body's thermostat is located in the hypothalamus.
- The anterior hypothalamus is responsible for reacting to increases in core temperature, while the posterior hypothalamus governs the body's responses to a decrease in temperature.
- An increase in core temperature results in the anterior hypothalamus initiating a series of physiological actions aimed at increasing heat loss. These actions include: (1) the commencement of sweating and (2) an increase in skin blood flow.
- Cold exposure results in the posterior hypothalamus promoting physiological changes that increase body heat production (shivering) and reduce heat loss (cutaneous vasoconstriction).

Thermal Events During Exercise

Now that an overview of how the hypothalamus responds to different thermal challenges has been presented, let's examine a brief scenario of the thermal events that occur during submaximal constant load exercise in a cool/moderate environment (i.e., low humidity and room temperature). Heat production increases during exercise due to muscular contraction and is directly proportional to the exercise intensity. The venous blood draining the exercising

Figure 12.6

Changes in metabolic energy production, evaporative heat loss, convective heat loss, and radiative heat loss during twenty-five minutes of submaximal exercise in a cool environment.

Figure 12.7

The relationship between metabolic rate and rectal temperature during constant load arm (•) and leg (■) exercise.

From M. Nelson, 1938, "Die Regulation der Korpertemperatur bei Muskelarbeit" in *Scandinavica Archives Physiology*, 79:193. Copyright ©1938 Blackwell Scientific Publications, Ltd., Oxford, England. Reprinted by permission.

muscle distributes the excess heat throughout the body core. As core temperature increases, thermal sensors in the hypothalamus sense the increase in blood temperature, and the thermal integration center in the hypothalamus compares this increase in temperature with the set-point temperature and finds a difference between the two (12, 25, 27). The response is to direct the nervous system to commence sweating and to increase blood flow to the skin (3, 29). These acts serve to increase body heat loss and minimize the increase in body temperature. At this point, the internal temperature reaches a new, elevated steady state level (see figure 12.6). Note that this new steady state core temperature does not represent a change in the set-point temperature, as occurs in fever (12, 25, 27, 45). Instead, the thermal regulatory center attempts to return the core temperature back to resting levels, but is incapable of doing so in the face of the sustained heat production associated with exercise.

Figure 12.6 also illustrates the roles of evaporation, convection, and radiation in heat loss during constant-load exercise in a moderate environment. Notice the constant but small role of convection and radiation in heat loss during this type of exercise. This is due to a constant temperature gradient between the skin and the room. In contrast, evaporation plays the most important role in heat loss during exercise in this type of environment (25, 27, 31).

During constant-load exercise the core temperature increase is directly related to the exercise intensity and is independent of ambient temperature over a wide range of conditions (i.e., 8°–29° C with low relative humidity) (30). This point is illustrated in figure 12.7. Notice the linear rise in core temperature

as the metabolic rate increases. The fact that it is the exercise intensity and not the environmental temperature that determines the rise in core temperature during exercise suggests that the method of heat loss during continuous exercise is modified according to ambient conditions (23, 30). This concept is presented in figure 12.8 which shows heat loss mechanisms during constant intensity exercise. Note that as the ambient temperature increases, the rate of convective and radiative heat loss decreases due to a decrease in the skin-to-room temperature gradient. This decrease in convective and radiative heat loss is matched by an increase in evaporative heat loss, and core temperature remains the same (see figure 12.8).

As mentioned previously, heat production increases in proportion to the exercise intensity. This point is illustrated in figure 12.9. Notice the linear increase in energy output (expenditure), heat production, and total heat loss as a function of exercise work rate. Further, note that convective and radiative heat loss does not increase as a function of exercise work rate. This is due to a relatively constant temperature gradient between the skin and the environment. In contrast, there is a consistent rise in evaporative heat loss with increments in exercise intensity. This observation reemphasizes the point that evaporation is the primary means of losing heat during exercise.

Figure 12.8

Heat exchange during exercise at different environmental temperatures. Notice the change in evaporative and convective/radiative heat loss as the environmental temperature increases. See text for discussion.

From M. Nelson, 1938, "Die Regulation der Korpertemperatur bei Muskelarbeit" in *Scandinavica Archives Physiology*, 79:193. Copyright © 1938 Blackwell Scientific Publications, Ltd., Oxford, England. Reprinted by permission.

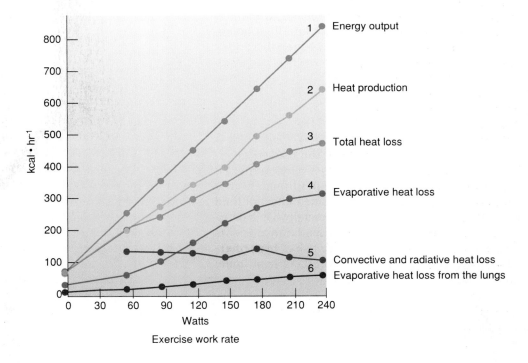

Figure 12.9

Heat exchange at rest and during cycle ergometer exercise at a variety of work rates. Note the steady increase in evaporative heat loss as a function of an increase in power output. In contrast, an increase in metabolic rate has essentially no influence on the rate of convective and radiative heat loss.

From M. Nelson, 1938, "Die Regulation der Korpertemperatur bei Muskelarbeit" in *Scandinavica Archives Physiology*, 79:193. Copyright © 1938 Blackwell Scientific Publications, Ltd., Oxford, England. Reprinted by permission.

Exercise in the Heat

Continuous exercise in a hot/humid environment poses a particularly stressful challenge to maintenance of normal body temperature and fluid homeostasis. High heat and humidity reduce the body's ability to lose heat by radiation/convection and evaporation, respectively. This inability to lose heat during exercise in a hot/humid environment results in a greater core temperature and a higher sweat rate (more fluid loss) when compared to the same exercise in a moderate environment (35–39, 41). This point is illustrated in figure 12.10. Notice the marked differences in sweat rates and core temperatures during exercise between the hot/humid conditions and the moderate environment. The combined effect of fluid loss and high core temperature generally has a detrimental effect on performance in endurance events (see chapter 24) and increases the risk of **hyperthermia** (large rise in core temperature) and heat injury (see A Closer Look 12.2).

Gender and Age Differences in Thermoregulation

Although controversy exists about the issue, most women appear to be less heat tolerant than men (32). Factors contributing to women's limited heat tolerance include lower sweat rates and generally a higher percentage of body fat than men (a high percentage of body fat reduces heat loss). However, when women and men are matched for the same degree of heat acclimatization and similar body compositions, the gender differences in the physiological responses to thermal stress are small (32).

Figure 12.10
Differences in core temperature and sweat rate during forty-five minutes of submaximal exercise in a hot/humid environment versus a cool environment.

Does aging impair one's ability to thermoregulate and exercise in the heat? This issue remains controversial, with some investigators suggesting that the ability to exercise in the heat deteriorates with old age (8) and still others suggesting that age per se does not limit an individual's ability to thermoregulate (7, 34).

Research Focus 12.1

Can Exercise Training in Sweat Clothing in Cool Conditions Promote Heat Acclimatization?

Athletes that train in cool environments often travel to warmer climates to compete. Without adequate heat acclimatization, these athletes will be at a disadvantage compared to athletes that have developed a high level of heat adaptation by training in a hot/humid environment. Therefore, a key question is, "Can training in sweat clothing in a cool environment promote heat acclimatization?" The answer to this question is yes but the magnitude of the heat acclimatization that is obtained by this method is generally less than the maximal level of acclimatization that can be achieved by daily training in a hot/humid environment (1,6a). Nonetheless, "artificial" heat training in sweat clothing in cool conditions appears to be better than attempting no heat acclimatization measures (6a). See reference 6a for a review on this topic.

However, recent studies examining temperature regulation during exercise in well conditioned old and young men show little difference in thermoregulation between these age groups (34). Based on these results it is tempting to speculate that deconditioning and a lack of heat acclimatization in older subjects may explain why some of the earlier studies reported a decrease in thermoregulation with age. More research is required to resolve this issue.

Heat Acclimatization

Regular exercise in a hot environment results in a series of physiological adjustments designed to minimize disturbances in homeostasis due to heat stress (this is referred to as heat acclimatization). The end result of heat acclimatization is a lower heart rate and core temperature during submaximal exercise (7). Although partial heat acclimatization can occur by training in a cool environment, it is essential that athletes exercise in a hot environment to obtain maximal heat acclimatization (1). Because an elevation in core temperature is the primary stimulus to promote heat acclimatization, it is recommended that the athlete perform strenuous interval training or continuous exercise at an intensity exceeding 50% of the athlete's $\dot{V}O_2$ max in order to promote higher core temperatures (33) (see Research Focus 12.1).

The primary adaptations that occur during heat acclimatization are an increased plasma volume, earlier onset of sweating, higher sweat rate, reduced salt loss in sweat, and a reduced skin blood flow (11, 40). It is interesting that heat adaptation occurs rapidly, with almost complete acclimatization being achieved by seven to fourteen days after the first exposure (3, 45).

Heat acclimatization results in a 10%–12% increase in plasma volume (4, 11). The increase in plasma volume is due to an increase in plasma proteins. This increased plasma volume maintains central blood volume, stroke volume, sweating capacity, and allows the body to store more heat with a smaller temperature gain.

Table 12.2	A Summary of the Primary Adaptations That Occur as a Result of Heat Acclimatization

1. Increased plasma volume
2. Earlier onset of sweating
3. Higher sweat rate
4. Reduced sodium chloride loss in sweat
5. Reduced skin blood flow

As stated previously, heat adaptation results in an earlier onset of sweating. This means that sweating begins rapidly after the commencement of exercise, which translates into less heat storage at the beginning of exercise and a lower core temperature. In addition, heat acclimatization may increase the sweating capacity almost threefold above the rate achievable prior to heat adaptation (40). Therefore, much more evaporative cooling is possible, which is a major advantage in minimizing heat storage during prolonged work. Finally, sweat losses of sodium and chloride are reduced following heat acclimatization due to an increased secretion of aldosterone (45). While this adaptation results in a reduction of electrolyte loss and aids in reducing electrolyte disturbances during exercise in the heat, it does not minimize the need to replace water loss, which is higher than normal (see chapters 23 and 24). A summary of heat-adaptive responses is presented in table 12.2.

The rate of decay of heat acclimatization is rapid, with reductions in heat tolerance occurring within a few days of inactivity (i.e., no heat exposure). In this regard, studies have shown that heat tolerance can decline significantly within seven days of no heat exposure and complete loss of heat tolerance can occur following twenty-eight days of no heat exposure (1). Therefore, repeated exposure to heat is required to maintain heat acclimatization (44).

in summary

- During prolonged exercise in a moderate environment, core temperature will increase gradually above the normal resting value and will reach a plateau at approximately thirty to forty-five minutes.
- During exercise in a hot/humid environment, core temperature does not reach a plateau, but will continue to rise. Long-term exercise in this type of environment increases the risk of heat injury.
- Heat acclimatization results in: (1) an increase in plasma volume, (2) an earlier onset of sweating during exercise, (3) a higher sweat rate, (4) a reduction in the amount of electrolytes lost in sweat, and (5) a reduction in skin blood flow.

Exercise in a Cold Environment

Exercise in a cold environment enhances an athlete's ability to lose heat and therefore greatly reduces the chance of heat injury. In general, the combination of metabolic heat production and warm clothing prevents the development of **hypothermia** (large decrease in core temperature) during short-term work on a cold day. However, exercise in the cold for extended periods of time (a long triathlon), or swimming in cold water, may overpower the body's ability to prevent heat loss, and hypothermia may result. In such cases, heat production during exercise is not able to keep pace with heat loss. This is particularly true during swimming in extremely cold water (e.g., < 15° C). Severe hypothermia may result in a loss of judgment, which increases the risk of further cold injury.

Individuals with a high percentage of body fat have an advantage over lean individuals when it comes to cold tolerance (16, 32). Large amounts of subcutaneous fat provide an increased layer of insulation from the cold. This additional insulation reduces the rate of heat loss and therefore improves cold tolerance. It is for this reason that women generally tolerate mild cold exposure better than men (32).

Participation in sports activities in the cold may present several other types of problems for the athlete. For example, hands exposed to cold weather become numb due to the reduction in the rate of neural transmission and reduced blood flow due to vasoconstriction. This results in a loss of dexterity and of course affects such skills as throwing and catching. In addition, exposed flesh is susceptible to frostbite, which may present a serious medical condition (4). Further details of the effects of a cold environment on performance will be presented in chapter 24.

Cold Acclimatization

In humans chronically exposed to cold (e.g., primitive societies, mountain climbers), there appears to be at least three physiological adaptations to cold exposure (8a, 15, 18). First, cold adaptation results in a reduction in the mean skin temperature at which shivering begins. That is, people who are cold acclimatized begin shivering at a lower skin temperature when compared to unacclimatized individuals. The explanation for this observation is that cold-acclimatized individuals maintain heat production with less shivering by increasing nonshivering thermogenesis. They increase the secretion of norepinephrine, which results in an increase in metabolic heat production (4, 5, 15).

A second physiological adjustment that occurs due to cold acclimatization is that cold-adjusted individuals are able to maintain a higher mean hand-and-foot temperature during cold exposure when compared to unacclimatized persons. Cold acclimatization apparently results in improved intermittent peripheral vasodilation to increase blood flow (and heat flow) to both the hands and feet.

The third and final physiological adaptation to cold is the improved ability to sleep in cold environments. Unacclimatized people, when attempting to sleep in cold environments, will often shiver so much that sleep is impossible (4). In contrast, cold-acclimatized individuals have the ability to sleep comfortably in cold environments due to their elevated level of nonshivering thermogenesis. The exact time course of complete cold acclimatization is not clear. However, subjects placed in a cold chamber begin to show signs of cold acclimatization after one week (33).

in summary

- Exercise in a cold environment enhances an athlete's ability to lose heat and therefore greatly reduces the chance of heat injury.
- Cold acclimatization results in three physiological adaptations: (1) improved ability to sleep in cold environments, (2) increased nonshivering thermogenesis, and (3) a higher intermittent blood flow to the hands and feet. The overall goal of these adaptations is to increase heat production and maintain core temperature, which will make the individual more comfortable during cold exposure.

study questions

1. Define the following terms: (1) *homeotherm*, (2) *hyperthermia*, and (3) *hypothermia*.
2. Why does a significant increase in core temperature represent a threat to life?
3. Explain the comment that the term *body temperature* is a misnomer.
4. How is body temperature measured during exercise?
5. Briefly, discuss the role of the hypothalamus in temperature regulation. How do the anterior hypothalamus and posterior hypothalamus differ in function?
6. List and define the four mechanisms of heat loss. Which of these avenues plays the most important part during exercise in a hot/dry environment?
7. Discuss the two general categories of heat production in people.
8. What hormones are involved in biochemical heat production?
9. Briefly, outline the thermal events that occur during prolonged exercise in a moderate environment. Include in your discussion information concerning changes in core temperature, skin blood flow, sweating, and skin temperature.
10. Calculate the amount of evaporation that must occur to remove 400 kcal of heat from the body.
11. How much heat would be removed from the skin if 520 ml of sweat evaporated during a thirty-minute period?
12. List and discuss the physiological adaptations that occur during heat acclimatization.
13. How might exercise in a cold environment affect dexterity in such skills as throwing and catching?
14. Discuss the physiological changes that occur in response to chronic exposure to cold.

suggested readings

Armstrong, L., and C. Maresh. 1991. The induction and decay of heat acclimatisation in trained athletes. *Sports Medicine* 12:302–12.

Dawson, B. 1994. Exercise training in sweating clothing in cool conditions to improve heat tolerance. *Sports Medicine* 17:233–44.

Doubt, T. 1991. Physiology of exercise in the cold. *Sports Medicine* 11:367–81.

Kenney, W., and J. Johnson. 1992. Control of skin blood flow during exercise. *Medicine and Science in Sport and Exercise* 24:303–12.

Mosely, P., and C. Gisolfi. 1993. New frontiers in thermoregulation and exercise. *Sports Medicine* 16:163–67.

references

1. Armstrong, L., and C. Maresh. 1991. The induction and decay of heat acclimatisation in trained athletes. *Sports Medicine* 12:302–12.
2. Åstrand, P., and K. Rodahl. 1986. *Textbook of Work Physiology*. New York: McGraw-Hill.
3. Brengelmann, G. 1977. Control of sweating and skin blood flow during exercise. In *Problems with Temperature Regulation during Exercise*, ed. E. Nadel. New York: Academic Press.
4. Brooks, G., and T. Fahey. 1987. *Fundamentals of Human Performance*. New York: Macmillian.
5. Cabanac, M. 1975. Temperature regulation. *Annual Review of Physiology* 37:415–39.
6. Clausen, T., C. Van Hardeveld, and M. Everts. 1991. Significance of cation transport in control of energy metabolism and thermogenesis. *Physiological Reviews* 71:733–74.
6a. Dawson, B. 1994. Exercise training in sweating clothing in cool conditions to improve heat tolerance. *Sports Medicine* 17:233–44.
7. Delamarche, P., J. Bittel, J. Lacour, and R. Flandrois. 1990. Thermoregulation at rest and during exercise in prepubertal boys. *European Journal of Applied Physiology* 60:436–40.
8. Dill D., and C. Consolazio. 1962. Responses to exercise as related to age and environmental temperature. *Journal of Applied Physiology* 17:64–69.
8a. Doubt, T. 1991. Physiology of exercise in the cold. *Sports Medicine* 11:367–81.
9. Epstein, Y. 1990. Heat intolerance: Predisposing factor or residual injury? *Medicine and Science in Sports and Exercise* 22:29–35.
10. Fox, S. 1993. *Human Physiology*. Dubuque, IA: Wm. C. Brown.
11. Gisolfi, C., and J. Cohen. 1979. Relationships among training, heat acclimation, and heat tolerance in men and women: The controversy revisited. *Medicine and Science in Sports* 11:56–59.
12. Gisolfi, C., and C. B. Wenger. 1984. Temperature regulation during exercise: Old concepts, new ideas. In *Exercise and Sport Science Reviews*, vol. 12, ed. R. Terjung, 339–72.
13. Guyton, A. C. 1991. *Textbook of Medical Physiology*. Philadelphia: W. B. Saunders.
14. Hole, J. 1993. *Human Anatomy and Physiology*. Dubuque, IA: Wm. C. Brown.
15. Hong, S., D. Rennie, and Y. Park. 1987. Humans can acclimatize to cold: A lesson from Korean divers. *News in Physiological Sciences* 2:79–82.
16. Horvath, S. 1981. Exercise in a cold environment. In *Exercise and Sport Science Reviews*, vol. 9, 221–63.
17. Hubbard, R. 1990. An introduction: The role of exercise in the etiology of exertional heatstroke. *Medicine and Science in Sports and Exercise* 22:2–5.

18. Iampietro, P., D. Bass, and E. Buskirk. 1959. Diurnal oxygen consumption and rectal temperature of men during cold exposure. *Journal of Applied Physiology* 10:398–403.

19. Johnson, J. 1992. Exercise and the cutaneous circulation. In *Exercise and Sport Science Reviews*, vol. 20, ed. J. Holloszy, 59–98.

20. Johnson, L. 1983. *Biology*. Dubuque, IA: Wm. C. Brown.

21. Kenney, W. 1988. Control of heat-induced cutaneous vasodilation in relation to age. *European Journal of Applied Physiology* 57:120–25.

22. Kenney, W., and J. Johnson. 1992. Control of skin blood flow during exercise. *Medicine and Science in Sport and Exercise* 24:303–12.

23. Kruk, B. et al. 1991. Comparison in men of physiological responses to exercise of increasing intensity at low and moderate ambient temperatures. *European Journal of Applied Physiology* 62:353–57.

24. McArdle, W., F. Katch, and V. Katch. 1991. *Exercise Physiology: Energy, Nutrition, and Human Performance.* Philadelphia: Lea & Febiger.

25. Nadel, E. 1979. Temperature regulation. In *Sports Medicine and Physiology*, ed. R. Strauss. Philadelphia: W. B. Saunders.

26. Nadel, E. 1988. Temperature regulation during prolonged exercise. In *Perspectives in Exercise Science and Sports Medicine: Prolonged Exercise*, eds. D. Lamb and R. Murray, 125–52. Indianapolis: Benchmark Press.

27. Nielson, B. 1969. Thermoregulation during exercise. *Acta Physicologica Scandanavica* (Suppl.) 323:10–73.

28. Nielson, B. 1990. Solar heat load: Heat balance during exercise in clothed subjects. *European Journal of Applied Physiology* 60:452–56.

29. Nielson, B. et al. 1990. Muscle blood flow and muscle metabolism during exercise and heat stress. *Journal of Applied Physiology* 69:1040–46.

30. Nielson, M. 1938. Die Regulation der Korpertemperatur bei Muskelarbeit. *Scandanavica Archives Physiology* 79:193.

31. Noble, B. 1986. *Physiology of Exercise and Sport.* St. Louis: C. V. Mosby.

32. Nunneley, S. 1978. Physiological responses of women to thermal stress: A review. *Medicine and Science in Sports and Exercise* 10:250–55.

33. Pandolf, K. 1979. Effects of physical training and cardiorespiratory fitness on exercise-heat tolerance: Recent observations. *Medicine and Science in Sports and Exercise* 11:60–65.

34. Pandolf, K. et al. 1988. Thermoregulatory responses of middle-aged men and young men during dry-heat acclimatization. *Journal of Applied Physiology* 65:65–70.

35. Powers, S., E. Howley, and R. Cox. 1982. A differential catecholamine response during prolonged exercise and passive heating. *Medicine and Science in Sports and Exercise* 6:435–39.

36. Powers, S., E. Howley, and R. Cox. 1982. Ventilatory and metabolic reactions to heat stress during prolonged exercise. *Journal of Sports Medicine and Physical Fitness* 22:32–36.

37. Powers, S., E. Howley, and R. Cox. 1985. Blood lactate concentrations during submaximal work under differing environmental conditions. *Journal of Sports Medicine and Physical Fitness* 25:84–89.

38. Rasch, W. et al. 1991. Heat loss from the human head during exercise. *Journal of Applied Physiology* 71:590–95.

39. Robinson, S. 1963. Temperature regulation during exercise. *Pediatrics* 32:691–702.

40. Sato, F. et al. 1990. Functional and morphological changes in the eccrine sweat gland with heat acclimation. *Journal of Applied Physiology* 69:232–36.

41. Stolwijk, J., B. Saltin, and A. Gagge. 1968. Physiological factors associated with sweating during exercise. *Aerospace Medicine* 39:1101–5.

42. Tikuisis, P., D. Bell, and I. Jacobs. 1991. Shivering onset, metabolic response, and convective heat transfer during cold air exposure. *Journal of Applied Physiology* 70:1996–2002.

43. Wenger, C. B. 1972. Heat evaporation of sweat: Thermodynamic considerations. *Journal of Applied Physiology* 32:456–59.

44. Williams, C., C. Wyndham, and J. Morrison. 1967. Rate of loss of acclimatization in summer and winter. *Journal of Applied Physiology* 22:21–26.

45. Wyndham, C. 1973. The physiology of exercise under heat stress. *Annual Review of Physiology* 35:193–220.

CHAPTER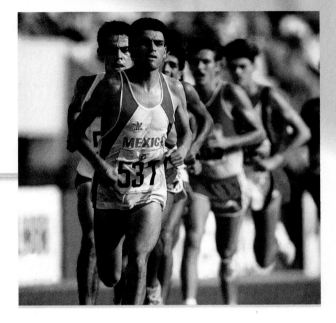

The Physiology of Training

Effect on $\dot{V}O_2$ Max,
Performance, Homeostasis,
and Strength

objectives

By studying this chapter, you should be able to do the following:

1. Explain the basic principles of training: overload and specificity.
2. Contrast cross-sectional with longitudinal research studies.
3. Indicate the typical change in $\dot{V}O_2$ max with endurance training programs, and the effect of the initial (pretraining) value on the magnitude of the increase.
4. State typical $\dot{V}O_2$ max values for various sedentary, active, and athletic populations.
5. State the formula for $\dot{V}O_2$ max using heart rate, stroke volume, and the a-$\bar{v}$ O_2 difference; indicate which of the variables is most important in explaining the wide range of $\dot{V}O_2$ max values in the population.
6. Discuss, using the variables identified in objective 5, how the increase in $\dot{V}O_2$ max comes about for the sedentary subject who participates in an endurance training program.
7. Define preload, afterload, and contractility, and discuss the role of each in the increase in the maximal stroke volume that occurs with endurance training.
8. Describe the changes in muscle structure that are responsible for the increase in the maximal a-$\bar{v}$ O_2 difference with endurance training.
9. Describe the underlying causes of the decrease in $\dot{V}O_2$ max that occurs with cessation of endurance training.

10. Describe how the capillary and mitochondrial changes that occur in muscle as a result of an endurance training program are related to the following adaptations to submaximal exercise:
    a. a lower O_2 deficit
    b. an increased utilization of FFA and a sparing of blood glucose and muscle glycogen
    c. a reduction in lactate and H^+ formation
    d. an increase in lactate removal
11. Discuss how changes in "central command" and "peripheral feedback" following an endurance training program can lower the heart rate, ventilation, and catecholamine responses to a submaximal exercise bout.
12. Contrast the role of neural adaptations with hypertrophy in the increase in strength that occurs with resistance training.

outline

Principles of Training   230
   Overload   230
   Specificity   231
Research Designs to Study
   Training   231
Endurance Training and $\dot{V}O_2$
   Max   231
   Training Programs and Changes in
     $\dot{V}O_2$ Max   232
$\dot{V}O_2$ Max: Cardiac Output and the
   Arteriovenous O_2
   Difference   232
   Stroke Volume   234
   Arteriovenous O_2 Difference   235

Detraining and $\dot{V}O_2$ Max   236
Endurance Training: Effects on
   Performance and
   Homeostasis   236
   Biochemical Adaptations and the
     Oxygen Deficit   237
   Biochemical Adaptations and the
     Plasma Glucose
     Concentration   239
   Biochemical Adaptations and Blood
     pH   240
   Biochemical Adaptations and
     Lactate Removal   241

Endurance Training: Links Between
   Muscle and Systemic
   Physiology   243
   Peripheral Feedback   243
   Central Command   244
Physiological Effects of Strength
   Training   245
Physiological Mechanisms Causing
   Increased Strength   246
   Neural Factors   246
   Muscular Enlargement   247
   Simultaneous Strength and
     Endurance Training   247

key terms

bradycardia
ejection fraction

overload
reversibility

specificity

 theme that has been used throughout this book is that there are automatic regulatory mechanisms operating at rest and during exercise to maintain homeostasis. Figure 13.1 identifies some of the variables that are maintained within narrow limits during exercise in spite of the tremendous demands placed on various tissues and organ systems. What has become clear is that participation in regular endurance exercise increases the cardiovascular system's ability to deliver blood to the working muscles, and increases the muscle's capacity to produce energy aerobically. These parallel changes result in less disruption of the internal environment during exercise. This, of course, leads to improved performance.

The purpose of this chapter is to tie together much of what has been presented previously, since most tissues and organ systems are either directly or indirectly affected by training programs. There is a need to discuss separately those physiological changes causing an increase in $\dot{V}O_2$ max from those associated with improvements in prolonged submaximal performance. $\dot{V}O_2$ max is most closely linked to the functional capacity of the cardiovascular system to deliver blood to the working muscles during maximal and supramaximal (>100% $\dot{V}O_2$ max) work, while maintaining mean arterial blood pressure. The ability to sustain long-term submaximal exercise is linked more to the maintenance of homeostasis due to specific structural and biochemical properties of working muscles (5, 28, 48). Finally, we will explore the physiology of strength development. Strength training causes adaptations in muscle that are potentially in conflict with those adaptations associated with running or cycling training programs. This raises

Figure 13.1
Homeostatic variables maintained within narrow limits in spite of the challenge presented by exercise.

questions about whether or not the effects of the two training programs actually interfere with each other. Before we begin a discussion of these topics, information about the principles of training and the design of research studies will be presented.

Principles of Training

The three principles of training are **overload, specificity,** and **reversibility.** These principles will be applied in chapters 16 and 17 for those training for fitness, and in chapters 21 and 22 for those training for performance.

Overload

Overload refers to the observation that a system or tissue must be exercised at a level beyond which it is presently accustomed in order for a training effect to occur. The system or tissue gradually adapts to this overload. This pattern of overload followed by adaptation continues until the system or tissue can no longer adapt. The typical variables that constitute the overload include the intensity, duration, and frequency (days per week) of exercise. The corollary of the overload principle, the principle of *reversibility*, simply indicates that the gains are quickly lost when the overload is removed.

Specificity

The training effect is *specific* to the muscle fibers involved in the activity. This may seem like an obvious statement in that one should not expect the arms to become trained during a ten-week jogging program. However, this also means that if an individual participates in a long, slow, distance running program that utilizes the slow-twitch muscle fibers, there is little or no training effect taking place in those fast-twitch fibers in the same muscle (28, 56a). A good example of specificity is found in a study in which subjects did either cycle or run training, but had their lactate threshold (LT) evaluated before and after training on both the cycle and treadmill. Run training increased the LT 58% and 20% for the treadmill and cycle, respectively. The cycle training increased the cycle LT 39%, with no measured improvement in the treadmill LT (43). Training effects were clearly specific to the type of training.

Specificity also refers to the types of adaptations occurring in muscle as a result of training. If a muscle is engaged in endurance types of exercise, the primary adaptations are in capillary and mitochondria number, which increase the capacity of the muscle to produce energy aerobically (28, 56). If a muscle is engaged in heavy resistive training, the primary adaptation is an increase in the quantity of the contractile proteins; the mitochondrial and capillary densities actually decrease (36). This high degree of specificity in the training effect is related to a point raised earlier, that one type of training may interfere with the adaptations to the other (see later discussion).

in summary

- The principle of overload states that for a training effect to occur a system or tissue must be challenged with an intensity, duration, or frequency of exercise to which it is unaccustomed. Over time the tissue or system adapts to this load. The reversibility principle is a corollary to the overload principle.
- The principle of specificity indicates that the training effect is limited to the muscle fibers involved in the activity. In addition, the muscle fiber adapts specifically to the type of activity: mitochondrial and capillary adaptations to endurance training, and contractile protein adaptations to resistive weight training.

Research Designs to Study Training

The effect of exercise training on various physiological systems has been studied using two different designs: cross-sectional and longitudinal. In cross-sectional studies the investigator examines groups differing in physical activity (e.g., cardiac patients, sedentary students, and world-class endurance athletes) and records the differences that exist in $\dot{V}O_2$ max, cardiac output, or fiber-type distribution. These studies are relatively inexpensive to conduct and provide good descriptive information about differences that exist among various populations. They are also useful in developing questions about how these differences came about, including hypotheses about the relative role of genetics versus training. Longitudinal studies examine *changes* in $\dot{V}O_2$ max, cardiac output, or fiber-type distribution occurring over the course of a training program. These studies control for the genetic factor since the same subject is repeatedly tested, and allow one to investigate the *rate* at which the variables respond to training or detraining. Longitudinal studies are expensive and difficult to conduct due to the potential for subjects dropping out and the demand for all equipment and procedures to be maintained constant at all testing points in the study. Due to these constraints, only small numbers of subjects are used in these studies. The investigator must take special care that the subjects are representative of the population, and that they do not alter other life-style patterns (diet, smoking, etc.) that might influence the outcome of the study (3).

As we mentioned in the introduction, the effects of training on $\dot{V}O_2$ max will be discussed separately from the effects on performance and homeostasis. The application of this information in the design of training programs for fitness and performance is found in chapters 16, 17, 21, and 22.

in summary

- Cross-sectional training studies contrast the physiological responses of groups differing in habitual physical activity (e.g., sedentary individuals versus runners).
- Longitudinal training studies examine the changes taking place over the course of a training program.

Endurance Training and $\dot{V}O_2$ Max

Maximal aerobic power, $\dot{V}O_2$ max, is a reproducible measure of the capacity of the cardiovascular system to deliver blood to a large muscle mass involved in dynamic work (48). Chapter 4 introduced this concept,

Table 13.1 $\dot{V}O_2$ Max Values Measured in Healthy and Diseased Populations

Population	Males	Females
Cross-country skiers	84	72
Distance runners	83	62
Sedentary: young	45	38
Sedentary: middle-aged adults	35	30
Post myocardial infarction patients	22	18
Severe pulmonary disease patients	13	13

Values are expressed in ml · kg^{-1} · min^{-1}.

Taken from Saltin and Åstrand (54), Åstrand and Rodahl (3), and Howley and Franks (29).

and chapters 9 and 10 showed how specific cardiovascular and pulmonary variables respond to graded exercise up to $\dot{V}O_2$ max. The following sections discuss the effect of endurance exercise programs on the increase in $\dot{V}O_2$ max and the physiological changes bringing about that increase.

Training Programs and Changes in $\dot{V}O_2$ Max

Endurance training programs that increase $\dot{V}O_2$ max involve a large muscle mass in dynamic exercise (e.g., running, cycling, swimming, or cross-country skiing) for twenty to sixty minutes per session, three to five times per week at an intensity of 50%–85% $\dot{V}O_2$ max (1). Details about how to design a training program for the average individual and the athlete are presented in chapters 16 and 21, respectively. While endurance training programs of two to three months duration cause an increase in $\dot{V}O_2$ max of about 15%, the range of improvement can be as low as 2%–3% for those who start the program with high $\dot{V}O_2$ max values (15), and as high as 30%–50% for those with low initial $\dot{V}O_2$ max values (15, 18, 27, 48, 53).

Table 13.1 shows that $\dot{V}O_2$ max can be less than 20 ml · kg^{-1} · min^{-1} in patients with severe cardiovascular and pulmonary disease, and more than 80 ml · kg^{-1} · min^{-1} in world-class distance runners and cross-country skiers. The extremely high $\dot{V}O_2$ max values measured in elite male and female endurance athletes have been ascribed to a genetic gift of a large cardiovascular capacity (3). Early work by Klissourus et al. (33) supported this idea with the observation that identical twins have very similar $\dot{V}O_2$ max values, while fraternal twins do not. Given that identical twins have identical genes, it was suggested that 93% of the variation in $\dot{V}O_2$ max values in the general population was due to genetics. On the surface, that high estimate appears to be consistent with the small changes in $\dot{V}O_2$ max that occur with the training programs just mentioned. However, serious

questions were raised about this conclusion. A recent examination of this question suggests that we need to revise that estimate downward to a figure somewhat closer to 40%–66% (7, 20). Although some scientists feel that these estimates are still too high (7a), it is clear that a genetic predisposition for possessing a high $\dot{V}O_2$ max value is still a prerequisite for values in the range of 60–80 ml · kg^{-1} · min^{-1}. Further, there is evidence that the sensitivity of the individual to the effect of a training program is also genetically determined (7, 45). That is, even when one controls for a variety of pretraining measures, there will still be a great deal of variation in the degree of improvement (6). Recent evidence points to differences in mitochondrial DNA as being important in the individual differences in $\dot{V}O_2$ max and its response to training (16).

Consistent with these lower estimates of the genetic contribution to $\dot{V}O_2$ max are the observations that training for two to three years (18), or participation in severe interval training (27) can increase $\dot{V}O_2$ max by as much as 44%. The results of the latter study showed a linear increase in $\dot{V}O_2$ max over ten weeks of training, whereas most studies show a leveling off of the $\dot{V}O_2$ max values after only a few weeks of training. The much larger increase in $\dot{V}O_2$ max with this ten-week training program was due to a much higher intensity, frequency, and duration than is usually used in endurance exercise programs. We'll next discuss what causes the $\dot{V}O_2$ max to increase as a result of an endurance exercise program.

in summary

- Endurance training programs that increase $\dot{V}O_2$ max involve a large muscle mass in dynamic activity for twenty to sixty minutes per session, three to five times per week, at an intensity of 50%–85% $\dot{V}O_2$ max.
- Although $\dot{V}O_2$ max increases an average of about 15% as a result of an endurance training program, the largest increases are associated with deconditioned or patient populations having very low pretraining $\dot{V}O_2$ max values.
- Genetic predisposition accounts for 40%–66% of one's $\dot{V}O_2$ max value. Very strenuous and/or prolonged training can increase $\dot{V}O_2$ max in normal sedentary individuals by more than 40%.

$\dot{V}O_2$ Max: Cardiac Output and the Arteriovenous O_2 Difference

Since oxygen uptake is the product of systemic blood flow (cardiac output) and systemic oxygen extraction (arteriovenous oxygen difference), changes in $\dot{V}O_2$ max

Table 13.2 Physiological Basis for Differences in $\dot{V}O_2$ Max in Different Populations

Population	$\dot{V}O_2$ max (ml · min⁻¹)	=	Heart Rate (beats · min⁻¹)	×	Stroke Volume (ℓ · beat⁻¹)	×	a-v̄ O_2 Difference (ml O_2 · ℓ⁻¹)
Athletes	6,250	=	190	×	.205	×	160
Normally active	3,500	=	195	×	.112	×	160
Mitral stenosis	1,400	=	190	×	.043	×	170

From L. B. Rowell, *Human Circulation Regulation During Physical Stress.* Copyright © 1986 Oxford University Press, New York N.Y. Reprinted by permission.

Table 13.3 Longitudinal Data on Changes in Maximal Oxygen Uptake

	$\dot{V}O_2$ max (ℓ · min⁻¹)	HR max (b · min⁻¹)	Stroke Volume (ml · beat⁻¹)	Cardiac Output (ℓ · min⁻¹)	a-v̄ O_2 Difference (ml · ℓ⁻¹)
Subject LM					
Before training	3.58	206	124	25.5	140
Four months	4.38	210	143	28.1	142
Eighteen months	4.53	205	149	30.5	149
Subject IS					
Before training	3.07	205	122	23.9	126
Four months	3.87	205	134	26.2	131
Thirty-two months	4.36	185	151	27.6	158
Fifty-one months	4.41	186	146	26.6	166

From B. Ekblom, "Effect of Physical Training on Oxygen Transport System in Man," in *Acta Physiologica Scandinavica.* Supplement 328. Copyright © 1969 Blackwell Scientific Publications, Ltd., Oxford, England. Reprinted by permission.

would have to be due to changes in one or more of the following variables on the right side of the equal sign.

$$\dot{V}O_2 \text{ max} = HR \text{ max} \times SV \text{ max} \times (\text{a-v̄ } O_2 \text{ difference}) \text{ max}$$

Cross-sectional comparisons of groups differing in their level of habitual physical activity have allowed scientists to identify the most important of these variables as the prime determinant of $\dot{V}O_2$ max. Such a comparison is presented in table 13.2, where values for $\dot{V}O_2$ max, maximal heart rate, maximal stroke volume, and the maximal a-v̄ O_2 difference are presented for three groups of subjects: mitral stenosis patients (heart valve problem limiting stroke volume), normally active subjects, and finally, world-class endurance athletes (48). The $\dot{V}O_2$ max is more than 100% greater for the normally active subjects compared to those with mitral stenosis, and again, almost 100% higher for the athletes as compared to the normally active subjects. What variable explains the tremendous differences in $\dot{V}O_2$ max values? Given that the maximal heart rate and the maximal a-v̄ O_2 difference were virtually identical for the three groups, the only variable explaining the difference in $\dot{V}O_2$ max is the maximal stroke volume (43 ml versus 112 ml versus 205 ml). Consistent with this, 68% of the variation in $\dot{V}O_2$ max between men and women was ascribed to left ventricular mass, a measure of heart size (30).

Longitudinal studies provide a slightly different picture of how training causes an increase in $\dot{V}O_2$ max. Generally, maximal heart rate either remains the same

or decreases with endurance training (18, 19, 48). As a result, the increase in $\dot{V}O_2$ max is shared between the increase in the stroke volume and the systemic a-v̄ O_2 difference. Studies reported by Saltin (53) in which young sedentary subjects trained for two to three months show that the sharing is about equal, half the gain due to SV changes and half to an increased oxygen extraction. In older men and women endurance training has been shown to increase $\dot{V}O_2$ max by 19% and 22%, respectively. However, while changes in stroke volume (+15%) accounted for most of the gain in $\dot{V}O_2$ max in the men, the entire increase in $\dot{V}O_2$ max in the women was due to an increase in the a-v̄ O_2 difference (56c). Similarly, when training is extended for years, the continued increase in $\dot{V}O_2$ max can be due to an increase in one factor more than the other. Data from Ekblom (18), shown in table 13.3, make this point. Subject LM's increase in $\dot{V}O_2$ max from the start of training was due primarily to an increase in stroke volume. The a-v̄ O_2 difference changed only 9 milliliters of O_2 per liter of blood over the eighteen months of training. In contrast, subject IS, whose $\dot{V}O_2$ max increased 44% over fifty-one months, showed no change in maximal cardiac output from sixteen to fifty-one months; the entire increase in $\dot{V}O_2$ max was due to an expanded a-v̄ O_2 difference. What causes the maximal stroke volume and the maximal arteriovenous oxygen difference to increase as a result of endurance training? The answers are provided in the next two sections.

in summary

- In young sedentary subjects approximately 50% of the increase in $\dot{V}O_2$ max due to training is related to an increase in maximal stroke volume (maximal heart rate remains the same), and 50% is due to an increase in the a-$\bar{v}$ O_2 difference.
- The large differences in $\dot{V}O_2$ max in the normal population (2 versus 6 liters/min) are due to differences in maximal stroke volume.

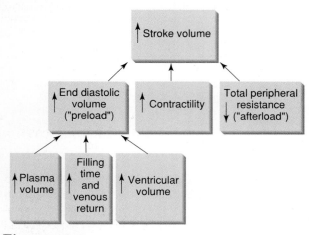

Figure 13.2
Factors increasing stroke volume.

Stroke Volume

Stroke volume is equal to the difference between end diastolic volume (EDV) and end systolic volume (ESV). Figure 13.2 summarizes the factors increasing stroke volume: an increase in EDV due to an increase in ventricle size or an increase in venous return ("preload"), an increase in myocardial contractility (the force of contraction at a constant muscle fiber length, with other factors controlled), and a decrease in resistance to blood flow out of the heart ("afterload"). Each of these will be discussed relative to the increase in the maximal stroke volume that occurs with endurance training.

End Diastolic Volume (EDV)

There is evidence that left ventricle size increases as a result of endurance training, with little change in ventricular wall thickness, while isometric exercises cause an increase in wall thickness, with little or no change in ventricular volume (17, 41, 47). This effect is believed to be due to the "volume loading" experienced by the heart *during exercise*. However, Rowell (48) raises the question that the increase in stroke volume that occurs with endurance training may simply be due to the chronic stretch of the myocardium *at rest* because of the increased filling time associated with the slower resting heart rate **(bradycardia)**. Plasma volume increases with endurance training. Experimental expansion of the plasma volume (200–300 ml) causes a 4% increase in $\dot{V}O_2$ max, and the

loss of plasma volume is the primary reason for the decrease in $\dot{V}O_2$ max in the first two weeks of detraining (11, 12). Overall, EDV increases as a result of an endurance training program, and according to the Frank-Starling mechanism (chapter 9), an increased stretch of the ventricle leads to an increase in stroke volume (48).

Cardiac Contractility

Cardiac contractility refers specifically to the strength of the cardiac muscle contraction when the fiber length (EDV), afterload (peripheral resistance), and heart rate are constant (since all affect contractility). While an acute exercise bout increases cardiac contractility due to the action of the sympathetic nervous system on the ventricle, it is difficult to conclude whether or not the inherent contractility of the heart changes with endurance training. The reason for this is that the factors that directly affect contractility (EDV, heart rate, and afterload) are themselves affected by endurance training (48). Blomqvist and Saltin (5) suggest that changes in contractility probably are not too important in explaining the increase in maximal stroke volume with endurance training. This was based on the observation that the fraction of the EDV ejected from the heart per beat **(ejection fraction)** is already so high in sedentary subjects prior to an endurance exercise program that there is not much to be gained by increasing contractility.

Afterload

Afterload refers to the peripheral resistance against which the ventricle is contracting as it tries to push a portion of the EDV into the aorta. If the heart contracts with the same force while the peripheral resistance decreases, a greater stroke volume will be realized. What is clear is that following an endurance training program, trained muscles offer less resistance to blood flow *during maximal work*. This decrease in resistance parallels the increase in maximal cardiac output so that mean arterial blood pressure is unchanged (MAP = $\dot{Q}$ × TPR). How does endurance training cause a lower resistance in the working muscle to facilitate a higher blood flow?

One might think that the increased blood flow through the trained muscle is due to an increase in the local factors (H^+, CO_2, etc.) associated with the higher work rates achieved after an endurance training program, but it is not. This can be seen in the following example. Prior to training, a subject takes a graded exercise test while maximal values for $\dot{V}O_2$ max and $\dot{Q}$ are measured. On another day the same subject takes an exercise test set at a work rate equal to 120% of the $\dot{V}O_2$ max achieved on the previous test and, of course, measures the same value for $\dot{V}O_2$ max. This supramaximal (>100% $\dot{V}O_2$ max) test should have caused a higher concentration of local factors in the working muscles that would have facilitated vasodilation and increased muscle blood flow. However, if this vasodilation were to happen with the cardiac output already at its maximal value, mean arterial blood pressure would fall, with dire consequences (48). How is this fall in blood pressure prevented?

When an additional muscle mass is recruited to do the supramaximal work rate, other vascular beds would have to be vasoconstricted by the sympathetic nervous system to maintain blood pressure. Since the renal and splanchnic vascular beds are already maximally constricted at maximal work, the only possibility is to vasoconstrict some vascular beds in already active muscle when additional muscle groups are recruited to do the supramaximal work (48). Consequently, the increase in muscle blood flow during the maximal exercise test following an endurance training program is due to a reduction in the sympathetic vasoconstrictor activity to the arterioles of the trained muscles. This occurs simultaneously with the increase in maximal cardiac output. This combination allows for the higher $\dot{V}O_2$ max at a constant mean arterial blood pressure, the homeostatic variable that appears to be closely regulated in maximal work (48).

Evidence supporting this explanation is found in studies where one-legged exercise is conducted. $\dot{V}O_2$ max measured during one-legged exercise on a cycle ergometer is equal to about 75%–80% of that measured during the regular two-legged test (10, 32). This is due to the greater arteriolar dilation and higher blood flow achieved in the working muscles during one-legged exercise. If the same degree of vasodilation were to occur in each leg when both were exercising maximally, the muscle's *capacity for blood flow* would exceed the heart's ability to provide it, and blood pressure would fall. To counter this tendency during maximal two-legged work, some of the muscle mass must be vasoconstricted to maintain blood pressure (32, 48). This is why the two-legged $\dot{V}O_2$ max value is not the sum of the $\dot{V}O_2$ max values of each leg. In conclusion, during maximal work with trained muscles following an endurance training program, there is a decrease in the resistance of that vascular bed to match the increase in maximal cardiac output to maintain blood pressure.

Arteriovenous O_2 Difference

Stroke volume causes 50% of the increase in $\dot{V}O_2$ max associated with an endurance exercise program in young sedentary subjects; O_2 extraction is responsible for the other 50%. The increase in the arteriovenous O_2 difference could be due to an elevation of the arterial oxygen content (higher hemoglobin or PO_2), or a decrease in the mixed venous oxygen content. Given that the hemoglobin concentration does not change with training and that the arterial PO_2 is usually sufficient to maintain arterial saturation of hemoglobin (chapter 10), the increase in the a-$\bar{v}$ O_2 difference is not due to an increase in the arterial O_2 content (48).

The increased capacity of the muscle to extract O_2 following training is believed to be due to the increase in capillary density, with the mitochondrial number being of secondary importance (5, 28, 48). The increase in capillary density in trained muscle accommodates the increase in muscle blood flow during maximal exercise, decreases the diffusion distance to the mitochondria, and slows the rate of blood flow to allow time for diffusion to take place.

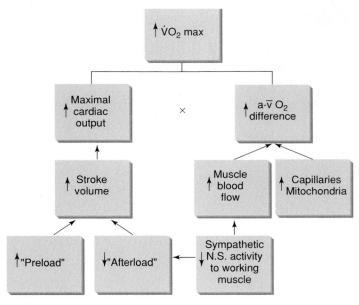

Figure 13.3
Summary of factors causing an increase in $\dot{V}O_2$ max with endurance training.

Changes in capillary density parallel changes in leg blood flow and $\dot{V}O_2$ max with training (48). The increases in mitochondria following endurance training favor O_2 transport from the capillary, and contribute to the expanded a-$\bar{v}$ O_2 differences. However, the capacity of the mitochondria to use O_2 far exceeds the capability of the heart to deliver O_2, making mitochondrial number *not* the factor limiting $\dot{V}O_2$ max (5, 28, 48). Figure 13.3 provides a summary of the factors causing an increase in $\dot{V}O_2$ max with an endurance training program.

in summary

- The training-induced increase in maximal stroke volume is due to both an increase in preload and a decrease in afterload.
  a. The increased preload is primarily due to an increase in end diastolic ventricular volume and the associated increase in plasma volume.
  b. The decreased afterload is due to a decrease in the arteriolar constriction in the trained muscles, increasing maximal muscle blood flow with no change in the mean arterial blood pressure.
- In young, sedentary subjects, 50% of the increase in $\dot{V}O_2$ max is due to an increase in the systemic a-$\bar{v}$ O_2 difference. The increased a-$\bar{v}$ O_2 difference is due to an increase in the capillary density of the trained muscles that is needed to accept the increase in maximal muscle blood flow. The greater capillary density allows for a sufficiently slow red blood cell transit time through the muscle, providing enough time for oxygen diffusion, which is facilitated by the increase in the number of mitochondria.

Figure 13.4

Time course of changes in $\dot{V}O_2$ max and associated cardiovascular variables with detraining.

From E. F. Coyle, et al., 1984, "Time Course of Loss of Adaptation after Stopping Prolonged Intense Endurance Training" in *Journal of Applied Physiology,* 57:1857-64. Copyright © 1984 American Physiological Society, Bethesda MD. Reprinted by permission.

Detraining and $\dot{V}O_2$ Max

When highly trained individuals stop training, $\dot{V}O_2$ max decreases over time. Why? Basically, because maximal cardiac output and oxygen extraction decrease. Figure 13.4 shows changes in maximal oxygen uptake, cardiac output, stroke volume, heart rate, and oxygen extraction over an 84-day period of no training (14). The initial decrease (first 12 days) in $\dot{V}O_2$ max was due entirely to the decrease in stroke volume, since the heart rate and a-$\bar{v}$ O_2 difference remained the same or increased. This sudden decrease in maximal stroke volume appears to be due to the rapid loss of plasma volume with detraining (11). When plasma volume is artificially restored by infusion, $\dot{V}O_2$ max increases toward pre-training values (11). This was confirmed in a recent study in which a 200–300 ml expansion of plasma volume was shown to increase $\dot{V}O_2$ max, even though the hemoglobin concentration was reduced (12). Figure 13.4 shows that between the 21st and 84th days of detraining, the decrease in $\dot{V}O_2$ max is due to the decrease in the a-$\bar{v}$ O_2 difference. This was associated with a decrease in muscle mitochondria; capillary density remained the same. The overall oxidative capacity of skeletal muscle was reduced, with Type IIa fibers decreasing from 43% to 26%, and IIb fibers increasing from 5% to 19% (13, 14). It is clear that changes in $\dot{V}O_2$ max, due to training or detraining are caused by changes in stroke volume and the capacity of the muscle to extract oxygen.

in summary

- The decrease in $\dot{V}O_2$ max with cessation of training is due to both a decrease in maximal stroke volume and a decrease in oxygen extraction, the reverse of what happens with training.

Endurance Training: Effects on Performance and Homeostasis

The ability to continue prolonged submaximal work is dependent on the maintenance of homeostasis during the activity. Endurance training results in a more rapid transition from rest to the steady-state metabolic requirement, a reduced reliance on the limited liver and muscle glycogen stores, and numerous cardiovascular and thermoregulatory adaptations that increase the chance that homeostasis will be maintained. Part of these training-induced adaptations are due to structural and biochemical changes in muscle, and we will discuss those in detail in the next few pages. However, a portion of these adaptations is related to factors external to the muscle. For example, in chapter 5 you saw how rapidly the plasma epinephrine and norepinephrine response to exercise was decreased with training. These hormones directly or indirectly affect numerous metabolic responses to exercise and may be involved in some of the adaptations to muscle associated with endurance training (44b). This needs to be stated at the beginning of this section because, while we focus on the link between changes in skeletal muscle and performance, there is clear evidence that some improvements in performance occur prior to structural or biochemical changes in skeletal muscle (22). This suggests that the initial metabolic adaptations to endurance training might consist of neural, or neural-hormonal-receptor adaptations, which are followed by structural adaptations. If so, this would not be unlike the adaptations to strength training (see later discussion).

In the introduction to this chapter we mentioned that the increase in performance following an endurance training program was due more to biochemical and structural changes in the trained skeletal muscle than to a small increase in $\dot{V}O_2$ max. Endurance training causes rather large changes in the biochemical and structural characteristics of the working muscles. The typical changes include increases in the number of mitochondria (up to fourfold for Type II fibers) and capillary density (28). The increase in mitochondria is associated with increases in the enzymes involved in oxidative metabolism: Krebs cycle, fatty-acid (β-oxidation) cycle, and the electron transport chain. Changes also occur in the "shuttle system" that is used for moving NADH from the cytoplasm, where it is produced in glycolysis, to the

| Table 13.4 | Succinate Dehydrogenase Activity in Thigh Muscle Fiber Types in Response to Conditioning and Deconditioning | | | |

Fitness Level	Range of $\dot{V}O_2$ max (ml · kg^{-1} · min^{-1})	Type I	Muscle Fiber Type Type IIa (μmol · g^{-1} · min^{-1})	Type IIb
Deconditioned	30–40	5.0	4.0	3.5
Sedentary	40–50	9.2	5.8	4.9
Conditioning (months)	45–55	12.1	10.2	5.5
Endurance athletes	>70	23.2	22.1	22.0

Adapted from Saltin and Gollnick (56a)

Figure 13.5

Time-course of training/detraining adaptations in mitochondrial content of skeletal muscle. Note that about 50 percent of the increase in mitochondrial content was lost after one week of detraining (a) and that all of the adaptation was lost after five weeks of detraining. Also, it took four weeks of retraining (b) to regain the adaptation lost in the first week of detraining.

mitochondria where it is used in the electron transport chain to produce ATP. Finally, changes occur in the type of LDH enzyme, which is involved in the conversion of pyruvate to lactate. It is the changes in these characteristics of muscle that "drive" or determine the overall physiological responses to a given submaximal exercise bout. Table 13.4 presents data on succinate dehydrogenase activity, a measure of the oxidative capacity of muscle, for each of the three major fiber types for people differing in fitness. An important observation is that the oxidative capacity is not different among the fibers of the endurance athlete. In contrast, these values are twice that of the Type I fibers of individuals who have been exercising for months, and four times that of sedentary individuals. How long does it take for these changes to occur?

It is a common experience for most individuals who do run, swim, or cycle training that a break of only two weeks can dramatically affect performance. This is due primarily to the changes in the mitochondria's oxidative enzymes (28b, 37a, 58). In fact, mitochondrial oxidative capacity undergoes rapid changes at the onset

and termination of exercise training. Figure 13.5 shows how quickly muscle mitochondria increase at the onset of training, doubling in about five weeks of training. However, only one week of detraining (shown by the letter "a") results in a loss of about 50 percent of what was gained during the five weeks of training (5a, 56c). Three to four weeks of retraining were required to achieve the former levels (shown by the letter "b" in figure 13.5). The old adage, "use it or lose it" is very true for the oxidative capacity of muscle (see A Closer Look 13.1). The following sections will describe how this greater capacity for oxidative metabolism results in less disruption of physiological (e.g., plasma glucose and H$^+$ concentrations) variables maintained by homeostatic mechanisms.

Biochemical Adaptations and the Oxygen Deficit

At the onset of exercise, ATP is converted to ADP and P$_i$ by the cross-bridges in order to develop tension. The increase in the ADP concentration in the cytoplasm is the immediate stimulus for ATP-producing systems to come into play to meet the ATP demands of the cross-bridges. Phosphocreatine responds immediately to this ATP need, followed by glycolysis and mitochondrial oxidative phosphorylation. The latter process provides all the ATP aerobically during the steady state phase of the work, with the mitochondrial oxygen consumption driven by the ADP concentration. Muscle cells with few mitochondria must have a high ADP concentration to stimulate the limited number of mitochondria to consume oxygen at a given rate (28). How does endurance training affect these oxygen uptake responses at the onset of submaximal steady state work?

The steady state $\dot{V}O_2$ measured during a submaximal work test is not affected by endurance training. The mitochondria are still consuming the same number of O$_2$ molecules per minute. What is different, due to the large increase in mitochondria, oxidative enzymes, and the number of capillaries per muscle fiber, is how the ATP-producing chore is shared among the mitochondria. Figure 13.7 shows schematically that if a muscle cell has only one mitochondrion, an increase of 100 units in the ADP concentration is needed for the muscle to consume 2.0 liters of O$_2$ per minute. After

Role of Exercise Intensity and Duration on Mitochondrial Adaptations

A muscle fiber's oxidative capacity can improve only if the muscle fiber is recruited during the exercise session. Figures 13.6a and 13.6b show changes in citrate synthase (CS) activity, a marker of mitochondrial oxidative capacity, due to exercise programs differing in duration (30, 60, and 90 minutes) and intensity (~55%, ~65%, and ~75% $\dot{V}O_2$ max). Figure 13.6a shows that CS activity increased in the red gastrocnemius (primarily Type IIa fibers) for all treatments, but the magnitude of the change was independent of the intensity and duration of the activity. In contrast, figure 13.6b shows that for the white gastrocnemius (primarily Type IIb fibers) CS activity increased due to both intensity and duration of activity. Why the difference? The Type IIa fibers were easily recruited by the lowest exercise intensity while very strenuous exercise was required to recruit the Type IIb fibers (44a). These observations support our understanding of the specificity of exercise—light to moderate exercise will improve or maintain the oxidative capacity of high oxidative fibers (Type I and Type IIa), while strenuous exercise is needed to change low oxidative (Type IIb) fibers (16a, 56d). Given the rapid loss of a muscle's oxidative capacity with cessation of training, it is no surprise that high-level endurance performances, which require the recruitment of Type IIb fibers, fall off quickly when training ceases.

Figure 13.6

Changes in citrate synthase activity with different intensities and durations of exercise.

training, when the number of mitochondria has doubled, the ADP concentration increases only half as much, since each mitochondrion needs only half the stimulation to take up 1.0 liter of O_2 per minute. The increase in the capillary density in the muscle cell after endurance training is a parallel change that supports this process. In essence, after an endurance training program, it takes less change in the ADP concentration to stimulate the mitochondria to take up the oxygen (28). Since less of a change in the ADP concentration is needed to stimulate the mitochondria, the rising ADP concentration at the onset of work (due to cross-bridges causing ATP $\rightarrow$ ADP + P_i) will cause oxidative phosphorylation to be activated earlier. This translates into a faster rise in the oxygen uptake curve at the onset of work, resulting in the steady state $\dot{V}O_2$ being achieved earlier (see figure 4.2) (25, 44). This faster rise in oxygen uptake at the onset of work means that the O_2 deficit is less: less creatine phosphate depletion and less lactate and H^+ formation (9a, 23).

The reductions in lactate and H^+ formation and phosphocreatine depletion are also linked to the lower ADP concentration in the muscle cell after the endurance training program. The lower ADP concentration results in less phosphocreatine depletion since the reaction for this is |ADP| + |PC| $\rightarrow$ |ATP| + |C|. The lower ADP concentration in the cell also results in less stimulation of glycolysis. Chapter 3 indicated that phosphofructokinase (PFK) is the enzyme in glycolysis that controls the rate at which glucose is metabolized, and that high levels of ADP and low levels of PC in the cell stimulate this enzyme to process glucose through the pathway. The reduced stimulation of glycolysis due to the lower ADP and higher PC concentrations following endurance training results in less reliance on anaerobic glycolysis to provide ATP at the onset of exercise (21, 23). The net result is a lower oxygen

Figure 13.7
Influence of mitochondria number on the change in the ADP concentration needed to increase the $\dot{V}O_2$.

Figure 13.8
Endurance training reduces the O_2 deficit at the onset of work.

deficit, less depletion of phosphocreatine, and a reduction in lactate and H^+ formation. Figure 13.8 shows that the biochemical adaptations following endurance training result in a faster rise in the oxygen uptake curve at the onset of work, with less disruption of homeostasis.

Biochemical Adaptations and the Plasma Glucose Concentration

Plasma glucose is the primary fuel of the nervous system and, as described in chapter 5, the majority of hormonal changes associated with fasting or exercise are aimed at maintaining this important homeostatic variable. How do the biochemical changes in muscle that occur as a result of endurance training help maintain the blood glucose concentration during prolonged submaximal exercise? The answer is again found in the increases in mitochondrial number and capillary density that occur with endurance training.

The increased number of mitochondria increases a muscle fiber's capacity to oxidize both carbohydrate and fat. However, the most dramatic change in muscle metabolism following training is the increased utilization of fat, and the sparing of carbohydrate. This is due to an improved capacity to take up FFA from the circulation, an increased ability to transport FFA from the cytoplasm to the mitochondria of the muscle, and an increase in the fatty-acid (β-oxidation) cycle enzymes

needed to degrade the FFA to acetyl-CoA units for the Krebs cycle (28). These points will now be discussed.

Transport of FFA into Muscle

Plasma FFA provide half the fat oxidized by muscle during exercise, and the uptake of FFA by muscle is proportional to the FFA concentration in the plasma (42). An enhanced mobilization of FFA would favor the maintenance of the plasma FFA concentration at a time when the muscle is using FFA at a faster rate. However, that does not occur and the plasma FFA concentration is actually lower following training (8, 37b). How does the endurance-trained muscle compensate for this? Plasma FFA must be transported from the capillary, across the cell membrane to the cytoplasm, and then into the mitochondria before oxidation can occur. It has been generally accepted that the first step, from capillary to cytoplasm, was accomplished by passive diffusion, and the higher the plasma FFA concentration, the greater the rate of FFA uptake by the cell. There is now evidence that the transport of FFA into the muscle cell involves a carrier molecule whose capacity to transport FFA can become saturated at high plasma FFA concentrations (55). Endurance training has been shown to increase the capacity to transport FFA such that a trained individual can transport more FFA at the same plasma FFA concentration, compared to an untrained individual (31a). This increased ability to transport FFA is facilitated by a greater capillary density in the trained muscle which slows the rate of blood flow past the cell membrane, allowing more time for the FFA to be transported into the cell (55).

Transport of FFA from the Cytoplasm to the Mitochondria

The FFA are transported from the cytoplasm to the mitochondria by carnitine transferase, an enzyme associated with the mitochondrial membrane. This enzyme catalyzes the reaction of FFA and the carrier molecule, carnitine, which moves quickly across the mitochondrial membrane where the reaction is reversed, yielding the FFA for oxidation. The increase in the mitochondrial number with endurance training increases the surface area of the mitochondrial membranes and the amount of carnitine transferase such that FFA can be transported at a faster rate from the cytoplasm to the mitochondria for oxidation (56a). The faster rate of transport from the cytoplasm to the mitochondria favors the movement of more FFA into the muscle cell from the plasma.

Mitochondrial Oxidation of FFA

The increase in mitochondria number increases the enzymes involved in FFA oxidation, specifically, the fatty-acid (β-oxidation) cycle. This results in an increased rate at which acetyl-CoA molecules are formed from FFA for entry to the Krebs cycle, where citrate (the first molecule in the cycle) is formed. The high citrate level inhibits PFK activity in the cytoplasm and therefore reduces carbohydrate metabolism (28).

in summary

- The combination of the increase in the density of capillaries and the number of mitochondria per muscle fiber increases the capacity to transport FFA from the plasma → cytoplasm → mitochondria.
- The increase in the enzymes of the fatty acid cycle increases the rate of formation of acetyl-CoA from FFA for oxidation in the Krebs cycle. This increase in fat oxidation in endurance-trained muscle spares both muscle glycogen and plasma glucose, the latter being a focal point of homeostatic regulatory mechanisms. These points are summarized in figure 13.9.

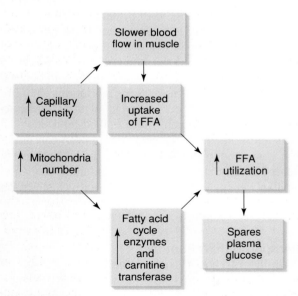

Figure 13.9
Increased mitochondria number and capillary density increase the rate of free-fatty-acid utilization, preserving plasma glucose.

Biochemical Adaptations and Blood pH

The pH of blood is maintained near 7.40 ± 0.02 at rest. As described in chapter 11, acute and long-term challenges to the pH are met by responses of both the pulmonary and renal systems. How does endurance training result in less disruption of the blood pH during submaximal work? The answer relates to the reduced lactate and H^+ formation following endurance training.

Lactate formation occurs when there is an accumulation of NADH and pyruvate in the cytoplasm of the cell where lactate dehydrogenase (LDH) is present:

$$[pyruvate] + [NADH] \rightarrow [lactate] + [NAD]$$
$$LDH$$

Anything that affects the concentration of pyruvate, NADH, or the type of LDH in the cell will affect the rate of lactate formation. We have already seen that the increased number of mitochondria can have a dramatic effect on pyruvate formation: the lower ADP concentration stimulates PFK less at the onset of work, and the increased capacity to use fats reduces the need for carbohydrate oxidation during prolonged work. If less carbohydrate is used, less pyruvate is formed. In addition, the increase in mitochondria number increases the chance that pyruvate will be taken up by the mitochondria for oxidation in the Krebs cycle, rather than being bound to LDH in the cytoplasm. All of these adaptations favor a lower pyruvate concentration and a reduction in lactate formation.

There are two additional biochemical changes in muscle due to endurance training that reduce lactate and, consequently, H^+ formation. The NADH produced during glycolysis can react with pyruvate, as shown in the above equation, or it can be transported into the mitochondrion to be oxidized in the electron transport chain to form ATP (chapter 3). Endurance training increases the malate-aspartate shuttle system, which transports NADH into the mitochondrion (28). If the NADH formed in glycolysis is more quickly transported to the mitochondria, there will be less lactate and H^+ formation. Lastly, endurance training causes a change in the type of LDH present in the muscle cell. This enzyme exists in five forms (isozymes): M_4, M_3H, M_2H_2, MH_3, and H_4. The H_4, or heart form of LDH, has a low affinity for the available pyruvate. Endurance training shifts the LDH toward the H_4 form, making lactate and H^+ formation less likely and the uptake of pyruvate by the mitochondria more likely. Figure 13.10 summarizes the effect these biochemical changes have on lactate formation and the production of H^+ during submaximal work.

Figure 13.10
Increased mitochondria number decreases lactate and H+ formation to maintain the blood pH.

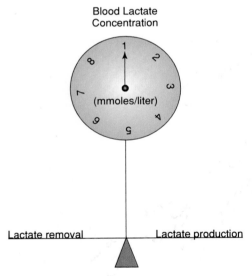

Figure 13.11
The resting blood lactate concentration is the result of a balance between lactate production and removal.

Biochemical Adaptations and Lactate Removal

Lactate accumulation in the blood is dependent on the balance between lactate production by working muscle and lactate removal by liver and other tissues. Figure 13.11 shows that the blood lactate concentration stays at 1 mmol/liter at rest and during light exercise when there is a balance between production and removal. As the exercise intensity increases, the blood lactate could rise due to an acceleration of lactate production, or to a reduction in the rate of removal by the liver and other tissues (9). As described in chapter 9, blood flow to nonworking muscles, kidney, liver, and GI tract decreases as exercise intensity increases, reducing the rate of lactate removal. How does endurance training affect blood flow to these tissues?

Endurance training causes an increase in the capillary density of the working muscles. This results in two changes favorable for oxygen transport to the mitochondria: a decrease in the distance from capillary to mitochondrion, and a decrease in the rate of blood flow through each capillary, allowing more time for the diffusion of oxygen to the mitochondria. As a result, the same submaximal work rate demands *less* blood flow to the working muscles after training. The muscle can extract more oxygen from each liter of blood (larger a-$\bar{v}O_2$ difference) to achieve the same steady state $\dot{V}O_2$, with a lower blood flow.

Since the cardiac output for a given submaximal work rate is unchanged or only slightly decreased after training (18), where is the blood flow now distributed that was formally going to the working muscles? Two vascular beds that receive an increase in blood flow following training are the liver and the kidneys. Since the liver is a major site for lactate removal for gluconeogenesis, the blood lactate level is lower following an endurance training program due in part to the liver's increased ability to remove lactate. Figure 13.13 summarizes these events.

Exercise and Resistance to Infection

We possess considerable knowledge about the effects of exercise on metabolism, cardiovascular function, and skeletal muscle structure. In contrast, we know little about how our immune system responds to exercise. This is due, in part, to the limited number of studies that have been done in which important factors that can affect resistance to infection have been controlled. These factors include (9b):

- Having a control group to account for temporal changes (circadian and seasonal) in immune function;
- Matching groups on the basis of psychological stressors which are known to affect immune function;
- Ensuring adequate dietary intake

In addition to these concerns, it has become clear that one cannot draw broad conclusions about the relationship of exercise to overall resistance to infection from observations of a single immune response (9b). In spite of these limitations there are some epidemiological and experimental studies on the effect of exercise on upper respiratory tract infections (URTI) that provide some guidance. Nieman's review (1994) of this topic suggests that the risk of URTI follows a "J"-shaped pattern relative to the amount and intensity of exercise as shown in figure 13.12.

The model suggests that moderate exercise lowers the risk of URTI, while excessive amounts of exercise increase the risk. Evidence for this model includes the following (41a, 56b):

- Six times as many runners experienced URTI following a marathon compared to nonparticipating runners;
- Runners training more than 96 km/wk had twice the risk of URTI as those doing only 32 km/wk;
- Races of only 5 km to 21.1 km do not seem to increase the risk of URTI in the week following the race;
- Those doing moderate exercise training (45 minutes of brisk walking, five days per week) experienced half as many days with URTI symptoms compared to a sedentary group;
- Elderly subjects who did 40 minutes of walking, 5 times per week had an incidence of URTI of only 21% compared to 50% for a sedentary control group.

In summary, moderate exercise training, and running races up to a half-marathon seem to be consistent with good or improved resistance to upper respiratory tract infections. Additional research is needed to determine the clinical importance of the changes in immune function with exercise, and the influence of exercise rehabilitation on patients with immunodeficiencies due to disease, medication, and aging (9b, 41a, 56b).

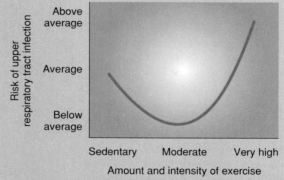

Figure 13.12

"J"-shaped model of relationship between varying amounts of exercise and risk of URTI. This model suggests that moderate exercise may lower risk of respiratory infection while excessive amounts may increase the risk (41a).

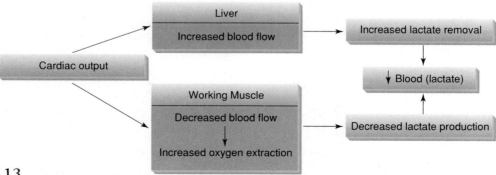

Figure 13.13

Effect of endurance training on the redistribution of blood flow and lactate removal during exercise at a fixed submaximal work load.

in summary

- Mitochondrial adaptations to endurance training include an increase in the enzymes involved in oxidative metabolism: Krebs cycle, fatty-acid (β-oxidation) cycle, and the electron transport chain.
- Those mitochondrial adaptations result in the following:
  a. a smaller O_2 deficit due to a more rapid increase in oxygen uptake at the onset of work
  b. an increase in fat metabolism that spares muscle glycogen and blood glucose
  c. a reduction in lactate and H^+ formation
  d. an increase in lactate removal

Endurance Training: Links Between Muscle and Systemic Physiology

We have just described the importance of the local changes occurring in endurance-trained muscle on the maintenance of homeostasis during prolonged submaximal work. However, these same changes are also related to the lower heart rate, ventilation, and catecholamine responses measured during submaximal work following an endurance training program. What is the link between the changes in muscle and the improved heart rate and ventilation responses to exercise?

The following endurance training study illustrates the importance of the trained muscle in the body's overall response to a submaximal work bout. In this study each subject's left and right leg was tested separately on a cycle ergometer at a submaximal work rate prior to and during an endurance training program. Heart rate and ventilation were measured at the end of the submaximal exercise test, and a blood sample was obtained to monitor changes in lactate, epinephrine, and norepinephrine. During the study each subject *trained only one leg* for thirteen sessions, fifteen minutes a session, at an exercise intensity causing a heart rate of 170 beats per minute. At the end of each week of training, the subject was tested at the same submaximal work rate used prior to starting the training program. This procedure allowed the investigator to determine how fast the "training effect" occurred. Figure 13.14 shows that heart rate, ventilation, blood lactate, and plasma epinephrine and norepinephrine responses decreased throughout the study. Results such as these have been used to support the idea that the cardiovascular, pulmonary, and sympathetic nervous systems have each adapted to the exercise. However, that may not be quite true. At the end of this training program the "untrained" leg was trained for five consecutive days at the same submaximal work rate used for the "trained leg." Physiological measurements were obtained during the exercise session on the first, third, and fifth days. If the cardiovascular, pulmonary, and sympathetic nervous systems had become "trained" as a result of the thirteen exercise sessions with the other leg, you might expect some "transfer" of the training effect when the untrained leg was tested. Interestingly, figure 13.14 shows that all the systems responded as if they had never been exposed to exercise (10). There was no transfer of the training effect from one leg to the other. This example shows that the heart rate, ventilation, and plasma catecholamine responses to prolonged submaximal exercise are determined, not by the specific adaptation of each organ or system, but by the training state of the specific muscle groups engaged in the exercise. How is this possible?

In chapter 10 the control of ventilation during exercise required a discussion of central and peripheral neural influences that could help explain the precise matching of ventilation to the increased oxygen demands of incremental exercise. This same approach will be taken here to explain how endurance training of specific muscle groups results in the decrease in cardiorespiratory and sympathetic nervous system responses to the same submaximal work rate. The output of the cardiovascular and respiratory control centers is influenced by input from higher brain centers, where the motor task originates, as well as from the muscles carrying out the task. A decrease in motor unit recruitment or a reduction in output from the receptors in the working muscles to the brain reduces these physiological responses to the work task. Following a brief summary of "peripheral" and "central" control mechanisms, an attempt will be made to show how both are involved in the reduced physiological responses to submaximal exercise.

Peripheral Feedback

Rowell (48) indicates that Zuntz and Geppert were the originators of the idea that reflexes in working muscles might control or "drive" cardiovascular or pulmonary systems in proportion to the metabolic rate. A number of receptors have been examined that respond to chemical or physical changes in muscle that might signify work rate. The involvement of the muscle spindle and Golgi tendon organ received considerable attention as possible sites for these reflexes, given their ability to monitor changes in muscle length and tension development, respectively. However, blocking the afferent nerves from these receptors did not eliminate specific cardiovascular responses to muscle tension development (40, 48). Attention has now been directed to small-diameter nerve fibers (group III and group IV fibers) that are responsive to both tension, temperature, and chemical changes in muscle. These fibers increase their rate of

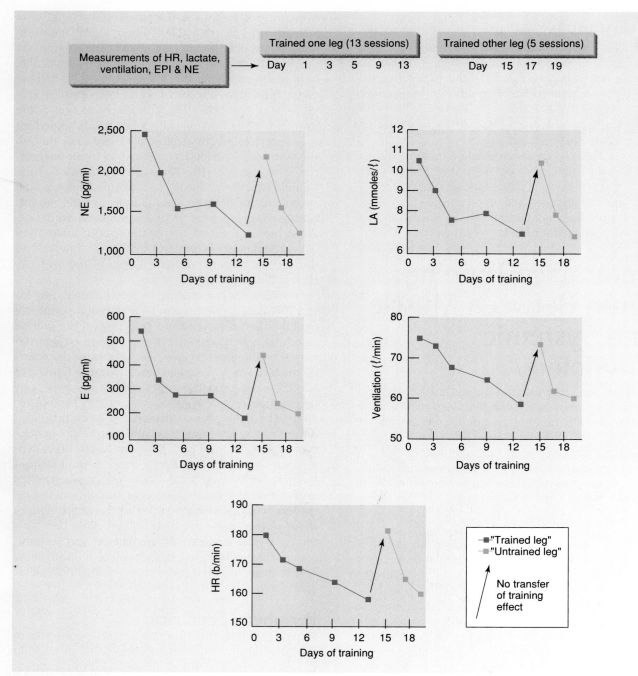

Figure 13.14
The lack of transfer of a training effect, indicating that the responses of the cardiovascular, pulmonary, and sympathetic nervous systems are more dependent on the trained state of the muscles involved in the activity than on some specific adaptation in those systems.

firing action potentials in proportion to changes in metabolic rate. Figure 13.15 shows schematically the neuronal circuitry for the reflex regulation of the cardiovascular and respiratory responses to exercise by these group III and group IV fibers.

Central Command

The general idea surrounding central control of the physiological response to exercise is presented in

figure 13.16. Higher brain centers (motor cortex, basal ganglia, cerebellum—see chapter 7) prepare to execute a motor task and send action potentials through lower brain centers and spinal nuclei to influence the cardiorespiratory and sympathetic nervous system responses to exercise. As more motor units are recruited to develop the greater tension needed to accomplish a work task, larger physiological responses are required to sustain the metabolic rate of

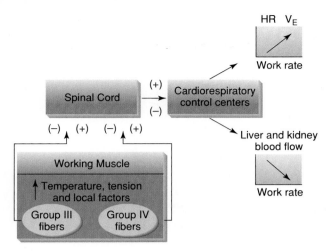

Figure 13.15
Peripheral control mechanisms in muscle influence the heart rate, ventilation, and kidney and liver blood flow responses to submaximal work.

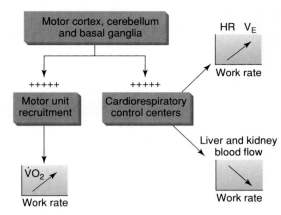

Figure 13.16
Central control of motor unit recruitment, heart rate, ventilation, and liver and kidney blood flow responses to submaximal work.

the muscles (39, 48). For example, if some muscle fibers are prevented from contracting, additional muscle fibers must be recruited to maintain tension. This generates higher heart rate responses to the work task (2). How are these peripheral and central controls related to the decreases in sympathetic nervous system activity, heart rate, and ventilation observed during submaximal exercise following an endurance training program?

The ability to perform a fixed submaximal exercise bout for a prolonged period of time is dependent on the recruitment of a sufficient number of motor units to meet the tension (work) requirements through oxidative phosphorylation. Prior to endurance training, more mitochondria-poor motor units must be recruited to carry out a work task at a given $\dot{V}O_2$. This results in a greater "central" drive to the cardiorespiratory control centers, which causes higher sympathetic nervous system, heart rate, and ventilation responses. The feedback from chemoreceptors at the untrained muscle would also stimulate the cardiorespiratory control center. With the increase in mitochondrial number following endurance training, local factors (H^+, adenosine compounds, etc.) do not change as much. This leads to less local stimulation of blood flow, and a reduced chemoreceptor input to the cardiorespiratory centers. In addition, the higher number of mitochondria allows the tension to be maintained with fewer motor units involved in the activity. This reduced "feed forward" input from the higher brain centers and reduced "feedback" from the muscle results in lower sympathetic nervous system output, heart rate, and ventilation responses to exercise (39, 48, 49).

in summary

- The biochemical changes in muscle due to endurance training influence the physiological responses to exercise. The reduction in "feedback" from chemoreceptors in the trained muscle and a reduction in the need to recruit motor units to accomplish a work task results in reduced sympathetic nervous system, heart rate, and ventilation responses to submaximal exercise.

Physiological Effects of Strength Training

The basic principles of training related to improving strength have been around for thousands of years, and Morpurgo's observation that gains in strength were associated with increases in muscle size was made almost one hundred years ago (4). Despite this history, most recent research on the effects of training has focused on $\dot{V}O_2$ max and endurance performance, possibly because of their link to the prevention and treatment of heart disease. However, times and circumstances change, and in the most recent update of the American College of Sports Medicine's position stand on exercise recommendations for health and fitness, strength training was included (1).

Before we begin, some terms need to be defined and some basic principles need to be restated. Muscular strength refers to the maximal force that a muscle or muscle group can generate and is commonly expressed as the one-repetition maximum or 1-RM, the maximum load that can be moved through a range of motion once in good form. Muscular endurance refers to the ability to make repeated contractions against a submaximal load. Consistent with our earlier discussion of training

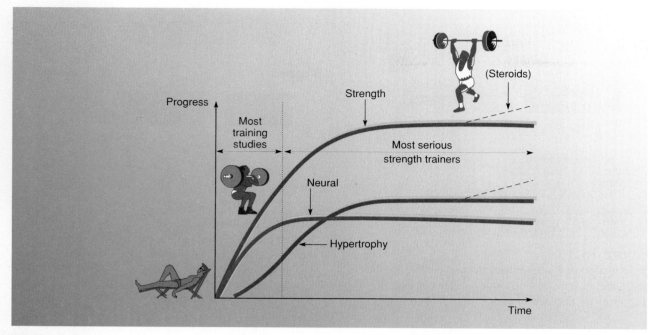

Figure 13.17
Relative roles of neural and muscular adaptations to resistance training.

and $\dot{V}O_2$ max, large individual differences exist in the response to strength training programs, and the percent gain in strength is inversely related to the initial strength (34). These observations imply a genetic limitation to the gains that can be realized due to training, similar to what we have seen for gains in $\dot{V}O_2$ max. Finally, the basic principles of training, overload and specificity, apply here as well. For example, high-resistance training (2–10 RM loads) results in gains in muscular strength; in contrast, low-resistance training (20+ RM loads) results in gains in muscular endurance, with less of a change in strength (34). What physiological changes occur with resistance training that result in improvements in muscular strength and endurance?

Physiological Mechanisms Causing Increased Strength

Chapter 8 described the roles that motor unit recruitment, stimulus frequency, and synchronous firing of motor units play in the development of muscle tension, as well as the fact that Type II motor units develop more tension than Type I motor units. In addition, we described how stimulatory (muscle spindle) and inhibitory (Golgi tendon organ) muscle reflexes affect tension development. These factors are very much involved in the improvement of strength with training.

Figure 13.17 provides a schematic to follow that will facilitate our discussion of muscular and neural factors related to gains in strength (50). In training studies

of short duration (8–20 weeks), neural adaptations related to learning, coordination, and the ability to recruit prime movers play a major role in the gain in strength. In contrast, in long-term training programs an increase in the size of the prime movers plays the major role in strength development. The role of anabolic steroids (see chapter 5) relates to this latter point (50). We will now consider neural and muscular factors in more detail.

Neural Factors

It has become clear that a portion of the gains in strength that occurs with training, especially early in a program, is due to neural adaptations and not an enlargement of muscle (50). Some of these observations show that neural adaptations to strength training are different from those that occur with running or cycling training. In figure 13.14 we showed that when one leg was trained on a cycle ergometer, the training effect did not "carry over" to the untrained leg. In contrast, when one arm is strength trained, a portion of the training effect is "transferred" to the other arm. In this case, the gain in strength in the trained arm was related to both muscle hypertrophy and an increased ability to activate motor units, while in the untrained arm the improvement was due solely to the latter factor—a neural adaptation (50). A recent study confirmed this when gains of muscular strength and endurance of a trained leg were transferred to the untrained leg (31). The neural adaptations related to strength training include an improved synchronization of motor unit firing and an improved ability to recruit motor units to enable a person to match the strength elicited by electrical stimulation (50).

As we age muscle strength declines, with most of the decline occurring after age fifty. The loss of strength is associated with the loss of muscle mass, due to a decrease in the number of both Type I and Type II fibers (see chapter 8). The loss of muscle fibers seems to be related to a neurological change at the level of a motor neuron, and whatever affects the motor neuron affects the fibers attached to it. What is promising about an otherwise dismal picture is that progressive resistance training programs for the elderly result in increases in muscle hypertrophy and strength, similar to what is observed for young people (21a, 21b). This has major ramifications for health care given the increase in the number of people classified as elderly (5b, 28a, 47a).

Muscular Enlargement

Recall that Type II muscle fibers develop slightly more specific tension (i.e., force/cross-sectional area) than Type I fibers (56a); however, an enlargement of either fiber results in gains in strength. Strength training causes an enlargement of both Type I and Type II fibers, with the latter changing more than the former (34, 57). However, bodybuilders who train with low intensity (high RM) and large volume workouts have smaller Type II fibers than powerlifters who train with heavy resistance (low RM) workouts (34, 57). It must be added that while bodybuilders have a higher percentage of slow-twitch fibers than elite powerlifters, there are questions about whether the difference is due to training or self-selection based on a genetic predisposition for success (57). Interestingly, differences between bodybuilders and powerlifters carry over to other muscular adaptations.

In contrast to the skeletal muscle adaptations that accompany running and cycling training, there is no increase in capillary density with heavy resistance training. As a result of the muscle's enlargement, capillary density actually decreases (34, 57). However, bodybuilders who use low resistance, high volume workouts show increases in the capillary to fiber ratio such that the capillary density is similar to that of nonathletes, despite the muscle enlargement. Short-term strength training programs do not change capillary density, but mitochondrial density is decreased in proportion to the degree of hypertrophy (57).

Hypertrophy and Hyperplasia

During normal human development, from birth until adulthood, muscle size increases manyfold, with no change in the number of muscle fibers—a true hypertrophy. It is therefore not surprising that muscle enlargement associated with strength training is also due to a hypertrophy of existing fibers, not the generation of new fibers (hyperplasia), an observation Morpurgo made almost one hundred years ago (4, 56a). However, a variety of observations have raised questions that perhaps *some* of the muscle enlargement due to training is the result of hyperplasia. Some studies report that elite body builders have more fibers per motor unit than the average person, raising the point that hyperplasia might occur with long-term training (35, 37). In addition, when resistance training resulted in a 24% increase in muscle mass but only an 11% increase in fiber cross-sectional area, scientists suggested that hyperplasia might have played a role in the muscle enlargement (38).

Simultaneous Strength and Endurance Training

At this point in the chapter it may have occurred to you that strength training might interfere with the adaptations associated with endurance training. For example, cycle training increases mitochondrial density, and strength training does the opposite. Does one type of training really interfere with the effects of the other? To date, a definite answer to this question is not available, nonetheless, let's examine studies on this issue.

In 1980, Hickson (24) showed that a 10-week combined strength and endurance training program resulted in similar gains in $\dot{V}O_2$ max compared to an endurance-only group, but there was some interference with the gains in strength. The strength-only group increased strength throughout the entire ten weeks, but the combined strength and endurance group showed a leveling off and a decrease in strength at 9 and 10 weeks. In contrast to this, when a 10-week (3-day-per-week) strength training program was added to a run-and-cycle training program *after* the group had leveled off in endurance performance, the group experienced a 30% gain in strength, but without hypertrophy. $\dot{V}O_2$ max was unaffected, but cycle time to exhaustion at 80% $\dot{V}O_2$ max was increased from 71 to 85 minutes. This suggests that strength training can improve the performance of prolonged heavy endurance exercise (26).

Sale et al. (52) found that relative to gains in strength (S) and endurance (E), when E-training was added to S-training (S + E), additional improvements occurred in *endurance* than were generated by S-training alone. However, strength measures were unaffected. When S-training was added to E-training (E + S), more gains were made in *strength* than were generated by E-training alone; endurance measures were unaffected. The authors concluded that concurrent S- and E-training did not interfere with S- or E-development in comparison to S- or E-training alone. They suggest that the effectiveness of added training may depend on a variety of factors, such as intensity, volume, and frequency of training, status of the subjects, and how the training modes are integrated. For example, when S- and E-training were done on the same days of the week, there was less strength development compared to when S- and E-training were done on different days (51).

This last point was reinforced in a study in which twelve subjects did two 7.5-week training programs—high resistance-low repetition (for improving strength), and low resistance-high repetition (for muscular endurance), with a 5.5-week pause between programs.

Six subjects did the endurance program first and the strength program second; the other six followed the opposite order. All major fiber types (I, IIa, IIb) increased in cross-sectional area after the first 7.5 weeks, independent of type of training. However, in the second 7.5 weeks, the strength program caused a further increase in the cross-sectional area of the Type I and IIb fibers, while a decrease occurred in those doing the endurance program (46).

in summary

- Increases in strength due to short-term (8–20 weeks) training are the result of neural adaptations, while gains in strength in long-term training programs are due to an increase in the size of the muscle.
- There is evidence both for and against the proposition that the physiological effects of strength training interfere with the physiological effects of endurance training.

study questions

1. Define the following principles of training: overload and specificity.
2. Give one example of a cross-sectional study and a longitudinal study.
3. What are typical $\dot{V}O_2$ max values for young men and women? Cardiac patients?
4. Given the formula for $\dot{V}O_2$ max using heart rate, stroke volume, and the a-$\bar{v}$ O_2 difference, which variable is most important in explaining the differences in $\dot{V}O_2$ max in different populations? Give a quantitative example.
5. Describe how the increase in $\dot{V}O_2$ max comes about for the sedentary subject who undertakes an endurance training program.
6. Explain the importance of preload, afterload, and contractility in the increase of the maximal stroke volume that occurs with endurance training.
7. What are the most important changes in muscle structure that are responsible for the increase in the maximal a-$\bar{v}$ O_2 difference that occurs with endurance training?
8. What causes the $\dot{V}O_2$ max to decrease following termination of an endurance training program?

9. Describe how the capillary and mitochondrial changes that occur in muscle as a result of an endurance training program are related to the following adaptations to submaximal exercise:
   a. a lower O_2 deficit
   b. an increased utilization of FFA and a sparing of blood glucose and muscle glycogen
   c. a reduction in lactate and H^+ formation
   d. an increase in lactate removal
10. Define "central command" and "peripheral feedback" and explain how changes in muscle as a result of endurance training can be responsible for the lower heart rate, ventilation, and catecholamine responses to a submaximal exercise bout.
11. In short-term training programs, what neural factors may be responsible for the increase in strength?
12. Contrast hyperplasia with hypertrophy, and explain the role of each in the increase in muscle size that occurs with long-term strength training.
13. Does strength training interfere with the physiological effects of endurance training?

suggested readings

Costill, P. L. 1986. *Inside Running*. Indianapolis: Benchmark Press.

Hargreaves, M. ed. 1995. *Exercise Metabolism*. Champaign, IL: Human Kinetics.

Komi, P. V. ed. 1992. *Strength and Power in Sport*. Champaign, IL: Human Kinetics.

references

1. American College of Sports Medicine. 1990. Position stand: The recommended quantity and quality of exercise for developing and maintaining cardiorespiratory and muscular fitness in healthy adults. *Medicine and Science in Sports and Exercise* 22:265–74.

2. Asmussen, E. et al. 1965. On the nervous factors controlling respiration and circulation during exercise. Experiments with curarization. *Acta Physiologica Scandinavica* 63:343–50.

3. Åstrand, P. O., and K. Rodahl. 1986. *Textbook of Work Physiology*. 3d ed. New York: McGraw-Hill.

4. Atha, J. 1981. Strengthening muscle. In *Exercise and Sport Science Reviews*, vol. 9, ed. D. I. Miller, 1–73. Philadelphia: The Franklin Institute Press.

5. Blomqvist, C. G., and B. Saltin. 1983. Cardiovascular adaptations to physical training. *Annual Review of Physiology* 45:169–89.

5a. Booth, F. W. 1977. Effects of endurance exercise on cytochrome c turnover in skeletal muscle. *Annals of the New York Academy of Science* 301:431–39.

5b. Booth, F. W., S. H. Weeden, and B. S. Tseng. 1994. Effect of aging on human skeletal muscle and motor function. *Medicine and Science in Sports and Exercise* 26:556–60.

6. Bouchard, C., M. R. Boulay, J-A. Simoneau, G. Lortie, and L. Pérusse. 1988. Heredity and trainability of aerobic and anaerobic performances: An update. *Sports Medicine* 5:69–73.

7. Bouchard, C. et al. 1986. Aerobic performance in brothers, dizygotic and monozygotic twins. *Medicine and Science in Sports and Exercise* 18:639–46.

7a. Bouchard, C., F. T. Dionne, J-A. Simoneau, and M. R. Boulay. 1992. Genetics of aerobic and anaerobic performances. In *Exercise and Sport Science Reviews*, vol. 20, ed. J. O Holloszy, 27–58. Baltimore: Williams & Wilkins.

8. Bransford, D. R., and E. T. Howley. 1979. Effects of training on plasma FFA during exercise. *European Journal of Applied Physiology* 41:151–58.

9. Brooks, G. A. 1985. Anaerobic threshold: Review of the concept and directions for future research. *Medicine and Science in Sports and Exercise* 17:22–31.

9a. Cadefau, J., H. J. Green, M. Ball-Burnett, and G. Jamieson. 1994. Coupling of muscle phosphorylation potential to glycolysis during work after short-term training. *Journal of Applied Physiology* 76:2586–93.

9b. Cannon, J. G. 1993. Exercise and resistance to infection. *Journal of Applied Physiology* 74:973–81.

10. Claytor, R. P. 1985. Selected cardiovascular, sympathoadrenal, and metabolic responses to one-leg exercise training. Ph. D. diss., The University of Tennessee, Knoxville.

11. Coyle, E. F., M. K. Hemmert, and A. R. Coggan. 1986. Effects of detraining on cardiovascular responses to exercise: Role of blood volume. *Journal of Applied Physiology* 60:95–99.

12. Coyle, E. F., M. K. Hopper, and A. R. Coggan. 1990. Maximal oxygen uptake relative to plasma volume expansion. *International Journal of Sports Medicine* 11:116–19.

13. Coyle, E. F., W. H. Martin III, S. A. Bloomfield, O. H. Lowry, and J. O. Holloszy. 1985. Effects of detraining on responses to submaximal exercise. *Journal of Applied Physiology* 59:853–59.

14. Coyle, E. F., W. H. Martin III, D. R. Sinacore, M. J. Joyner, J. M. Hagberg, and J. O. Holloszy. 1984. Time course of loss of adaptations after stopping prolonged intense endurance training. *Journal of Applied Physiology: Respiratory, Environmental and Exercise Physiology* 57:1857–64.

15. Cronan, T. L., and E. T. Howley. 1974. The effect of training on epinephrine and norepinephrine excretion. *Medicine and Science in Sports* 6:122–25.

16. Dionne, F. T., L. Turcotte, M-C. Thibault, M. R. Boulay, J. S. Skinner, and C. Bouchard. 1989. Mitochondrial DNA sequence polymorphism, $\dot{V}O_2$ max, and response to endurance training. *Medicine and Science in Sports and Exercise* 23:177–85.

16a. Dudley, G. A., W. M. Abraham, and R. L. Terjung. 1982. Influence of exercise intensity and duration on biochemical adaptations in skeletal muscle. *Journal of Applied Physiology* 53:844–50.

17. Ehsani, A. A., J. M. Hagberg, and R. C. Hickson. 1978. Rapid changes in left ventricular dimensions and mass in response to physical conditioning. *American Journal of Cardiology* 42:52–56.

18. Ekblom, B. 1969. Effect of physical training on oxygen transport system in man. *Acta Physiologica Scandinavica* (Suppl.) 328:1–45.

19. Ekblom, B. et al. 1968. Effect of training on circulatory responses to exercise. *Journal of Applied Physiology* 24:518–28.

20. Fagard, R., E. Bielen, and A. Amery. 1991. Heritability of aerobic power and anaerobic energy generation during exercise. *Journal of Applied Physiology* 70:357–62.

21. Favier, R. J. et al. 1986. Endurance exercise training reduces lactate production. *Journal of Applied Physiology* 61:885–89.

21a. Fiatarone, M. A. et al. 1990. High-intensity strength training in nonagenarians: effects on skeletal muscle. *JAMA* 263:3029–34.

21b. Fiatarone, M. A. et al. 1994. Exercise training and nutritional supplementation for physical frailty in very elderly people. *New England Journal of Medicine* 330:1769–75.

22. Green, H. J., S. Jones, M. E. Ball-Burnett, D. Smith, J. Livesey, and B. W. Farrance. 1991. Early muscular and metabolic adaptations to prolonged exercise training in humans. *Journal of Applied Physiology* 70:2032–38.

23. Hagberg, J. M. et al. 1980. Faster adjustment to and recovery from submaximal exercise in the trained state. *Journal of Applied Physiology: Respiratory, Environmental and Exercise Physiology* 48:218–24.

24. Hickson, R. C. 1980. Interference of strength development by simultaneously training for strength and endurance. *European Journal of Applied Physiology* 45:255–63.

25. Hickson, R. C., H. A. Bomze, and J. O. Holloszy. 1978. Faster adjustment of O_2 uptake to the energy requirement of exercise in the trained state. *Journal of Applied Physiology: Respiratory, Environmental and Exercise Physiology* 44:877–81.

26. Hickson, R. C., B. A. Dvorak, E. M. Gorostiaga, T. T. Kurowski, and C. Foster. 1977. Linear increase in aerobic power induced by a strenuous program of endurance exercise. *Journal of Applied Physiology: Respiratory, Environmental and Exercise Physiology* 42:372–76.

27. ———. 1988. Potential for strength and endurance training to amplify endurance performance. *Journal of Applied Physiology* 65:2285–90.

28. Holloszy, J. O., and E. F. Coyle. 1984. Adaptations of skeletal muscle to endurance exercise and their metabolic consequences. *Journal of Applied Physiology: Respiratory, Environmental and Exercise Physiology* 56:831–38.

28a. Hopp, J. F. 1993. Effects of age and resistance training on skeletal muscle: A review. *Physical Therapy* 73:361–73.

28b. Houmard, J. A. et al. 1992. Effect of short-term training cessation on performance measures in distance runners. *International Journal of Sports Medicine* 13:572–76.

29. Howley, E. T., and B. D. Franks. 1986. *Health/Fitness Instructor's Handbook*. Champaign, IL: Human Kinetics.

30. Hutchinson, P. L., K. J. Cureton, H. Outz, and G. Wilson. 1991. Relationship of cardiac size to maximal oxygen uptake and body size in men and women. *International Journal of Sports Medicine* 12:369–73.

31. Kannus, P. et al. 1992. Effect of one-legged exercise on the strength, power and endurance of the contralateral leg: A randomized, controlled study using isometric and concentric isokinetic training. *European Journal of Applied Physiology* 64:117–26.

31a. Kiens, B. et al. 1993. Skeletal muscle substrate utilization during submaximal exercise in man: Effect of endurance training. *Journal of Physiology* (London) 469:459–78.

32. Klausen, K. et al. 1982. Central and regional circulatory adaptations to one-leg training. *Journal of Applied Physiology: Respiratory, Environmental and Exercise Physiology* 52:976–83.

33. Klissouras, V. 1971. Heritability of adaptive variation. *Journal of Applied Physiology* 31:338–44.

34. Kraemer, W. J., M. R. Deschenes, and S. J. Fleck. 1988. Physiological adaptations to resistance exercise: Implications for athletic conditioning. *Sports Medicine* 6:246–56.

35. Larsson, L., and P. A. Tesch. 1986. Motor unit fibre density in extremely hypertrophied skeletal muscles in man: Electrophysiological signs of muscle fibre hyperplasia. *European Journal of Applied Physiology* 55:130–36.

36. MacDougall, J. D. 1986. Morphological changes in human skeletal muscle following strength training and immobilization. In *Human Muscle Power*, eds. N. L. Jones, N. McCartney, and A. J. McComas, chap. 17, 269–85. Champaign, IL: Human Kinetics.

37. MacDougall, J. D., D. G. Sale, S. E. Alway, and J. R. Sutton. 1984. Muscle fiber number in biceps brachii bodybuilders and control subjects. *Journal of Applied Physiology: Respiratory, Environmental and Exercise Physiology* 57:1399–1403.

37a. Madsen, K. et al. 1993. Effects of detraining on endurance capacity and metabolic changes during prolonged exhaustive exercise. *Journal of Applied Physiology*. 75:1444–51.

37b. Martin, W. H. et al. 1993. Effect of endurance training on plasma free fatty acid turnover and oxidation during exercise. *American Journal of Physiology* 265: E708–14.

38. Mikesky, A. E., C. J. Giddings, W. Matthews, and W. J. Gonyea. 1991. Changes in muscle fiber size and composition in response to heavy-resistance exercise. *Medicine and Science in Sports and Exercise* 23:1042–49.

39. Mitchell, J. H. 1990. Neural control of the circulation during exercise. *Medicine and Science in Sports and Exercise* 22:141–54.

40. Mitchell, J. H., and R. F. Schmidt. 1983. Cardiovascular reflex control by afferent fibers from skeletal muscle receptors. In *Handbook of Physiology: The Cardiovascular System. Peripheral Circulation and Organ Blood Flow*, eds. J. T. Shepherd, F. M. Abbound, and S. R. Geiger, 623–58. Bethesda, MD: American Physiological Society.

41. Morganroth, J. et al. 1975. Comparative left ventricular dimensions in trained athletes. *Annals of Internal Medicine* 82:521–24.

41a. Nieman, D. C. 1994. Exercise, infection, and immunity. *International Journal of Sports Medicine* 15:S131–S141.

42. Paul, P. 1975. Effects of long-lasting physical exercise and training on lipid metabolism. In *Metabolic Adaptation to Prolonged Physical Exercise*, eds. H. Howald and J. R. Poortmans, 156–87. Switzerland: Birkhauser Verlag Basel.

43. Pierce, E. F., A. Weltman, R. L. Seip, and D. Snead. 1990. Effects of training specificity on the lactate threshold and $\dot{V}O_2$ peak. *International Journal of Sports Medicine* 11:267–72.

44. Powers, S. K., S. Dodd, and R. E. Beadle. 1985. Oxygen uptake kinetics in trained athletes differing in $\dot{V}O_2$ max. *European Journal of Applied Physiology* 54:306–8.

44a. Powers, S. K. et al. 1994. Influence of exercise and fiber type on antioxidant enzyme activity in rat skeletal muscle. *American Journal of Physiology* 266: R375–80.

44b. Powers, S. K. et al. 1995. Role of beta-adrenergic mechanisms in exercise training-induced metabolic changes in respiratory and locomotor muscle. *International Journal of Sports Medicine* 16:13–18.

45. Prud'Homme, D. et al. 1984. Sensitivity of maximal aerobic power to training is genotype-dependent. *Medicine and Science in Sports and Exercise* 16:489–93.

46. Ratzin, C. G., A. L. Dickinson, and S. P. Ringel. 1990. Skeletal muscle fiber area alterations in two opposing modes of resistance-exercise training in the same individual. *European Journal of Applied Physiology* 61:37–41.

47. Rerych, S. K. et al. 1980. Effects of exercise training on left ventricular function in normal subjects: A longitudinal study by radionuclide angiography. *American Journal of Cardiology* 45:244–52.

47a. Rogers, M. J., and W. J. Evans. 1993. Changes in skeletal muscle with aging: Effects of exercise training. In *Exercise and Sport Science Reviews*, vol. 21, ed. J. O. Holloszy, 65–102. Baltimore: Williams & Wilkins.

48. Rowell, L. B. 1986. *Human Circulation-Regulation during Physical Stress*. New York: Oxford University Press.

49. Rowell, L. B., and D. S. O'Leary. 1990. Reflex control of the circulation during exercise: Chemoreflexes and mechanoreflexes. *Journal of Applied Physiology* 69:407–18.

50. Sale, D. G. 1988. Neural adaptation to resistance training. *Medicine and Science in Sports and Exercise* 20:S135–S145.

51. Sale, D. G., I. Jacobs, J. D. MacDougall, and S. Garner. 1990. Comparison of two regimens of concurrent strength and endurance training. *Medicine and Science in Sports and Exercise* 22:348–56.

52. Sale, D. G., J. D. MacDougall, I. Jacobs, and S. Garner. 1990. Interaction between concurrent strength and endurance training. *Journal of Applied Physiology* 68:260–70.

53. Saltin, B. 1969. Physiological effects of physical conditioning. *Medicine and Science in Sports* 1:50–56.

54. Saltin, B., and P. O. Åstrand. 1967. Maximal oxygen uptake in athletes. *Journal of Applied Physiology* 23:353–58.

55. ———. 1993. Free fatty acids and exercise. *American Journal of Clinical Nutrition* 57 (Suppl): 752S–758S.

56. Saltin, B. et al. 1977. Fiber types and metabolic potentials of skeletal muscles in sedentary man and endurance runners. *Annals of the New York Academy of Science* 301:3–29.

56a. Saltin, B., and P. D. Gollnick. 1983. Skeletal muscle adaptability: Significance for metabolism and performance. In *Handbook of Physiology*, eds. L. D. Peachey, R. H. Adrian, and S. R. Geiger, Section 10: Skeletal Muscle, chap. 19. Baltimore: Williams & Wilkins.

56b. Shephard, R. J., and P. N. Shek. 1995. Exercise, aging, and immune function. *International Journal of Sports Medicine* 16:1–6.

56c. Spina, R. J., et al. 1993. Differences in cardiovascular adaptations to endurance exercise training between older men and women. *Journal of Applied Physiology* 75:849–55.

56d. Terjung, R. L. 1995. Muscle adaptations to aerobic training. *Sports Science Exchange*. vol. 8, no. 1. Barrington, IL: Gatorade Sports Science Institute.

57. Tesch, P. A. 1988. Skeletal muscle adaptations consequent to long-term heavy resistance exercise. *Medicine and Science in Sports and Exercise* 20:S132–S134.

58. Wibom, R. et al. 1992. Adaptations of mitochondrial ATP production in human skeletal muscle to endurance training and detraining. *Journal of Applied Physiology* 73:2004–10.

Physiology of Health and Fitness

14

Patterns in Health and Disease

Epidemiology and Physiology

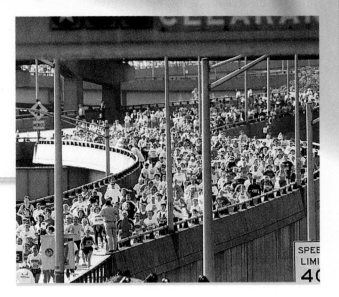

objectives

By studying this chapter, you should be able to do the following:

1. Define or describe the science of epidemiology.
2. Contrast infectious with degenerative diseases as causes of death.
3. Identify the three major categories of risk factors and examples of specific risk factors in each.
4. Compare the epidemiologic triad with the web of causation as models to study infectious and degenerative diseases, respectively.
5. Describe the difference between primary and secondary risk factors for coronary heart disease (CHD).
6. Describe the steps an epidemiologist must follow to show that a risk factor is causally connected to a disease.
7. Describe the hypothesis linking resistance to insulin as a cause of hypertension.

outline

Epidemiology   255
Coronary Heart Disease   258
  Physical Inactivity as a Risk
    Factor   259
Physiology   261
Synthesis   262

key terms

atherosclerosis
degenerative diseases
epidemiologic triad

epidemiology
infectious diseases
primary risk factor

secondary risk factor
web of causation

n many areas of inquiry scientists look for connections between facts (e.g., cigarette smoking and lung cancer), and try to determine whether the linkage is a causal one, or is due simply to chance. This chapter will describe the way two scientific disciplines, epidemiology and physiology, go about the business of moving from simple observations to the point of establishing that events are causally connected. Such a process allows us to understand the manner in which a disease develops and points the way toward intervention programs.

Epidemiology

In the mid 1850s in London there was a major outbreak of cholera, a disease characterized by vomiting and diarrhea that can lead to death (24). Although it was generally accepted in the medical community of that time that the disease was caused by "bad air" derived from decaying organic matter, Dr. John Snow thought otherwise. He systematically contacted the families of those who had died of cholera and found an association between the source of their drinking water and the death rate. People supplied by the Southwark water company experienced a cholera death rate of 5.0 per 1,000 population, compared to a rate of 0.9 per 1,000 for those supplied by other water companies (6, 24). About 100 years later, a study of British doctors showed a linear increase in lung cancer with the average number of cigarettes smoked per day. These studies are examples of the science of epidemiology in action. In the first case, Snow looked for connections between an environmental factor (water supply) and a communicable disease (cholera) by studying subgroups of the London population. The second study built on clinical observations linking a behavior (smoking) to a chronic disease (lung cancer) to see if the two might be causally connected.

Epidemiology is defined as the "study of the distribution and determinants of health-related states or events in specified populations, and the application of this study to control of health problems" (17). Epidemiology is used in a number of different ways:

- to establish cause—it is important to know whether the cause of a disease is due to genetic or environmental factors, or more likely, an interaction between the two (e.g., smoking and lung cancer). This can lead to strategies to prevent the disease (e.g., don't smoke).
- to trace the natural history of a disease—epidemiologists try to understand the normal course of a disease from a healthy state to a presymptomatic stage that leads to clinical signs and symptoms and finally, to death or recovery. The progress of the disease can be detected and treated at any stage, but the effectiveness of the treatment can only be determined if the natural history of the disease, in the absence of treatment, is known.
- to describe the health status of populations—by knowing the total burden of disease in a population, health authorities can establish priorities in the use of health-care dollars to have the greatest benefit.
- to evaluate an intervention—studies are done to determine the success or failure of programs established to prevent or treat a disease (6).

One of the major goals of epidemiology is to prevent and control diseases by understanding what causes them, but it is easier said than done, even for infectious diseases (6). Figure 14.1 describes an epidemiological model called the **epidemiologic triad** that shows connections between the environment, agent, and host that cause disease (11). If we use the cholera example mentioned earlier, the bacteria *vibrio*

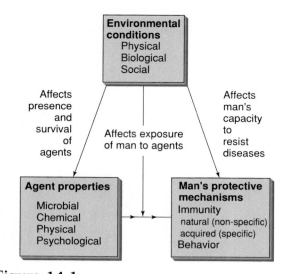

Figure 14.1

Epidemiologic triad: an epidemiologic model showing the interaction of the environment, host, and agent as a cause of disease.

cholerae is the agent that was transmitted via a poorly treated water supply (environment) to the population (host). The model also indicates that social factors such as poor housing and malnutrition can decrease natural protective mechanisms and make the host more susceptible to disease. In the cholera example the disease was controlled by making the drinking water safe. An important point to recognize is that disease control was achieved decades before the bacteria that causes cholera was discovered (6).

in summary

- Epidemiology is the study of the distribution and determinants of health states and the use of this information in the control of disease.
- Disease control can be achieved by: (1) destroying or removing the agent at its source, (2) altering the environment to reduce transmission of the agent, or improving the host's resistance to the agent, and (3) altering the host's behaviors such as improved nutrition, immunization, and exercise (11).

Over the last 100 years attention has shifted from **infectious diseases** (e.g., tuberculosis and pneumonia) as the major causes of death to **degenerative diseases** such as cancer and cardiovascular diseases. Table 14.1 shows the latter diseases to account for the vast majority of all deaths in the United States, with cardiovascular diseases being the leading causes of death. The problem of establishing the cause of a disease is much more difficult when dealing with chronic, degenerative diseases such as cardiovascular disease

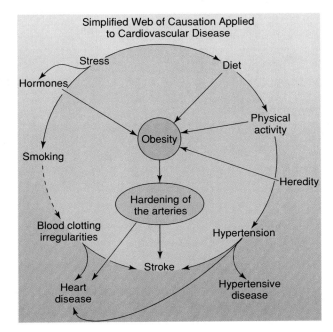

Figure 14.2

Web of causation: an epidemiologic model showing the complex interaction of risk factors associated with the development of chronic degenerative diseases such as cardiovascular diseases.

Table 14.1	Leading Causes of Death in the United States: 1991 Final Mortality
Causes	**Total Number of Deaths**
1. Diseases of heart and blood vessels	926,061
2. Cancer	514,657
3. Chronic obstructive pulmonary diseases	90,650
4. Accidents	83,347
5. Pneumonia and influenza	77,860

Based on material from 1995 *Heart and Stroke Facts*. Copyright © 1994 American Heart Association, Dallas, TX.

because genetic, environmental, and behavioral factors are involved in a very complex manner. The difficulty of establishing "cause" in these complex diseases is best described by another epidemiologic model called the **web of causation** (18, 24). Figure 14.2 shows how a combination of genetic, environmental, and behavioral factors can interact to cause cardiovascular diseases (24, 25). Trying to tease out the effect that one factor has on another, and on the final disease process is a difficult task that makes work in epidemiology interesting and challenging. The factors in the web of causation are positively associated with the development of cardiovascular diseases, but are not sufficient in and of themselves to cause them. These factors are called "risk factors" and they play a major role in prevention programs aimed at reducing disease and premature death associated with degenerative diseases. This has led to public health programs to educate the population about risk factors and the need for each of us to take personal responsibility for our health (6, 14).

in summary

- Epidemiologists show that the major causes of death in the United States are degenerative diseases such as heart disease and cancer. The development and progress of these diseases are affected by the interaction of environmental and behavioral risk factors.

In 1979 the surgeon general of the United States published a report, *Healthy People* (26), indicating that even though degenerative diseases have more complex causes than infectious diseases, the onset of these diseases can be delayed or prevented

MAJOR RISK FACTOR CATEGORIES

Inherited/Biological	Environmental	Behavioral
Age	Physical: air, water, noise, unsafe highways	Smoking
Gender	Socioeconomic: income, housing, employment, status, education	Poor nutrition
Race	Family: divorce, death of loved one, children leaving	Drinking alcohol
Susceptibility to disease		Inactivity
		Overuse of medication
		Fast driving/no seat belt
		Pressure to succeed

Figure 14.3

Major categories of risk factors with examples of each.

Source: U.S. Department of Health, Education, and Welfare, 1979, *Healthy People: The Surgeon General's Report on Health Promotion and Disease Prevention.*

(26). Figure 14.3 shows the three major risk factor categories associated with health and disease, with specific risk factors identified under each. While some diseases (hemophilia and sickle-cell anemia) are primarily inherited, the vast majority of diseases result from an interaction of genetics and the individual's environment (26). The *inherited/biological factors* include age, gender, race, and the ease with which one might develop a disease. Nothing can be done about these risk factors; they are fixed and some people simply have a higher risk of certain degenerative diseases than others. However, what has become clear over the past forty years is the fact that *environmental and behavior risk factors* are most influential in the early onset of degenerative diseases or death. Fortunately, these risk factors are most susceptible to change, and this brings us back to the issue of personal responsibility as a major force determining one's well-being. Personal responsibility means more than getting sufficient exercise, or eating the proper foods. There is a need for people to speak out for clean air and water, to support community-wide blood pressure and serum cholesterol screenings, and to not drink and drive. To expand on this risk factor concept we will focus on coronary heart disease.

Coronary Heart Disease

Coronary heart disease (CHD) is associated with a gradual narrowing of the arteries serving the heart due to a thickening of the inner lining of the artery. This process, **atherosclerosis,** is the leading contributor to heart attack and stroke deaths (3, 10a). It is now widely accepted that some people are at a greater risk of developing CHD than others. Our understanding of the risks associated with atherosclerotic disease is based primarily on the epidemiological investigation conducted in Framingham, Massachusetts (10a). When this study began in 1949,

cardiovascular disease already accounted for 50 percent of all deaths in the United States. The Framingham study is an observational prospective (longitudinal) study designed to determine how those who develop cardiovascular disease differ from those who do not. Approximately 5,000 men and women were examined every other year and measures such as blood pressure, electrocardiographic abnormalities, serum cholesterol, smoking, and body weight were obtained. The investigators were then able to relate the different measures to the progression of the coronary heart disease (10a). Early in the study, investigators found that about 20 percent of the population experienced a heart attack before sixty years of age, and of them, 20 percent resulted in sudden death. The natural history of this disease indicated that prevention was an important goal, and the Framingham Study is recognized for identifying the risk factors to predict subsequent disease and allow early intervention (14).

The Framingham Study found that the risk of CHD increases with the number of cigarettes smoked, the degree to which the blood pressure is elevated, and the quantity of cholesterol in the blood (14). In addition, the overall risk of CHD increases with the number of risk factors; that is, a person who has a systolic blood pressure of 160 mm Hg, a serum cholesterol of 250 mg/dl, and smokes more than a pack of cigarettes a day has about six times the risk of CHD as a person who has only one of these risk factors (10). It is important to remember that risk factors interact with each other to increase the overall risk of CHD. This has implications for prevention as well as treatment. In this regard, getting a hypertensive patient to quit smoking confers more immediate benefit than any antihypertensive drug (14). Further, regular physical activity reduces the risk of CHD, even in those who smoke and are hypertensive (see chapter 16).

Dr. Henry J. Montoye, Professor Emeritus at The University of Wisconsin (Madison) and former president of the American College of Sports Medicine, spent most of his professional life studying the relationship of physical activity to health. He was a principal investigator in the Tecumseh (Michigan) Community Health Study, a large epidemiological investigation (19). In this community of about 10,000

people he was able to document occupational and leisure-time activity, and how they varied with job classification (professional, semi-skilled, etc.) and age. He was also able to establish population-based norms for a step test, and show how electrocardiographic and metabolic responses to a graded treadmill test varied with age. This information, coupled with measurements of serum cholesterol,

blood pressure, and body composition allowed him to address the links between fitness, fatness, and physical activity—a theme that permeated his professional career. His extensive contributions to the research literature was recognized when he received the Scholar Award the first time it was offered by the American Alliance of Health, Physical Education, Recreation, and Dance.

in summary

- Risk factors can be divided into three categories: genetic/biological, environmental, and behavioral.
- The risk factors of smoking, high cholesterol, and hypertension interact to magnify the risk of CHD. Similarly, elimination of one of them causes a disproportionate reduction in the risk of CHD.

After looking at the web of causation for cardiovascular disease in figure 14.2 one can understand how difficult it is to determine whether an observed association between a risk factor and a disease is a causal one, or is due simply to chance. To facilitate the process of determining cause, epidemiologists apply the following guidelines (6):

- Temporal association—Does the cause precede the effect?
- Plausibility—Is the association consistent with other knowledge?
- Consistency—Have similar results been shown in other studies?
- Strength—What is the strength of the association (relative risk) between the cause and the effect? Relative risk is sometimes expressed as the ratio of the risk of disease among those exposed to the factor to the risk of those unexposed. The greater the ratio, the stronger the association.
- Dose-response relationship—Is increased exposure to the possible cause associated with increased effect?
- Reversibility—Does removal of the possible cause lead to a reduction of the disease risk?

- Study design—Is the evidence based on strong study design?
- Judging the evidence—How many lines of evidence lead to the conclusion?

Physical Inactivity as a Risk Factor

The concern about whether a risk factor is causally related to cardiovascular disease has special significance for physical activity. For many years physical inactivity was believed to be only weakly associated with heart disease and was not given much attention as a public health concern. However, in the late 1980s and early 1990s that changed rather dramatically. In 1987, Powell et al. (20a) did a systematic review of the literature dealing with the role of physical activity in the primary prevention of coronary heart disease, and applied the above guidelines relative to causation. They found that the majority of studies indicated that the level of physical activity predated the onset of CHD, thus meeting the temporal requirement. They also found a dose-response relationship in that as physical activity increased, the risk of CHD decreased, and the association was stronger in the better studies. The latter results met the consistency and study design criteria for causality. The review found the association to be plausible given the role of physical activity in improving glucose tolerance, increasing fibrinolysis (breaking of clots), and reducing blood pressure. The investigators calculated the relative risk of CHD due to inactivity to be about 1.9, meaning that sedentary individuals had about twice the chance of experiencing CHD compared to physically active individuals. The relative risk was similar to smoking (2.5), high serum cholesterol (2.4), and high blood pressure (2.1). When the authors controlled for smoking, blood pressure, cholesterol, age, and sex (all of which are associated with CHD), the association of physical activity

The risk factors associated with CHD have typically been divided into **primary** or major and **secondary** or contributing, where primary means that a factor in and of itself increases the risk of CHD, and secondary means that a certain factor increases the risk of CHD only if one of the primary factors is already present, or that its significance has not been precisely determined (10). Lists of risk factors have evolved over time as more epidemiological evidence has accumulated showing the association between various behaviors or characteristics and CHD. The following list of risk factors represents the current thinking of the American Heart Association (3). As was mentioned earlier, although some risk factors (e.g., age, gender, and genetics) cannot be changed, the majority of the risk factors can be altered to reduce the risk of CHD.

It should be noted that the American College of Sports Medicine (ACSM) (1) lists diabetes and one of the subfractions of cholesterol (high-density lipoprotein cholesterol [HDL-C]) as additional risk factors. There is

Primary		Secondary
Can't be Changed	*Can be Changed*	
Heredity	Cigarette smoking	Diabetes
Male sex	High serum cholesterol	Obesity
Increasing age	High blood pressure	Stress
	Physical inactivity	

good evidence that the risk of CHD is lower for those with higher concentrations of HDL-C, and the ratio of total cholesterol to HDL-C is viewed as a better index of risk than total cholesterol alone (14). In fact, the ACSM considers HDL-C to be a "negative risk factor" when levels exceed 60 mg/dl. Further, the American Heart Association lists obesity as a secondary or contributing risk factor, despite the body of evidence that points to it as a primary risk factor (15, 21). Lastly, you may have noticed that a high-fat diet is not even cited on the list of risk factors for CHD. The reason for this is that the detrimental effect of a high-fat diet is already represented in the obesity and serum cholesterol risk factors. However, it is generally believed

that a reduction in dietary fat would reduce the risk of CHD in the American population (see chapter 18).

As we have come to understand that physical inactivity, diet, and stress are risk factors for obesity, glucose intolerance (diabetes), hypertension, and high serum cholesterol, we have developed a new and potent view of how to intervene. Health promotion programs deal directly with physical inactivity, diet, and stress to prevent the primary risk factors and obesity from occurring. In addition, the major nonpharmacological treatment of these primary risk factors revolves around recommendations for a low-fat diet (see chapter 18), regular physical activity (see chapter 16), and stress reduction (5, 7, 8).

and CHD remained, indicating that physical activity was an independent risk factor for CHD (2).

In order to estimate the real impact a risk factor may have on a population, epidemiologists try to balance the relative risk with the number of people in the population that have the risk factor. This balancing act is summed up in the calculation of the *population attributable risk* for each risk factor (9). Figure 14.4 describes the relative risk for selected risk factors and the percent of the population affected. Given the large number of people who are inactive, changes in physical activity habits have a great potential to reduce CHD (see chapter 16).

Figure 14.4

Percentages of U.S. population at risk for recognized risk factors related to coronary heart disease and risk ratio for each risk factor.

Risk factor:	High blood pressure	Serum cholesterol	Cigarette smoking	Physical inactivity
Risk ratio:	2.1	2.4	2.5	1.9
Risk levels:	≥150 mm HG vs <130 mm HG	≥268 mg/dl vs <218 mg/dl	1 pk/day vs No smoking	No activity vs 3 times/wk, 20 minutes

Physiology

Epidemiologists are not the only scientists interested in looking at potential relationships between variables in an attempt to have a greater understanding of what causes cardiovascular disease. Physiologists study how tissues and organs function to maintain homeostasis and try to uncover the source of a problem when homeostasis is not maintained. A good example of a failure to maintain homeostasis is hypertension, a problem that affects more than 50 million Americans (3). Interestingly, investigators have found that hypertension does not generally occur in isolation. It is not uncommon for hypertensive individuals to also have multiple metabolic abnormalities such as:

- obesity—especially abdominal obesity
- insulin resistance—tissues do not take up glucose easily when stimulated with insulin, and muscle is the primary site of the insulin resistance
- dyslipidemia—abnormal levels of triglycerides

The fact that these abnormalities often occur as a group suggests a common underlying cause that might give us a better understanding of the disease processes associated with hypertension. The coexistence of insulin resistance, dyslipidemia, and hypertension has been called Syndrome X (22) and the Metabolic Cardiovascular Syndrome (20); those who add obesity to the model call it the Deadly Quartet (16).

Figure 14.5 shows hypothesized connections between and among these abnormalities. The central focus of the model is on insulin resistance, with skeletal muscle being the predominant tissue involved. Insulin resistance is commonly associated with obesity, especially upper body (abdominal) obesity (16, 20). However, as the arrows in figure 14.5 indicate, insulin resistance can be caused by a combination of genetic and environmental influences independent of obesity (12, 22). Insulin resistance is characterized by a reduced ability to take up glucose at a given insulin concentration. In response to this resistance the pancreas secretes more insulin to promote blood glucose uptake into tissues in order to return the blood glucose concentration to normal. If the pancreas cannot secrete

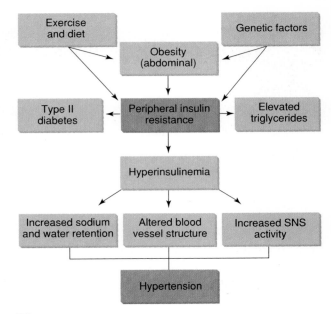

Figure 14.5

The insulin-resistance and hypertension hypothesis: Syndrome X.

sufficient insulin, the blood glucose will remain elevated and a condition known as Type II diabetes results. A drug may be required to stimulate the pancreas to secrete additional insulin to correct the problem (see chapter 17).

When the pancreas secretes additional insulin to deal with the insulin resistance the plasma insulin level becomes elevated (hyperinsulinemia); this can elevate blood pressure and lead to hypertension. Figure 14.5 shows that elevated insulin levels can:

- increase sympathetic nervous system (SNS) activity leading to elevation of epinephrine and norepinephrine levels which can increase heart rate, stroke volume, and increase blood pressure. The elevated E and NE levels can also interfere with insulin release from the pancreas and interfere with glucose uptake at the tissue, which aggravates the problem (see chapter 5),
- increase sodium and water retention which increases plasma volume and blood pressure, and
- increase the proliferation of smooth muscle cells in small blood vessels which can increase resistance to blood flow and drive up blood pressure.

Figure 14.5 also shows the connection between insulin resistance and altered blood lipids. Individuals with insulin resistance and/or abdominal obesity tend to have a higher free fatty acid (FFA) level which can lead to an increase in plasma triglycerides. The higher FFA level could be due to the inability of

Although you are familiar with the connection of muscle fiber type to performance (see chapters 8 and 19), a recent review by Dr. David Bassett, Jr. summarized potential links between fiber type and cardiovascular disease risk factors (4):

- Mean arterial blood pressure is higher in subjects with a high percentage of Type II fibers, and hypertension is associated with a lower capillary density in skeletal muscle.
- Insulin resistance is related to the capillary density of

skeletal muscle; those with fewer capillaries (high percentage of Type II fibers) experience greater insulin resistance.
- Obesity, especially, upper body obesity, is related to a high percentage of Type II fibers.

These facts suggest a strong connection between fiber type and risk factors, and when coupled with the observation that exercise training has little effect on the Type I/Type II muscle fiber distribution, one may wonder about the role exercise plays

in preventing or treating these risk factors. All is not lost. As pointed out by Bassett, endurance training causes increases in both capillary density and the ability of muscle to use fat as a fuel, and Type II muscle fibers take on characteristics similar to those found in Type I muscle fibers. Lastly, exercise increases the sensitivity of the muscle to insulin such that less insulin is needed to control the blood glucose level. The importance of exercise in the prevention of (and as a non-pharmacological treatment for) obesity, hypertension, and insulin resistance is enhanced by such findings.

insulin to suppress FFA (22), or the abdominal obesity, which is associated with an increased ability to mobilize FFA (16).

In this model the scientists hypothesized that the cause of hypertension is the insulin resistance, with skeletal muscle being the primary tissue involved. An alternative hypothesis has been offered to what may now be viewed as the chicken and egg question, that is, "Which comes first?" It has been proposed that it is the hypertension that causes the insulin resistance and not the reverse. In contrast to the Syndrome X model, others suggest that hypertension causes a decrease in the small blood vessels in muscle leading to a reduction in the delivery of glucose and insulin, both of which are needed to have normal glucose uptake (13). In addition, they propose that muscle fiber type is linked to hypertension (see A Closer Look 14.3).

Independent of whether the insulin resistance precedes or follows the hypertension, there is considerable evidence that exercise can benefit individuals with insulin resistance. This may be due to increases in the capillary density or oxidative capacity of muscle that occurs with exercise training (chapter 13), or an increase in glucose transporters in muscle (chapter 5). As the model indicates, two of the most important factors related to insulin resistance are physical activity (exercise) and obesity. These latter issues will be discussed in detail in chapters 16 and 18, respectively.

in summary

- The Deadly Quartet model describes potential causative connections between and among obesity, peripheral insulin resistance, hypertension, and dyslipidemia.
- The insulin resistance is located primarily in skeletal muscle, being greater in Type II muscles with their limited capillary supply.
- Exercise can both directly and indirectly decrease the risk of CHD by influencing obesity, insulin resistance, and hypertension.

Synthesis

A common theme coming from both the web of causation for cardiovascular disease and the Deadly Quartet is the importance of dealing with obesity through appropriate physical activity and nutrition. Following the publication of *Healthy People* in 1979 (26), the U.S. Department of Health and Human Services published *Promoting Health/Preventing Disease: Objectives for the Nation* (27), and most recently, *Healthy People* 2000 (28). The health objectives listed in these reports were based on the analysis of health problems in the United States and a recognition of what can be done to reduce their

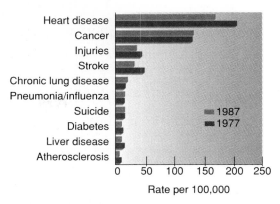

Figure 14.6

Changes in the leading causes of death—1977 compared to 1987.

Source: *Healthy People 2000: National Health Promotion and Disease Prevention Objectives*. U.S. Department of Health and Human Services, 1991.

magnitude. Figure 14.6 shows that progress was made during the 1980s in reducing the death rates from three of the leading causes of death among Americans: heart disease, stroke, and unintentional injury. The decrease in the death rate from heart disease (40%) and stroke (50%) since 1970 was related to the decline in cigarette smoking, increased blood pressure monitoring and control, and increased awareness of blood cholesterol levels and dietary fat intake (28). The *Healthy People* 2000 objectives were established to continue the improvement in

health-related behaviors to further reduce the death rate and improve our quality of life. While it is beyond the scope of this chapter to go into the specific objectives, we feel that some detail concerning the nutrition and exercise objectives is appropriate.

The focus of the objectives associated with physical activity and fitness is on the reduction in heart disease deaths and the number of overweight children and adults. Recommendations for physical activity include daily school-related physical activity for children, and company and community-based programs for all. Another objective is directed at increasing the number of physicians providing information about the proper quantity of exercise needed for health benefits. The proper intensity, duration, and frequency of exercise to bring about desired health benefits will be discussed in detail in chapter 16. There is an appropriate overlap in the nutrition objectives with those mentioned for heart disease and obesity. However, additional attention is directed at cancer and iron deficiency anemia. The nutrition objectives indicate a need to decrease fat and salt intake, and to increase complex carbohydrate intake. The dietary guidelines associated with these objectives will be discussed in chapter 18. The need to educate the public about proper food selection and the role of diet and exercise in weight control was clearly spelled out. The objectives also specified a need for better labeling of foods and for an increase in the number of schools and workplaces following the *Dietary Guidelines for Americans*.

study questions

1. There is a sudden increase in the number of birth defects in one section of a large city. Describe what an epidemiologist might do to determine what is causing this problem.

2. Why is a web of causation model needed to study the causes of degenerative diseases, in contrast to infectious diseases.

3. Physical inactivity was long considered only a secondary risk factor. What "proof" did investigators have to offer to convince the scientific community otherwise?

4. What is the difference between primary and secondary risks for coronary heart disease (CHD)? Why does a high-fat diet not appear as a risk factor for CHD?

5. Draw a diagram of the hypothesized connections between and among obesity, insulin resistance, hypertension, and dyslipidemia. Indicate the primary site of insulin resistance, and explain how exercise training might reduce this problem.

suggested readings

Bouchard, C., R. J. Shephard, T. Stevens, eds. 1994. *Physical Activity, Fitness, and Health*. Champaign, IL: Human Kinetics.

Dawber, Thomas R. 1980. *The Framingham Study*. Cambridge, MA: Harvard University Press.

references

1. American College of Sports Medicine. 1995. ACSM's *Guidelines for Exercise Testing and Prescription*. 5th ed. Baltimore: William & Wilkins.

2. American Heart Association. 1992. Statement on exercise. *Circulation* 86:340–44.

3. ———. 1994. *1995 Heart and Stroke Facts: Statistical Supplement*. Dallas, TX.

4. Bassett, D. R., Jr. 1994. Skeletal muscle characteristics: Relationships to cardiovascular risk factors. *Medicine and Science in Sports and Exercise* 26:957–66.

5. Bassett, D. R., Sr., and A. J. Zweifler. 1990. Risk factors and risk factor management. In *Clinical Ischemic Syndromes*, eds. G. B. Zelenock, L. D. D'Alecy, J. C. Fantone III, M. Shalfer, and J. C. Stanley, 15–46. St. Louis: C. V. Mosby.

6. Beaglehole, R., R. Bonita, and T. Kjellström. 1993. *Basic Epidemiology*. Geneva: World Health Organization.

7. Bouchard, C., R. J. Shephard, T. Stevens, J. R. Sutton, and B. D. McPherson. 1990. Exercise, fitness, and health: The consensus statement. In *Exercise, Fitness, and Health*, eds. C. Bouchard, R. J. Shephard, T. Stevens, J. R. Sutton, and B. D. McPherson, 3–28. Champaign, IL: Human Kinetics.

8. Brown, D. R. 1990. Exercise, fitness and mental health. In *Exercise, Fitness, and Health*, eds. C. Bouchard, R. J. Shephard, T. Stevens, J. R. Sutton, and B. D. McPherson. 607–26. Champaign, IL: Human Kinetics.

9. Caspersen, C. J. 1989. Physical activity epidemiology: Concepts, methods, and applications to exercise science. In *Exercise and Sport Science Reviews*, vol. 17, ed. K. B. Pandolf, 423–73. Baltimore: Williams & Wilkins.

10. Caspersen, C. J., and G. W. Heath. 1988. The risk factor concept of coronary heart disease. In *Resource Manual for Guidelines for Graded Exercise Testing and Prescription*, eds. S. N. Blair, P. Painter, R. R. Pate, L. K. Smith, and C. B. Taylor, 111–25. Philadelphia: Lea & Febiger.

10a. Dawber, T. R. 1980. *The Framingham Study*. Cambridge, MA: Harvard University Press.

11. Farmer, R., and D. Miller. 1991. *Lecture Notes on Epidemiology and Public Health Medicine*. Boston: Blackwell Scientific Publications, 107–11.

12. Ferrannini, E., S. M. Haffner, and M. P. Stern. 1990. Essential hypertension: An insulin-resistant state. *Journal Cardiovascular Pharmacology* 45 (Suppl. 5):S18–S25.

13. Julius, S., T. Gudbrandsson, K. Jamerson, and O. Andersson. 1992. The interconnection between sympathetics, microcirculation, and insulin resistance in hypertension. *Blood Pressure* 1:9–19.

14. Kannel, W. B. 1990. Contributions of the Framingham study to preventive cardiology. *Journal of the American College of Cardiology* 15:206–11.

15. Kannel, W. B., and T. Gordon. 1979. Physiological and medical concomitants of obesity: The Framingham study. In *Obesity in America*, 125–43. U.S. Department of Health, Education, and Welfare. NIH Publication No. 79–359.

16. Kaplan, N. M. 1989. The deadly quartet. *Archives Internal Medicine* 149:1514–20.

17. Last, J. M. 1988. *A dictionary of epidemiology*, 2nd edition. New York: Oxford University Press.

18. MacMahon, B., and T. F. Pugh. 1970. *Epidemiology*. Boston: Little, Brown and Company.

19. Montoye, H. J. 1975. *Physical activity and health: An epidemiologic study of an entire community*. Englewood Cliffs, NJ: Prentice-Hall, Inc.

20. Pollare, T. 1989. *Hypertension as One Part of a Metabolic Cardiovascular Syndrome*. Princeton, NJ: Squibb Corporation.

20a. Powell, K E. et al. 1987. Physical activity and the incidence of coronary heart disease. *Annual Review of Public Health* 8:253–87.

21. Rabkin, S. W., F. A. L. Mathewson, and Ping-hwa Hsu. 1977. Relation of body weight to development of ischemic heart disease in a cohort of young North American men after a 26-year observation period: The Manitoba study. *The American Journal of Cardiology* 39:452–58.

22. Reaven, G. M. 1988. Role of insulin resistance in human disease. *Diabetes* 37:1595–1607.

23. Rocchini, A. P. 1991. Insulin resistance and blood pressure regulation in obese and nonobese subjects. *Hypertension* 17:837–42.

24. Rockett, I. H. R. 1994. Population and health: An introduction to epidemiology. *Population Bulletin* 49(no. 3), 1–48.

25. Stallones, R. A. 1966. *Public Health Monograph 76* Washington, D.C.:U.S. Government Printing Office, p. 52.

26. U.S. Department of Health, Education and Welfare. 1979. *Healthy People: The Surgeon General's Report on Health Promotion and Disease Prevention*. Washington, D.C.: U.S. Government Printing Office. Stock No. 017-001-00416-2.

27. U.S. Department of Health and Human Services. Fall 1980. *Promoting Health/Preventing Disease: Objectives for the Nation*. Washington, D.C.: U.S. Government Printing Office.

28. ———. 1991. *Healthy People 2000: National Health Promotion and Disease Prevention Objectives*. Washington, D.C.: U.S. Government Printing Office.

Work Tests to Evaluate Cardiorespiratory Fitness

objectives

By studying this chapter, you should be able to do the following:

1. Identify the sequence of steps in the procedures for evaluating cardiorespiratory fitness (CRF).
2. Describe one maximal and one submaximal field test used to evaluate CRF.
3. Explain the rationale underlying the use of distance runs as estimates of CRF.
4. Identify the common measures taken during a graded exercise test (GXT).
5. Describe changes in the ECG that may take place during a GXT in subjects with ischemic heart disease.
6. List three criteria for having achieved $\dot{V}O_2$ max.
7. Estimate $\dot{V}O_2$ max from the last stage of a GXT and list the concerns about the protocol that may affect that estimate.
8. Estimate $\dot{V}O_2$ max by extrapolating the HR/$\dot{V}O_2$ relationship to the person's age-adjusted maximal HR.
9. Describe the problems with the assumptions made in the extrapolation procedure used in objective 8, and name the environmental and subject variables that must be controlled to improve such estimates.

10. Identify the criteria used to terminate the GXT.
11. Explain why there are so many different GXT protocols and why the rate of progression through the test is of concern.
12. Describe the YMCA's procedure to set the rate of progression on a cycle ergometer test.
13. Estimate $\dot{V}O_2$ max with the Åstrand and Ryhming nomogram given a data set for the cycle ergometer or step.

outline

Testing Procedures   266
  Screening   266
  Resting and Exercise
    Measures   268
Field Tests for Estimating
    CRF   268
  Maximal Run Tests   268
  Walk Tests   270
  Canadian Home Fitness
    Test   270

Graded Exercise Tests:
    Measurements   271
  Heart Rate   271
  Blood Pressure   272
  ECG   272
  Rating of Perceived
    Exertion   272
  Termination Criteria   273

$\dot{V}O_2$ Max   273
  Estimation of $\dot{V}O_2$ Max from Last
    Work Rate   274
  Estimation of $\dot{V}O_2$ Max from
    Submaximal HR
    Response   274
Graded Exercise Test:
    Protocols   275
  Treadmill   277
  Cycle Ergometer   278
  Step Test   281

angina pectoris
arrhythmia
conduction disturbances

double product
dyspnea
field test

myocardial ischemia
ST segment depression

n chapter 14 we discussed the risk factors that limit health and contribute to coronary heart disease (CHD). One of those risk factors was a sedentary life-style. According to *Healthy People 2000: National Health Promotion and Disease Prevention Objectives* there is a need to increase physical activity to improve cardiorespiratory function (CRF). This implies that changes in CRF can be measured. While most scientists believe that the function of the cardiorespiratory system is represented best by the measurement of $\dot{V}O_2$ max, others feel that the monitoring of heart rate (HR) and blood pressure (BP) at several submaximal work rates provides a more sensitive indicator of changes in CRF (38). You are already familiar with the use of a graded exercise test (GXT) to measure $\dot{V}O_2$ max; this chapter picks up on that theme and discusses the types of tests used to evaluate CRF. The type of test used depends on the fitness of the person being tested, the purpose of the test (experimental or epidemiological investigation), and the facilities, equipment, and personnel available to conduct the test. The choice of the GXT would be different for a young healthy child as compared to a sixty-year-old person with coronary heart disease (CHD) risk factors. The GXT might be used as a CRF test prior to entry into a fitness program, or it could be used as a diagnostic test by a cardiologist who evaluates a twelve-lead electrocardiogram for evidence of heart disease. Clearly, the type of personnel and equipment, and of course the cost, would be very different in these two situations. Given such diversity, how should the testing process begin?

Testing Procedures

Figure 15.1 shows a sequence of steps in a "decision tree," leading to participation in a fitness program. The first step in the evaluation of CRF is to identify those who might need a physician's clearance prior to taking an exercise test or participating in an exercise program. These procedures include obtaining written informed consent from the potential participant, a review of the person's health history, the administration of selected resting physiological measures, and the use of submaximal or maximal GXTs (38). The exercise test can be stopped by the subject at any time, and the tester

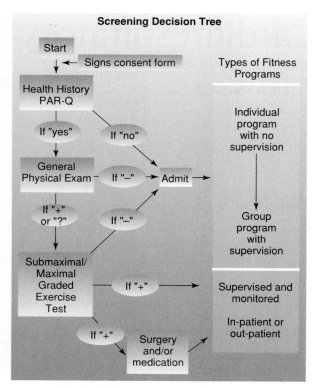

Figure 15.1

Decision tree in the evaluation of cardiorespiratory fitness.

has the right to terminate any of the procedures if the subject displays abnormal responses or experiences symptoms suggestive of an inappropriate adaptation to the GXT (3). Depending on the outcome at each of these steps, the person might be admitted to a fitness program with little or no supervision, or referred for additional tests that might lead to an exercise program in which the participants are monitored and supervised.

Screening

In chapter 14 we indicated the role that risk factors play in an overall profile of health status with regard to CHD. The health histories used to screen people for GXTs or fitness programs can be as simple as the Physical Activity Readiness Questionnaire (PAR-Q) shown in figure 15.2, or a detailed form such as the PAR$_X$

PHYSICAL ACTIVITY READINESS QUESTIONNAIRE (PAR-Q)*
A Self-administered Questionnaire for Adults

PAR-Q & YOU

PAR-Q is designed to help you help yourself. Many health benefits are associated with regular exercise, and the completion of PAR-Q is a sensible first step to take if you are planning to increase the amount of physical activity in your life.

For most people physical activity should not pose any problem or hazard. PAR-Q has been designed to identify the small number of adults for whom physical activity might be inappropriate or those who should have medical advice concerning the type of activity most suitable for them.

Common sense is your best guide in answering these few questions. Please read them carefully and check the ☞ YES or NO opposite the question if it applies to you.

YES NO

☐ ☐ 1. Has your doctor ever said you have heart trouble?

☐ ☐ 2. Do you frequently have pains in your heart and chest?

☐ ☐ 3. Do you often feel faint or have spells of severe dizziness?

☐ ☐ 4. Has a doctor ever said your blood pressure was too high?

☐ ☐ 5. Has your doctor ever told you that you have a bone or joint problem such as arthritis that has been aggravated by exercise, or might be made worse with exercise?

☐ ☐ 6. Is there a good physical reason not mentioned here why you should not follow an activity program even if you wanted to?

☐ ☐ 7. Are you over age 65 and not accustomed to vigorous exercise?

If You Answered

YES to one or more questions

If you have not recently done so, consult with your personal physician by telephone or in person BEFORE increasing your physical activity and/or taking a fitness test. Tell him what questions you answered YES on PAR-Q, or show him your copy.

Programs

After medical evaluation, seek advice from your physician as to your suitability for:
- unrestricted physical activity, probably on a gradually increasing basis.
- restricted or supervised activity to meet your specific needs, at least on an initial basis. Check in your community for special programs or services.

NO to all questions

If you answered PAR-Q accurately, you have reasonable assurance of your present suitability for:
- A GRADUATED EXERCISE PROGRAM—A gradual increase in proper exercise promotes good fitness development while minimizing or eliminating discomfort.
- AN EXERCISE TEST—Simple tests of fitness (such as the Canadian Home Fitness Test) or more complex types may be undertaken if you so desire.

Postpone

If you have a temporary minor illness, such as a common cold.

* Developed by the British Columbia Ministry of Health. Conceptualized and critiqued by the Multidisciplinary Advisory Board on Exercise (MABE). Reference PAR-Q Validation Report, British Columbia Ministry of Health, May, 1978.
* Produced by the British Columbia Ministry of Health and the Department of National Health & Welfare.

Figure 15.2

Physical Activity Readiness Questionnaire (PAR-Q). A self-administered questionnaire for adults.

Developed by British Columbia Ministry of Health, conceptualized and critiqued by the Multidisciplinary Advisory Board on Exercise (MABE). Reference PAR-Q Validation Report, British Columbia Ministry of Health, May 1978. Produced by the British Columbia Ministry of Health and the Department of National Health and Welfare.

which highlights absolute and relative contraindications for participating in exercise (see appendix D). An additional question added to various modifications of the PAR-Q asks about medications that might affect a person's response to exercise (e.g., an insulin-dependent diabetic or a cardiac patient taking the beta adrenergic blocker, propranolol) (26, 69). These forms are used to determine if a person needs consultation with a physician before taking a GXT, or before entering a fitness program.

Resting and Exercise Measures

Following the screening, measurements of heart rate and blood pressure are taken at rest prior to the exercise test. Additional measurements such as a blood sample for serum cholesterol, and an electrocardiogram (ECG) may also be obtained, with the latter one a necessity if the GXT is to be a diagnostic test. The exercise tests used to evaluate CRF may require a submaximal or maximal effort by the subject. They may be conducted in a lab containing sophisticated equipment, or on a running track with nothing more complicated than a stop watch. In a submaximal GXT, HR is measured at each stage of the test that progresses from light work (~3 METs) to a predetermined end point such as 70%–85% of predicted maximal heart rate. A treadmill, cycle ergometer, or a bench can be used to impose the work rates, and these tests will be described in detail in subsequent sections. Instead of stopping the submaximal GXT at some predetermined end point (70%–85% maximal HR), the GXT can be taken to the point of volitional exhaustion, or to where specific signs (ECG or BP changes) or symptoms like chest pain **(angina pectoris)** or breathlessness **(dyspnea)** occur. In these cases CRF is based on the last work rate achieved. However, there are some maximal tests of CRF that are not "graded" and for which physiological measurements are not made during the test [e.g., Cooper's 12-minute or 1.5-mile run (19), and the AAHPERD's 1-mile run (2)]. These latter **field tests** will now be considered in more detail, along with the Canadian Home (Aerobic) Fitness Test (71), and a 1-mile walk test (46). This will be followed by a discussion of GXTs using the treadmill, cycle ergometer, and bench step.

---

in summary

- The steps to follow prior to conducting an exercise test to evaluate CRF include:
  a. signing of a consent form,
  b. screening, and
  c. obtaining Resting HR and BP as well as Cholesterol and ECG measures.

Field Tests for Estimating CRF

Maximal Run Tests

Some field tests for CRF involve a measurement of how far a person can run in a set time (twelve to fifteen minutes), or how fast a person can run a set distance (one to two miles). The advantages of such field tests include their moderately high correlation with $\dot{V}O_2$ max, the use of a natural activity, the large numbers of people who can be tested at one time, and the low cost. The disadvantages of using field tests include the difficulty of monitoring physiological responses, the importance that motivation plays in the outcome, and the fact that the test is not graded but is a maximal effort. These field tests should be used only after a person has progressed through a program of exercise at lower intensities. The most popular field test for adults is Cooper's 12-minute or 1.5-mile run (19), and for school children, the AAHPERD's 1-mile walk/run (2). The aim is to determine the average velocity that can be maintained over the time or distance. These tests represent evolutionary changes from the original work of Balke (10) who showed that running tests of ten to twenty minutes provide reasonable estimates of $\dot{V}O_2$ max. The basis for the field tests is the linear relationship that exists between $\dot{V}O_2$ (ml $\cdot$ kg^{-1} $\cdot$ min^{-1}) and running speed, as shown in chapter 6. The duration of ten to twenty minutes represents a compromise that attempts to maximize the chance that the person is running at a speed demanding 90%–95% $\dot{V}O_2$ max, and minimize the contribution of energy coming from anaerobic sources. In distance runs of five minutes or less, anaerobic sources would provide relatively large amounts of energy, and $\dot{V}O_2$ max would probably be overestimated.

The method of calculating the $\dot{V}O_2$ when the running speed is known was described in detail in A Closer Look 6.2, and the formula is presented here again:

$$\dot{V}O_2 = 0.2 \text{ (ml} \cdot \text{kg}^{-1} \cdot \text{min}^{-1} \text{ per m} \cdot \text{min}^{-1})$$
$$+ 3.5 \text{ (ml} \cdot \text{kg}^{-1} \cdot \text{min}^{-1})$$

This formula provides reasonable estimates of $\dot{V}O_2$ max for adults, but would underestimate values for young children because of their relatively poor economy of running (23). On the other hand, this formula would overestimate the value for $\dot{V}O_2$ max for those who walk, since the net cost of walking is half that of running (see A Closer Look 6.1):

$$\dot{V}O_2 = 0.1 \text{ (ml} \cdot \text{kg}^{-1} \cdot \text{min}^{-1} \text{ per m} \cdot \text{min}^{-1})$$
$$+ 3.5 \text{ (ml} \cdot \text{kg}^{-1} \cdot \text{min}^{-1})$$

A Closer Look 15.1

Cardiovascular Fitness Standards for Children

The best way to evaluate fitness in children has been a concern for educators and scientists for most of this century (63a). The most recent controversy has revolved around the question of what kind of standards to use in making judgments about a child's level of fitness. Normative standards such as percentile scores have traditionally been used to describe where a child stands relative to his or her peers. (e.g., 75th percentile). The current thinking, especially for health-related fitness tests (one-mile walk/run test and the skinfold test) is that criterion-reference standards might be more appropriate. Criterion-reference standards attempt to describe the minimum level of fitness consistent with good health, independent of what percentile that might be in a normative data set. For example, Blair (13a) showed that in adults, $\dot{V}O_2$ max values associated with a low risk of disease were not that high, e.g., $\geq$35 ml $\cdot$ kg^{-1} $\cdot$ min^{-1} for men and $\geq$30 ml $\cdot$ kg^{-1} $\cdot$ min^{-1} for women 20–39 years of age. This information was used in setting the criterion-reference standards for the Fitnessgram®, the fitness evaluation program developed by the Institute for Aerobics Research. $\dot{V}O_2$ max standards were set at 42 ml $\cdot$ kg^{-1} $\cdot$ min^{-1} for boys 5–17 years of age. For girls the values were set at 40 ml $\cdot$ kg^{-1} $\cdot$ min^{-1} for ages 5–9 years of age, with a decrease of 1 ml $\cdot$ kg^{-1} $\cdot$ min^{-1} per year until age 14, where the 35 ml $\cdot$ kg^{-1} $\cdot$ min^{-1} value held until age 17 years. After the criterion-reference standards were set, the designers of the test had to translate those ml $\cdot$ kg^{-1} $\cdot$ min^{-1} values into equivalent one-mile run times—the actual test the children would take. The test designers had to consider the % $\dot{V}O_2$ max the children would perform at during the run, and the fact that economy of running improves with age. These steps, while complicated, have led to standards that are now used nationwide to classify children as to whether they have a sufficient level of cardiorespiratory fitness consistent with a low risk of disease (21).

While Cooper (19) provides categories of $\dot{V}O_2$ max values by age and sex (see table 15.1), estimates of $\dot{V}O_2$ max based on distance runs are most useful when compared over time for the same individual, rather than between individuals. Variation in economy of running, motivation, and other factors makes such comparisons of estimated $\dot{V}O_2$ max values between individuals unreasonable (6, 70). In this light, distance swim and bicycle riding tests provide useful information about changes in an individual's CRF over time, even though estimates of $\dot{V}O_2$ max are not available (18, 20).

The formulas used for estimating $\dot{V}O_2$ max from a 12-minute run are not very useful for prepubescent children since their economy of running is less than that of an adult (23). Investigators (48) worked around this problem by testing first, second, and third grade boys and girls with 800-, 1,200-, and 1,600-meter runs, and related performance to the measured $\dot{V}O_2$ max scores. They found the 1,600-meter run was the best predictor with good test/retest reliability (r = 0.82 to 0.92) in children who were given instruction on paced running (48). While performance in a run test is obviously a function of $\dot{V}O_2$ max, both running economy and the ability to run at a high % $\dot{V}O_2$ max also play a role (see chapter 21). It has been shown in young children of six to eleven years of age that % $\dot{V}O_2$ max is more closely related to performance of the 1-mile walk/run than is $\dot{V}O_2$ max (55)

$\dot{V}O_2$ max (ml $\cdot$ kg^{-1} $\cdot$ min^{-1}) estimated in an endurance run test is influenced by cardiovascular function and body fatness. It has been shown that differences in estimated $\dot{V}O_2$ max values between males and females can be explained, in part, by differences in % body fat (20a, 23, 75). In a 12-minute run test, performance was decreased 89 meters when body weight was experimentally increased by 5% to simulate an additional 5% fat (22). One should expect, then, that with a combined exercise and weight reduction program, CRF will increase due to both an increase in cardiovascular function and a decrease in % body fat. In table 15.1 categories for $\dot{V}O_2$ max values are adjusted for age due to the observation that in the general population $\dot{V}O_2$ max decreases with age. However, recent studies (39, 42, 78) have shown that $\dot{V}O_2$ max does not decrease as fast in individuals who maintain their physical activity program and body weight. This observation provides additional rationale for a regular evaluation of CRF to keep track of small changes before they become big changes.

Table 15.1 Men's and Women's Aerobics Fitness Classifications

Men's

Category	Age (Years)					
	13–19	20–29	30–39	40–49	50–59	60+
1. Very Poor	<35.0*	<33.0	<31.5	<30.2	<26.1	<20.5
2. Poor	35.0–38.3	33.0–36.4	31.5–35.4	30.2–33.5	26.1–30.9	20.5–26.0
3. Fair	38.4–45.1	36.5–42.4	35.5–40.9	33.6–38.9	31.0–35.7	26.1–32.2
4. Good	45.2–50.9	42.5–46.4	41.0–44.9	39.0–43.7	35.8–40.9	32.3–36.4
5. Excellent	51.0–55.9	46.5–52.4	45.0–49.4	43.8–48.0	41.0–45.3	36.5–44.2
6. Superior	>56.0	>52.5	>49.5	>48.1	>45.4	>44.3

*Values for oxygen uptake in $ml \cdot kg^{-1} \cdot min^{-1}$

Women's

Category	Age (Years)					
	13–19	20–29	30–39	40–49	50–59	60+
1. Very Poor	<25.0*	<23.6	<22.8	<21.0	<20.2	<17.5
2. Poor	25.0–30.9	23.6–28.9	22.8–26.9	21.0–24.4	20.2–22.7	17.5–20.1
3. Fair	31.0–34.9	29.0–32.9	27.0–31.4	24.5–28.9	22.8–26.9	20.2–24.4
4. Good	35.0–38.9	33.0–36.9	31.5–35.6	29.0–32.8	27.0–31.4	24.5–30.2
5. Excellent	39.0–41.9	37.0–40.9	35.7–40.0	32.9–36.9	31.5–35.7	30.3–31.4
6. Superior	>42.0	>41.0	>40.1	>37.0	>35.8	>31.5

*Values for oxygen uptake in $ml \cdot kg^{-1} \cdot min^{-1}$

Data from Kenneth H. Cooper, 1977. *The Aerobics Way*. New York: Bantam Books, Inc.

Walk Tests

An alternative to the maximal run tests used to evaluate CRF is a 1-mile walk test in which the HR is monitored during the test (46). The equation used to predict $\dot{V}O_2$ max was based on one population of men and women, aged 30 to 69, and was then validated on another comparable population. The subject walks as fast as possible for one mile on a flat, measured track, and HR is measured at the end of the last lap. The following equation can be used to estimate $\dot{V}O_2$ max ($ml \cdot kg^{-1} \cdot min^{-1}$):

$$\dot{V}O_2 \text{ max} = 132.853 - 0.0769 \text{ (wt)}$$
$$- 0.3877 \text{ (age)} + 6.315 \text{ (sex)} - 3.2649 \text{ (time)}$$
$$- 0.1565 \text{ (HR)}$$

where (wt) is body weight in pounds, (age) is in years, (sex) equals 0 for female and 1 for male, (time) is in minutes and hundredths of minutes, and (HR) is in $beats \cdot min^{-1}$ measured at the end of the last quarter mile.

This test appears to fill a void in the field tests available to estimate $\dot{V}O_2$ max since it uses a common activity and requires the simple measurement of

HR. As a participant's fitness improves, the time required for the mile and/or the HR response decreases, increasing the estimated $\dot{V}O_2$ max. A similar study using a 2-kilometer walk test supports this proposition (62).

Canadian Home Fitness Test

In contrast to the Cooper 1.5-mile run test and the 1-mile walk test, which require an all-out effort, the Canadian Home Fitness Test (CHFT) is a submaximal step test that uses the lowest two 8-inch steps found in a conventional staircase (63). The stepping cadence in this test is maintained by a long-playing record or audio tape. Prior to the test the person completes the Physical Activity Readiness Questionnaire (PAR-Q) (figure 15.2) to determine if he or she should proceed. The first stage of the test requires the individual to step for three minutes at a rate equivalent to 65%–70% of the average $\dot{V}O_2$ max of the next oldest age group (remember $\dot{V}O_2$ max generally decreases with age). An immediate ten-second recovery pulse is counted, and if it does not exceed the maximum allowable, another three-minute step test at 65%–70% of the average $\dot{V}O_2$ max of the person's

Table 15.2 Physical Fitness Evaluation Chart for the Canadian Home Fitness Test

10-Second Pulse Rate

Age (yr)	After First Three Minutes of Exercise	After Second Three Minutes of Exercise
15–19	If 30 or more, stop. You have an undesirable personal fitness level.	If 27 or more, you have a minimum personal fitness level. If 26 or less, you have the recommended personal fitness level.
20–29	If 29 or more, stop. You have an undesirable personal fitness level.	If 26 or more, you have a minimum personal fitness level. If 25 or less, you have the recommended personal fitness level.
30–39	If 28 or more, stop. You have an undesirable personal fitness level.	If 25 or more, you have a minimum personal fitness level. If 24 or less, you have the recommended personal fitness level.
40–49	If 26 or more, stop. You have an undesirable personal fitness level.	If 24 or more, you have a minimum personal fitness level. If 23 or less, you have the recommended personal fitness level.
50–59	If 25 or more, stop. You have an undesirable personal fitness level.	If 23 or more, you have a minimum personal fitness level. If 22 or less, you have the recommended personal fitness level.
60–69	If 24 or more, stop. You have an undesirable personal fitness level.	If 23 or more, you have a minimum personal fitness level. If 22 or less, you have the recommended personal fitness level.

From R. J. Shephard, et al., "Development of the Canadian Home Fitness Test," originally published in *Canadian Medical Association Journal*, 114:675–79, 1976. Copyright © 1976 Canadian Medical Association, Ottawa, Canada. Reprinted by permission

own age group is completed. Another pulse rate is then taken. Table 15.2 shows how physical fitness can be estimated as "undesirable, minimum, or recommended" (71). $\dot{V}O_2$ max can be estimated from the CHFT results (12, 41, 72).

in summary

- Field tests for CRF use natural activities such as walking, running, and stepping in which large numbers of people can be tested at low cost. However, for some, physiological responses are difficult to measure, and motivation plays an important role in the outcome.
- VO_2 max estimates from all-out run tests are based on the linear relationship between running speed and the oxygen cost of running.
- The Canadian Home Fitness Test is a step test that uses conventional 8-inch steps to evaluate cardiorespiratory fitness.

Graded Exercise Tests: Measurements

Cardiorespiratory fitness is commonly measured using a treadmill, cycle ergometer, or a stepping bench. These tests are usually incremental, in which the work rate changes every two to three minutes until the subject reaches some predetermined end point, or when some pathological sign or symptom occurs. These GXTs can be maximal or submaximal, and the variables measured during the test can be as simple as HR and BP, or as complex as $\dot{V}O_2$; it depends on the purpose of the test, and the facilities, equipment, and personnel involved (36). What follows is a brief summary of common measurements made during a GXT.

Heart Rate

Heart rate can be measured by palpation of the radial or carotid artery, using a stethoscope with the microphone on the chest wall, or by using surface electrodes that transmit the signal to an oscilloscope, electrocardiograph, or a monitor that can display heart rate directly. In palpating the carotid artery, care must be taken not to use too much pressure, since this could slow the HR by way of the baroreceptor reflex. However, when people are trained in this procedure, reliable measurements can be obtained (63, 68). Heart rate is measured over a fifteen- to thirty-second time period *during* steady state exercise to obtain a reliable estimate of the HR. If using a *post-exercise* HR as an indication of the HR during exercise, the HR should be measured for ten seconds within the first fifteen seconds after stopping exercise because the HR changes rapidly at this time. The ten-second count is multiplied by six to express the HR in beats $\cdot$ min^{-1}(68).

Blood Pressure

Blood pressure is measured by auscultation as described in chapter 9. It is important to use the proper cuff size and a sensitive stethoscope to obtain correct values at rest and during work. In addition, if using an aneroid sphygmomanometer, it is important to calibrate it on a regular basis against the mercury sphygmomanometer (44). During the walking or cycling exercise test (BP cannot be reliably measured during a running test), the microphone of the stethoscope is placed below the cuff and over an area where the sound is the loudest (in many cases this will be in the intramuscular space on the medial side of the arm). The subject should not be holding onto the handlebar of the cycle or treadmill during the measurement. The first Korotkoff sound is taken as systolic BP, and the fourth sound (change in tone or muffling) is taken as diastolic BP (64). The HR can also be measured if the pressure is maintained just above the diastolic value. The following procedure can be used to obtain the HR and BP values during an exercise test: pump up cuff above the point where the pulse disappears, decrease pressure slowly (<5 mm Hg per second), and obtain systolic BP; decrease quickly to a value above resting diastolic BP and count HR for fifteen seconds; slowly decrease pressure and obtain the diastolic reading.

ECG

GXTs are used to diagnose CHD because exercise causes the heart to work harder and challenges the coronary arteries' ability to deliver sufficient blood to meet the oxygen demand of the myocardium. An estimate of the work (and O_2 demand) of the heart is the **double product**—the product of the HR and the systolic BP (45, 61). As you already know, HR and systolic BP increase with exercise intensity such that myocardial oxygen demand increases throughout the test. The ECG is used as an indicator of the ability of

Figure 15.3
Three types of ST segment depression.

From A. D. Martin, "ECG and Medications" in E. T. Howley and B. D. Franks, *Health/Fitness Instructor's Handbook*. Copyright © 1986 Human Kinetics Publishers, Inc., Champaign IL. Used by permission.

the heart to function normally during these times of imposed work. During exercise the ECG can be measured with a single bipolar lead (e.g., CM$_5$), however, a full twelve-lead arrangement is preferred (3). The ECG is evaluated for arrhythmias, conduction disturbances, and myocardial ischemia. **Arrhythmias** are irregularities in the normal electrical rhythm of the heart that can be localized to the atria (e.g., atrial fibrillation), the AV node (e.g., premature junctional contraction), or in the ventricles (e.g., premature ventricular contractions—PVCs). **Conduction disturbances** describe a defect in which depolarization is slowed or completely blocked (e.g., first degree AV block, or bundle branch block). **Myocardial ischemia** is defined as an inadequate perfusion of the myocardium relative to the metabolic demand of the heart. Since oxygen uptake by the myocardium is almost completely flow dependent, a flow limitation indicates an oxygen insufficiency. A *symptom* of myocardial ischemia is angina pectoris, which is pain or discomfort caused by a temporary ischemia; the pain could be located in the center of the chest, neck, jaw, shoulders, or radiate to the arms and hands (51). A *sign* associated with myocardial ischemia is a depression of the ST segment on the electrocardiogram (chapter 9). Figure 15.3 shows three types of **ST segment depression.** People with upsloping or horizontal ST segment depression have similar life expectancies, but the prognosis for those with downsloping ST segment is worse (25). Interested readers are referred to Dubin's introductory text on ECG analysis (see Suggested Readings), and Ellestad's text on exercise electrocardiography (25).

Rating of Perceived Exertion

Another common measurement made at each stage of the GXT is Borg's (14) Rating of Perceived Exertion (RPE). Table 15.3 lists his original and revised scales.

Table 15.3 Rating of Perceived Exertion Scales

Original Rating Scale		Revised Rating Scale	
6		0	Nothing at all
7	Very, very light	0.5	Very, very light (just noticeable)
8		1	Very light
9	Very light	2	Light (weak)
10		3	Moderate
11	Fairly light	4	Somewhat hard
12		5	Heavy (strong)
13	Somewhat hard	6	
14		7	Very heavy
15	Hard	8	
16		9	
17	Very hard	10	Very, very heavy (almost max)
18		•	Maximal
19	Very, very hard		
20			

From: G. A. U. Borg. "Psychological Bases of Physical Exertion" in *Medicine and Science in Sports and Exercise*, 14:377–81, 1982. Copyright © 1982 American College of Sports Medicine, Indianapolis IN. Reprinted by permission.

Table 15.4 General Indications for Stopping an Exercise Test in Apparently Healthy Adults*

1. Onset of angina or angina-like symptoms
2. Significant drop (20 mm Hg) in systolic blood pressure or a failure of the systolic blood pressure to rise with an increase in exercise intensity
3. Excessive rise in blood pressure: systolic pressure >260 mm Hg or diastolic pressure > 115 mm Hg
4. Signs of poor perfusion: lightheadedness, confusion, ataxia, pallor, cyanosis, nausea, or cold and clammy skin
5. Failure of heart rate to increase with increased exercise intensity
6. Noticeable change in heart rhythm
7. Subject requests to stop
8. Physical or verbal manifestations of severe fatigue
9. Failure of the testing equipment

*Assumes that testing is nondiagnostic and is being performed without direct physician involvement or electrocardiographic monitoring.

From ACSM-ACSM *Guidelines for Exercise Testing and Prescription*, 5th ed. Copyright © 1995 Williams & Wilkins, A Waverly Company. Reprinted by permission.

The original scale used the rankings 6–20 to approximate the HR values from rest to maximum (60–200). The revised scale represents an attempt to provide a ratio scale of the RPE values. The RPE scores are good indicators of subjective effort and provide a quantitative way to track a person's progress through a GXT or an exercise session (16, 17, 32). This is helpful in knowing when a subject is approaching exhaustion, and the values can be used in prescribing exercise intensity (see chapter 16).

Termination Criteria

The reasons for stopping a GXT vary with the type of population being tested and the purpose of the test. Table 15.4, from the ACSM's *Guidelines for Exercise Testing and Prescription*, is appropriate for nondiagnostic GXTs in apparently healthy adults (3).

in summary

- Typical measurements obtained during a graded exercise test include heart rate, blood pressure, ECG, and rating of perceived exertion.
- Specific signs (e.g., fall in systolic pressure with an increase in work rate) and symptoms (e.g., dizziness) are used to stop GXTs.

$\dot{V}O_2$ Max

The measurement of $\dot{V}O_2$ max represents the standard against which any estimate of CRF is compared (see chapters 6 and 20 for procedures). $\dot{V}O_2$ increases with increasing loads on a GXT until the maximal capacity of the cardiorespiratory system is reached; attention to detail is crucial if one is to obtain accurate values (53). Commonly used criteria for having achieved $\dot{V}O_2$ max include a leveling off of the $\dot{V}O_2$ (<150 ml · kg^{-1} · min^{-1} or < 2.1 ml · kg^{-1} · min^{-1}) even though a higher work rate is achieved (77), a post-exercise blood lactate level of >8 mmoles · liter^{-1} (5), and the R exceeding 1.15 (40). While many subjects will meet these criteria, some, especially the elderly (74), children (5), and postcoronary (43) subjects, will not. In addition, one should not expect a subject to meet all three of these standards (43, 74). For example, in one study (74) 20 percent of the women subjects who met the "leveling off" criterion did not even achieve an R of 1.00! The R values have been shown to vary with age and the training status of the subjects (1). In general, these criteria are useful because they give the investigator an objective indicator of the subject's effort. However, subjects should not be expected to meet all the criteria on any single test (36a).

$\dot{V}O_2$ max is a very reproducible measure on subjects tested with the same test protocol on the same piece of equipment. The value for $\dot{V}O_2$ max does not seem to be dependent on whether the test is a continuous GXT or a discontinuous GXT as long as it is

In P. O. Åstrand's classic study on the $\dot{V}O_2$ max of children, he was confronted with a problem—only 50 percent of the children achieved a leveling off in $\dot{V}O_2$ when the work rate was increased to maximum levels. This led Åstrand to look for an alternative indicator that the children had, in fact, achieved $\dot{V}O_2$ max. The children had completed one test per day over a period of three to four weeks, with a day or two break between tests. A blood sample was taken a few minutes after each exercise test to measure the blood lactate concentration. In the children who experienced a plateau in $\dot{V}O_2$, he found that the lactate concentration ranged from 6.7–10.1 mM when the $\dot{V}O_2$ curves leveled off, with the average being 7.9–8.4 mM. He then compared the $\dot{V}O_2$ max values of boys and girls who had experienced a leveling off in $\dot{V}O_2$ with those who had achieved a high lactate level, but not a leveling off in $\dot{V}O_2$. The average $\dot{V}O_2$ max was the same for both groups. Based on these observations, Åstrand used the elevated blood lactate value and the subjective stress of the subject to select the highest $\dot{V}O_2$ value as the subject's $\dot{V}O_2$ max when a plateau was not observed (5).

conducted with the same work instrument (27, 52, 76). However, when $\dot{V}O_2$ max values are compared across protocols, some systematic differences appear (9). The highest value for $\dot{V}O_2$ max is usually measured with a running test up a grade on a treadmill, followed by a walking test up a grade on a treadmill, and then on a cycle ergometer. In American populations, walk test protocols yield values about 6% lower than those for a run test (52), while cycle test protocols yield values about 10%–11% lower than those for a run test (28, 52). Europeans show only a 5%–7% difference in this latter comparison (9, 35). An arm ergometer test will yield values equal to about 70% of the $\dot{V}O_2$ max measured with the legs (30, 67). It is important to recognize these differences when comparing one test to another, or when comparing the same subject over time with different ergometers. These differences among tests have led to the convention to call $\dot{V}O_2$ max the value measured on a graded running test; $\dot{V}O_2$ peak is the term used to describe the highest $\dot{V}O_2$ achieved on walk, cycle, or arm ergometer protocol (66). However, these terms can cause confusion when applied to highly trained athletes, such as cyclists, as they have higher $\dot{V}O_2$ max values when measured on a cycle, compared to a treadmill (76a). The actual measurement of $\dot{V}O_2$ max is crucial for research studies and in some clinical settings. However, it is unreasonable to suggest actual measurement of $\dot{V}O_2$ max as the standard to use as a measure of CRF in exercise programs.

Estimation of $\dot{V}O_2$ Max from Last Work Rate

Given the complexity and cost of the procedures involved in the measurement of $\dot{V}O_2$ max, it is no surprise that in many fitness and clinical settings $\dot{V}O_2$ max is estimated with equations that allow calculation of $\dot{V}O_2$ max from the last work rate achieved on the GXT. The equations for estimating the oxygen cost of running and walking outlined in chapter 6 allow such calculations and, in general, the estimates are reasonable (57, 58). What is important in the use of these equations is that the work test is suited to the individual. If the increments in the GXT from one stage to the next are too large relative to a person's CRF, or if the time for each stage is so short that a person might not be able to achieve the steady state oxygen requirement for that stage, then the equations will overestimate the person's $\dot{V}O_2$ max (29, 34, 57). As described in chapter 4, poorly fit individuals take longer to achieve the steady state at moderate to heavy work rates, and this increases the chance of an overestimation of $\dot{V}O_2$ max when using these formulas. This suggests that a more conservative protocol be used for low-fit individuals to allow them to reach a steady state at each stage. A recommended procedure is to use only the last completed stage of a test. However, independent of the proper matching of the protocol with the individual, it must be remembered that these are only *estimations*.

Estimation of $\dot{V}O_2$ Max from Submaximal HR Response

Another common procedure used with GXT protocols is to estimate $\dot{V}O_2$ max on the basis of the subject's HR response to a variety of submaximal work rates (31). In these tests the HR is plotted against work rate (or estimated $\dot{V}O_2$) until the termination criterion of 70%–85% of age-adjusted maximal HR is reached. Figure 15.4 shows the HR response for a twenty-year-old who has taken a submaximal GXT on a cycle ergometer. Heart rate was measured at each work rate until a value equal to 85% of estimated maximal HR was reached (170 b · min^{-1}). A line was drawn through the HR points and extrapolated to the estimated maximal HR, which is

Figure 15.4

Estimation of $\dot{V}O_2$ max from heart rate values measured during a series of submaximal work rates on a cycle ergometer. The test was stopped when the subject reached 85% of maximal HR. A line is drawn through the HR points measured during the test and is extrapolated to the age-adjusted estimate of maximal HR. Another line is dropped from that point to the x-axis, and the $\dot{V}O_2$ max is identified.

calculated by subtracting age from 220. Another line is dropped from that point to the x-axis, and the work rate or $\dot{V}O_2$ (in this case, 2.7 $\ell \cdot min^{-1}$) that would have been achieved if the individual had worked until maximal HR was reached is recorded (31). While this is a simple and commonly used procedure to estimate $\dot{V}O_2$ max, it has several potential problems.

The first problem relates to the formula used for estimating the maximal HR. These estimates have a standard deviation (SD) of about 11 $b \cdot min^{-1}$ (49). A twenty year old's maximal HR might be estimated to be 200 $b \cdot min^{-1}$, but if a person were out at ±2 SD, the value would be 178 or 222 $b \cdot min^{-1}$. For those who do maximal testing, one will occasionally observe subjects having *measured* maximal HRs ±20 $b \cdot min^{-1}$ away from their age-adjusted estimate of maximal heart rate. Taking this as an example, what if the subject in figure 15.4 had a true maximal HR of only 180 $b \cdot min^{-1}$ instead of the estimated 200 $b \cdot min^{-1}$? The estimated $\dot{V}O_2$ max would be an overestimation of the correct value.

Further, a submaximal end point such as 85% of estimated maximal heart rate may be very light work for one individual and maximal work for another. The reason for this is related to the estimate of maximal heart rate (220 – age) mentioned earlier. If a thirty-year-old individual has a real maximum heart rate of 160 $b \cdot min^{-1}$ and the GXT takes the person to 85% of estimated maximal HR (220 – 30 = 190; 85% of 190 = 161 $b \cdot min^{-1}$), then the person would be taken to maximal HR.

Another problem with submaximal GXT protocols using the HR response as the primary indicator of fitness is that any variable that affects submaximal heart rate will affect the slope of the HR/$\dot{V}O_2$ line and, of course, the estimate of $\dot{V}O_2$ max. These variables would include: eating prior to the test, dehydration,

elevated body temperature, temperature and humidity of the testing area, emotional state of the subject, medications that affect HR, and previous physical activity (7, 70). Clearly, many environmental variables must be controlled if one is to use such protocols to estimate $\dot{V}O_2$ max.

Despite these problems, this estimate of $\dot{V}O_2$ max is useful in providing appropriate feedback to participants in fitness programs. Following training, the HR response to any fixed submaximal work rate is lower, suggesting an increase in $\dot{V}O_2$ max when the HR/$\dot{V}O_2$ line is drawn through those HR points to the age-adjusted maximal HR. In this case, because the same individual is being tested over time, the 220 – age formula introduces only a constant and unknown error that will not affect the projection of the HR/$\dot{V}O_2$ line. Further, the low cost and ease of measurement make it a good test that can be used for education and motivation (69).

in summary

- The measurement of $\dot{V}O_2$ max is the gold standard measure of cardiorespiratory fitness.
- $\dot{V}O_2$ max can be estimated based on the final work rate achieved in a graded exercise test.
- $\dot{V}O_2$ max can be estimated from heart rate responses to submaximal exercise by extrapolating the relationship to the subject's age-adjusted estimate of maximal heart rate. Careful attention to environmental factors that can affect the heart rate response to submaximal exercise is an important aspect of the procedures for these tests.

Graded Exercise Test: Protocols

The GXT protocols can be either submaximal or maximal, depending on the end points used to stop the test. The choice of the GXT should be based on the population (athletes, cardiac patients, children), purpose (estimate CRF, measure $\dot{V}O_2$ max, diagnose CHD), and cost (equipment and personnel) (36, 38). This section will discuss the selection of the test based on these factors and provide examples of common GXT protocols.

When choosing a GXT protocol, the population being tested must be considered, given that the last stage in a GXT for cardiac patients might not even be a warm-up for a young athletic subject. Test protocols should vary in terms of the initial work rate, how large the increment in work rate will be between stages, and the duration of each stage. In general, the GXT for a sedentary subject might start at 2–3 METs (1 MET = 3.5 $ml \cdot kg^{-1} \cdot min^{-1}$), and progress at about 1 MET per stage,

Table 15.5   Treadmill Protocols

A—Protocol for Poorly Fit Subjects (60)

Stage*	METs	Speed (mph)	% Grade
1	2.5	2	0
2	3.5	2	3.5
3	4.5	2	7.0
4	5.5	2	10.5
5	6.5	2	14.0
6	7.5	2	17.5
7	8.5	3	12.5
8	9.5	3	15.0
9	10.5	3	17.5

*Stage lasts three minutes

B—Protocol for Normal, Sedentary Subjects (11)

Stage*	METs	Speed (mph)	% Grade
1	4.3	3	2.5
2	5.4	3	5.0
3	6.4	3	7.5
4	7.4	3	10.0
5	8.5	3	12.5
6	9.5	3	15.0
7	10.5	3	17.5
8	11.6	3	20.0
9	12.6	3	22.5

*Stage lasts two minutes

C—Protocol for Young, Active Subjects (15)

Stage*	METs	Speed (mph)	% Grade
1	5	1.7	10
2	7	2.5	12
3	9.5	3.4	14
4	13	4.2	16
5	16	5.0	18

*Stage lasts three minutes

D—Protocol for Very Fit Subjects (7)

Stage*	METs	Speed (mph)	% Grade
1	12.9/18	7/10	2.5
2	14.1/19.8	7/10	5.0
3	15.3/21.5	7/10	7.5
4	16.5/23.2	7/10	10.0
5	17.7/24.9	7/10	12.5

*Stage lasts two minutes; vigorous warm-up precedes test.

with each stage lasting two to three minutes to allow enough time for a steady state to be reached. For young active subjects, the initial work rate might be 5 METs, with increments of 2–3 METs per stage (64). Table 15.5 shows four well-known treadmill protocols and the populations for which they are suited. The National Exercise and Heart Disease protocol (60) is usually used with poorly-fit subjects, with the work rate increasing only 1 MET each three minutes. The Standard Balke protocol (11) starts at about 4 METs and progresses 1 MET each two minutes, and is suitable for most average sedentary adults. The Bruce protocol for young, active subjects (15) starts at about 5 METs and progresses at 2–3 METs per stage. This protocol includes walking and running up a grade, and is not suitable for those at the low end of the fitness continuum. The last protocol shown is used by the fit and athletic populations, with the speed dependent on the fitness of the subject (7).

As mentioned earlier, one of the most common approaches used in estimating $\dot{V}O_2$ max is to take the final stage in the test and apply the formula for converting grade and speed to $\dot{V}O_2$ in ml · kg^{-1} · min^{-1}. Nagle et al. (59) and Montoye et al. (57) have shown that apparently healthy individuals reach the new steady state requirement by approximately 1.5 minutes of each stage up to moderately heavy work. These formulas give reasonable estimates of CRF if the test has been suited to the individual (34, 57). However, if the increments in the stages are too large, or if the time at each stage is too short, then the person might not be able to reach the oxygen requirement associated with that stage of the GXT. In these cases the formulas will overestimate the subject's $\dot{V}O_2$ max. This problem is more common with low-fit individuals and suggests that the more conservative tests be used to estimate the $\dot{V}O_2$ max based on grade and speed achieved.

in summary

- When selecting a GXT, the population being tested must be considered. The initial work rate and the rate of change of work rate need to accommodate the capabilities of the population.

Treadmill

Treadmill GXT protocols can accommodate everyone, from those least fit to those most fit, and use the natural activities of walking and running. Treadmills set the pace for the subject and provide the greatest potential load on the cardiovascular system. However, they are expensive, not portable, and make some measurements (BP and blood sampling) difficult (70). As mentioned previously, the type of treadmill test does influence the magnitude of the measured $\dot{V}O_2$ max, with the graded running test giving the highest value, the running test at 0% grade the next highest, and the walking test protocols the lowest (9, 52). There are also some limitations in the types of measurements that can be made, depending on whether walking or running is used. For example, during running tests measurement of BP is not possible, and there is more potential for artifact in the ECG tracing.

In order for estimates of $\dot{V}O_2$ to be obtained from grade and speed considerations, the grade and speed settings must be correct (36). In addition, the subject must follow instructions carefully and not hold onto the treadmill railing during the test. If this is not done, estimates of $\dot{V}O_2$ max based on either the HR/$\dot{V}O_2$ extrapolation procedure, or the use of the formula that uses the last speed/grade combination achieved will not be reasonable (6, 65). For example, when a subject who was walking on a treadmill at 3.4 mph and 14% grade held onto the railing, the HR decreased 17 b · min^{-1} (6). This would result in an overestimation of the $\dot{V}O_2$ max using

Data:

Subject: male, age = 45 years Estimated HR max = 175 b/min 85% HR max = 149 b/min	% grade	HR (b/min)
	0	100
	2.5	102
	5.0	108
	7.5	110
	10.0	123
	12.5	136
	15.0	149

% Grade	0.0	2.5	5.0	7.5	10.0	12.5	15.0	17.5	20.0
METs	3.3	4.4	5.4	6.4	7.4	8.4	9.5	10.5	11.6

Figure 15.5

Estimation of $\dot{V}O_2$ max from the heart rate values measured during different stages of a treadmill test.

From E. T. Howley and B. D. Franks, *Health/Fitness Instructor's Handbook.* Copyright © 1986 Human Kinetics Publishers, Inc., Champaign IL. Used by permission.

either of the submaximal procedures just mentioned, and special equations would have to be developed if holding onto the handrail were allowed (54). Finally, with the treadmill there is no need to make adjustments to the $\dot{V}O_2$ calculation due to differences in body weight. Treadmill tests require the subject to carry his or her own weight, and the $\dot{V}O_2$ is therefore proportional to body weight (56).

In the following example of a submaximal GXT, a forty-five-year-old male takes a Balke Standard Protocol (3 mph, 2.5% each two minutes) and the test is terminated at 85% of age-adjusted maximal HR (149 b · min^{-1}). Heart rate was measured in the last thirty seconds of each stage, and $\dot{V}O_2$ max was estimated by the HR/$\dot{V}O_2$ extrapolation to age-adjusted maximal HR (175 b · min^{-1}). Figure 15.5 shows the plot of the HR response at each stage, and the extrapolation to the person's estimated maximal heart rate. In the early stages of the test the HR does not increase in a predictable manner with increasing grade. This may be due to the changes in stroke volume that occur early in upright work (see chapter 9). The beginning stages also act as a warm-up and adjustment period for the subject. The HR response is usually quite linear between 110 b · min^{-1} and 85% maximal HR (8). The HR/$\dot{V}O_2$ line is extrapolated to 175 b · min^{-1}, and a vertical line is dropped to the x-axis where the estimated $\dot{V}O_2$ max is identified: 11.6 METs, or 40.6 ml · kg^{-1} · min^{-1}.

Recently a single-stage submaximal treadmill test has been validated for use with low-risk subjects who are likely to have average values for ~$\dot{V}O_2$ max (24). In this test the treadmill is set at 0% grade, and a walking speed is set between 2 and 4.5 mph to elicit a heart rate between 50% and 70% of age-adjusted maximal HR. Following this 4-minute warm-up the grade is elevated to 5% for 4 minutes. HR is measured in the last minute and used with speed (S in mph), age (A in years), and gender (G, with female = 0 and male = 1) in the following regression equation to predict $\dot{V}O_2$ max.

$$\dot{V}O_2 \text{ max} = 15.1 + 21.8 \text{ (S)} - 0.327 \text{ (HR)} - 0.263$$
$$(S \times A) + 0.00504 \text{ (HR} \times A) + 5.98 \text{ (G)}$$

Cycle Ergometer

Cycle ergometers are portable, moderately priced work instruments that allow measurements to be made easily, however, they are self-paced and result in some localized fatigue (70). On mechanically braked cycle ergometers (e.g., Monark) the work rate can be increased by increasing the pedal rate or the resistance on the flywheel. Generally, the pedal rate is maintained constant during a GXT at a rate suitable to the populations being tested: 50–60 rpm for the low to average fit, and 70–100 for the high fit and competitive cyclists (33). The pedal rate is maintained by having the subject pedal to a metronome, or by providing some other source of feedback (visual analog or digital display of the rpm). The load on the wheel is increased in a sequential fashion to systematically overload the cardiovascular system. The starting work rate and the increment from one stage to the next is dependent on the fitness of the subject and the purpose of the test. The $\dot{V}O_2$ can be estimated from a formula that gives reasonable estimates of the $\dot{V}O_2$ up to work rates of about 1,200 kgm $\cdot$ min^{-1} (38):

$$\dot{V}O_2 \text{ (ml} \cdot \text{min}^{-1}) = 2 \text{ ml} \cdot \text{kgm}^{-1} \times \text{kgm} \cdot \text{min}^{-1}$$
$$+ 300 \text{ ml} \cdot \text{min}^{-1}$$

The cycle ergometer is different from the treadmill in that the body weight is supported by the seat, and the work rate is dependent only on the crank speed and the load on the wheel. This means that for a small person the relative $\dot{V}O_2$ at any work rate is higher than for a big person. For example, if the work rate is 900 kgm $\cdot$ min^{-1}, the estimated $\dot{V}O_2$ is 2,100 ml $\cdot$ min^{-1}; this represents a relative $\dot{V}O_2$ of 35 ml $\cdot$ kg$^-$ $\cdot$ min^{-1} for a 60-kg person, and only 23 ml $\cdot$ kg^{-1} $\cdot$ min^{-1} for a 90-kg person. In addition, the increments in the work rate, by demanding a fixed increase in the $\dot{V}O_2$ (e.g., an increment of 150 kgm $\cdot$ min^{-1} is equal to a $\dot{V}O_2$ change of 300 ml $\cdot$ min^{-1}), forces a small and unfit subject to make larger cardiovascular adjustments than a large or high-fit subject. These facts have been taken into consideration by the American College of Sports Medicine (3) and the YMCA (31) in recommending submaximal GXT protocols. The idea is to provide a means of obtaining a variety of HR responses to several submaximal work rates in a way that reduces the duration of the test.

Directions:

1. Set the first work load at 150 kgm $\cdot$ min^{-1} (0.5 kp).
2. If the HR in the 3rd minute is
   - less than (<) 80, set the second load at 750 kgm (2.5 kp);
   - 80 to 89, set the second load at 600 kgm (2.0 kp);
   - 90 to 100, set the second load at 450 kgm (1.5 kp);
   - greater than (>) 100, set the second load at 300 kgm (1.0 kp).
3. Set the third and fourth (if required) loads according to the loads in the columns below the second loads.

Figure 15.6

The Y's Way to Physical Fitness protocol used to select work rates for submaximal cycle ergometer tests.

From Lawrence A. Golding, et al., *The Complete Guide to Fitness Testing and Instruction*, 3d ed. Copyright © 1989 YMCA of the USA, 101 N. Wacker Drive, Chicago IL 60606. Reprinted by permission.

Figure 15.6 shows the different "routes" followed in the YMCA protocol depending on the subject's HR response to a work rate of 150 kgm $\cdot$ min^{-1}. The YMCA protocol makes use of the observation that the relationship between $\dot{V}O_2$ and HR is a linear one between 110 and 150 b $\cdot$ min^{-1}. For this reason the YMCA protocol requires the subject to work only one more work rate past the one that yields a HR $\geq$ 110 b $\cdot$ min^{-1}. As a general recommendation for all cycle ergometer tests, seat height is adjusted so that the knee is slightly bent when the foot is at the bottom of the pedal swing and parallel to the floor; the seat height is recorded for later testing. In the YMCA protocol each stage lasts three minutes and heart rate values are obtained in the last thirty seconds of the second and third minutes. If the difference in HR is <5 b $\cdot$ min^{-1} between the two time periods, a steady state is assumed; if not, an additional minute is added to that stage. A line then connects the two HR values and is extrapolated to the subject's estimated maximal HR. A vertical line is dropped to the x-axis and the estimated $\dot{V}O_2$ max value is obtained as described for the submaximal treadmill protocol.

Subject: female, age = 30 years Estimated HR max = 190 b/min 85% HR max = 162 b/min	Data: Work rate (kpm/min)	Heart rate (b/min)
	150	103
	300	115
	450	128

Figure 15.7

Example of the YMCA protocol used to estimate $\dot{V}O_2$ max.

From E. T. Howley and B. D. Franks, *Health/Fitness Instructor's Handbook.* Copyright © 1986 Human Kinetics Publishers, Inc., Champaign IL. Used by permission.

Figure 15.7 shows the YMCA protocol for a thirty-year-old female. The first work rate chosen was 150 kgm · min⁻¹, and a heart rate of 103 b · min⁻¹ was measured. Following the YMCA protocol, the next loads were 300 and then 450 kgm · min⁻¹, and the measured HR values were 115 and 128 b · min⁻¹, respectively. A line was drawn through the two HR points greater than 110 b · min⁻¹, and extrapolated to 190 b · min⁻¹. The estimated $\dot{V}O_2$ max for this woman was approximately 2.7 liters · min⁻¹.

In addition to this extrapolation procedure for estimating $\dot{V}O_2$ max, Åstrand and Ryhming (8) provide a method that requires the subject to complete one work rate of approximately six minutes, demanding a HR between 125 and 170 b · min⁻¹. These investigators observed that at 50% $\dot{V}O_2$ max males had an average HR of 128, and females, 138 b · min⁻¹, and at 70% $\dot{V}O_2$ max the average HRs were 154 and 164 b · min⁻¹, respectively. These data were collected on young men and women, ages eighteen to thirty. The basis for the test is that if you know from a HR response that a person is at 50% $\dot{V}O_2$ max at a work rate equal to 1.5 ℓ · min⁻¹, then the estimated $\dot{V}O_2$ max would be twice that, or 3.0 ℓ · min⁻¹. A nomogram (see figure 15.8) is used to estimate the $\dot{V}O_2$ max based on the subject's HR response to one six-minute work rate. Because maximal HR decreases with increasing age, and the data were collected on young subjects, Åstrand (4) established correction factors to multiply the estimated $\dot{V}O_2$ max values taken from the nomogram in order to correct for the lower maximal HR.

Siconolfi et al. (73) presented a submaximal cycle ergometer test for epidemiological investigations that is a modification of the YMCA protocol that uses the Åstrand and Ryhming (8) nomogram. It is presented here because the advantages of this test include (1) the requirement that the subject achieve only 70% of the estimated maximal HR and (2) the procedure was validated on men and women of ages twenty to seventy years. Men over age thirty-five and all women start the test at 150 kgm · min⁻¹, and the work rate is increased that amount each two minutes until a HR ≥70% of estimated maximal HR is achieved; the subject continues for two or more minutes until a steady state HR is measured. Men under age thirty-five begin at 300 kgm · min⁻¹ and increase that amount each two minutes as above. However, when the HR is between 60% and 70% of maximal HR, the work rate is increased only 150 kgm · min⁻¹. The Åstrand and Ryhming (8) nomogram is used as before (without the age correction), and the estimated $\dot{V}O_2$ max values are used in the following equations (73):

For males:
$$\dot{V}O_2 \text{ (liters} \cdot \text{min}^{-1}) = 0.348 (X_1) - 0.035 (X_2) + 3.011$$
For females:
$$\dot{V}O_2 \text{ (liters} \cdot \text{min}^{-1}) = 0.302 (X_1) - 0.019 (X_2) + 1.593$$

where $X_1 = \dot{V}O_2$ max from Åstrand and Ryhming nomogram, and $X_2 =$ age in years. The test yields acceptable estimates of $\dot{V}O_2$ max and puts the subject under less stress by requiring that a HR of only 70% of the age-adjusted maximal HR be achieved.

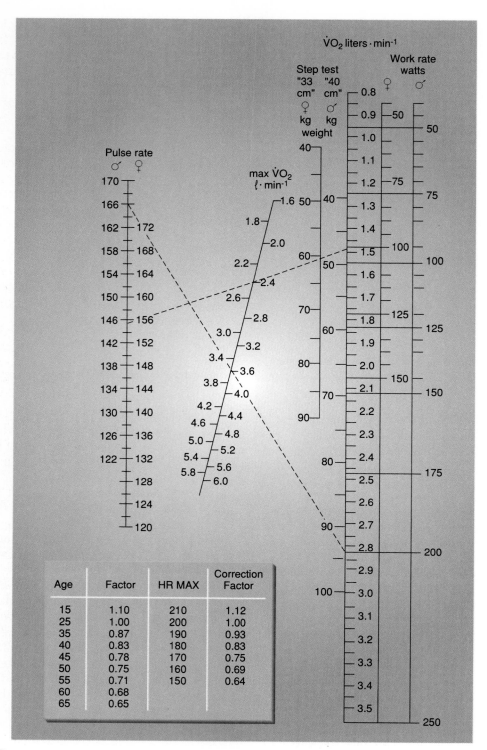

Figure 15.8

Nomogram for the estimation of $\dot{V}O_2$ max from submaximal HR values measured on either a cycle ergometer or step test. For the cycle ergometer the work rate in watts (1 watt = 6.1 kgm · min^{-1}) is shown on the two right-most columns, one for men and one for women. The results of a cycle ergometer test for a man who worked at 200 watts is shown. A dashed line is drawn between the 200-watt work rate and the HR value of 166 measured during the test. The estimated $\dot{V}O_2$ max is 3.6 liters · min^{-1}. The step test uses a rate of 22.5 lifts · min^{-1}, and two different step heights, 33 cm for women and 40 cm for men. The step test scale lists body weight for the subject and the results of a test on a 61-kg woman are shown. A dashed line is drawn between the 61 kg on the 33-cm scale and the HR value of 156 b · min^{-1} measured during the test. The estimated $\dot{V}O_2$ max is 2.4 liters · min^{-1}. These estimates of $\dot{V}O_2$ max are influenced by the person's maximal HR, which is known to decrease with age. A correction factor chosen from the accompanying table corrects these $\dot{V}O_2$ max values when either the maximal HR or age is known. Simply multiply the $\dot{V}O_2$ value by the correction factor.

Subject: female, age = 60 years	Data:	
Estimated HR max = 160 b/min	Step rate (lifts/min)	Heart rate (b/min)
85% HR max = 136 b/min	15	112
	21	124
	27	136

Figure 15.9

Use of a step test to predict $\dot{V}O_2$ max from a series of submaximal HR responses.

From E. T. Howley and B. D. Franks, *Health/Fitness Instructor's Handbook.* Copyright © 1986 Human Kinetics Publishers, Inc., Champaign IL. Used by permission.

Step Test

A step-test protocol is used to estimate $\dot{V}O_2$ max in the same way that treadmill and cycle ergometer protocols are used. The step test does not require expensive equipment, the step height does not have to be calibrated, everyone is familiar with the stepping exercise, and the energy requirement is proportional to body weight, as is the treadmill (50). The work rate can be increased by increasing the step height while keeping the cadence the same, or by increasing the cadence while keeping the step height the same. The step height can be varied with a hand-cranking device (59) or by using a series of wooden steps with increments in step height of 10 cm. The rate of stepping is established with a metronome, and the stepping cadence has four counts: up, up, down, down. The subjects must step all the way up and down in time with the metronome. Figure 15.9 shows the results of a step test on a sixty-year-old female. In this step test the height of the step was kept

constant at 16 centimeters and the rate of stepping increased 6 lifts · min^{-1} each two minutes. The line drawn through the HR points is extrapolated to the estimated maximal HR, 160 b · min^{-1}, and a line is dropped to the horizontal axis to estimate the $\dot{V}O_2$ max.

The Åstrand and Ryhming (8) nomogram (figure 15.8) also accommodates a step test, using a rate of 22.5 lifts per minute (metronome = 90) and step heights of 40 cm for men and 33 cm for women. The principle is the same as described for their cycle ergometer protocol.

The recent introduction of step ergometers (i.e., StairMaster 4000) allows a graded exercise test to be conducted in a manner similar to that of a treadmill. The work rates seem to be independent of step rate, while the HR responses are slightly higher than those measured on the treadmill at any $\dot{V}O_2$ (37). Such a test has been shown to measure changes in $\dot{V}O_2$ max that result from either treadmill or step-ergometer training, indicating more commonality than specificity among step and treadmill tests (13).

In summary, there are a variety of tests that can be used to estimate CRF. The usefulness of a test is a function of both the accuracy of the measurement and the ability to repeat the test on a routine basis to evaluate changes in CRF over time. It is this latter point that decreases the need that the test be able to estimate the true $\dot{V}O_2$ max to the nearest ml · kg^{-1} · min^{-1}. In effect, if a person is taking a submaximal GXT on a regular basis and the HR response to a fixed work rate is decreasing over time, one can reasonably conclude that the person is making progress in the intended direction, independent of how accurate the estimate of $\dot{V}O_2$ max is.

in summary

- $\dot{V}O_2$ max can be estimated with the extrapolation procedure using the treadmill, cycle ergometer, or step.
- The subject must follow directions carefully and environmental conditions must be controlled if the estimate of $\dot{V}O_2$ max is to be reasonable and reproducible.

study questions

1. What is the sequence of steps used in evaluating cardiorespiratory fitness?
2. What is a health or cardiac risk inventory? Name one currently in use and explain its purpose.
3. A forty-year-old man runs 1.5 miles (2,415 meters) in ten minutes. What is his estimated $\dot{V}O_2$ max? Is his value "normal"?
4. Draw an example of ST segment depression and describe its significance in the diagnosis of heart disease.
5. You are monitoring a GXT in which $\dot{V}O_2$ max is measured. How would you know if a person achieved $\dot{V}O_2$ max?
6. Given the following information collected during a treadmill test on a fifty-year-old man, estimate his $\dot{V}O_2$ max.

Work Rate	Heart Rate
3 METs	110
5 METs	125
7 METs	140

7. Given the assumption that the formula, 220 − age, can be used to estimate maximal heart rate, how far off could you be in your estimate of $\dot{V}O_2$ max in question 6?

8. What information do you gain by monitoring the RPE during a GXT?

9. List five reasons for stopping a GXT.

10. Should you use the same GXT protocol on all subjects? Why or why not?

suggested readings

American College of Sports Medicine. 1995. *ACSM's Guidelines for Exercise Testing and Prescription*. 5th ed. Baltimore: Williams & Wilkins.

Dubin, D. 1974. *Rapid Interpretation of EKGs*. 3d ed. Tampa, FL: Cover.

Pollock, M. L., and J. H. Wilmore. 1990. *Exercise in Health and Disease*. 2d ed. Philadelphia: W. B. Saunders.

references

1. Aitken, J. C., and J. Thompson. 1988. The respiratory $\dot{V}CO_2/\dot{V}O_2$ exchange ratio during maximum exercise and its use as a predictor of maximum oxygen uptake. *European Journal of Applied Physiology* 57:714–19.

2. American Alliance for Health, Physical Education, Recreation and Dance. 1988. *Physical Best*. Reston, VA.

3. American College of Sports Medicine. 1995. *ACSM's Guidelines for Exercise Testing and Prescription*. 5th ed. Baltimore: Williams & Wilkins.

4. Åstrand, I. 1960. Aerobic work capacity in men and women with special reference to age. *Acta Physiologica Scandinavica* 49 (Suppl.) 169.

5. Åstrand, P. O. 1952. *Experimental Studies of Physical Working Capacity in Relation to Sex and Age*. Copenhagen: Manksgaard.

6. ———. 1984. Principles of ergometry and their implications in sports practice. *International Journal of Sports Medicine* 5:102–5.

7. Åstrand, P. O., and K. Rodahl. 1986. *Textbook of Work Physiology*. New York: McGraw-Hill.

8. Åstrand, P. O., and I. Ryhming. 1954. A nomogram for calculation of aerobic capacity (physical fitness) from pulse rate during submaximal work. *Journal of Applied Physiology* 7:218–21.

9. Åstrand, P. O., and B. Saltin. 1961. Maximal oxygen uptake and heart rate in various types of muscular activity. *Journal of Applied Physiology* 16:977–81.

10. Balke, B. 1963. A simple field test for assessment of physical fitness. *Civil Aeromedical Research Institute Report* 63–66.

11. ———. 1970. Advanced exercise procedures for evaluation of the cardiovascular system. Monograph. Milton, WI: The Burdick Corporation.

12. Bell, D. G., I. Jacobs, and S. W. Lee. 1992. Blood lactate response to the Canadian Aerobic Fitness Test (CAFT). *Canadian Journal of Sport Science* 17:1, 14–18.

13. Ben-Ezra, and R. Verstraete. 1991. Step ergometry: Is it task-specific training? *European Journal of Applied Physiology* 63:261–64.

13a. Blair, S. N., H. W. Kohl III, R. S. Paffenbarger, Jr., D. G. Clark, K. H. Cooper, and L. W. Gibbons. 1990. Physical fitness and all-cause mortality. *Journal of the American Medical Association* 262:2395–2401.

14. Borg, G. A. U. 1982. Psychological bases of physical exertion. *Medicine and Science in Sports and Exercise* 14:377–81.

15. Bruce, R. A. 1972. Multi-stage treadmill tests of maximal and submaximal exercise. In *Exercise Testing and Training of Apparently Healthy Individuals: A Handbook for Physicians*. 32–34. New York: American Heart Association.

16. Carton, R. L., and E. C. Rhodes. 1985. A critical review of the literature on ratings scales for perceived exertion. *Sports Medicine* 2:198–222.

17. Chow, R. J., and J. H. Wilmore. 1984. The regulation of exercise intensity by ratings of perceived exertion. *Journal of Cardiac Rehabilitation* 4:382–87.

18. Conley, D. S., K. J. Cureton, D. R. Dengel, and P. G. Weyand. 1991. Validation of the 12-min swim as a field test of peak aerobic power in young men. *Medicine and Science in Sports and Exercise* 23:766–73.

19. Cooper, K. H. 1977. *The Aerobic Way*. New York: Bantam.

20. Cooper, M., and K. H. Cooper. 1972. *Aerobics for Women*. New York: Evans.

20a. Cureton, K. J., L. D. Hensley, and A. Tiburzi. 1979. Body fatness and performance differences between men and women. *Research Quarterly* 50:333–40.

21. Cureton, K. J., and G. L. Warren. 1990. Criterion-referenced standards for youth health-related fitness tests: A tutorial. *Research Quarterly for Exercise and Sport* 61:7–19.

22. Cureton, K. J. et al. 1978. Effect of experimental alterations in excess weight on aerobic capacity and distance running performance. *Medicine and Science in Sports* 10:194–99.

23. Daniels, J. et al. 1978. Differences and changes in $\dot{V}O_2$ among young runners 10–18 years of age. *Medicine and Science in Sports* 10:200–203.

24. Ebbeling, C. B., A. Ward, E. M. Puleo, J. Widrick, and J. M. Rippe. 1991. Development of a single-stage submaximal treadmill walking test. *Medicine and Science in Sports and Exercise* 23:966–73.

25. Ellestad, M. 1995. *Stress Testing: Principles and Practice*. 4th ed. Philadelphia: F. A. Davis.

26. *Exercise and Your Heart*. 1981. U.S. Department of Health and Human Services. NIH Publication, No. 81-1677.

27. Falls, H., and L. D. Humphrey. 1973. A comparison of methods for eliciting maximal oxygen uptake for college women during treadmill walking. *Medicine and Science in Sports* 5:239–41.

28. Faulkner, J. A. et al. 1971. Cardiovascular responses to submaximum and maximum effort cycling and running. *Journal of Applied Physiology* 30:457–61.

29. Foster, C. et al. 1984. Prediction of oxygen uptake during exercise testing in cardiac patients and health volunteers. *Journal of Cardiac Rehabilitation* 4:537–42.

30. Franklin, B. A. 1985. Exercise testing, training and arm ergometry. *Sports Medicine* 2:100–119.

31. Golding, L. A., C. R. Myers, and W. E. Sinning. 1989. *The Y's Way to Physical Fitness*. Champaign, IL: Human Kinetics.

32. Gutmann, M. C. et al. 1981. Perceived exertion-heart rate relationship during exercise testing and training of cardiac patients. *Journal of Cardiac Rehabilitation* 1:52–59.

33. Hagberg, J. M. et al. 1981. Effect of pedaling rate on submaximal exercise responses of competitive cyclists. *Journal of Applied Physiology* 51:447–51.

34. Haskell, W. L. et al. 1982. Factors influencing estimated oxygen uptake during exercise testing soon after myocardial infarction. *American Journal of Cardiology* 50:299–304.

35. Hermansen, L., and B. Saltin. 1969. Oxygen uptake during maximal treadmill and bicycle exercise. *Journal of Applied Physiology* 26:31–37.

36. Howley, E. T. 1988. Exercise testing laboratory. In *Resource Manual for Guidelines for Exercise Testing and Prescription*, ed. S. N. Blair et al., chap. 47. Philadelphia: Lea & Febiger.

36a. Howley, E. T., D. R. Bassett, Jr., and H. G. Welch. 1995. Criteria for maximal oxygen uptake—review and commentary. *Medicine and Science in Sports and Exercise* 27:1292–1301.

37. Howley, E. T., D. L. Colacino, and T. C. Swensen. 1992. Factors affecting the oxygen cost of stepping on an electronic stepping ergometer. *Medicine and Science in Sports and Exercise* 24:1055–58.

38. Howley, E. T., and B. D. Franks. 1992. *Health/Fitness Instructor's Handbook*. 2d ed. Champaign, IL: Human Kinetics.

39. Howley, E. T., H. J. Montoye, and F. J. Nagle. 1986. Minimal change in $\dot{V}O_2$ max with age in active subjects who maintain body weight. *Medicine and Science in Sports and Exercise* 18:521.

40. Issekutz, B., N. C. Birkhead, and K. Rodahl. 1962. The use of respiratory quotients in assessment of aerobic power capacity. *Journal of Applied Physiology* 17:47–50.

41. Jette, M. et al. 1976. The Canadian Home Fitness Test as a predictor of aerobic capacity. *Canadian Medical Association Journal* 114:680–83.

42. Kasch, F. W., J. L. Boyer, S. P. Van Camp, L. S. Verity, and J. P. Wallace. 1990. The effects of physical activity and inactivity on aerobic power in older men (a longitudinal study). *The Physician and Sportsmedicine* 18:73–83.

43. Kavanagh, T., and R. J. Shephard. 1976. Maximal exercise tests on "postcoronary" patients. *Journal of Applied Physiology* 40:611–18.

44. Kirkendall, W. M. et al. 1980. Recommendations for human blood pressure determination by sphygmomanometers. *Circulation* 62:1146A–1155A.

45. Kitamura, K. et al. 1972. Hemodynamic correlates of myocardial oxygen consumption during upright exercise. *Journal of Applied Physiology* 32:516.

46. Kline, G. M. et al. 1987. Estimation of $\dot{V}O_2$ max from a one-mile track walk, gender, age, and body weight. *Medicine and Science in Sports and Exercise* 19:253–59.

47. Kohl, H. W., L. W. Gibbons, N. F. Gordon, and S. N. Blair. 1990. An empirical evaluation of the ACSM guidelines for exercise testing. *Medicine and Science in Sports and Exercise* 22:533–39.

48. Krahenbuhl, G. S. et al. 1978. Field testing of cardiorespiratory fitness in primary school children. *Medicine and Science in Sports and Exercise* 10:208–13.

49. Londeree, B. R., and M. L. Moeschberger. 1984. Influence of age and other factors on maximal heart rate. *Journal of Cardiac Rehabilitation* 4:44–49.

50. Margaria, R., P. Aghemo, and E. Rovelli. 1965. Indirect determination of maximal $\dot{V}O_2$ consumption in man. *Journal of Applied Physiology* 20:1070–73.

51. Martin, A. D. 1986. ECG and medications. In *Health/Fitness Instructor's Handbook*, eds. E. T. Howley and B. D. Franks, chap. 12. Champaign, IL: Human Kinetics.

52. McArdle, W. D., F. I. Katch, and G. S. Pechar. 1973. Comparison of continuous and discontinuous treadmill and bicycle tests for max $\dot{V}O_2$. *Medicine and Science in Sports and Exercise* 5:156–60.

53. McConnell, T. R. 1988. Practical considerations in the testing of $\dot{V}O_2$ max in runners. *Sports Medicine* 5:57–68.

54. McConnell, T. R., and B. A. Clark. 1987. Prediction of maximal oxygen consumption during handrail-supported treadmill exercise. *Journal of Cardiopulmonary Rehabilitation* 7:324–31.

55. McCormack, W. P., K. J. Cureton, T. A. Bullock, and P. G. Weyand. 1991. Metabolic determinants of 1-mile run/walk performance in children. *Medicine and Science in Sports and Exercise* 23:611–17.

56. Montoye, H. J., and T. Ayen. 1986. Body size adjustment for oxygen requirement in treadmill walking. *Research Quarterly for Exercise and Sport* 57:82–84.

57. Montoye, H. J. et al. 1985. The oxygen requirement for horizontal and grade walking on a motor-driven treadmill. *Medicine and Science in Sports and Exercise* 17:640–45.

58. Montoye, H. J., T. Ayen, and R. A. Washburn. 1986. The estimation of $\dot{V}O_2$ max from maximal and sub-maximal measurements in males, age 10–39. *Research Quarterly for Exercise and Sport* 57:250–53.

59. Nagle, F. J., B. Balke, and J. P. Naughton. 1965. Gradational step tests for assessing work capacity. *Journal of Applied Physiology* 20:745–48.

60. Naughton, J. P., and R. Haider. 1973. Methods of exercise testing. In *Exercise Testing and Exercise Training in Coronary Heart Disease*, eds. J. P. Naughton, H. K. Hellerstein, and L. C. Mohler, 79–91. New York: Academic Press.

61. Nelson, R. R. et al. 1974. Hemodynamic predictors of myocardial oxygen consumption during static and dynamic exercise. *Circulation* 50:1179–89.

62. Oja, P., R. Laukkanen, M. Pasanen, T. Tyry, and I. Vuori. 1991. A 2-km walking test for assessing the cardiorespiratory fitness of healthy adults. *International Journal of Sports Medicine* 12:356–62.

63. Oldridge, N. B., W. L. Haskell, and P. Single. 1981. Carotid palpation, coronary heart disease and exercise rehabilitation. *Medicine and Science in Sports and Exercise* 13:6–8.

63a. Park, R. J. 1989. Measurement of physical fitness: A historical perspective. Washington, D.C.: U.S. Department of Health and Human Services, Public Health Service.

64. Pollock, M. L., and J. H. Wilmore. 1990. *Exercise in Health and Disease.* 2d ed. Philadelphia: W. B. Saunders.

65. Ragg, K. E. et al. 1980. Errors in predicting functional capacity from a treadmill exercise stress test. *American Heart Journal* 100:581–83.

66. Rowell, L. B. 1974. Human cardiovascular adjustments to exercise and thermal stress. *Physiology Reviews* 54:75–159.

67. Sawka, M. N. et al. 1983. Determination of maximal aerobic power during upper-body exercise. *Journal of Applied Physiology: Respiration, Environmental, and Exercise Physiology* 54:113–17.

68. Sedlock, D. A. et al. 1983. Accuracy of subject-palpated carotid pulse after exercise. *The Physician and Sportsmedicine* 11(4):106–16.

69. Sharkey, B. J. 1984. *Physiology of Fitness.* 2d ed. Champaign, IL: Human Kinetics.

70. Shephard, R. J. 1984. Tests of maximal oxygen uptake: A critical review. *Sports Medicine* 1:99–124.

71. Shephard, R. J., D. A. Bailey, and R. L. Mirwald. 1976. Development of the Canadian home fitness test. *Canadian Medical Association Journal* 114:675–79.

72. Shephard, R. J., S. Thomas, and I. Weller. 1991. The Canadian home fitness test: 1991 Update. *Sports Medicine* 11:358–66.

73. Siconolfi, S. F. et al. 1982. Assessing $\dot{V}O_2$ max in epidemiologic studies: Modification of the Åstrand-Ryhming test. *Medicine and Science in Sports and Exercise* 14:335–38.

74. Sidney, K. H., and R. J. Shephard. 1977. Maximum and submaximum exercise tests in men and women in the seventh, eighth, and ninth decades of life. *Journal of Applied Physiology* 43:280–87.

75. Sparling, P. B., and K. J. Cureton. 1983. Biological determinants of the sex difference in 12-minute run performance. *Medicine and Science in Sports and Exercise* 15:218–23.

76. Stamford, B. A. 1976. Step increments versus constant load tests for determination of maximal oxygen uptake. *European Journal of Applied Physiology* 35:89–93.

76a. Strømme, S. B., F. Ingjer, and H. D. Meen. 1977. Assessment of maximal aerobic power in specifically trained athletes. *Journal of Applied Physiology* 42:833–37.

77. Taylor, H. L., E. R. Buskirk, and A. Henschel. 1955. Maximal oxygen intake as an objective measure of cardiorespiratory performance. *Journal of Applied Physiology* 8:73–80.

78. Wallace, J. P. 1983. Physical conditioning: Intervention in aging cardiovascular function. In *Intervention in the Aging Process, Part A: Quantitation, Epidemiology, and Clinical Research,* ed. A. R. Liss, 307–23.

16

Exercise Prescriptions for Health and Fitness

objectives

By studying this chapter, you should be able to do the following:

1. Characterize physical inactivity as a coronary heart disease risk factor comparable to smoking, hypertension, and high serum cholesterol.

2. Contrast "exercise" with "physical activity"; explain how both relate to a lower risk of CHD and improvement in cardiorespiratory fitness (CRF).

3. Describe the "Exercise Lite" program recommended by the American College of Sports Medicine and the Centers for Disease Control and Prevention to improve the health status of U.S. adults.

4. Explain what "screening" and "progression" mean for a person wishing to initiate an exercise program.

5. Identify the optimal frequency, intensity, and duration of activity associated with improvements in CRF; why is more not necessarily better than less?

6. Calculate a target heart rate range by either the heart rate range or percent of maximal HR methods.

7. Explain why the appropriate sequence of physical activity for sedentary persons is walk → walk/jog → jog → games.

8. Explain how the target heart rate (THR) helps adjust exercise intensity in times of high heat, humidity, or while at altitude.

outline

Prescription of Exercise   286
  Dose-Response   287
  Physical Activity and Health   287
General Guidelines for Improving Fitness   289
  Screening   289
  Progression   289
  Warm-Up, Stretch, and Cool-Down, Stretch   290

Exercise Prescription for CRF   290
  Frequency   290
  Duration   290
  Intensity   291
Sequence of Physical Activity   292
  Walking   292
  Jogging   293
  Games and Sports   294

Strength Training   294
Environmental Concerns   295

key terms

dose
effect (response)

exercise
physical activity

physical fitness
target heart rate (THR) range

n chapter 14 we discussed a variety of risk factors related to cardiovascular and other diseases. Physical inactivity had long been considered only a secondary risk factor in the development of CHD—that is, an inactive life-style would increase a person's risk for CHD only if other primary risk factors were present. However, as explained in chapter 14, this is no longer the case. Recent studies (24, 25, 34, 38) suggest that physical inactivity is a primary risk factor for coronary heart disease (CHD), similar to smoking, hypertension, and high serum cholesterol. These studies also show that regular vigorous physical activity is instrumental in reducing the risk of CHD in those who smoke or are hypertensive (26). Based on this growing body of evidence the American Heart Association recognized physical inactivity as a primary or major risk factor (3). Finally, recent epidemiological studies show that increases in physical activity (26a) and fitness (6a) are associated with a reduced death rate from all causes as well as from CHD. This means that physical activity should be used along with other therapies to reduce the risk of CHD in those possessing other risk factors. Consequently, there is little disagreement that regular physical activity is a necessary part of a healthy life-style. The only question is, how much?

Before we answer this question we need to distinguish among the terms: physical activity, exercise, and fitness. **Physical activity** is defined as any form of muscular activity. Therefore physical activity results in the expenditure of energy proportional to muscular work, and is related to **physical fitness. Exercise** represents a subset of physical activity that is planned, with a goal of improving or maintaining fitness (7). These distinctions, while subtle, are important to understand in our discussion of the role of physical activity as a part of a healthy life-style. For example, there is no question that a planned exercise program will improve $\dot{V}O_2$ max, and that a higher $\dot{V}O_2$ max is associated with a lower death rate (6). However, we must emphasize that physical activity, including that done at a low intensity, is beneficial. The reduction in the risks of CHD due to the latter types of activity may be mediated through changes in the distribution of cholesterol, or an increase in fibrinolysis (clot dissolving) activity (14b). It should be no surprise that the American College of Sports Medicine, in the ACSM's *Guidelines for Exercise Testing and Prescription*, states the need for low-intensity exercise (e.g., brisk walking) throughout the life span (2). Such a recommendation is consistent with exposing the general population to low-risk physical activity to achieve health-related benefits aimed at reducing cardiovascular and metabolic diseases. In contrast to this general recommendation for everyone, there is a need to follow a variety of guidelines in prescribing moderate to strenuous exercise that is aimed at improving $\dot{V}O_2$ max. In this chapter we will address both concerns.

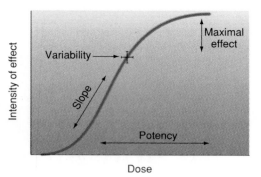

Figure 16.1

The relationship between the dose of a drug (expressed as the log of the dose) and the effect.

Data from L. S. Goodman and A. Gilman, eds., 1975, *The Pharmacological Basis of Therapeutics*. New York: Macmillan Publishing Company.

in summary

- Physical inactivity has been classified as a primary risk factor for coronary heart disease.
- Physical activity can reduce the overall risk for those who smoke or who are hypertensive.
- Those who increase their physical activity and/or cardiorespiratory fitness have a lower death rate from all causes compared to those who remain sedentary.

Prescription of Exercise

The concern about the proper **dose** of exercise needed to bring about a desired **effect (response)** is similar to the physician's need to know the type and quantity of a drug needed, as well as the time frame over which it must be taken, to cure a disease. Clearly, there is a difference in what is needed to cure a headache compared to what is needed to cure tuberculosis. In the same way there is no question that the dose of physical activity needed to achieve high level running performance is different from that required to improve a health-related outcome (e.g., lower blood pressure) or fitness (e.g., an increase in $\dot{V}O_2$ max). This dose-response relationship for medications is described in figure 16.1.

- *Potency.* The potency of a drug is a relatively unimportant characteristic of a drug in that it makes little difference whether the effective dose of a drug is 1 μg or 100 mg as long as it can be administered in an appropriate dosage. Applied to exercise, walking four miles is as effective in expending calories as running two miles (11b).
- *Slope.* The slope of the curve gives some information about how much of a change in effect is obtained from a change in dose. Some physiological measures change quickly for a given dose of exercise, while some

Section Two Physiology of Health and Fitness

health-related effects require the application of exercise over many months to see a desired outcome (11b).

- *Maximal effect.* The maximal effect (efficacy) of a drug varies with the type of drug. For example, morphine can relieve pain of all intensities while aspirin is effective against only mild to moderate pain (11b). Similarly, strenuous exercise can cause an increase in $\dot{V}O_2$ max as well as modify risk factors, while light-to-moderate exercise can change risk factors with only a minimal impact on $\dot{V}O_2$ max (an important point we will return to later).

- *Variability.* The effect of a drug varies between individuals, and within individuals depending on the circumstances. The intersecting brackets in figure 16.1 indicate the variability in the dose required to bring about a particular effect, and the variability in the effect associated with a given dose (11b). For example, gains in $\dot{V}O_2$ max due to endurance training show considerable variation, even when the initial $\dot{V}O_2$ max value is controlled for (11a).

- *Side effect.* A last point worth mentioning that can also be applied to our discussion of exercise prescription is that no drug produces a single effect (11b). The spectrum of effects might include adverse (side) effects that limit the usefulness of the drug (e.g., for exercise the side effects might include increased risk of injury or sudden death).

In contrast to drugs that individuals stop taking when a disease is cured, there is a need to engage in some form of physical activity throughout one's life to experience the health-related and fitness effects.

Dose-Response

The exercise dose is usually characterized by the intensity, frequency, duration, and type of activity. The intensity can be described in terms of:

- % $\dot{V}O_2$ max,
- % maximal heart rate,
- rating of perceived exertion, and
- the onset of blood lactate accumulation (the lactate threshold).

The frequency could include:

- number of days per week and
- number of times per day.

The duration of exercise for each exercise session can be given as the:

- number of minutes of exercise,
- total kilocalories (kcal) expended, and
- total kcals expended per kilogram body weight.

The type of exercise relates to whether resistance exercises or cardiovascular endurance exercises are used in the training program. For the latter, we would also distinguish among the effects of walking vs. jogging/running, vs. swimming. Although we know a considerable amount about the role that each of these variables may play in a gain in $\dot{V}O_2$ max, little is known about the minimum or optimal quantities of each variable related to health outcomes (14a).

The response (effect) generated by a particular dose of exercise can include changes in $\dot{V}O_2$ max, resting blood pressure, insulin sensitivity, body weight (percent fat), and depression. Haskell (14, 14a) provided an important insight into how we should rethink our understanding of cause and effect when we study how a dose of physical activity is related to the responses, physical fitness, and health. Physical activity could bring about favorable changes by:

- improving fitness (especially cardiovascular fitness) and thereby, improving health, or
- improving fitness and health simultaneously and separately, or
- improving fitness, but not a specific health outcome, or
- improving some specific health outcome, but not fitness.

It has become clear that improvements in a variety of health-related concerns are not dependent on an increase in $\dot{V}O_2$ max. This is important and provides a transition to our next section.

in summary

- An exercise dose reflects the interaction of the intensity, frequency, and duration of exercise.
- The cause of the health-related response may be related to an improvement in $\dot{V}O_2$ max or may act through some other mechanism, making health-related outcomes and gains in $\dot{V}O_2$ max independent of each other.

Physical Activity and Health

The issue of the proper dose of exercise to bring about a desired effect is a crucial one in the prescription of exercise for both prevention and rehabilitation. Over the past two decades we have learned that the proper dose differs greatly, depending on the outcome. For example, an improvement in some health-related variable (e.g., resting blood pressure) might be accomplished with an exercise intensity lower than that required to achieve an increase in $\dot{V}O_2$ max. In addition, the frequency with which the exercise must be taken to have the desired effect varies with the intensity and the duration of the session (see later discussion).

Figure 16.2

Proposed dose-response relationships between amount of exercise performed/week at 60% to 70% maximum work capacity and changes in blood pressure (BP) and insulin sensitivity (curve to the left side), which appear most sensitive to exercise, maximum oxygen consumption ($\dot{V}O_2$max) and resting heart rate which are parameters of physical fitness (middle curve), and lipid changes such as high density lipoprotein (HDL) (right hand curve).

Certain physiological variables respond very quickly to a "dose" of exercise. For example, we have shown how rapidly the sympathetic nervous system, blood lactate, and heart rate (chapter 13) adapt to exercise training, taking only days to see changes in response. In contrast to these rapid responses to exercise training, a variety of physiological variables such as the capillary number change more slowly. Similarly, when Haskell describes the potential association between physical activity and health he distinguishes between short-term (acute) and long-term (training) responses (14a). The following terms are used to describe the patterns of responses in the weeks following the initiation of a dose of exercise:

- acute responses—occur with one or several exercise bouts but does not improve further
- rapid responses—benefits occur early and plateau
- linear—gains are made continuously over time
- delayed—occurs only after weeks of training

The need for such distinctions can be seen in figure 16.2 which shows proposed dose-response relationships between physical activity, defined as minutes of exercise per week at 60% to 70% of maximal work capacity, and a variety of physiological responses (19a): (1) blood pressure and insulin sensitivity are most responsive to exercise, (2) changes in $\dot{V}O_2$ max

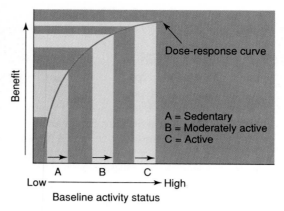

Figure 16.3

The dose-response curve represents the best estimate of the relationship between physical activity (dose) and health benefit (response). The lower the baseline physical activity status, the greater will be the health benefit associated with a given increase in physical activity (arrows A, B, and C).

Data from R. R. Pate, et al., 1995, "Physical Activity and Public Health" in *Journal of the American Medical Association*, 273:402–407. Chicago, IL: American Medical Association.

and resting heart rate are intermediate, and (3) serum lipid changes such as high density lipoprotein (HDL) are delayed.

By this time it should be clear that it is difficult to provide a single exercise prescription that addresses all issues related to prevention and/or treatment of various diseases. However, in spite of this difficulty, there has been a pressing need to spell out a general exercise recommendation to improve the health status of all U.S. adults. The American College of Sports Medicine and the Center for Disease Control and Prevention responded to this need by publishing the "Exercise Lite" guidelines. Their guidelines are based on a comprehensive review of the literature dealing with health-related aspects of physical activity. The dose-response curve in figure 16.3 summarizes their findings. By having the most sedentary group move up to the "A" level of physical activity shown in figure 16.3, the greatest gains in health-related benefits can be realized. It is recommended that **every U.S. adult should accumulate thirty minutes or more of moderate-intensity (3–6 METs) physical activity on most, preferably all, days of the week.** This recommendation is based on the finding that caloric expenditure and total time of physical activity are associated with reduced cardiovascular disease and mortality. Further, doing the activity in intermittent bouts as short as eight to ten minutes is a suitable way of meeting the thirty-minute goal (1a, 26b). However, recent studies question some of the underlying assumptions associated with this recommendation (see A Closer Look 16.1).

Moderate vs. Vigorous Activity

Two sets of guidelines are provided in this chapter: the "Exercise Lite" proposal from ACSM/CDC aimed at getting the most sedentary adults up and moving, and the ACSM position stand on what is needed to increase or maintain $\dot{V}O_2$ max. The former is based on the evidence indicating that the number of calories expended or the number of minutes of activity is the crucial ingredient associated with lower rates of health-related problems and death from all causes. However, a recent paper based on the same Harvard Alumni Health Study challenges some of that thinking (21a). Their data suggest that death from all causes is most clearly linked to vigorous (≥ 6 METs) rather than nonvigorous (< 6 METs) activity. The authors wondered if the reduction in the death rate from all causes was related to an improvement in $\dot{V}O_2$ max, which is brought about more by vigorous than nonvigorous physical activity. In any event, the evidence reinforces the need for more people to be physically active, and where possible, to achieve a moderate level of cardiovascular fitness, which has been shown by itself to be related to a lower death rate from all causes (6).

in summary

- The basis of the "Exercise Lite" recommendation is that the health-related benefits of physical activity may be more related to the total number of calories expended than the intensity of exercise.
- The focus of the "Exercise Lite" exercise prescription is for light-to-moderate activity to be done most, if not all, days of the week for a total of thirty minutes a day.

General Guidelines for Improving Fitness

An increase in moderate physical activity is an important goal related to a reduction in health-related problems. These benefits occur at a point where the overall risk associated with physical activity is relatively small. However, even though the risk of cardiac arrest in habitually active men is higher *during vigorous activity*, the overall (rest + exercise) risk of cardiac arrest in vigorously active men is only 40 percent of the risk in sedentary men (37). Lastly, there is a growing body of evidence indicating that achievement of an average to high level of cardiorespiratory fitness ($\dot{V}O_2$ max) confers additional health benefits, as well as increasing the capacity of the individual to engage in a broad range of recreational activities. The purpose of this section is to review the general guidelines for exercise programs aimed at increasing $\dot{V}O_2$ max. In chapter 13 the concepts of overload and specificity were presented relative to the adaptations that take place with different training programs. While these principles apply here, what is important to remember is that little exercise is needed to achieve a health-related effect. This stands in marked contrast to the intensity of exercise needed to achieve performance goals (see chapter 21).

in summary

- In previously sedentary subjects, small changes in physical activity result in large health benefits with only minimal risk.
- Strenuous exercise increases the risk of a heart attack during the activity, but reduces the overall (rest + exercise) risk of such an event.
- Moderate to high levels of cardiorespiratory fitness reduce the risk of death from all causes.

Screening

The first thing to do, if not already done in the evaluation of CRF, is to carry out some form of health status screening to decide who should begin an exercise program and who should obtain further consultation with a physician (see chapter 15 for details).

Progression

The emphasis in any health-related exercise program is to do too little rather than too much. By starting slowly and progressing from the easily accomplished activities to those that are more difficult, the chance of causing muscle soreness and of aggravating old injuries is reduced. The emphasis on slow-to-moderate walking as the primary activity early in the fitness program is consistent with this recommendation, and the participant must be educated not to move too quickly into the more demanding activities. Once the person can walk about four miles without fatigue, the progression to a walk-jog and jogging program is a reasonable recommendation (19).

Figure 16.4

Effects of increasing the frequency, duration, and intensity of exercise on the increase in $\dot{V}O_2$ max in a training program. This figure demonstrates the increasing risk of orthopedic problems due to exercise sessions that are too long, or conducted too many times per week. The probability of cardiac complications increases with exercise intensity beyond that recommended for improvements in cardiorespiratory fitness.

Warm-Up, Stretch, and Cool-Down, Stretch

Prior to the actual activity used in the exercise session, a variety of very light exercises and stretches are done to improve the transition from rest to the exercise state. The emphasis at the onset of an exercise session is to gradually increase the level of activity until the proper intensity is reached. Stretching exercises to increase the range of motion of the joints involved in the activity, as well as specific stretches to increase the flexibility of the lower back, are included in the warm-up. At the end of the activity session, about five minutes of cool-down activities—slow walking and stretching exercises—are recommended to gradually return HR and BP toward normal. This part of the exercise session is viewed as important in reducing the chance of a hypotensive episode after the exercise session (19).

Exercise Prescription for CRF

The exercise program includes dynamic large muscle activities such as walking, jogging, running, swimming, cycling, rowing, and dancing. The CRF training effect of exercise programs is dependent on the proper frequency, duration, and intensity of the exercise sessions. An exercise program conducted three to five times per week, for twenty to sixty minutes per session, at an intensity of about 50%–85% $\dot{V}O_2$ max, has been shown to cause appropriate CRF effects (1, 2). The combination of duration and intensity should result in the expenditure of about 200–300 kcal per session, and is consistent with achieving weight loss goals and reducing the risk factors associated with CHD (1, 2, 14b, 27, 28).

Frequency

Improvements in CRF increase with the frequency of exercise sessions, with two sessions being the minimum, and the gains in CRF leveling off after three to four sessions per week (2, 41). Gains in CRF can be achieved with a two-day-per-week program, but the intensity has to be higher than the three-day-per-week program, and participants might not achieve weight loss goals (28). The schedule of three to four days per week includes a day off between sessions and reduces the scheduling problems associated with planned exercise programs. Figure 16.4 shows that higher frequencies are associated with higher rates of injuries (11, 30).

Duration

The duration has to be viewed together with intensity, in that the total work accomplished per session (200–300 kcal) seems to be the most important variable associated with improvements in CRF once the minimal threshold of intensity is achieved (2). This is important given that many sedentary persons could more easily accomplish an exercise session of low intensity and long duration than the reverse, and achieve the health-related benefits of physical activity with minimal risk. For example, an 80-kg (176 lb) person walking at about 3.5 mph would consume O_2 at the rate of 1 liter per minute. Given 5 kcal per liter of O_2, the person is using 5 $kcal \cdot min^{-1}$, and sixty minutes of walking would be required to expend 300 kcal. As the intensity of exercise increases, the duration needed to expend 300 kcal decreases. Figure 16.4 shows that doing strenuous exercise (75% $\dot{V}O_2$ max) for more than thirty minutes per session increases the risk of orthopedic problems.

Intensity

Intensity describes the overload on the cardiovascular system that is needed to bring about a training effect. Improvements in CRF occur when the intensity is between 50%–85% $\dot{V}O_2$ max. The intensity threshold for a training effect for those at the low end of the CRF continuum is about 50% $\dot{V}O_2$ max, when coupled with the right duration. Those at the top end of the CRF continuum can work at 85% $\dot{V}O_2$ max to achieve their goals. For most people, 60%–80% $\dot{V}O_2$ max seems to be a range sufficient to achieve CRF goals (1, 2). It appears that in order for this information to be useful, the exercise leader has to know the energy requirements ($\dot{V}O_2$) of all the fitness activities so that a correct match can be made between the activity and the participant. Fortunately, because of the linear relationship between exercise intensity and HR, the exercise intensity can be set by using the HR values equivalent to 60%–80% $\dot{V}O_2$ max. The range of heart rate values associated with the exercise intensity needed to have a CRF training effect is called the **target heart rate (THR) range.** How do you determine the THR range?

Direct Method

Figure 16.5 shows the HR response of a twenty-year-old subject during a maximal GXT on a treadmill. The subject's $\dot{V}O_2$ max was 12 METs, so that 60% and 80% $\dot{V}O_2$ max is equal to about 7.2 and 9.6 METs, respectively. A line is drawn from each of these work rates up to the HR/$\dot{V}O_2$ line, and over to the y-axis where the HR values equivalent to these work rates are obtained. These HR values, 138–164 b · min^{-1}, represent the THR range, the proper intensity for a CRF training effect (1, 19).

Indirect Methods

The THR range can also be estimated by some simple calculations, knowing that the relationship between HR and $\dot{V}O_2$ is linear. The heart rate reserve, or Karvonen method of calculating a THR range has three simple steps (20, 21):

1. Subtract resting HR from maximal HR to obtain HR reserve (HRR).
2. Take 60% and 80% of the HRR.
3. Add each HRR value to resting HR to obtain the THR range.

For example:

1. If a subject has a maximal HR of 200 b · min^{-1} and a resting HR of 60 b · min^{-1}, then the HRR is 140 b · min^{-1} (200 − 60).
2. 60% × 140 b · min^{-1} = 84 b · min^{-1} and 80% × 140 b · min^{-1} = 112 b · min^{-1}.
3. 84 b · min^{-1} + 60 b · min^{-1} = 144 b · min^{-1} 112 b · min^{-1} + 60 b · min^{-1} = 172 b · min^{-1}. The THR range is 144 − 172 b · min^{-1}.

Figure 16.5

Target heart rate range determined from the results of an exercise stress test. The heart rate values measured at work rates equal to 60% and 80% $\dot{V}O_2$ max constitutes the THR range.

This method gives reasonable estimates of the exercise intensity because 60%–80% of the HRR is equal to about 60%–80% $\dot{V}O_2$ max (31).

The other indirect method of calculating the THR range is the *percentage of maximal* HR method. In this method you simply take 70% and 85% of maximal HR to obtain the THR range. In the following example the subject has a maximal HR of 200 b · min^{-1}. The THR range for this person is 140–170 b · min^{-1} (70% × 200 = 140 b · min^{-1}; 85% × 200 = 170 b · min^{-1}). Seventy percent of maximal HR is equal to about 55% $\dot{V}O_2$ max, and 85% of maximal HR is equal to about 75% $\dot{V}O_2$ max, both within the intensity range needed for CRF gains (15, 16, 17, 22).

Table 16.1 lists the relationship between % $\dot{V}O_2$ max, % HRR, and % maximal HR. The intensity of exercise can be prescribed by the direct method, or by either of the indirect methods. Both of the indirect methods require knowledge of the maximal HR. If the maximal HR is measured during a maximal GXT, use it in the calculations. However, if you have to use the age-adjusted estimate of maximal HR (220 − age), remember the potential error, with the standard deviation of the estimate equal to ±11 b · min^{-1}. The estimated THR range is a guideline for exercise intensity and is meant to be used with other information (abnormal symptoms or signs) to determine if the exercise intensity is reasonable.

In this regard, Borg's RPE scale can be used in prescribing exercise intensity for apparently healthy persons. Exercise perceived as "somewhat hard," 12–14 on the original RPE scale (4 on the new RPE scale), approximates 70%–85% of maximal HR (1, 5, 10, 12, 13,

Table 16.1 Relationship of Percent of HR Max, HRR[a], and %$\dot{V}O_2$ Max

% Max $\dot{V}O_2$	% HRR	% Max HR
50	50	66
55	55	70
60	60	74
65	65	77
70	70	81
75	75	85
80	80	88
85	85	92
90	90	96

[a]HRR is the difference between max HR and resting HR.

From E. T. Howley and B. D. Franks, *Health/Fitness Instructor's Handbook*, 2d ed. Copyright © 1992 Human Kinetics Publishers, Inc., Champaign IL. Used by permission. Based on data from Londeree and Ames (22) and Pollock and Wilmore (31).

31). The RPE scale is helpful because the participant learns to associate the THR range with a certain whole-body perception of effort, decreasing the need for frequent pulse rate measurements. The RPE scale has been shown to have a high test-retest reliability (9), and is closely linked to the % $\dot{V}O_2$ max and lactate threshold, independent of the mode of exercise and fitness of the subject (18, 35, 36). Remember, the intensity threshold needed to achieve CRF goals is lower for the less fit, and vice versa.

in summary

- A sedentary person needs to go through a health status screening prior to participating in exercise.
- Exercise programs for previously sedentary persons should start with low-intensity activities (walking), and the person should not progress until he or she can walk about four miles comfortably.
- The optimal characteristics of an exercise program are: intensity = 60%–80% $\dot{V}O_2$ max; frequency = three to four times per week; duration = minutes needed to expend about 200–300 kcal.
- The THR range, taken as 60%–80% HRR, or 70%–85% of maximal HR, is a reasonable estimate of the proper exercise intensity.
- The intensity threshold for a training effect is low (≤50% $\dot{V}O_2$ max) for the deconditioned, and high (≥80% $\dot{V}O_2$ max) for the very fit.

In order to determine if the subject is in the THR range during the activity, HR should be checked immediately after stopping, taking a ten-second pulse count within the first fifteen seconds. The pulse can be taken at the radial artery or the carotid artery; if the latter is used, the participant should use only light pressure, since heavy pressure can actually slow the HR (19, 31).

The proper intensity, frequency, and duration of exercise needed to have a CRF training effect were discussed in the previous section. It is important that sedentary individuals start slowly before exercising at the recommended intensities specified in the THR range. The next section provides some directions to make that transition.

Sequence of Physical Activity

The old adage that you should "walk before you run" is consistent with the way exercise should be recommended to sedentary persons, be they young or old. Once the person demonstrates an ability to do prolonged walking without fatigue, then controlled fitness exercises conducted at a reasonable intensity (THR) can be introduced. After that, and depending on the interest of the participant, a variety of fitness activities that are more game-like can be included. This section will deal with this sequence of activities that can lead to a fit life (19).

Walking

The primary activity to recommend to someone who has been sedentary for a long period of time is walking. This recommendation is consistent with the introductory material on health benefits, and deals with the issue of injuries associated with more strenuous physical activity. In addition, there is good reason to believe that some subjects, especially the obese and the elderly, may use walking as their primary form of exercise. The emphasis at this stage is to simply get people active by providing an activity that can be done anywhere, anytime, and with anyone, young or old. In this way, the number of possible interfering factors that can result in the discontinuance of the exercise is reduced.

The person should choose comfortable shoes that are flexible, offer a wide base of support, and have a fitted heel cup. There are a great number of "walking" shoes available, but a special pair of shoes is not usually required. The emphasis is on getting started; if walking becomes a "serious" activity, or leads to hiking, then the investment would be reasonable. If weather is not to interfere with the activity, then proper selection of clothing is necessary. The participant should wear light, loose-fitting clothing in warm weather, and layers of wool or polypropylene in cold weather. For those who cannot bear the extremes in temperature and humidity out of doors, various shopping malls provide a controlled environment with a smooth surface. Walkers

Walking Program

Rules:

1. Start at a level that is comfortable for you.
2. Be aware of new aches or pains.
3. Don't progress to the next level if you are not comfortable.
4. Monitor your heart rate and record it.
5. It would be healthful to walk at least every other day.

Stage	Duration	Heart rate	Comments
1	15 min	_____	_____
2	20 min	_____	_____
3	25 min	_____	_____
4	30 min	_____	_____
5	30 min	_____	_____
6	30 min	_____	_____
7	35 min	_____	_____
8	40 min	_____	_____
9	45 min	_____	_____
10	45 min	_____	_____
11	45 min	_____	_____
12	50 min	_____	_____
13	55 min	_____	_____
14	60 min	_____	_____
15	60 min	_____	_____
16	60 min	_____	_____
17	60 min	_____	_____
18	60 min	_____	_____
19	60 min	_____	_____
20	60 min	_____	_____

Reprinted, by permission, from B. D. Franks and E. T. Howley, 1989, *Fitness Leader's Handbook*, Champaign IL: Human Kinetics Publishers), 136. This form may be copied by the fitness leader for distribution to participants.

should choose the areas in which they walk with care in order to avoid damaged streets, high traffic zones, and poorly lighted areas. Safety is important in any health-related exercise program (19).

A walking program is presented in A Closer Look 16.2 (19). The steps are rather simple in that progression to the next stage does not occur unless the individual feels comfortable at the current stage. The HR should be recorded as described above, but the emphasis is not on achieving the THR. Later on in the walking program when higher walking speeds are used, the THR zone will be attained. Remember that walking, in spite of not being very strenuous by the THR zone scale, when combined with long duration is an effective part of a weight control and CHD risk factor reduction program (25, 32). Walking is an activity that many people find they can do every day, providing many opportunities to expend calories.

Jogging

Jogging begins when a person moves at a speed and form that results in a period of flight between foot strikes; this may be 3 or 4 mph, or 6 or 7 mph,

depending on the fitness of the individual. As described in chapter 6, the net energy cost of jogging/running is about twice that of walking (at slow to moderate speeds), and requires a greater cardiovascular response. This is not the only reason for the jogging program to follow a walking program; there is also more stress on joints and muscles due to the impact forces that must be tolerated during the push off and landing of jogging (8).

The emphasis at the start of a jogging program is to make the transition from the walking program in such a way as to minimize the discomfort associated with the introduction of any new activity. This is accomplished by beginning with a jog-walk-jog program that eases the person into jogging by mixing in the lower energy cost and trauma associated with walking. The jogging speed is set according to the THR, with the aim to stay at the low end of the THR zone at the beginning of the program. As the participant adapts to jogging, the HR response for any jogging speed will decrease and jogging speed will have to be increased to stay in the THR zone. This is the primary marker that a training effect is taking place. A Closer Look 16.3

A Closer Look 16.3

Jogging Program

Rules:

1. Complete the Walking Program before starting this program.
2. Begin each session with walking and stretching.
3. Be aware of new aches and pains.
4. Don't progress to the next level if you are not comfortable.
5. Stay at the low end of your THR zone; record your heart rate for each session.
6. Do the program on a work-a-day, rest-a-day basis.

Stage 1
Jog 10 steps, walk 10 steps. Repeat five times and take your heart rate. Stay within THR zone by increasing or decreasing walking phase. Do 20–30 minutes of activity.

Stage 2
Jog 20 steps, walk 10 steps. Repeat five times and take your heart rate. Stay within THR zone by increasing or decreasing walking phase. Do 20–30 minutes of activity.

Stage 3
Jog 30 steps, walk 10 steps. Repeat five times and take your heart rate. Stay within THR zone by increasing or decreasing walking phase. Do 20–30 minutes of activity.

Stage 4
Jog 1 minute, walk 10 steps. Repeat three times and take your heart rate. Stay within THR zone by increasing or decreasing walking phase. Do 20–30 minutes of activity.

Stage 5
Jog 2 minutes, walk 10 steps. Repeat two times and take your heart rate. Stay within THR zone by increasing or decreasing walking phase. Do 30 minutes of activity.

Stage 6
Jog 1 lap (400 meters, or 440 yards) and check heart rate. Adjust pace during run to stay within the THR zone. If heart rate is still too high, go back to the Stage 5 schedule. Do 6 laps with a brief walk between each.

Stage 7
Jog 2 laps and check heart rate. Adjust pace during run to stay within the THR zone. If heart rate is still too high, go back to Stage 6 activity. Do 6 laps with a brief walk between each.

Stage 8
Jog 1 mile and check heart rate. Adjust pace during the run to stay within THR zone. Do 2 miles.

Stage 9
Jog 2–3 miles continuously. Check heart rate at the end to ensure that you were within THR zone.

Reprinted, by permission, from B. D. Franks and E. T. Howley, 1989, *Fitness Leader's Handbook*, Champaign IL: Human Kinetics Publishers), 137. This form may be copied by the fitness leader for distribution to participants.

presents a jogging program with some simple rules to follow. Special attention is made to completing the walking program first, staying in the THR zone, and not progressing to the next level if the participant is not comfortable with the current level. Jogging is not for everyone, and for those who are obese, or have ankle, knee, or hip problems, it might be a good activity to avoid. Two activities that reduce such stress are cycling (stationary or outdoor) and swimming (19). More on exercise for special populations will be presented in the next chapter.

Games and Sports

As a person becomes accustomed to exercising in the THR range while jogging, swimming, or cycling, more uncontrolled activities can be introduced that require higher levels of energy expenditure, but do so in a more intermittent fashion. Games (paddleball, racquetball, squash), sports (basketball, soccer), and various forms of exercise to music can keep a person's interest and make it more likely that the person will maintain a physically active life. These activities should be built on a walk-and-jogging base to reduce the chance that the participant will make poor adjustments to the activity. In addition, by having the habit of walking or jogging (swimming or cycling), the participant will still be able to maintain his or her habit of physical activity when there is no one to play with or lead the class. In contrast to jogging, cycling, or swimming, it will be more difficult to stay in the THR range with these intermittent activities. It is more likely that the HR will move from below the threshold value to above the top end of the THR from time to time. This is a normal response to activities that are intermittent in nature. It must be stressed, however, that when playing games it is important that the participants have some degree of skill and be reasonably well matched. If one is much better than the other, neither will have a good workout (23).

Strength Training

The focus in this chapter has been on training to improve cardiorespiratory fitness. In its most recent position stand on the issue of exercise and fitness, the American College of Sports Medicine has added strength training, one goal of which is to maintain lean body mass. The latter variable is important in maintaining energy balance over the life span (see chapter 18 for details). Strength is also essential to allow individuals to do the activities of daily living comfortably and safely. The recommendation is for dynamic resistance exercises requiring a full range of motion at an intensity that would cause fatigue in ten to twelve repetitions. A minimum of eight to ten different exercises should be done to involve the major muscle groups, and the routine should be performed at least twice a week. The exercise can be done using resistance-training equipment, or could include traditional calisthenics in which body weight is the resistance (1). The interested reader is referred to a recent review of the health- and performance-related benefits of resistance training (39).

Environmental Concerns

It is important that the participant be educated about the effects of extreme heat and humidity, altitude, and cold on the adaptation to exercise. The THR range acts as a guide in that it provides feedback to the participant about the interaction of the environment and the exercise intensity. As the heat and humidity increase, there is an increased need to circulate additional blood to the skin to dissipate the heat. As altitude increases,

there is less oxygen bound to hemoglobin and the person must pump more blood to the muscles to have the same oxygen delivery. In both of these situations the HR response to a fixed work bout will be higher. To counter this tendency and stay in the THR range, the subject should decrease the work rate. Exercise in most cold environments can be refreshing and safe if a person plans in advance and dresses accordingly. However, there are some temperature/wind combinations that should be avoided because of the inability to adapt to them. As mentioned previously, some people simply plan exercise indoors (shopping malls, health spas, home exercise) during those occasions so that their routine is not interrupted. These environmental factors will be considered in more detail in chapter 24.

in summary

- The THR acts as a guide to adjust exercise intensity in adverse environments such as high temperature and humidity, or altitude.
- A decrease in exercise intensity will counter the effects of high environmental temperature and humidity to allow one to stay in the target HR zone.

study questions

1. What are the practical implications of classifying physical inactivity as a primary risk factor?
2. From a public health standpoint, why is there so much attention paid to increasing a sedentary person's physical activity by a small amount rather than recommending strenuous exercise?
3. What is the risk of cardiac arrest for someone who participates in a regular physical activity program?
4. What is the difference between "exercise" and "physical activity"?
5. List the optimal frequency, intensity, and duration of exercise needed to achieve an increase in cardiorespiratory function.
6. For a person with a maximal heart rate of 180 b · min^{-1} and a resting heart rate of 70 b · min^{-1}, calculate a target heart rate range by the Karvonen method and the percent of maximal HR method.
7. Recommend an appropriate progression of activities for a sedentary person wishing to become fit.
8. Why is it important to monitor heart rate frequently during exercise in heat, humidity, and at altitude?

suggested readings

Howley, E. T., and B. Don Franks. 1992. *Health/Fitness Instructor's Handbook*. 2d edition. Champaign, IL: Human Kinetics.

Nieman, D. C. 1990. *Fitness and Sports Medicine: An Introduction*. Palo Alto, CA: Bull.

Pollock, M. L. and J. H. Wilmore. 1990. *Exercise in Health and Disease*. 2d edition. Philadelphia: W. B. Saunders.

references

1. American College of Sports Medicine. 1990. Position stand: The recommended quantity and quality of exercise for developing and maintaining cardiorespiratory and muscular fitness in healthy adults. *Medicine and Science in Sports and Exercise* 22:265–74.

1a. ———. 1993. Summary statement: Workshop on physical activity and public health. *Sports Medicine Bulletin* 28:7.

2. ———. 1995. *ACSM's Guidelines for Exercise Testing and Prescription*. Baltimore: Williams & Wilkins.

3. American Heart Association. 1992. Statement on exercise. *Circulation* 86:340–44.

4. Badenhop, D. T. et al. 1983. Physiologic adjustments to higher- or lower-intensity exercise in elders. *Medicine and Science in Sports and Exercise* 15:496–502.

5. Birk, T. J., and C. A. Birk. 1987. Use of ratings of perceived exertion for exercise prescription. *Sports Medicine* 4:1–8.

6. Blair, S. N., H. W. Kohl III, R. S. Paffenbarger, Jr., D. G. Clark, K. H. Cooper, and L. W. Gibbons. 1989. Physical fitness and all-cause mortality. *Journal of the American Medical Association* 262:2395–2401.

6a. Blair, S. N. et al. 1995. Changes in physical fitness and all-cause mortality. *Journal of the American Medical Association* 273:1093–98.

7. Caspersen, C. J., K. E. Powell, and G. M. Christenson. 1985. Physical activity, exercise, and physical fitness: Definitions and distinctions for health-related research. *Public Health Reports* 100:126–31.

8. Cavanagh, P. R. 1980. *The Running Shoe Book*. Mountain View, CA: Anderson World.

9. Ceci, R., and P. Hassmen. 1991. Self-monitored exercise at three different RPE intensities in treadmill and field running. *Medicine and Science in Sports and Exercise* 23:732–38.

10. Chow, R. J., and J. H. Wilmore. 1984. The regulation of exercise intensity by ratings of perceived exertion. *Journal of Cardiac Rehabilitation* 4:382–87.

11. Dehn, M. M., and C. B. Mullins. 1977. Physiologic effects and importance of exercise in patients with coronary artery disease. *Cardiovascular Medicine* 2:365.

11a. Dionne, F. T. et al. 1991. Mitochondrial DNA sequence polymorphism, $\dot{V}O_2$ max, and response to endurance training. *Medicine and Science in Sports and Exercise* 23:177–85.

11b. Goodman, L. S., and A. Gilman (eds). 1975. *The Pharmacological Basis of Therapeutics*. New York: Macmillan Publishing Company, Inc.

12. Gutmann, M. C. et al. 1981. Perceived exertion-heart rate relationship during exercise testing and training in cardiac patients. *Journal of Cardiac Rehabilitation* 1:52–59.

13. Hage, P. 1981. Perceived exertion: One measure of exercise intensity. *The Physician and Sportsmedicine* 9(9):136–43.

14. Haskell, W. L. 1985. Physical activity and health: Need to define the required stimulus. *American Journal of Cardiology* 55:4D–9D.

14a. ———. 1994. Dose-response issues from a biological perspective. In *Physical Activity, Fitness, and Health*, eds. C. Bouchard, R. J. Shephard, and T. Stevens. 1030–39. Champaign, IL: Human Kinetics Publishers, Inc.

14b. Haskell, W. L., H. J. Montoye, and D. Orenstein. 1985. Physical activity and exercise to achieve health-related physical fitness components. *Public Health Reports* 100:202–12.

15. Hellerstein, H. K., and R. Ader. 1971. Relationship between percent maximal oxygen uptake (% max $\dot{V}O_2$) and percent maximal heart rate (% MHR) in normals and cardiacs (ASHD). *Circulation* 43–44 (Suppl. II):76.

16. Hellerstein, H. K. et al. 1973. Principles of exercise prescription for normals and cardiac subjects. In *Exercise Training in Coronary Heart Disease*, eds. J. P. Naughton and H. K. Hellerstein, 129–67. New York: Academic Press.

17. Hellerstein, H. K., and B. A. Franklin. 1984. Exercise testing and prescription. In *Rehabilitation of the Coronary Patient* 2d ed., N. K. Wenger and H. K. Hellerstein, 197–284. New York: John Wiley & Sons.

18. Hetzler, R. K., R. L. Seip, S. H. Boutcher, E. Pierce, D. Snead, and A. Weltman. 1991. *Medicine and Science in Sports and Exercise* 23:88–92.

19. Howley, E. T., and B. D. Franks. 1992. *Health/Fitness Instructor's Handbook*. 2d ed. Champaign, IL: Human Kinetics.

19a. Jennings, G. L. et al. 1991. What is the dose-response relationship between exercise training and blood pressure? *Annals of Medicine* 23:313–18.

20. Karvonen, J., and T. Vuorimaa. 1988. Heart rate and exercise intensity during sports activities: Practical application. *Sports Medicine* 5:303–12.

21. Karvonen, M. J., E. Kentala, and O. Mustala. 1957. The effects of training heart rate: A longitudinal study. *Annales of Medicinae Experimentalis et Biologiae Fenniae* 35:307–15.

21a. Lee, I-M., C. Hsieh, and R. S. Paffenbarger. 1995. Exercise intensity and longevity in men. *Journal of the American Medical Association* 273:1179–84.

22. Londeree, B. R., and S. A. Ames. 1976. Trend analysis of the % $\dot{V}O_2$ max – HR regression. *Medicine and Science in Sports* 8:122–25.

23. Morgans, L. F. et al. 1987. Heart rate responses during singles and doubles tennis competition. *The Physician and Sportsmedicine* 15(7):67–74.

24. Paffenbarger, R. S., and W. E. Hale. 1975. Work activity and coronary heart mortality. *New England Journal of Medicine* 292 (March 13):545–50.

25. Paffenbarger, R. S., R. T. Hyde, and A. L. Wing. 1986. Physical activity, all cause mortality, and longevity of college alumni. *New England Journal of Medicine* 314 (March 6):605–13.

26. ———. 1990. Physical activity and physical fitness as determinants of health and longevity. In *Exercise, Fitness and Health*, eds. C. Bouchard, R. J. Shephard, T. Stevens, J. R. Sutton, and B. D. McPherson, 33–48. Champaign, IL: Human Kinetics.

26a. Paffenbarger, R. S. et al. 1993. The association of changes in physical-activity level and other lifestyle characteristics with mortality among men. *New England Journal of Medicine* 328:538–45.

26b. Pate, R. R. et al. 1995. Physical activity and public health. *Journal of the American Medical Association* 273:402–7.

27. Pollock, M. L. 1978. How much exercise is enough? *The Physician and Sportsmedicine* 6:50–64.

28. Pollock, M. L. et al. 1972. Effect of training two days per week at different intensities on middle-aged men. *Medicine and Science in Sports* 4:192–97.

29. Pollock, M. L. et al. 1975. Effects of mode of training on cardiovascular functions and body composition of adult men. *Medicine and Science in Sports and Exercise* 7:139–45.

30. Pollock, M. L. et al. 1977. Effects of frequency and duration of training on attrition and incidence of injury. *Medicine and Science in Sports* 9:31–36.

31. Pollock, M. L., and J. H. Wilmore. 1990. *Exercise in Health and Disease* 2d ed. Philadelphia: W. B. Saunders.

32. Porcari, J. P., C. B. Ebbling, A. Ward, P. S. Freedson, and J. M. Rippe. 1989. Walking for exercise testing and training. *Sports Medicine* 8:189–200.

33. Powell, K. E., and R. S. Paffenbarger. 1985. Workshop on epidemiologic and public health aspects of physical activity and exercise: A summary. *Public Health Reports* 100:118–26.

34. Powell, K. E., P. D. Thompson, and C. J. Caspersen. 1987. Physical activity and the incidence of coronary heart disease. *Annals Review of Public Health* 8:253–87.

35. Robertson, R. J. et al. 1990. Cross-modal exercise prescription at absolute and relative oxygen uptake using perceived exertion. *Medicine and Science in Sports and Exercise* 22:653–59.

36. Seip, R. L. et al. 1991. Perceptual responses and blood lactate concentration: Effect of training state. *Medicine and Science in Sports and Exercise* 23:80–87.

37. Siscovick, D. S. et al. 1984. The incidence of primary cardiac arrest during vigorous exercise. *New England Journal of Medicine* 311:874–77.

38. Siscovick, D. S. et al. 1984. Habitual vigorous exercise and primary cardiac arrest: Effect of other risk factors on the relationship. *Journal of Chronic Disease* 37:625–31.

39. Stone, M. H., S. J. Fleck, N. T. Triplett, and W. J. Kraemer. 1991. Health- and performance-related potential of resistance training. *Sports Medicine* 11:210–31.

40. U.S. Department of Health and Human Services. 1990. *Healthy People 2000: National Health Promotion and Disease Prevention Objectives.* Washington, D.C.: U.S. Government Printing Office.

41. Wenger, H. A., and G. J. Bell. 1984. The interactions of intensity, frequency and duration of exercise training in altering cardiorespiratory fitness. *Sports Medicine* 3:346–56.

CHAPTER

17

Exercise for Special Populations

objectives

By studying this chapter, you should be able to do the following:

1. Describe the difference between Type I and Type II diabetes.

2. Contrast how a diabetic responds to exercise when blood glucose is "in control," compared to when it is not.

3. Explain why exercise may complicate the life of a Type I diabetic, while being a recommended and primary part of a Type II diabetic's life-style.

4. Describe the changes in diet and insulin that might be made prior to a diabetic undertaking an exercise program.

5. Describe the sequence of events leading to an asthma attack, and how cromolyn sodium and β-adrenergic agonists act to prevent and/or relieve an attack.

6. Describe the cause of exercise-induced asthma, and how one may deal with this problem.

7. Contrast chronic obstructive pulmonary disease (COPD) with asthma in terms of causes, prognosis, and the role of rehabilitation programs in a return to "normal" function.

8. Identify the types of patient populations that one might see in a cardiac rehabilitation program, and the types of medications that these individuals may be taking.

9. Contrast the type of exercise test used for cardiac populations with the test used for the apparently healthy population.

10. Describe the physiological changes in the elderly that result from an endurance-training program.

11. Describe the guidelines for exercise programs for pregnant women.

outline

Diabetes   300
   Exercise and the Diabetic   301
Asthma   304
   Causes   304
   Prevention/Relief of
      Asthma   304
   Exercise-Induced
      Asthma   305

Chronic Obstructive Pulmonary
   Disease   307
   Testing and Training   307
Hypertension   308
Cardiac Rehabilitation   309
   Population   309
   Testing   309
   Exercise Programs   309

Elderly   310
Pregnancy   312

arrhythmias	diabetic coma	myocardial infarction (MI)
beta receptor agonist (β_2-agonist)	immunotherapy	nitroglycerin
coronary artery bypass graft surgery (CABGS)	insulin shock	percutaneous transluminal coronary angioplasty
cromolyn sodium	ketosis	theophylline
	mast cell	

hapter 16 presented some recommendations for planning an appropriate exercise program for the apparently healthy individual. Exercise has also been used as a primary nonpharmacological intervention for a variety of problems such as obesity and mild hypertension, and as a normal part of therapy for the treatment of diabetes and coronary heart disease. This chapter will discuss the special concerns that must be addressed when exercise is used for populations with specific diseases, disabilities, or limitations. However, the student of exercise science should recognize that this information is introductory in nature. More detailed accounts are cited throughout the chapter.

Diabetes

Diabetes is a major health problem in the United States. More than 12 million have the disease and it is the third largest cause of death by disease. Diabetes injures and kills indirectly by causing blindness, kidney disease, heart disease, stroke, and peripheral vascular disease (3). Diabetics are divided into two distinct groups on the basis of whether or not the diabetes is caused by lack of insulin (Type I), or a resistance to insulin (Type II). Type I, insulin-dependent diabetes, develops primarily in young persons, and is associated with viral (flu-like) infections. The warning signs, which develop quickly, consist of (3):

- frequent urination/unusual thirst,
- extreme hunger,
- rapid weight loss, weakness and fatigue, and
- irritability, nausea, and vomiting.

Since Type I diabetics do not produce adequate insulin, they are dependent on exogenous (injected) insulin to maintain the blood glucose concentration within normal limits. Type II, noninsulin-dependent, diabetes develops more slowly and later in life than does Type I diabetes. Type II diabetes represents about 90 percent of all diabetics (7), and is primarily linked to upper-body or android obesity. The increased mass of fat tissue results in a resistance to insulin, which is usually available in adequate amounts within the body. However, some Type II diabetics may require injectable insulin or an oral medication that stimulates the pancreas to produce additional insulin. The primary treatment of Type II diabetics includes diet and exercise to reduce body weight and to help control plasma glucose. Table 17.1 summarizes the differences between Type I and Type II diabetics (7, 12).

in summary

- Type I, or insulin-dependent, diabetes develops early in life and represents 10 percent of the diabetic population.
- Type II, or insulin-resistant, diabetes occurs later in life and is associated with upper-body or android obesity. Diet and exercise are important parts of the treatment program for Type II diabetes to achieve weight loss and improved insulin sensitivity.

Table 17.1 Summary of the Differences Between Type I and Type II Diabetes

Characteristics	Type I Insulin-Dependent	Type II Noninsulin-Dependent
Another name	Juvenile-onset	Adult-onset
Proportion of all diabetics	~10%	~90%
Age at onset	<20	>40
Development of disease	Rapid	Slow
Family history	Uncommon	Common
Insulin required	Always	Common, but not always
Pancreatic insulin	None, or very little	Normal or higher
Ketoacidosis	Common	Rare
Body fatness	Normal/lean	Generally obese

From Berg (7) and Cantu (12).

Figure 17.1

Effect of prolonged exercise on blood glucose and ketone body levels in normal subjects, diabetics in "control," and diabetics taking an inadequate amount of insulin (ketosis).

From M. Berger, et al., 1977, "Metabolic and Hormonal Effects of Muscular Exercise in Juvenile Type Diabetics" in *Diabetologia*, 13:355–65. Copyright © 1977 Springer-Verlag, New York NY. Reprinted by permission.

Exercise and the Diabetic

In chapter 5 we indicated that exercise increases the rate at which glucose leaves the blood. In this way exercise has been viewed as a useful part of the treatment to maintain blood glucose control for the diabetic. However, this beneficial effect of exercise is dependent on whether or not the diabetic is in reasonable "control" before exercise begins. Control means that the blood glucose concentration is close to normal. Figure 17.1 shows the effect of a prolonged exercise bout on diabetics who were in control versus those who had not taken an adequate amount of insulin. A lack of insulin causes **ketosis,** a metabolic acidosis resulting from the accumulation of too many ketone bodies (short-chain fatty acids). The Type I diabetic who was in control shows a decrease in plasma glucose toward normal values during exercise, suggesting better control. On the other hand, those Type I diabetics who did not inject an adequate amount of insulin before exercise show an increase in plasma glucose (5). Why the difference in response? The controlled diabetic has sufficient insulin such that glucose can be taken up into muscle during exercise, and counter the normal increase in glucose release from the liver due to the action of catecholamines and glucagon (see chapter 5). In contrast, the diabetic with inadequate insulin experiences only a small increase in glucose utilization by muscle, but has the normal increase in glucose release from the liver. This, of course, causes an elevation of the plasma glucose, resulting in a hyperglycemia (67a).

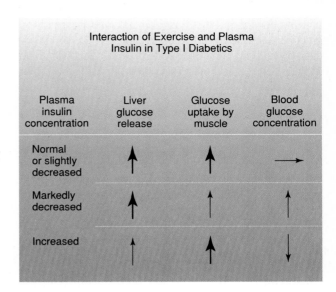

Figure 17.2

Effect of varied plasma insulin levels in Type I diabetics on glucose homeostasis during exercise.

Figure 17.2 summarizes these effects and adds one more (51). If an insulin-dependent diabetic starts exercise with too much insulin, the rate at which plasma glucose is used by muscle is accelerated, while glucose release from the liver is decreased. This causes a very dangerous hypoglycemic response. This information is crucial to understanding how to prescribe exercise for diabetics. Because the importance of exercise as a part of a treatment plan is different for Type I and Type II diabetics, we will discuss each type separately. The reader is referred to Campaigne and Lampman's *Exercise in the Clinical Management of Diabetes* for a detailed presentation on this topic.

Type I Diabetes

For many years exercise was one part of the treatment for Type I diabetes, with insulin and diet being the other two (35). However, as mentioned earlier, if a diabetic is not in control prior to exercise, the ability to maintain a reasonable plasma glucose concentration may be compromised. Further, exercise programs, by themselves, have not been shown to improve control of blood glucose (3a). The greatest concern is not the hyperglycemia and ketosis that can lead to **diabetic coma** when too little insulin is present; rather it is the possibility of hypoglycemia, which can lead to **insulin shock.** Richter and Galbo (51) and Kemmer and Berger (35) point out the difficulties a Type I diabetic has starting an exercise program: the person must maintain a regular exercise schedule in terms of intensity, frequency, and duration, as well as altering diet and insulin. Such regimentation is difficult for some to follow, and given the variability in how a diabetic's blood glucose might respond to exercise on a day-to-day basis, the use of exercise as a primary tool in maintaining metabolic control has been diminished (3a). Because metabolic control can be achieved by altering insulin and diet based on self-monitored blood glucose, exercise complicates this picture (35, 51). However, considering the importance of physical activity in an individual's life, and the effect of regular activity on CHD risk factors, a Type I diabetic should not be discouraged from participation in regular exercise—if there are no complications (35, 51).

The Type I diabetic should have a careful medical exam prior to starting an exercise program. If the diabetic is over the age of thirty-five, has renal disease, or has had diabetes for ten years or more, a graded diagnostic exercise test is recommended. This recommendation is based on the observation that strenuous exercise may accelerate or worsen retina, kidney, or peripheral nerve damage that is already present. The concern for the retina is related to the higher blood pressures developed during exercise, while the concern for the kidney is related to the decrease in blood flow to that organ with increasing intensities of exercise. The peripheral nerve damage may block signals coming from the foot such that serious damage may occur before it is perceived. Proper shoes for exercise, as well as the choice of the activity, are important (11a, 20).

The primary concern to address when exercise is prescribed for the Type I diabetic is the avoidance of hypoglycemia. This is achieved through careful self-monitoring of the blood glucose concentration before, during, and after exercise, and varying carbohydrate intake and insulin depending on the exercise intensity and duration, and the fitness of the individual:

- Before exercise, if the blood glucose concentration is ≤80–100 mg/dl, carbohydrates should be consumed. If it is above 250 mg/dl, exercise should be delayed until it is below 250 mg/dl.
- One should not exercise at the time of peak insulin action, which varies with the type of insulin (short- or intermediate-acting, continuous infusion). The insulin should be injected in a nonexercising muscle group or into a skinfold, and the quantity of insulin injected is usually decreased, the extent depending on the type of insulin.
- Glucose should be monitored frequently during exercise (every fifteen minutes for beginners, and less often for experienced participants), immediately after exercise, and at four to five hours after exercise.
- Additional carbohydrate should be consumed during recovery from exercise. Hypoglycemia might occur following exercise if this is not done since dietary carbohydrate is also being used to replace the depleted muscle glycogen store.

The exercise prescription for the Type I diabetic must also consider other problems associated with this disease: autonomic neuropathy, peripheral neuropathy, retinopathy, and nephropathy. Individuals with autonomic nervous system dysfunction may have abnormal heart rate and blood pressure responses to exercise. Those with peripheral nerve damage may experience pain, impaired balance, weakness, and decreased proprioception. Damage to the retina is common in diabetics, and is aggravated by increased blood pressure or any jarring action directed at the head. Finally, kidney damage is also a common experience for those with Type I diabetes. This can lead to altered blood pressure responses that can affect the retina (11a). It should be no surprise that the exercise prescription for the diabetic must address these problems, if they are present. Recommendations include (11a):

- performing a submaximal exercise test and setting the exercise intensity in terms of heart rate and rating of perceived exertion (RPE) responses based on the blood pressure response to the test,
- using nonweight-bearing, low-impact activities (e.g., water exercise, cycling),
- avoiding heavy weight lifting and the Valsalva maneuver to minimize the blood pressure response. Light weight lifting is acceptable when blood pressure responses are normal,
- drinking more fluid and carrying a readily available form of carbohydrate and adequate identification, and
- exercising with someone who can help in an emergency.

In conclusion, although exercise may not be viewed as a primary factor in maintaining the blood glucose concentration in the normal range, the fact that Type I diabetics who stay physically active have fewer diabetic complications is reason enough to pursue the active life (22a).

in summary

- A sedentary Type I diabetic has to juggle diet and insulin to achieve control of the blood glucose concentration. An exercise program may complicate matters, and therefore exercise is not viewed as a primary means of achieving "control." In spite of this, the diabetic is encouraged to participate in a regular exercise program to experience its health-related benefits.
- The diabetic may have to increase carbohydrate intake and/or decrease the amount of insulin *prior to* activity to maintain the glucose concentration close to normal *during* the exercise. The extent of these alterations is dependent on a number of factors, including the intensity and duration of the physical activity, the blood glucose concentration prior to the exercise, and the physical fitness of the individual.

Type II Diabetes

As mentioned earlier, Type II diabetes occurs later in life, and the patients have a variety of risk factors in addition to their diabetes: hypertension, high cholesterol, obesity, and inactivity (9, 66). There is some epidemiological evidence that Type II diabetes is linked to a lack of physical activity and low fitness, independent of obesity (35a). In contrast to the insulin-dependent diabetic whose life may be more complicated (in terms of blood glucose control) at the start of an exercise program, exercise is a primary recommendation for the Type II diabetic to help deal with both the obesity that is usually present, as well as to help control blood glucose. The combination of exercise and diet may be sufficient, and eliminate the need for insulin or the oral medication used to stimulate insulin secretion (12, 18, 23a). Because Type II diabetics represent about 90 percent of the whole population of diabetics, and because it occurs later in life (after forty years of age), it is not uncommon to see such individuals in adult fitness programs. It is important for clear communication to exist between the participant and the exercise leader, in order to reduce the chance of a "surprise" hypoglycemic response.

Noninsulin-dependent diabetics do not experience the same fluctuations in blood glucose during exercise as do the Type I diabetics (20); however, those taking oral medication to stimulate insulin secretion may have to decrease their dosage to maintain a normal blood glucose concentration (51). The exercise prescription for the Type II diabetic is similar to that described in chapter 16 for improving $\dot{V}O_2$ max: dynamic aerobic activity, done at 70% to 85% maximal heart rate, for 20–60 minutes, 3 to 5 times per week (3b, 11a, 73). Strength training with light weights is also recommended (11a, 60a). However, some important distinctions need to be mentioned.

- The frequency should be as high as 5 to 7 times per week to promote a sustained increase in insulin sensitivity and to facilitate weight loss and weight maintenance.
- There is little to gain by working at or above the top end of the intensity recommendation. Those exercising at 50% $\dot{V}O_2$ max experience the same improvement in insulin sensitivity as those exercising at 70% $\dot{V}O_2$ max (10a).

As with all exercise programs for deconditioned individuals, it is more important to do too little than too much at the start of a program. By starting with light activity and gradually increasing the duration, exercise can be done each day. This will provide an opportunity to learn how to maintain adequate control of blood glucose while minimizing the chance of a hypoglycemic response. In addition, a "habit" of exercise will develop that is crucial if one is to realize the benefits, since the exercise-induced increase in insulin sensitivity does not last long (52, 66). Further,

the combination of intensity, frequency, and duration mentioned above has been shown to directly benefit those with borderline hypertension, a condition often associated with Type II diabetes. Consistent with the recommendations for the Type I diabetic, clear identification and a readily available source of carbohydrate should be carried along in any exercise session. In addition, it would be much safer for a diabetic to exercise with someone who could help out if a problem occurred.

Exercise is only one part of the treatment; diet is the other. The American Diabetes Association (4) states five goals related to nutrition therapy for the diabetic:

- maintain near-normal blood glucose levels by balancing diet and insulin,
- achieve optimal serum lipid levels,
- provide adequate calories to attain reasonable weight,
- prevent long-term complications associated with diabetes, and
- improve overall health through optimal nutrition, using the Dietary Guidelines for Americans and the Food Guide Pyramid (see chapter 18) as guides.

The emphasis in achieving optimal nutrition is through a low-fat (<30%), high-carbohydrate diet to achieve nutrient goals for protein, vitamins, and minerals. The low-fat diet has been shown to be useful in achieving weight-loss and blood lipid goals as well as diabetic control (4). The Type II diabetic secures a variety of benefits from proper exercise and dietary practices: lower body fat and weight (see chapter 18), increased HDL cholesterol, increased sensitivity to insulin (decreasing the need), improved capacity for work, and an improved self-concept (7, 36, 66). These physiological changes should not only improve the prognosis of the Type II diabetic as far as control of blood glucose is concerned, but reduce the overall risk associated with coronary heart disease (51).

in summary

- Type II diabetics have a variety of risk factors in addition to their diabetes, including hypertension, high cholesterol, obesity, and inactivity.
- An exercise prescription emphasizing low-intensity, long-duration activity that is done almost every day will maximize the benefits related to insulin sensitivity and weight loss.
- The dietary recommendation is for a low-fat diet, similar to what is recommended for all Americans for good health, with the additional goals of achieving normal serum glucose and lipid levels.

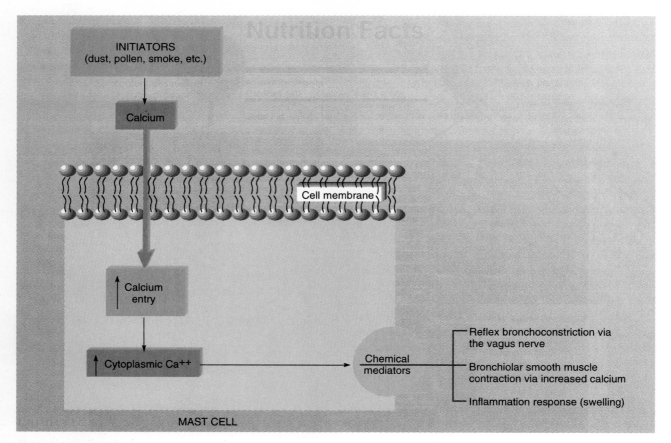

Figure 17.3
Proposed mechanism by which an asthma attack is initiated.

Asthma

Asthma is a respiratory problem characterized by a shortness of breath accompanied by a wheezing sound. It is due to a contraction of the smooth muscle around the airways, a swelling of the mucosal cells, and a hypersecretion of mucous. The asthma can be caused by an allergic reaction, exercise, aspirin, dust, pollutants, and emotion, and can be divided into the following categories (43):

- Extrinsic Asthma—allergen induced, mediated by an immune system reaction
- Intrinsic Asthma—no allergic cause found
- Aspirin-Induced Asthma—10 percent of all asthmatics
- Mixed Asthma—caused by more than one factor

Causes

An asthma attack is the result of an orderly sequence of events that can be initiated by a wide variety of factors. These events are important if we are to understand how certain medications prevent or relieve the asthmatic attack. Figure 17.3 summarizes these events. The focus of attention is on the **mast cell,** one of the cells that is part of tissue in the bronchial tubes. It is believed that a variety of factors such as dust, chemicals, antibodies,

and exercise initiate an asthma attack by increasing Ca^{++} influx into the mast cell, causing a release of chemical mediators such as histamine, and a special chemical that attracts white blood cells. The mediators, in turn, trigger the following effects:

- increase smooth muscle contraction (via an elevation of Ca^{++} in the muscle cell) leading to bronchoconstriction,
- initiate a bronchoconstrictor reflex via the vagus nerve, and
- cause an inflammation response (swelling of tissue).

Given that the vast majority of people do not experience an asthmatic attack while being exposed to the above factors, a "sensitivity" or hyperirritability of the respiratory tract is a necessary prerequisite (43).

Prevention/Relief of Asthma

There are a variety of steps that can be taken to prevent the occurrence of an asthmatic attack, and to provide relief should one occur. If a person is sensitive (allergic) to something, then simple avoidance of the allergen will prevent the problem. If a person cannot avoid contact with the allergen, **immunotherapy** may be helpful in making the person less sensitive to the allergen while being treated.

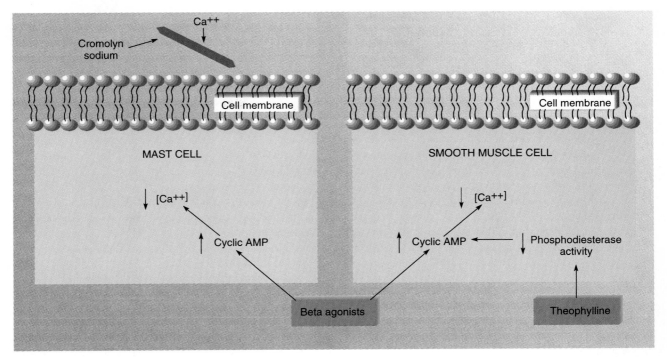

Figure 17.4
Mechanisms by which beta agonists, cromolyn sodium, and theophylline block the events that initiate or maintain an asthma attack.

Drugs have been developed to deal with the mast cell, which is a focal point in the asthmatic response, as well as the bronchiolar smooth muscle that causes the decrease in airway diameter. **Cromolyn sodium** inhibits the chemical mediator release from the mast cell, probably by interfering with Ca^{++} influx into the cell. **Beta receptor agonists (β_2-agonist)** decrease chemical mediator release as well as cause relaxation of bronchiolar smooth muscle by decreasing the Ca^{++} concentration in mast and smooth muscle cells. This effect is brought about through increased adenylate cyclase activity leading to an elevation of cytoplasmic cyclic AMP (see chapter 5). Finally, **theophylline,** a caffeine-like drug, aids in bronchiolar smooth muscle relaxation by inhibiting phosphodiesterase, the enzyme that inactivates cyclic AMP. The result is a higher cyclic AMP and lower Ca^{++} concentration in the cell. The effects of these drugs are summarized in figure 17.4. The net result is that both the inflammation response and the constriction of bronchiolar smooth muscle are blocked.

Exercise-Induced Asthma

A form of asthma that may be of particular interest to the reader is exercise-induced asthma (EIA). The asthmatic attack is caused by exercise and can occur five to fifteen minutes (Early Phase) or four to six hours (Late Phase) after exercise. Approximately 80 percent of asthmatics experience EIA, versus only 3 percent–4 percent of the nonallergic population (65). What is interesting is that 61 percent of the 1984 U.S. Olympic team members with EIA won an Olympic medal. Furthermore, if one compares 1988 Olympic athletes who experienced EIA with the athletes who did not, one finds no difference in the percentage who won medals (34, 44, 65). Clearly, if anyone wondered whether or not EIA can be controlled, those results should dispel any doubts.

Numerous causes of EIA have been identified over the past 100 years. These included cold air, hypocapnia (low PCO_2), respiratory alkalosis, and specific intensities and durations of exercise. The focus of attention is now on the *cooling and drying* of the respiratory tract that occurs when large volumes of dry air are breathed during the exercise session (17, 39b, 56). Respiratory heat loss is related primarily to the rate of ventilation, with the humidity and the temperature of the inspired air being of secondary and tertiary importance. As you remember from chapter 10, when dry air is taken into the lungs it is moistened and warmed as it moves through the respiratory airways. In this way moisture is evaporated from the surface of the airways, which is therefore cooled.

The proposed mechanism for how EIA is initiated takes us back to the mast cell mentioned earlier. When dry air removes water from the surface of the mast cell, an increase in osmolarity occurs. This increase in osmolarity triggers the influx of Ca^{++} that leads to the increased release of chemical mediators and the narrowing of the airways (17, 33, 56). This hypothesis has received strong support from data showing the EIA can be prevented when warm humidified air is breathed. What kind of circumstances bring on EIA?

Screening for Asthma

Asthma is the leading cause of chronic illness and the most common respiratory disorder in children (16a). Concern has been expressed about the need for screening programs early in life to identify those with a high risk of developing asthma. Jones and Bowen (28a) measured peak expiratory flow rate before and after an all-out run in children from ten primary schools. Over a six year follow-up period they compared children who had a negative result with those who had a positive result (a decrease in peak expiratory flow rate of ≥15%) due to the exercise test. Of the 864 children not known to have asthma, 60 had a positive test result. A follow-up of 55 of these 60 children showed 32 had developed clinically recognizable asthma six years later. These children also had a significantly higher prevalence of respiratory illnesses. Such field tests have much to offer in gaining control over this disease.

The probability of an exercise-induced bronchospasm is related to the type of exercise, the time since the previous bout of exercise, the interval since medication was taken, and the temperature and humidity of the inspired air (56). It has been known since the late 1600s that certain types of exercise cause an attack more readily than others. Running was observed to cause more attacks than cycling or walking which, in turn, caused more than swimming. Interestingly, this old observation still finds support in studies in which the temperature and the humidity of the inspired air are controlled. Running still caused more severe attacks than did swimming, even with oxygen consumption and ventilation matched (56).

Generally, EIA is precipitated more with strenuous, long-duration exercise than the reverse (33, 56). One way to deal with this is to do short-duration exercise (<5 min) at low to moderate intensities. Further, when an exercise session occurs within sixty minutes of a previous EIA attack, the degree of bronchospasm is reduced (17). This suggests that a warm-up within an hour of more strenuous exercise would reduce the severity of an attack, and there is good evidence to support that proposition (41a).

There was special concern for the athletes of the 1984 Olympic Games, given the pollution in Los Angeles, which can aggravate an EIA attack (47). As mentioned before, the fact that 61 percent of the athletes who experienced EIA won Olympic medals suggests that procedures for preventing EIA with medication are generally established. Voy (65) reports that a simple questionnaire identified 90 percent of the athletes with EIA, even though only 52 percent were receiving treatment prior to the Olympics (see A Closer Look 17.1). The medications mentioned earlier were used to manage the condition to allow the athletes to go "all out."

In a majority of cases EIA can be prevented when β_2-agonists are used prior to athletic performance (10b). Cromolyn sodium is also effective in inhibiting the early- and late-phase responses, and can be used in conjunction with a β_2-agonist (39a). The asthmatic who is simply participating in a fitness program should also follow a medication plan to *prevent* the occurrence of an EIA attack. The exercise session should include the conventional warm-up, with mild to moderate activity planned in five minute segments. Swimming is better than other types of exercise, given that air above the water tends to be warmer and contains more moisture. A scarf or face mask can be used when exercising outdoors in cold weather to help trap moisture. The participant should carry an inhaler with a β_2-agonist and use it at the first sign of wheezing (1, 22). As with the diabetic, the buddy system is a good plan to follow in case a major attack occurs.

in summary

- An asthmatic attack is brought on when an agent causes an increased influx of Ca^{++} into a mast cell in the respiratory tract, which, in turn, triggers the release of chemical mediators. These chemical mediators cause a reflex and calcium-mediated constriction of bronchiolar smooth muscle along with an increase in secretions into the airways.
- Cromolyn sodium and β-adrenergic agonists act to prevent this by preventing the entry of Ca^{++} into the mast cell, and by increasing the level of cyclic AMP in the mast and smooth muscle cells, respectively.
- Cooling and drying of the respiratory tract lead to an increase in the osmolarity of the fluid on the surface of a mast cell. This event is believed to be the central factor in the initiation of the asthmatic attack during exercise. Exercise of short duration, preceded by a warm-up, appears to reduce the chance of an attack. Drugs should be used prior to exercise to prevent an attack, and β-adrenergic agonists should be carried along in case one occurs.

Table 17.2 Guide to Grading Disability of COPD Patient (Based on 40-Year-Old Man)

Grade	Cause of Dyspnea	FEV_1 (% Predicted)	Max $\dot{V}O_2$ ($ml \cdot min^{-1} \cdot kg^{-1}$)	Exercise Max $\dot{V}_E$ ($\ell \cdot min^{-1}$)	Blood Gases
1	Fast walking and stair climbing	>60	>25	Not limiting	Normal $PaCO_2$, SaO_2
2	Walking at normal pace	<60	<25	>50	Normal $PaCO_2$; SaO_2 above 90% at rest and with exercise
3	Slow walking	<40	<15	<50	Normal $PaCO_2$; SaO_2 below 90% with exercise
4	Walking limited to less than one block	<40	<7	<30	Elevated $PaCO_2$; SaO_2 below 90% at rest and with exercise

From J. S. Skinner, *Exercise Testing and Exercise Prescription of Special Cases.* Copyright © 1987 Lea & Febiger. A Waverly Company, Baltimore MD. Reprinted by permission.

Chronic Obstructive Pulmonary Disease

Chronic obstructive pulmonary diseases (COPD) cause a reduction in airflow that can have a dramatic effect on daily activities. These diseases include chronic bronchitis, emphysema, and bronchial asthma, either alone or in combination. These diseases are distinct from the exercise-induced asthma discussed earlier in that the airway obstruction remains in spite of continuous medication (15). Chronic bronchitis is characterized by a persistent production of sputum due primarily to a thickened bronchial wall with excess secretions. In emphysema the elastic recoil of alveoli and bronchioles is reduced and those pulmonary structures are enlarged (10, 55). The patient with developing COPD cannot perform normal activities without experiencing dyspnea, but, tragically, by the time this occurs the disease is already well advanced (10). COPD is characterized by a decreased ability to exhale, and because of the narrowed airways, a "wheezing" sound is made. The person with COPD experiences a decreased capacity for work, which may influence employment, but he/she may also experience an increase in psychological problems, including anxiety (regarding the simple act of breathing) and depression (related to a loss of sense of self-worth).

It should be no surprise then that treatment of COPD includes more than simple medication and oxygen-inhalation therapy. A typical COPD rehabilitation program focuses on the goal of the patient's ability for self-care. To achieve that goal a number of medical and support personnel are recruited to deal with the various manifestations of the disease process (44, 61). The COPD patient receives education about the different ways to deal with the disease, including breathing exercises, ways to approach the activities of daily living at home, and how to handle work-related problems. The latter can be so affected that new on-the-job responsibilities may have to be assigned, or if the person cannot meet the requirements, retirement may be the only outcome. In order to help deal with these problems, counseling by psychologists and clergy may be needed for patient and family. The extent of these problems is directly related to the severity of the disease. Those with minimal disease may require the help of only a few of the professionals just mentioned, while others with severe disease may require the assistance of all. It is therefore important to understand that the rehabilitation program is very individualized (44, 61).

Testing and Training

The consistent recommendation for anyone with known disease is to have a complete medical exam, including exercise testing, prior to beginning an exercise program. This is especially true for COPD patients because the severity of the disease varies greatly. Common tests used to classify COPD patients include the FEV_1, (the maximum volume of air that can be moved in one second), a graded exercise test to evaluate $\dot{V}O_2$ max, maximum exercise ventilation, and changes in the arterial blood gases, PO_2 and PCO_2. Table 17.2 shows a 4-point scale used to grade the level of disability (29). It should be clear that there are great differences between those with a $\dot{V}O_2$ max greater than 25 $ml \cdot kg^{-1} \cdot min^{-1}$, and those with a $\dot{V}O_2$ max less than 7 $ml \cdot kg^{-1} \cdot min^{-1}$. You might also look to the left side of the table to see how little exertion is required of those at Grade 4 to bring on the sensation of dyspnea, and to the far right to see what happens to the blood gases. It is obvious that exercise programming varies with the severity of the disease. While those with a Grade 1 disability can follow the normal exercise prescription process, those with a Grade 4 disability are probably in respiratory and cardiovascular failure. Goals for the latter group are very pragmatic: ability to do home or work activities, ability to climb two flights of stairs, and so on, and these activities might require supplemental oxygen or inspiratory pressure support (10, 29, 34a, 44). A wide range of exercises (e.g., walking, cycling, swimming, games, resistance training, breathing exercises) can be used to improve the patient's functional capacity (13, 15, 29). What is clear is that the success of the program depends on a good match of the patient's limitations with the appropriate exercises. Generally, COPD patients achieve an increase in exercise tolerance without dyspnea and an increase in the sense of well-being, but without a reversal of the disease process (13, 29, 34a, 44, 55). The changes in the psychological variables are very important in the long run, given that the person's willingness to continue the exercise program is a major factor determining the rate of decline during the course of the disease.

in summary

- Chronic obstructive pulmonary disease (COPD) includes chronic asthma, emphysema, and bronchitis. These latter two diseases create changes in the lung that are irreversible and result in a gradual deterioration of function.
- Rehabilitation is a multidisciplinary approach involving medication, breathing exercises, dietary therapy, exercise, and counseling. The programs are individually designed due to the severity of the illness, and the goals are very pragmatic in terms of the events of daily living and work.

Hypertension

As mentioned in chapter 14, the risk of coronary heart disease (CHD) increases with increases in resting values of systolic and diastolic blood pressure (30). Hypertension, defined as systolic pressure of ≥140 mm Hg or diastolic pressure of ≥90 mm Hg, is a major health problem in the United States involving over 50 million people (31). Special attention is now being focused on those with mild to moderate hypertension: diastolic pressure between 90 and 105 mm Hg, and/or systolic pressure between 140 and 180 mm Hg (2). These individuals represent the majority of all hypertensives, and account for most of the morbidity and mortality associated with hypertension (23). Although there is little disagreement that medication should be used to deal with hypertension when blood pressure values are greater than 180/105 mm Hg, many believe that nonpharmacological approaches should be used for those with mild or borderline hypertension (2, 6, 24, 30, 31, 72). The reasons nonpharmacological approaches are recommended include the possibility of side effects due to medication, and the counterproductive behavioral changes associated with classifying a person as a "patient" (24).

Generally, the person with mild hypertension should have a physical exam to identify potential underlying problems, as well as the presence of other risk factors. Kannel (30) indicates that while medication might be used to control blood pressure when multiple risk factors (smoking, high cholesterol, inactivity, etc.) are present, the simple act of stopping smoking confers more immediate benefit against the overall risk of CHD than any medication. It is within this context that a nonpharmacological intervention program focuses on the use of exercise and diet to control blood pressure and establish behaviors that favorably influence other aspects of health (6, 24).

Dietary recommendations to control blood pressure include a reduction in sodium intake for those sensitive to excess sodium, and in caloric intake for those who are overweight. Kaplan's (31) review indicates that salt restriction results in an average reduction in systolic and diastolic blood pressures of 5 and 3 mm Hg, while a 1-kg weight loss is associated with a 1.6 and 1.3 mm Hg reduction, respectively. Endurance exercise is associated with a 10 mm Hg reduction in resting blood pressure in hypertensive individuals, however, the magnitude of the reduction is inversely related to the pretraining blood pressure (2, 18a, 24). While all hypertensive individuals don't respond to endurance exercise in this way, exercise is recommended for all since other changes occur to reduce the risk of CHD, even if blood pressure is not reduced (24). The question is, how much exercise?

The standard American College of Sports Medicine exercise prescription for improving $\dot{V}O_2$ max (see chapter 16) is also effective in reducing blood pressure in previously hypertensive individuals. In addition, endurance exercise at lower intensities (40%–70% $\dot{V}O_2$ max) has also been shown to reduce blood pressure (2, 24). Lower intensity exercise should be done frequently and for durations long enough to result in the expenditure of a large number of calories. Gordon et al. (23) suggest a goal of 14–20 kcal/kg per week (about 980 to 1440 kcal for a 70 kg person). There is, of course, no reason why the exercise program could not be accompanied by improvements in other life-style behaviors such as smoking cessation, low-fat diet, and weight reduction. For those on medication, blood pressure should be checked frequently so that the medication regime can be altered by the physician, if necessary.

in summary

- Exercise can be used as a nonpharmacological intervention for those with hypertension. Exercise recommendations include light to vigorous activity (40%–85% $\dot{V}O_2$ max), done three or more days per week, and for twenty to sixty minutes per session. For those on medication, blood pressure should be checked frequently.

Cardiac Rehabilitation

Exercise training is now an accepted part of the therapy used to restore an individual who has some form of coronary heart disease (CHD). The details of how to structure such programs, from the first steps taken after being confined to a bed to the time of returning to work and beyond, are spelled out clearly in books such as ACSM's *Guidelines for Exercise Testing and Prescription* (2a), Pollock and Wilmore's *Exercise in Health and Disease* (50), and Wenger and Hellerstein's *Rehabilitation of the Coronary Patient* (68). This brief section will simply comment on various aspects of such programs.

Population

The persons served by cardiac rehabilitation programs include those who have experienced angina pectoris, myocardial infarctions (MI), coronary artery bypass graft surgery (CABGS), and angioplasty (19). Angina pectoris is the chest pain related to ischemia of the ventricle due to occlusion of one or more of the coronary arteries. The symptoms occur when the work of the heart (estimated by the double product: systolic blood pressure × HR) exceeds a certain value. **Nitroglycerin** is used to prevent an attack and/or relieve the pain by relaxing the smooth muscle in veins to reduce venous return and the work of the heart (40). Angina patients may also be treated with a beta blocker like propranolol (Inderal®) to reduce the HR and/or blood pressure such that the angina symptoms occur at a later stage into work. Exercise training supports this drug effect: as the person becomes trained, the HR response at any work rate is reduced. This allows the individual to take on more tasks without experiencing the chest pain.

Myocardial infarction (MI) patients have actual heart damage (loss of ventricular muscle) due to a prolonged occlusion of one or more of the coronary arteries. The degree to which left ventricular function is compromised is dependent on the mass of the ventricle permanently damaged. These patients are usually on medications to reduce the work of the heart (β-blocker), and control the irritability of the heart tissue so that dangerous **arrhythmias** (irregular heart rhythms) do not occur. Generally, these patients experience a training effect similar to those who do not have an MI (19).

Coronary artery bypass graft surgery (CABGS) patients have had surgery to bypass one or more blocked coronary arteries. In this procedure, a blood vessel from the patient is sutured onto the existing coronary arteries above and below the blockage. The success of the surgery is dependent on the amount of heart damage that existed prior to surgery, as well as the success of the revascularization itself. In those who had chronic angina pectoris prior to CABGS, most find a relief of symptoms, with 50 percent to 70

percent having no more pain. Generally, with an increased blood flow to the ventricle there is an improvement in both left ventricular function and the capacity for work (69). These patients benefit from systematic exercise training because most are deconditioned prior to surgery as a result of activity restrictions related to chest pain. In addition, exercise improves the chance that the blood vessel graft will remain open (50a). Finally, the cardiac rehabilitation program helps the patient differentiate angina pain from chest wall pain related to the surgery. The overall result is a smoother and less traumatic transition back to normal function.

Some CHD patients undergo **percutaneous transluminal coronary angioplasty** to open occluded arteries. In this procedure the chest is not opened; instead, a balloon-tipped catheter (a long slender tube) is inserted into the coronary artery where the balloon is inflated to push the plaque back toward the arterial wall. These patients tend not to have as severe disease as those who undergo CABGS (62).

Testing

The testing of patients with CHD is much more involved than that presented for the apparently healthy person in chapter 15. There are classes of CHD patients for whom exercise or exercise testing is inappropriate and dangerous (2a). The PAR_x screening form in appendix D lists some absolute and relative contraindications for exercise. For those who can be tested, a 12-lead ECG is monitored at discrete intervals during the GXT, while a variety of leads are displayed continuously on an oscilloscope. Blood pressure, RPE, and various signs or symptoms are also noted. The criteria for terminating the GXT goes well beyond achieving a certain percentage of maximal HR, focusing instead on various pathological signs (e.g., ST-segment depression) and symptoms, such as angina pectoris. On the basis of the response to the GXT the person may be referred for additional testing, such as the use of radioactive molecules to evaluate perfusion (^{201} thallium) and the capacity of the ventricle to eject blood (^{99} technetium), or direct angiography, in which a dye that is opaque to X-rays is injected into the coronary arteries to determine the blockage directly (50). The results of all the tests are used to classify the individual as a low, intermediate, or high risk patient. The resulting classification has a major impact on deciding whether or not to use exercise as a part of the rehabilitation process and, if exercise is appropriate, determines the type and format of the exercise program (2a).

Exercise Programs

Cardiac rehabilitation includes a "Phase I" inpatient exercise program that is used to help the patients make the transition from the cardiovascular event (e.g., a myocardial infarction that put them in the hospital) to the time of discharge from the hospital. The specific signs and symptoms exhibited by the patient are used to determine whether the patient should be placed in an exercise program, and if so, when to terminate the exercise session (2a). Once the patient is discharged from the hospital, a "Phase II" program can be started. This program resembles the one mentioned earlier for apparently healthy persons in that warm-up with stretching, endurance, and strengthening exercises, and cool-down activities are included. However, the CHD patients, who are generally very deconditioned ($\dot{V}O_2$ max of ~20 ml · kg^{-1} · min^{-1}), require only light exercise to achieve their THR. In addition, because these patients are on a wide variety of medications that may decrease maximal heart rate, the THR zone is determined from their GXT results; the 220 − age formula cannot be used. The patients usually begin with intermittent low intensity exercise (one minute on, one minute off) using a variety of exercises to distribute the total work output over a larger muscle mass. In time the patient increases the duration of the work period for each exercise. The strengthening exercises emphasize a low resistance and high repetition format to involve the major muscle groups; free and machine weights can be used in a circuit program format (2a, 64). Given that CABGS and post-MI patients have had direct damage to their hearts, the exercise should facilitate, not interfere with, the healing process. As you might guess, given the nature of the patient and the risk involved, cardiac rehabilitation programs take place in hospitals and clinics where there is direct medical supervision and the capacity to deal with emergencies, should they occur. After a patient completes an eight- to twelve-week "Phase II" program, the person may continue in a "Phase III" program away from the hospital where there is less supervision, except for the ability to respond to an emergency (2a, 50). What are the benefits of such programs to the patient with CHD?

Effects

There is no question that CHD patients have improved cardiovascular function as a result of an exercise program. This is shown in higher $\dot{V}O_2$ max values, higher work rates achieved without ischemia as shown by angina pectoris or ST-segment changes, and an increased capacity for prolonged submaximal work (50, 68). The improved lipid profile (lower total cholesterol and higher HDL cholesterol) is a function of more than the exercise alone, given that weight loss and the saturated fat content of the diet can modify these variables (5, 46). It must be mentioned that a cardiac rehabilitation program should not be viewed simply as an exercise program. It is a multi-intervention effort involving exercise, medication, diet, and counseling.

in summary

- Cardiac rehabilitation programs include a wide variety of patients, including those having angina pectoris, bypass surgery, myocardial infarctions, and angioplasty. These patients may be taking nitroglycerin to control angina symptoms, β-blockers to reduce the work of the heart, or anti-arrhythmia medications to control dangerous heart rhythms.
- The exercise tests for CHD patients include a 12-lead ECG, and are used for referral to other tests. Exercise programs bring about large changes in functional capacity in these populations due to their low starting point. The programs are gradual and are based on their entry-level exercise tests and other clinical findings.

Elderly

Maximal aerobic power decreases in the average population after the age of twenty at the rate of about 1 percent per year. A recent report by Kasch et al. (32) shows that not only can this decline be interrupted by a physical activity program, but middle-aged men who maintain their activity and body weight show half the expected decrease in $\dot{V}O_2$ max over a twenty-year period. This is consistent with an analysis of cross-sectional and longitudinal data showing that the decrease in $\dot{V}O_2$ max with age is related to a decrease in physical activity and an increase in percent body fat (27a). Unfortunately, the vast majority of people experience a steady decline in $\dot{V}O_2$ max so that by sixty years of age their ability to engage comfortably in normal activities is reduced. This initiates a vicious cycle that leads to lower and lower levels of cardiorespiratory fitness, which may not allow them to perform daily tasks. In turn, this affects the elderly's quality of life and independence, which may necessitate reliance on others (58). A physical activity program is useful, not only in dealing with this downward spiral of cardiorespiratory fitness, but with the osteoporosis that is related to the sudden hip fractures that can lead to more inactivity and death (58).

Osteoporosis is a loss of bone mass that primarily affects women over fifty years of age and is responsible for 1.2 million fractures annually. Type I osteoporosis is related to vertebral and distal radius fractures in fifty- to sixty-five year olds, and is eight times more common in women than men. Type II osteoporosis, found in those aged seventy and above, results in hip, pelvic, and distal humerus fractures and is twice as common in women (28). The problem is more common in women over age fifty due to menopause and the lack of estrogen. Estrogen treatment, instituted

Exercise and the Elderly: The Training Effect

Over the past fifteen years a substantial body of knowledge has accumulated documenting the capacity of the elderly to experience a training effect similar to what has been observed in younger men and women. This has major ramifications when one considers the increase in the number of elderly in our population and the need to maintain their health status and independence for as long as possible. Data on the effect of exercise on the elderly have been obtained from cross-sectional studies comparing older athletes to their sedentary counterparts and from longitudinal studies in which training programs have been carried out over many months. A brief summary of each follows (25).

Cross-sectional studies have shown that, in contrast to older sedentary individuals, endurance-trained older athletes have

- higher $\dot{V}O_2$ max values and have half the expected decrease in $\dot{V}O_2$ max due to age,

- higher HDL cholesterol, and lower triglycerides, total, and LDL cholesterol,
- enhanced glucose tolerance and insulin sensitivity, and
- greater strength, reaction time and a lower risk of falling.

These comparisons could be biased due to the potential for a strong genetic factor that might drive an individual to pursue an active life. In contrast, longitudinal studies compare a trained group to a control group over many months to see how each changes; this minimizes the concerns raised in the cross-sectional studies. The results from these studies parallel those mentioned above. Endurance training:

- increases $\dot{V}O_2$ max and the kinetics of oxygen uptake in a manner similar to younger individuals, but more time may be required for the training effect to occur (5a). The increase in $\dot{V}O_2$ max is

due to both peripheral (skeletal muscle) and central (cardiovascular) adaptations (61a). Interestingly, the training effect can be brought about by lower intensities of exercise than required for younger subjects.
- causes favorable changes in blood lipids, but the changes seem to be linked to a reduction in body fatness, rather than exercise, per se,
- lowers blood pressure to the same degree as shown for younger hypertensives,
- improves glucose tolerance and insulin sensitivity, and
- increases or maintains muscular strength and bone density. It must be added that resistance-training results in large increases in strength which may play an important role in reducing the risk of falls.

early in menopause, may prevent bone loss. If estrogen is used years after menopause, lost bone cannot be replaced, but existing bone can be maintained (37). Given that prevention is better than treatment, attention is focused on adequate dietary calcium (26) and exercise throughout life (58).

Dietary calcium is important in preventing and treating osteoporosis. While the daily calcium requirement is 800 mg · d^{-1}, no group of adult women meets that standard (45). In an attempt to prevent osteoporosis, attention is directed at young women (under twenty-five) to maximize bone growth. The calcium requirement is set to 1200 mg/day to accomplish that.

Bone structure is maintained by the force of gravity (upright posture), and the lateral forces associated with muscle contraction. Weight-bearing activities (walking, jogging) are better than bicycling and swimming for maintaining spine and hip mineral, but for the low fit or those with previous fractures these latter activities are recommended (58). Further, it may be safer to stay with a walking program rather than move to a

jogging program because of the higher incidence of injuries associated with the latter program (49). While we may know the exercise prescription needed to achieve cardiorespiratory fitness, we do not have the prescription for preventing osteoporosis (60). However, two to three hours of exercise a week may reduce the expected rate of bone mineral loss with age (16b, 58).

As is true for any special population, a complete medical exam is a reasonable recommendation to help discover problems or the presence of a combination of risk factors that might affect decisions about entry into an exercise program (2a). There is no question that the elderly, like their younger counterparts, exhibit a specificity and an adaptability to training, be it for strength or endurance (16, 24, 49). Consequently, the exercise program should provide endurance, flexibility, and strength activities within the capacity of the population of elderly being served in order to make improvements in these fitness components (63). The potential benefits are clearly worth the time and energy invested (see A Closer Look 17.2).

In conclusion, the use of exercise programs for the elderly improves cardiorespiratory fitness and helps to maintain the integrity of bone. When this is coupled with the opportunity for socialization, it is easy to see why exercise is an important part of life from youth to old age.

in summary

- The "normal" deterioration of physiological function with age can be attenuated or reversed with regular endurance and strength training. The benefits of participation in a regular exercise program include an improved risk factor profile (e.g., higher HDL and lower LDL cholesterol, improved insulin sensitivity, higher $\dot{V}O_2$ max, and lower blood pressure), but the training effects may take longer to realize.
- The guidelines for exercise training programs for the elderly are similar to those who are younger, emphasizing the need for a medical exam and screening for risk factors. The effort required to bring about the training effect may be less than for younger individuals.

Pregnancy

Pregnancy places special demands on a woman due to the developing fetus' needs for calories, protein, minerals, vitamins, and of course, the physiologically stable environment needed to process these nutrients. It is against this background that the implementation of a fitness program must be evaluated. In much the same way that a diabetic, asthmatic, or cardiac patient would initiate an exercise program, the pregnant woman should begin with a thorough medical examination by her physician to rule out complications that would make exercise inappropriate, and to provide specific information about signs or symptoms to watch for during the course of the pregnancy. Examples of absolute contraindications for aerobic exercise during pregnancy include Type I diabetes, history of two or more spontaneous abortions, multiple pregnancy, smoking, and excessive alcohol intake. Relative contraindications include a history of premature labor, anemia, obesity, Type II diabetes, and very low fitness prior to pregnancy (71). Clearly, to protect mother and fetus, a consultation with a physician is a reasonable recommendation prior to the initiation of an exercise program.

Interestingly, compared to our knowledge of how diabetics, asthmatics, and cardiac patients respond to exercise training, we are now only beginning to understand how the mother and fetus respond to such a program (12a, 70, 71a). In general, the following describe the major cardiovascular and metabolic adaptations to pregnancy compared to the nonpregnant state (70):

- Blood volume increases 40 percent to 50 percent.
- Oxygen uptake is slightly higher at rest and during submaximal exercise.
- Oxygen cost of weight-bearing exercise is markedly increased.
- Heart rates are higher at rest and during submaximal exercise.
- Cardiac output is higher at rest and during submaximal exercise for the first two trimesters; in the third trimester cardiac output is lower and the potential for arterial hypotension is greater.

In spite of all these changes, moderate exercise does not appear to interfere with oxygen delivery to the fetus, and the heart rate response of the fetus shows no signs of distress. The fetal heart rate increases with the intensity and duration of exercise, and gradually returns to normal during postexercise recovery (70, 71a). Cardiac output has been shown to be higher at 26 weeks gestation during submaximal exercise than at 8 weeks following delivery. The fact that the a-$\bar{v}$ O_2 difference was lower suggests that the higher cardiac output was distributed to other vascular beds (e.g., the uterus) and muscle blood flow was maintained (54, 71a). Since absolute $\dot{V}O_2$ max (ℓ/min) doesn't change much over the course of a pregnancy (39), what happens when exercise training is done during pregnancy?

In general, there is evidence that estimated $\dot{V}O_2$ max (in ℓ/min) is increased as a result of training in previously sedentary pregnant women, while relative $\dot{V}O_2$ max (ml $\cdot$ kg^{-1} $\cdot$ min^{-1}) is maintained or increased slightly, despite the weight gain (71a). What is interesting is that when well-conditioned recreational athletes trained throughout and following their pregnancy, absolute $\dot{V}O_2$ max was increased as long as 36–44 weeks after delivery compared to a "control" group of women who maintained training and did not become pregnant (14). This suggests that the combination of pregnancy and training resulted in adaptations greater than could be achieved by training alone. What are reasonable recommendations to follow when a pregnant woman wishes to exercise?

There has been limited research in this area. Guidelines have been developing over the past decade, with disagreement voiced among specialists in obstetrics and gynecology (11, 21). In an earlier set of guidelines from the American College of Obstetricians and Gynecologists, fixed criteria (e.g., don't exercise over an HR of 140 b/min) were provided with the emphasis on taking a conservative approach to exercise prescription. The most recent guidelines, see table 17.3, recognize that research support for such restrictions does not exist (1a). The guidelines emphasize the need to avoid doing exercise in the supine position after the first trimester and to modify intensity according to

Table 17.3 Recommendations for Exercise in Pregnancy and Postpartum

There are no data in humans to indicate that pregnant women should limit exercise intensity and lower target heart rates because of potential adverse effects. For women who do not have any additional risk factors for adverse maternal or perinatal outcome, the following recommendations may be made:

1. During pregnancy, women can continue to exercise and derive health benefits even from mild-to-moderate exercise routines. Regular exercise (at least three times per week) is preferable to intermittent activity.

2. Women should avoid exercise in the supine position after the first trimester. Such a position is associated with decreased cardiac output in most pregnant women; because the remaining cardiac output will be preferentially distributed away from splanchnic beds (including the uterus) during vigorous exercise, such regimens are best avoided during pregnancy. Prolonged periods of motionless standing should also be avoided.

3. Women should be aware of the decreased oxygen available for aerobic exercise during pregnancy. They should be encouraged to modify the intensity of their exercise according to maternal symptoms. Pregnant women should stop exercising when fatigued and not exercise to exhaustion. Weight-bearing exercises may, under some circumstances, be continued at intensities similar to those prior to pregnancy throughout pregnancy. Non-weight-bearing exercises such as cycling or swimming will minimize the risk of injury and facilitate the continuation of exercise during pregnancy.

4. Morphologic changes in pregnancy should serve as a relative contraindication to types of exercise in which loss of balance could be detrimental to maternal or fetal well-being, especially in the third trimester. Further, any type of exercise involving the potential for even mild abdominal trauma should be avoided.

5. Pregnancy requires an additional 300 kcal/d in order to maintain metabolic homeostasis. Thus, women who exercise during pregnancy should be particularly careful to ensure an adequate diet.

6. Pregnant women who exercise in the first trimester should augment heat dissipation by ensuring adequate hydration, appropriate clothing, and optimal environmental surroundings during exercise.

7. Many of the physiologic and morphologic changes of pregnancy persist four to six weeks postpartum. Thus, prepregnancy exercise routines should be resumed gradually based on a woman's physical capability.

From American College of Obstetricians and Gynecologists: Recommendation for Exercise in Pregnancy and Postpartum. Technical Bulletin No. 189. Washington DC, ACOG, © 1994. Reprinted with permission.

symptoms and not push on to exhaustion. Weight-supported activities are encouraged due to the lower risk of injury, and attention is focused on the need for hydration to maintain body temperature in the normal range associated with exercise. The latter recommendation is different from earlier guidelines to limit the increase in maternal body temperature to 38° C. Research suggests that normal exercise-induced increases in body temperatures carry little risk to the fetus (12a, 70). Although heart rate has been used to set exercise intensity, the fact that the relationship between heart rate and $\dot{V}O_2$ may change over the course of pregnancy suggests that the rating of perceived exertion (RPE) may be a better choice (2a). Finally, concern has been expressed that exercise leaders for these programs receive special instruction to enhance the safety and benefits of the exercise program (38).

in summary

- A pregnant woman should consult with her physician before starting an exercise program.
- Endurance exercise can be done during pregnancy without complication to mother and fetus.

study questions

1. What is the difference between Type I and Type II diabetes?

2. If a Type I diabetic does not take an adequate amount of insulin, what happens to the blood glucose concentration during prolonged exercise? Why?

3. If exercise is helpful in controlling blood glucose, how could it complicate the life of a Type I diabetic?

4. Provide general recommendations regarding changes in insulin and diet for diabetics who engage in exercise.

5. How is exercise-induced asthma triggered, and how do medications reduce the chance of an attack?

6. Why are exercise and diet recommended as nonpharmocological treatments for those with borderline hypertension?

7. What is COPD, and where does exercise fit in as a part of a rehabilitation program?

8. What are angina pectoris, CABGS, and angioplasty?

9. What additional measurements are made during a GXT of a cardiac patient, as compared to an apparently healthy individual?

10. How do the elderly respond to exercise training compared to younger subjects?

11. What are the concerns about exercise during pregnancy, and what are the guidelines recommended for a pregnant woman who wishes to begin an exercise program?

suggested readings

Campaigne, B. N., and R. M. Lampman. 1994. *Exercise in the Clinical Management of Diabetes.* Champaign, IL: Human Kinetics Publishers.

Pollock, M. L., and J. H. Wilmore. 1990. *Exercise in Health and Disease.* 2d ed. Philadelphia: W. B. Saunders.

Wenger, N. K., and H. K. Hellerstein. 1984. *Rehabilitation of the Coronary Patient.* 2d ed. New York: John Wiley & Sons.

references

1. Afrasiabi, R., and S. L. Spector. 1991. Exercise-induced asthma. *The Physician and Sportsmedicine* 19:49–62.

1a. American College of Obstetricians and Gynecologists. 1994. Exercise during pregnancy and the postpartum period. (Technical Bulletin #189). Washington, D.C.:ACOG.

2. American College of Sports Medicine. 1993. Position stand: Physical activity, physical fitness, and hypertension. *Medicine and Science in Sports and Exercise.* 25:i–x.

2a. ———. 1995. *ACSM's Guidelines for Exercise Testing and Prescription.* 5th ed. Baltimore: Williams & Wilkins.

3. American Diabetes Association. 1985. *Fact Sheet on Diabetes.* Alexandria, VA.

3a. ———. 1990. Diabetes and exercise: Position statement. *Diabetes Care.* 13:804–5.

3b. ———. 1990. Exercise and NIDDM. *Diabetes Care* 13:785–89.

4. ———. 1994. Position statement: Nutritional recommendations and principles for people with diabetes mellitus. *Diabetes Care* 17:519–22.

5. American Heart Association Committee Report. 1982. Rationale of the diet-heart statement of the American Heart Association. *Nutrition Today* (Sept./Oct.):16–20; (Nov./Dec.):15–19.

5a. Babcock, M., D. H. Paterson, and D. A. Cunningham. 1994. Effects of aerobic endurance training on gas exchange kinetics of older men. *Medicine and Science in Sports and Exercise.* 26:447–52.

6. Bassett, D. R., and A. J. Zweifler. 1990. Risk factors and risk factor management. In *Clinical Ischemic Syndromes,* eds. G. B. Zelenock, L. G. D'Alecy, J. C. Fantone III, M. Shlafer, and J. C. Stanley, 15–46. St. Louis: C. V. Mosby.

7. Berg, K. E. 1986. *Diabetic's Guide to Health and Fitness.* Champaign, Il.: Life Enhancement Publications.

8. Berger et al. 1977. Metabolic and hormonal effects of muscular exercise in juvenile type diabetics. *Diabetologia* 13:355–65.

9. Berger, M., and F. W. Kemmer. 1990. Discussion: Exercise, fitness and diabetes. In *Exercise, Fitness, and Health,* eds. C. Bouchard, R. J. Shephard, T. Stevens, J. R. Sutton, and B. D. McPherson, 491–95. Champaign, IL: Human Kinetics.

10. Berman, L. B., and J. R. Sutton. 1986. Exercise and the pulmonary patient. *Journal of Cardiopulmonary Rehabilitation* 6:52–61.

10a. Braun, B., M. B. Zimmermann, and N. Kretchmer. 1995. Effects of exercise intensity on insulin sensitivity in women with non-insulin-dependent diabetes mellitus. *Journal of Applied Physiology* 78:300–306.

10b. Brysasco, V., and E. Crimi. 1994. Allergy and sports: Exercise-induced asthma. *International Journal of Sports Medicine* 15:S184–S186.

11. Caldwell, F., and T. Jopke. 1985. Questions and answers: ACSM 1985. *The Physician and Sportsmedicine* 13(8):145–51.

11a. Campaigne, B. N., and R. M. Lampman. 1994. *Exercise in the Clinical Management of Diabetes* Champaign, IL: Human Kinetics Publishers.

12. Cantu, D. C. 1982. *Diabetes and Exercise* Ithaca, NY: Movement Publications.

12a. Carpenter, M. W. 1994. Physical activity, fitness, and health of the pregnant mother and fetus. In *Physical Activity, Fitness, and Health,* eds. C. Bouchard, R. J. Shephard, and T. Stephens, 967–79. Champaign, IL: Human Kinetics Publishers.

13. Carter, R., J. C. Coast, and S. Idell. 1992. Exercise training in patients with chronic obstructive pulmonary disease. *Medicine and Science in Sports and Exercise* 24:281–91.

14. Clapp, J. F. III, and E. Capeless. 1991. The $\dot{V}O_2$ max of recreational athletes before and after pregnancy. *Medicine and Science in Sports and Exercise* 23:1128–33.

15. Cox, N. J. M., C. L. A. van Herwaarden, H. Folgering, and R. A. Binkhorst. 1988. Exercise and training in patients with chronic obstructive lung disease. *Sports Medicine* 6:180–92.

16. Cress, M. E., D. P. Thompson, J. Johnson, F. W. Kasch, R. G. Cassens, E. Smith, and J. C. Agre. 1991. Effect of training on $\dot{V}O_2$ max, thigh strength, and muscle morphology in septuagenarian women. *Journal of Applied Physiology* 23:752–58.

16a. Cypcar, D., and R. F. Lemanske. 1994. Asthma and exercise. *Clinics in Chest Medicine* 15:351–68.

16b. Drinkwater, B. L. 1994. Physical activity, fitness, and osteoporosis. In *Physical Activity, Fitness, and Health,* eds. C. Bouchard, R. J. Shephard, and T. Stephens, 724–36. Champaign, IL: Human Kinetics Publishers.

17. Eggleston, P. A. 1986. Pathophysiology of exercise-induced asthma. *Medicine and Science in Sports and Exercise* 18:318–21.

18. Ekoe, J-M. 1989. Overview of diabetes mellitus and exercise. *Medicine and Science in Sports and Exercise* 21:353–55.

18a. Fagard, R. H., and C. M. Tipton. 1994. Physical activity, fitness, and hypertension. In *Physical Activity, Fitness, and Health,* eds. C. Bouchard, R. J. Shephard, and T. Stephens, 633–55. Champaign, IL: Human Kinetics Publishers.

19. Franklin et al. 1986. Exercise prescription of the myocardial infarction patient. *Journal of Cardiopulmonary Rehabilitation* 6:62–79.

20. Franz, M. J. 1987. Exercise and the management of diabetes mellitus. *Journal of the American Dietetic Association* 87:872–80.

21. Gauthier, M. M. 1986. Guidelines for exercise during pregnancy: Too little or too much. *The Physician and Sportsmedicine* 14(4):162–69.

22. Gerhard, H., and E. N. Schachter. 1980. Exercise-induced asthma. *Postgraduate Medicine* 67:91–102.

22a. Giacca, A., Z. Q. Shi, E. B. Marliss, B. Zinman, and M. Vranic. 1994. Physical activity, fitness, and Type I diabetes. In *Physical Activity, Fitness, and Health*, eds. C. Bouchard, R. J. Shephard, and T. Stephens, 656–68. Champaign, IL: Human Kinetics Publishers.

23. Gordon, N. F., C. B. Scott, W. J. Wilkinson, J. J. Duncan, and S. N. Blair. 1990. Exercise and mild hypertension: Recommendations for adults. *Sports Medicine* 10:390–404.

23a. Gudat, U., M. Berger, and P. J. Lefèbvre. 1994. Physical activity, fitness, and non-insulin-dependent diabetes mellitus. In *Physical Activity, Fitness, and Health*, eds. C. Bouchard, R. J. Shephard, and T. Stephens, 669–83. Champaign, IL: Human Kinetics Publishers.

24. Hagberg, J. M. 1990. Exercise, fitness, and hypertension. In *Exercise, Fitness, and Health*, eds. C. Bouchard, R. J. Shephard, T. Stevens, J. R. Sutton, and B. D. McPherson, 455–66. Champaign, IL: Human Kinetics.

25. ———. 1994. Physical activity, fitness, health, and aging. In *Physical Activity, Fitness, and Health*, eds. C. Bouchard, R. J. Shephard, and T. Stephens, 993–1005. Champaign, IL: Human Kinetics Publishers.

25a. Hagberg, J. M., J. E. Graves, M. Limacher, D. R. Woods, S. H. Leggett, C. Cononie, J. J. Gruber, and M. L. Pollock. 1989. Cardiovascular responses of 70- to 79-yr-old men and women to exercise training. *Journal of Applied Physiology* 66:2589–94.

26. Heaney, R. P. 1987. The role of calcium in prevention and treatment of osteoporosis. *The Physician and Sportsmedicine* 15(11):83–88.

27. Hedlund, L. R., and J. C. Gallagher. 1987. The effects of fluoride on osteoporosis. *The Physician and Sportsmedicine* 15(11):111–18.

27a. Jackson, A. et al. 1995. Changes in aerobic power of men, ages 25–70 yr. *Medicine and Science in Sports and Exercise* 27:113–20.

28. Johnston, C. C., and C. Slemenda. 1987. Osteoporosis: An overview. *The Physician and Sportsmedicine* 15(11):65–68.

28a. Jones, A., and M. Bowen. 1994. Screening for childhood asthma using an exercise test. *British Journal of General Practice* 44:127–31.

29. Jones, N. L., L. B. Berman, P. D. Bartkiewicz, and N. B. Oldridge. 1987. Chronic obstructive respiratory disorders. In *Exercise Testing and Exercise Prescription for Special Cases*, ed. J. S. Skinner, 175–87. Philadelphia: Lea & Febiger.

30. Kannel, W. B. 1990. Contribution of the Framingham study to preventive cardiology. *Journal of the American College of Cardiology* 15:206–11.

31. Kaplan, N. M. 1994. *Clinical Hypertension.* 6th ed. Baltimore: Williams & Wilkins.

32. Kasch, F. W., J. L. Boyer, S. P. Van Camp, L. S. Verity, and J. P. Wallace. 1990. The effect of physical activity and inactivity on aerobic power in older men (a longitudinal study). *The Physician and Sportsmedicine* 18:73–83.

33. Katz, R. M. 1986. Prevention with and without the use of medications for exercise-induced asthma. *Medicine and Science in Sports and Exercise* 18:331–33.

34. Katz, R. M. 1987. Coping with exercise-induced asthma in sports. *The Physician and Sportsmedicine* 15 (July):100–112.

34a. Keilty, S. E., J. Ponte, T. A. Fleming, and J. Moxham. 1994. Effect of inspiratory pressure support on exercise tolerance and breathlessness in patients with severe stable chronic obstructive pulmonary disease. *Thorax* 49:990–94.

35. Kemmer, F. W., and M. Berger. 1983. Exercise and diabetes mellitus: Physical activity as a part of daily life and its role in the treatment of diabetic patient. *International Journal of Sports Medicine* 4:77–88.

35a. Kriska, A. M., S. N. Blair, and M. A. Pereira. 1994. The potential role of physical activity in the prevention of non-insulin-dependent diabetes mellitus: The epidemiological evidence. In *Exercise and Sports Sciences Reviews*, ed. J. O. Holloszy, Vol. 22, 121–43. Baltimore: Williams & Wilkins.

36. Lampman, R. M., and D. E. Schteingart. 1991. Effects of exercise training on glucose control, lipid metabolism, and insulin sensitivity in hypertriglyceridemia and non-insulin dependent diabetes mellitus. *Medicine and Science in Sports and Exercise* 23:703–12.

37. Lindsay, R. 1987. Estrogen and osteoporosis. *The Physician and Sportsmedicine* 15(11):105–8.

38. Lokey, E. A., Z. V. Tran, C. L. Wells, B. C. Myers, and A. C. Tran. 1991. Effects of physical exercise on pregnancy outcomes: A meta-analytic review. *Medicine and Science in Sports and Exercise* 23:1234–39.

39. Lotgering, F. K., M. B. van Doorn, P. C. Struijk, J. Pool, and H. C. S. Wallenburg. 1991. Maximal aerobic exercise in pregnant women: Heart rate, O_2 consumption, CO_2 production, and ventilation. *Journal of Applied Physiology* 70:1016–23.

39a. Mahler, D. A. 1993. Exercise-induced asthma. *Medicine and Science in Sports and Exercise* 25:554–61.

39b. Makker, H. K., and S. T. Holgate. 1994. Mechanisms of exercise-induced asthma. *European Journal of Clinical Investigation* 24:571–85.

40. Martin, A. D. 1986. ECG and medications. In *Health/Fitness Instructor's Handbook*, eds. E. T. Howley and B. D. Franks, 185–98. Champaign, IL: Human Kinetics.

41. McCarthy, P. 1989. Wheezing or breezing through exercise-induced asthma. *The Physician and Sportsmedicine* 17:125–30.

41a. McKenzie, D. C., S. L. McLuckie, and D. R. Stirling. 1994. The protective effects of continuous and interval exercise in athletes with exercise-induced asthma. *Medicine and Science in Sports and Exercise* 26:951–56.

42. McMurray, R. G., and V. L. Katz. 1990. Thermoregulation in pregnancy: Implications for exercise. *Sports Medicine* 10:146–58.

43. Middleton, E. 1980. A rational approach to asthma therapy. *Postgraduate Medicine* 67:107–23.

44. Miracle, V. A. 1986. Pulmonary exercise program: A model for pulmonary rehabilitation. *Journal of Cardiopulmonary Rehabilitation* 6:368–71.

45. National Research Council, National Academy of Sciences. 1989. *Recommended Dietary Allowances.* Washington, D.C.: National Academy Press.

46. *Physician and Sportsmedicine.* 1987. A Roundtable: Physiological adaptations to chronic endurance exercise training in patients with coronary artery disease. *Physician and Sportsmedicine* 15(9): 129–56.

47. Pierson et al. 1986. Implications of air pollution effects on athletic performance. *Medicine and Science in Sports and Exercise* 18:322–27.

48. Pivarnik, J. M., W. Lee, and J. F. Miller. 1991. Physiological and perceptual responses to cycle and treadmill exercise during pregnancy. *Medicine and Science in Sports and Exercise* 23:470–75.

49. Pollock, M. L., J. F. Carroll, J. E. Graves, S. H. Leggett, R. W. Braith, M. Limacher, and J. M. Hagberg. 1991. Injuries and adherence to walk/jog and resistance programs in the elderly. *Medicine and Science in Sports and Exercise* 23:1194–1200.

50. Pollock, M. L., and J. H. Wilmore. 1990. *Exercise in Health and Disease.* 2d edition. Philadelphia: W. B. Saunders.

50a. Quaglietti, S., and V. F. Froelicher. 1994. Physical activity and cardiac rehabilitation for patients with coronary heart disease. eds. C. Bouchard, R. J. Shephard, and T. Stephens. 591–608. Champaign, IL: Human Kinetics Publishers.

51. Richter, E. R., and H. Galbo. 1986. Diabetes, insulin and exercise. *Sports Medicine* 3:275–88.

52. Rogers, M. A. 1989. Acute effects of exercise on glucose tolerance in non-insulin-dependent diabetes. *Medicine and Science in Sports and Exercise* 21:362–68.

53. Sady, S. P., M. W. Carpenter, M. A. Sady, B. Haydon, B. Hoegsberg, E. M. Cullinane, P. D. Thompson, and D. R. Coustan. 1988. Prediction of $\dot{V}O_2$ max during cycle exercise in pregnant women. *Journal of Applied Physiology* 65:657–61.

54. Sady, S. P., M. W. Carpenter, P. D. Thompson, M. A. Sady, B. Haydon, and D. R. Coustan. 1989. Cardiovascular responses to cycle exercise during and after pregnancy. *Journal of Applied Physiology* 66:336–41.

55. Shephard, R. J. 1976. Exercise and chronic obstructive lung disease. In *Exercise and Sport Sciences Reviews,* vol. 4, eds. J. Keogle and R. S. Hutton, 263–96. California: Journal Publishing Affiliates.

56. Sly, R. M. 1986. History of exercise-induced asthma. *Medicine and Science in Sports and Exercise* 18:314–17.

57. Smith, E. L. 1984. Special considerations in developing exercise programs for the older adult. In *Behavioral Health: A Handbook of Health-Enhancement and Disease Prevention,* ed. J. D. Matarazzo, 525–46. New York: John Wiley & Sons.

58. Smith, E. L., and C. Gilligan. 1987. Effects of inactivity and exercise on bone. *The Physician and Sportsmedicine* 15(11):91–102.

59. Smith, E. L., and K. G. Stoedefalke. 1978. *Aging and Exercise.* Copyright: Author.

60. Snow-Harter, C., and R. Marcus. 1991. Exercise, bone mineral density, and osteoporosis. In *Exercise and Sport Sciences Reviews,* vol. 19, ed. J. O. Holloszy, 351–88. Baltimore: Williams & Wilkins.

60a. Soukup, J. T., and J. E. Kovaleski. 1993. A review of the effects of resistance training for individuals with diabetes mellitus. *Diabetes Education* 19:307–12.

61. Stockdale-Woolley, R., M. C. Haggerty, and P. M. McMahon. 1986. The pulmonary rehabilitation program at Norwalk Hospital. *Journal of Cardiopulmonary Rehabilitation* 6:505–18.

61a. Tate, C. A., M. F. Hyek, and G. E. Taffet. 1994. Mechanism for the responses of cardiac muscle to physical activity in old age. *Medicine and Science in Sports and Exercise* 26:561–67.

62. Tommaso, C. L., M. Lesch, and E. H. Sonnenblick. 1984. Alterations in cardiac function in coronary heart disease, myocardial infarction, and coronary bypass surgery. In *Rehabilitation of the Coronary Patient,* eds. N. K. Wenger and H. K. Hellerstein, 41–66. New York: John Wiley & Sons.

63. Van Camp, S., and J. L. Boyer. 1989. Exercise guidelines for the elderly (part 2 of 2). *The Physician and Sportsmedicine* 17:83–88.

64. Verrill, D., E. Shoup, G. McElveen, K. Witt, and D. Bergey. 1992. Resistive exercise training in cardiac patients: Recommendations. *Sports Medicine* 13:171–93.

65. Voy, R. O. 1986. The U.S. Olympic Committee experience with exercise-induced bronchospasm. 1984. *Medicine and Science in Sports and Exercise* 18:328–30.

66. Vranic, M., and Wasserman, D. 1990. Exercise, fitness, and diabetes. In *Exercise, Fitness, and Health,* eds. C. Bouchard, R. J. Shephard, T. Stevens, J. R. Sutton, and B. D. McPherson, 467–90. Champaign, IL: Human Kinetics.

67. Wallberg-Henriksson, H. 1989. Acute exercise: Fuel homeostasis and glucose transport in insulin-dependent diabetes mellitus. *Medicine and Science in Sports and Exercise* 21:356–61.

67a. ———. 1992. Exercise and diabetes mellitus. In *Exercise and Sport Sciences Reviews,* vol. 20, ed. J. O. Holloszy, 339–68. Baltimore: Williams & Wilkins.

68. Wenger, N. K., and H. K. Hellerstein. 1984. *Rehabilitation of the Coronary Patient.* 2d ed. New York: John Wiley & Sons.

69. Wenger, N. K., and J. W. Hurst. 1984. Coronary bypass surgery as a rehabilitative procedure. In *Rehabilitation of the Coronary Patient,* eds. N. K. Wenger and H. K. Hellerstein, 115–32. New York: John Wiley & Sons.

70. Wolfe, L. A., I. K. M. Brenner, and M. F. Mottola. 1994. Maternal exercise, fetal well-being and pregnancy outcome. In *Exercise and Sport Sciences Reviews,* vol. 22, ed. J. O. Holloszy, 145–94. Baltimore: Williams & Wilkins.

71. Wolfe, L. A., P. Hall, K. A. Webb, L. Goodman, M. Monga, and M. J. McGrath. 1989. Prescription of aerobic exercise during pregnancy. *Sports Medicine* 8:273–301.

71a. Wolfe, L. A., P. J. Ohtake, M. F. Mottola, and M. J. McGrath. 1989. Physiological interactions between pregnancy and aerobic exercise. In *Exercise and Sports Sciences Reviews,* vol. 17, ed. K. B. Pandolf, 295–351. Baltimore: Williams & Wilkins.

72. World Hypertension League. 1991. Physical exercise in the management of hypertension: A consensus statement by the World Hypertension League. *Journal of Hypertension* 9:283–87.

73. Young, J. C. 1995. Exercise Prescription for individuals with metabolic disorders. *Sports Medicine* 19:44–53.

CHAPTER 18

Body Composition and Nutrition for Health

By studying this chapter, you should be able to do the following:

1. Identify the U.S. Dietary Goals relative to (a) carbohydrates and fats as a percent of energy intake, (b) salt and cholesterol, and (c) saturated and unsaturated fats.
2. Contrast the Dietary Goals with the Dietary Guidelines.
3. Describe what is meant by the term *Recommended Dietary Allowance* (RDA), and how the RDA relates to the Daily Value (DV) used in food labeling.
4. List the classes of nutrients.
5. Identify the fat- and water-soluble vitamins, describe what toxicity is, and which class of vitamins is more likely to cause this problem.
6. Contrast major minerals with trace minerals, and describe the role of calcium, iron, and sodium in health and disease.
7. Identify the primary role of carbohydrates, the two major classes, and the recommended changes in the American diet to improve health status.
8. Identify the primary role of fat, and the recommended changes in the American diet to improve health status.
9. List the food groups and major nutrients represented in the Food Guide Pyramid.
10. Describe the Exchange System of planning diets, and how it differs from the Food Guide Pyramid.
11. Describe the limitation of the height/weight table in determining body composition.
12. Provide a brief description of the following methods of measuring body composition: isotope dilution, photon absorptiometry, potassium-40, hydrostatic (underwater weighing), dual energy x-ray absorptiometry, near infrared interactance, radiography, ultrasound, nuclear magnetic resonance, total body electrical conductivity, bioelectrical impedance analysis, and skinfold thickness.
13. Describe the two-component model of body composition and the assumptions made about the density values for the fat-free mass and the fat mass; contrast this with the multicomponent model.
14. Explain the principle underlying the measurement of whole body density with underwater weighing, and why one must correct for residual volume.
15. Explain why there is an error of ±2.0% in the calculation of percent body fat with the underwater weighing technique.
16. Explain how a sum of skinfolds can be used to estimate a percent body fatness value.
17. List the recommended percent body fatness values for health and fitness for males and females, and explain the concern for both high and low values.
18. Discuss the reasons why the average weight at any height (fatness) has increased while deaths from cardiovascular diseases have decreased.
19. Distinguish between obesity due to hyperplasia of fat cells and that due to hypertrophy of fat cells.
20. Describe the roles of genetics and environment in the development of obesity.
21. Explain the set point theory of obesity, and give an example of a physiological and behavioral control system.
22. Describe the pattern of change in body weight and caloric intake over the adult years.
23. Discuss the changes in body composition when weight is lost by diet alone versus diet plus exercise.
24. Describe the relationship of the fat-free mass and caloric intake to the BMR.
25. Define thermogenesis and explain how it is affected by both short- and long-term overfeeding.
26. Describe the effect of exercise on appetite and body composition.
27. Explain quantitatively why small differences in energy expenditure and dietary intake are important in weight gain over the years.

outline

Nutritional Goals   318
Standards of Nutrition   319
Classes of Nutrients   320
   Water   320
   Vitamins   321
   Minerals   323
   Carbohydrates   327
   Fats   328
   Protein   328

Meeting the Guidelines and
   Achieving the Goals   329
   Food Group Plans   329
   Evaluating the Diet   329
Body Composition   331
   Methods of Measuring Body
     Composition   331
   Two-Component System of Body
     Composition   335

Body Fatness for Health and
   Fitness   338
Obesity and Weight Control   339
   Obesity   339
Diet, Exercise, and Weight
   Control   342
   Energy and Nutrient Balance   342
   Diet and Weight Control   343
   Energy Expenditure and Weight
     Control   344

key terms

anorexia nervosa
basal metabolic rate (BMR)
bulimia nervosa
cholesterol
Daily Value (DV)
deficiency
Dietary Guidelines for Americans
elements
energy wasteful systems
ferritin
food records

HDL cholesterol
hemosiderin
high-density lipoproteins (HDL)
LDL cholesterol
lipoprotein
low-density lipoproteins (LDL)
major minerals
nutrient density
osteoporosis
provitamin

Recommended Dietary Allowances
   (RDA)
resting metabolic rate (RMR)
thermogenesis
toxicity
trace elements
transferrin
twenty-four-hour recall
underwater weighing
U.S. Dietary Goals
whole body density

hapter 14 described factors that limit health and fitness. These included hypertension, obesity, and elevated serum cholesterol. These three risk factors are linked to an excessive consumption of salt, total calories, and dietary fat, respectively. Clearly, knowledge of nutrition is essential to our understanding of health-related fitness. While chapters 3 and 4 described the metabolism of carbohydrates, fats, and proteins, this chapter will focus on the type of diet that should provide them. The first part of the chapter will present the nutritional goals for our nation, the nutrition standards and what they mean, a summary of the six classes of nutrients, and a way to evaluate our present diets and meet our nutritional goals. The second part of the chapter will discuss the role of exercise and diet in altering body composition. Nutrition related to athletic performance is covered in chapter 23.

Nutritional Goals

The American Heart Association has focused our attention on the role of diet in the elevation of serum cholesterol, obesity, and the development of hypertension (1a). Diet has also been linked to colon cancer and diabetes. In response to these problems a U.S. Senate Select Committee on Nutrition and Human Needs recruited experts to comment on and formulate **U.S. Dietary Goals** that would deal with diet-related problems (144). These goals, published in 1977, included the following:

- Increase carbohydrate intake to represent 55%–60% of caloric intake.
- Decrease fat consumption to 30% of caloric intake.
- Decrease saturated fat intake to represent only 10% of caloric intake; increase polyunsaturated and monounsaturated fats to approximately 10% of caloric intake.
- Reduce cholesterol intake to 300 mg per day.
- Reduce sugar consumption to account for only 15% of total calories.
- Reduce salt consumption by about 50%–85% to approximately 3 gm per day.

In order to achieve these goals the following changes in food selection and preparation were suggested:

- Increase the intake of fruits, vegetables, and whole grains.
- Increase consumption of poultry and fish, and decrease intake of meat.
- Decrease intake of foods high in fat, and partially substitute polyunsaturated fat for saturated fat.

- Substitute nonfat milk for whole milk.
- Decrease consumption of butter fat, eggs, and other high-cholesterol sources.
- Decrease consumption of sugar and foods high in sugar content.
- Decrease consumption of salt and foods high in salt content.

Not everyone agreed with these specific quantitative goals and the strong statements that were made about the role of diet in the prevention and treatment of disease. The select committee subsequently published responses of scientists and medical doctors who disagreed with the stated dietary goals (143). The revised document encouraged weight reduction to attain "ideal weight," and recommended a reduction in the use of alcohol.

In 1980 the U.S. Departments of Agriculture (141) published **Dietary Guidelines for Americans.** Rather than provide specific quantities to achieve for fat, cholesterol, salt, and carbohydrates as did the *Goals*, the *Guidelines* are more general statements aimed at people in good health. The following 1990 update of those guidelines shows little change over the previous five years (142).

- Eat a variety of foods.
- Maintain healthy weight.
- Choose a diet low in fat, saturated fat, and cholesterol.
- Choose a diet with plenty of vegetables, fruits, and grain products.
- Use sugars only in moderation.
- Use salt and sodium only in moderation.
- If you drink alcoholic beverages, do so in moderation.

These guidelines will be expanded in the following sections dealing with the essential nutrients, body composition, and weight control.

in summary

- The U.S. government established a set of *Dietary Goals* to improve health status: increase carbohydrates to 55%–60% of total calories, decrease fat intake to 30% of total calories (with saturated fat being only 10%), decrease dietary cholesterol to 300 mg per day, reduce sugar consumption to 15% of total calories, and decrease salt consumption to about 3 gm per day.
- A series of *Dietary Guidelines*, focusing on a high-carbohydrate, low-fat choices were provided to meet the *Dietary Goals*.

Standards of Nutrition

Food provides the carbohydrates, fats, protein, minerals, vitamins, and water needed for life. The quantity of each nutrient thought to meet the needs of practically all healthy persons is stated in the **Recommended Dietary Allowances (RDA)** found in appendix E. The values for each nutrient vary due to gender, body size, whether or not long-bone growth is taking place, pregnancy, and lactation (105). Given the fact that individuals differ in their need for each nutrient, some requiring more than the average and others less, the standards were set high enough to meet the needs of almost everyone (97.5% of the population), and also account for inefficient utilization by the body (105). For some vitamins and minerals the data used to set standards for specific population groups were considered inadequate, so values for these nutrients are referred to as "Estimated Safe and Adequate Intakes" rather than RDAs (see appendix F). The RDA does not set standards for carbohydrate and fat intake, but recommendations about these nutrients will be discussed shortly.

The RDA for caloric intake (energy) is not set at the same level as for the nutrients. Instead, the RDA for energy was simply set to meet the *average* caloric intake of each group (women, men, children, etc.) to reduce the chance that someone would gain weight while meeting the standard. The values for energy intake listed in appendix G assume an average level of physical activity (105), but, as we will discuss in more detail later in this chapter, there are many overweight individuals who may require less energy than is recommended due to their low metabolic rate and sedentary life-style. However, if an individual is consuming the RDA for energy and still gains weight, the person might increase his or her physical activity to achieve the desired weight rather than cut back on intake. The higher caloric intake will increase the chance that the person will meet the RDA for all the nutrients. How do you know how much of the RDA you have achieved?

The **Daily Value (DV)** is a standard used in nutritional labeling. For the essential nutrients (protein, vitamins, and minerals) the DVs are called Reference Daily Intakes (RDIs), and represent the highest 1968 RDA standard for any age or gender, except for pregnant and lactating women (58a). In addition, the food label contains important information about the calorie and fat content of the food. For example, if one serving of a product provides 50% of the DV for fat, it contains 50% of the total amount of fat recommended for one day (based on a 2000 calorie diet). Figure 18.1 provides an example of a food label; the following points are highlighted:

- serving size information,
- total calories and fat calories,

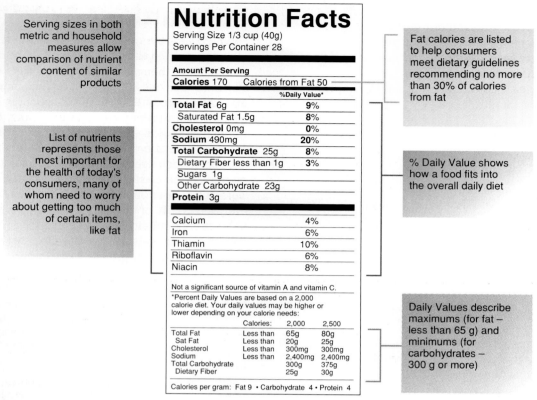

Serving sizes in both metric and household measures allow comparison of nutrient content of similar products

List of nutrients represents those most important for the health of today's consumers, many of whom need to worry about getting too much of certain items, like fat

Fat calories are listed to help consumers meet dietary guidelines recommending no more than 30% of calories from fat

% Daily Value shows how a food fits into the overall daily diet

Daily Values describe maximums (for fat — less than 65 g) and minimums (for carbohydrates — 300 g or more)

Nutrition Facts

Serving Size 1/3 cup (40g)
Servings Per Container 28

Amount Per Serving

Calories 170   Calories from Fat 50

%Daily Value*

Total Fat 6g	9%
Saturated Fat 1.5g	8%
Cholesterol 0mg	0%
Sodium 490mg	20%
Total Carbohydrate 25g	8%
Dietary Fiber less than 1g	3%
Sugars 1g	
Other Carbohydrate 23g	
Protein 3g	

Calcium	4%
Iron	6%
Thiamin	10%
Riboflavin	6%
Niacin	8%

Not a significant source of vitamin A and vitamin C.

*Percent Daily Values are based on a 2,000 calorie diet. Your daily values may be higher or lower depending on your calorie needs:

	Calories:	2,000	2,500
Total Fat	Less than	65g	80g
Sat Fat	Less than	20g	25g
Cholesterol	Less than	300mg	300mg
Sodium	Less than	2,400mg	2,400mg
Total Carbohydrate		300g	375g
Dietary Fiber		25g	30g

Calories per gram: Fat 9 • Carbohydrate 4 • Protein 4

Figure 18.1
An example of a food label.

- total fat grams, saturated fat grams, cholesterol, and the percent of DV for each (based on a 2,000 calorie diet),
- total carbohydrate and its sources, and
- the percent of the DV for vitamins and minerals; sodium is given special attention.

in summary

- The Recommended Dietary Allowance (RDA) is the quantity of a nutrient that will meet the needs of almost all healthy persons.
- The Daily Value (DV) is a standard used in nutritional labeling.

Classes of Nutrients

There are six classes of nutrients: water, vitamins, minerals, carbohydrates, fats, and proteins. In the following sections each nutrient will be described briefly and the primary food sources of each will be identified.

Water

Water is absolutely essential for life. While we can go without food for weeks, we would not survive long without water. The body is 50%–75% water, depending on age and body fatness, and a loss of only 3%–4% of body water adversely affects aerobic performance.

Larger losses can lead to death (101, 154). Under normal conditions without exercise, water loss equals about 2,500 ml/day, with most lost in urine (36). However, as higher environmental temperatures and heavy exercise are added, the water loss increases dramatically to 6–7 liters per day (59).

Under normal conditions the 2,500 ml of water per day is replaced with beverages (1,500 ml), solid food (750 ml), and the water derived from metabolic processes (250 ml) (36). Most people are surprised by the large volume of water contributed by "solid" food until they consider the following percentages of water in "solid" food: baked potato—75%, canned peas—77%, lettuce—96% (36). A general recommendation under ordinary circumstances is to consume 1 to 1.5 ml of water per kcal of energy expenditure (105). However, to avoid potential problems associated with dehydration, one should drink water *before and during* exercise; thirst is not an adequate stimulus to achieve water balance (see chapter 23).

Water weight can fluctuate depending on the body stores of carbohydrate and protein. Water is involved in the linkage between glucose molecules in glycogen and amino acid molecules in protein. The ratio is about 2.7 gms of water per gm of carbohydrate, and if an individual stores 454 gms (1 lb) of carbohydrate, body weight would increase by 3.7 lbs. Of course, when one diets and depletes this carbohydrate store, the reverse occurs. This results in an apparent weight loss of 3.7 lbs when only 1,816 kcal (454 gm of carbohydrate times 4 kcal/gm) have been lost. More on this later.

Vitamins

Vitamins were introduced in chapter 3 as organic catalysts involved in metabolic reactions. They are needed in small amounts and are not "used up" in the metabolic reactions. However, they are degraded (metabolized) like any biological molecule and must be replaced on a regular basis to maintain body stores. Several vitamins are in a precursor, or **provitamin,** form in foods, and are converted to the active form in the body. Beta-carotene, the most important of the provitamin A compounds, is a good example. A chronic lack of certain vitamins can lead to **deficiency** diseases, and an excess of others can lead to a **toxicity** condition (36). In our presentation, vitamins will be divided into the fat-soluble and water-soluble groups.

Fat-Soluble Vitamins

The fat-soluble vitamins include A, D, E, and K. These vitamins can be stored in large quantities in the body; thus a deficiency state takes longer to develop than for water-soluble vitamins. However, because of their solubility, so much can be stored that a toxicity condition can occur. Vitamin D is regarded as the most toxic. It is possible to achieve a level of toxicity with only four to five times the recommended dietary allowance (36, 105). Toxicity, of course, is far from a health-related goal. Table 18.1 summarizes the

Table 18.1	Key Information About the Vitamins				
Vitamin	RDA for Healthy Adults Ages 19–50	Major Dietary Sources	Major Functions	Signs of Severe, Prolonged Deficiency	Signs of Extreme Excess
Fat-Soluble					
A	Females: 800 RE[a] Males: 1,000 RE[a]	Fat-containing and fortified dairy products; liver; provitamin carotene in orange and deep green fruits and vegetables	Vitamin A is a component of rhodopsin; carotenoids can serve as antioxidants; retinoic acid affects gene expression; still under intense study	Night blindness, keratinization of epithelial tissues, including the cornea of the eye (xeropthalmia) causing permanent night blindness; dry scaling skin; increased susceptibility to infection	*Preformed vitamin A:* damage to liver, bone; headache, irritability, vomiting, hair loss, blurred vision *13-cis retinoic acid:* some fetal defects *Carotenoids:* yellowed skin
D	<25 years: 10 µg >25 years: 5 µg	Fortified and full-fat dairy products, egg yolk (diet often not as important as sunlight exposure)	Promotes absorption and use of calcium and phosphorus	Rickets (bone deformities) in children; osteomalacia (bone softening) in adults	Calcium deposition in tissues leading to cerebral, CV, and kidney damage
E	Females: 8 α-tocopherol equivalents Males: 10 α-tocopherol equivalents	Vegetable oils and their products; nuts, seeds	Antioxidant to prevent cell membrane damage; still under intense study	Possible anemia and neurological effects	Generally nontoxic, but at least one type of intravenous infusion led to some fatalities in premature infants; may worsen clotting defect in vitamin K deficiency
K	Females: <25: 60 µg >25: 65 µg Males: <25: 70 µg >25: 80 µg	Green vegetables; tea	Aids in formation of certain proteins, especially those for blood clotting	Defective blood coagulation causing severe bleeding on injury	Liver damage and anemia from high doses of the synthetic form menadione

Continued

[a]RE = retinol equivalents. (Because many food composition tables still list the vitamin A activity of foods as IU, it may be helpful to recognize that previous RDAs for vitamin A were 5000 IU [men] and 4000 IU [women].)

Table 18.1 continued

Vitamin	RDA for Healthy Adults Ages 19–50	Major Dietary Sources	Major Functions	Signs of Severe, Prolonged Deficiency	Signs of Extreme Excess
Water-Soluble Thiamin (B-1)	Females: 1.1 mg Males: 1.5 mg	Pork, legumes, peanuts, enriched or whole grain products	Coenzyme used in energy metabolism	Nerve changes, sometimes edema, heart failure; beriberi	Generally nontoxic, but repeated injections may cause shock reaction
Riboflavin (B-2)	Females: 1.3 mg Males: 1.7 mg	Dairy products, meats, eggs, enriched grain products, green leafy vegetables	Coenzyme used in energy metabolism	Skin lesions	Generally nontoxic
Niacin	Females: 15 niacin equivalents Males: 19 niacin equivalents	Nuts, meats; provitamin tryptophan in most proteins	Coenzyme used in energy metabolism	Pellagra (multiple vitamin deficiencies including niacin)	Flushing of face, neck, hands; potential liver damage
B-6	Females: 1.6 mg Males: 2.0 mg	High-protein foods in general	Coenzyme used in amino acid metabolism	Nervous, skin, and muscular disorders; anemia	Unstable gait, numb feet, poor hand coordination
Folic Acid	Females: 180 μg Males: 200 μg	Green vegetables, orange juice, nuts, legumes, grain products	Coenzyme used in DNA and RNA metabolism; single carbon utilization	Megaloblastic anemia (large, immature red blood cells); GI disturbances	Masks vitamin B-12 deficiency; interferes with drugs to control epilepsy
B-12	2 μg	Animal products	Coenzyme used in DNA and RNA metabolism; single carbon metabolism	Megaloblastic anemia; pernicious anemia when due to inadequate intrinsic factor; nervous system damage	Thought to be nontoxic
Pantothenic acid	4–7 mg[b]	Animal products and whole grains; whidely distributed in foods	Coenzyme used in energy metabolism	Fatigue, numbness, and tingling of hands and feet	Generally nontoxic; occasionally causes diarrhea
Biotin	30–100 μg[b]	Widely distributed in foods	Coenzyme used in energy metabolism	Scaly dermatitis	Thought to be nontoxic
C (ascorbic acid)	60 mg	Fruits and vegetables, especially broccoli, cabbage, cantaloupe, cauliflower, citrus fruits, green pepper, kiwi fruit, strawberries	Functions in synthesis of collagen; is an antioxidant; aids in detoxification; improves iron absorption; still under intense study	Scurvy; petechiae (minute hemorrhages around hair follicles); weakness; delayed wound healing; impaired immune response	GI upsets, confounds certain lab tests

[b]Estimated Safe and Adequate Daily Dietary Intake in 1989 RDAs.

From *Nutrition for Living* Fourth Edition, by Christian & Gregor. Copyright © 1994 Benjamin/Cummings Publishing Company, Menlo Park, CA. Reprinted by permission.

information on these vitamins, including RDA, dietary sources, function, and signs associated with deficiency or excess.

Water-Soluble Vitamins

The water-soluble vitamins include vitamin C and the B vitamins: thiamin (B-1), riboflavin (B-2), niacin, pyridoxine (B-6), folic acid, B-12, pantothenic acid, and biotin. Most are involved in energy metabolism. You have already seen the role of niacin, as NAD, and riboflavin, as FAD, in the transfer of energy in the Krebs cycle and electron transport chain. Thiamin (as thiamine pyrophosphate) is involved in the removal of CO_2 as pyruvate enters the Krebs cycle. Vitamin B-6, folic acid, B-12, pantothenic acid, and biotin are also involved as coenzymes in metabolic reactions. Vitamin C is involved in the maintenance of bone, cartilage, and connective tissue. Table 18.1 summarizes the information on these vitamins, including the RDA, function, dietary sources, and signs associated with deficiency or excess (36).

in summary

- The fat-soluble vitamins include A, D, E, and K. These can be stored in the body in large quantities and a toxicity can develop.
- The water-soluble vitamins include thiamin, riboflavin, niacin, B-6, folic acid, B-12, pantothenic acid, biotin, and C. Most of these are involved in energy metabolism. Vitamin C is involved in the maintenance of bone, cartilage, and connective tissue.

Minerals

Minerals are the chemical **elements,** other than carbon, hydrogen, oxygen, and nitrogen, associated with the structure and function of the body. We have already seen the importance of calcium in bone structure and in the initiation of muscle contraction, iron in O_2 transport by hemoglobin, and phosphorus in ATP. Minerals are important inorganic nutrients and are divided into two classes: (1) **major minerals** and (2) **trace elements.** The major minerals include calcium, phosphorous, magnesium, sulfur, sodium, potassium, and chloride, with whole-body quantities ranging from 35 gm for magnesium to 1,050 gm for calcium in a 70-kg man (36). The trace elements include iron, iodine, fluoride, zinc, selenium, copper, cobalt, chromium, manganese, molybdenum, arsenic, nickel, and vanadium. There are only 4 gm of iron and 0.0009 gm of vanadium in a 70-kg man. Like vitamins,

some minerals taken in excess (e.g., iron and zinc) can be toxic. The following sections will focus attention on calcium, iron, and sodium.

Calcium

Calcium (Ca^{++}) and phosphorus combine with organic molecules to form the teeth and bones. The bones are a "store" of calcium that helps to maintain the plasma Ca^{++} concentration when dietary intake is inadequate (see parathyroid hormone in chapter 5). Bone is constantly turning over its calcium and phosphorus, so diet must replace what is lost. If the diet is deficient in calcium for a long period of time, loss of bone, or **osteoporosis,** can occur. This weakening of the bone due to the loss of calcium and phosphorus from its structure is more common in women than in men, is accelerated at menopause, and is directly related to the higher rate of hip fractures in women. Three major factors are implicated: dietary calcium intake, inadequate estrogen, and lack of physical activity (63, 105, 119, 120).

There is concern that the increase in osteoporosis in our society is related to an inadequate calcium intake. While the RDA for calcium is 800 mg/day, no group of adult women meets the standard (105). The focus of attention has shifted to those under twenty-five years of age, where the goal is to maximize the chance for each individual to realize her genetically programmed peak bone mass (105). To achieve that goal, the RDA is set at 1,200 mg/day for women under 25 years of age. While menopause is the usual cause of a reduced secretion of estrogen, young, extremely active female athletes are experiencing this problem associated with amenorrhea (29, 35). The decrease in estrogen secretion is associated with the acceleration of osteoporosis. Estrogen therapy, with or without calcium supplementation, has been used successfully in menopausal women to reduce the rate of bone loss (103, 105). A third approach to deal with osteoporosis is based on the observation that exercise slows the rate of bone loss (2, 22, 64, 100, 109, 119). This has been shown in runners (22), as well as tennis players (100), and is viewed as an important reason for recommending regular moderate exercise in the elderly (see chapter 17).

Iron

Iron is an important part of hemoglobin and myoglobin, as well as the cytochromes of the electron transport chain. To remain in iron balance, the RDA is set at 10 mg/day for an adult male and 15 mg/day for an adult female; the higher amount is needed to replace that which is lost in the menses. A 70-kg man has about 2,500 mg of iron in hemoglobin, 150 mg in myoglobin, 6–8 mg in enzymes, and about 3 mg bound to **transferrin,** the iron-transporting protein in plasma. In addition to this, iron is stored as **ferritin** or **hemosiderin** in the liver, spleen, and bone marrow. The serum ferritin concentration is a sensitive measure of iron status. Each microgram (μg) of ferritin per liter of serum indicates the presence of 10 mg of stored iron (36, 58a, 62).

In spite of the higher need for iron, American women take in only 11 mg/day, while men take in 16 mg/day (36). This is due to higher caloric intakes in males than females. Since there are only 6 mg of iron per 1,000 kcal of energy in the American diet, a woman consuming 2,000 kcal/day would take in only 12 mg of iron. The male, consuming about 3,000 kcal/day, takes in 18 mg (62, 154). The diet provides iron in two forms, heme (ferrous) and nonheme (ferric). Heme iron, found primarily in meats, fish, and organ meats, is absorbed better than nonheme iron, which is found in vegetables. However, the absorption of nonheme iron can be increased by the presence of meat, fish, and vitamin C (36, 62, 154).

Anemia is a condition in which the hemoglobin concentration is low: less than 13 g/dl in men and less than 12 g/dl in women. This can be the result of blood loss (e.g., blood donation or bleeding), or a lack of vitamins or minerals in the diet. The most common cause of anemia in North America is a lack of dietary iron (36). In fact, iron deficiency is the most common nutrient deficiency. In iron deficiency anemia more than hemoglobin is affected. The iron bound to transferrin in the plasma is reduced and serum ferritin (an indicator of iron stores) is low (62). While children aged one to five, adolescents, young adult women, and the elderly are more apt to develop anemia, it also occurs in competitive athletes. This latter point will be discussed in detail in chapter 23.

Sodium

Sodium is directly involved in the maintenance of the resting membrane potential and the generation of action potential in nerves (chapter 7) and muscles (chapter 8). In addition, sodium is the primary electrolyte determining the extracellular fluid volume. If sodium stores fall, the extracellular volume, including plasma, is decreased. This could cause major problems related to the maintenance of the mean arterial blood pressure (chapter 9) and body temperature (chapter 12).

The problem in our society is not with sodium stores that are too small, but just the opposite. Americans consume about 11–12 grams of salt each day, equal to a sodium intake of 3.9–4.3 gm of sodium per day (salt is 39% sodium by weight) (105). While an RDA for sodium was not stated, the National Research Council's report, Diet and Health, (104) suggested that salt intake be limited to 6 gm per day (2.4 gm of sodium). This is consistent with the concerns raised by the American Heart Association (1a) that excess sodium intake can lead to hypertension in genetically susceptible individuals. In concert with this is one of the Dietary Guidelines for Americans, namely, to avoid too much sodium. The following suggestions were made relative to that guideline (142):

- Use salt sparingly, if at all, in cooking and at the table.
- When planning meals, consider that fresh and plain frozen vegetables prepared without salt are lower in sodium than canned ones.
- Cereals, pasta, and rice cooked without salt are lower in sodium than ready-to-eat cereals.
- Milk and yogurt are lower in sodium than most cheeses.
- Fresh meat, poultry, and fish are lower in sodium than most canned and processed ones.
- Most frozen dinners and combination dishes, packaged mixes, canned soups, and salad dressings contain a considerable amount of sodium. So do condiments, such as soy and other sauces, pickles, olives, catsup, and mustard.
- Use salted snacks, such as chips, crackers, pretzels, and nuts, sparingly.
- Check labels for the amount of sodium in foods. Choose those lower in sodium most of the time.

Those involved in athletic competition, strenuous exercise, or work in the heat must be concerned about adequate sodium replacement. Generally, because these individuals consume more kcal of food (containing more sodium), this is usually not a problem. More on this in chapter 23.

The previous sections have focused attention on three minerals—calcium, iron, and sodium—because of their relationship to current medical and health-related problems. A summary of each of the minerals, their function, and food sources is presented in table 18.2.

Table 18.2   Key Information About Many Essential Minerals

Mineral	RDA for Healthy Adults Ages 19–50	Major Dietary Sources	Major Functions	Signs of Severe, Prolonged Deficiency	Signs of Extreme Excess
Major Minerals					
Calcium	1,200 mg for ages 19–24; 800 mg for 25 and older	Milk, cheese, dark green vegetables, legumes	Bone and tooth formation; blood clotting; nerve transmission	Stunted growth; perhaps less bone mass	Depressed absorption of some other minerals; perhaps kidney damage
Phosphorus	1,200 mg for ages 19–24; 800 mg for 25 and older	Milk, cheese, meat, poultry, whole grains	Bone and tooth formation; acid-base balance; component of coenzymes	Weakness; demineralization of bone	Depressed absorption of some minerals
Magnesium	Females: 280 mg Males: 350 mg	Whole grains, green leafy vegetables	Component of enzymes	Neurological disturbances	Neurological disturbances
Sulfur	(Provided by sulfur amino acids)	Sulfur amino acids in dietary proteins	Component of cartilage, tendon, and proteins	(Related to protein deficiency)	Excess sulfur amino acid intake leads to poor growth; liver damage
Sodium	(no formal recommen-dation)	Salt, soy sauce, cured meats, pickles, canned soups, processed cheese	Body water balance; nerve function	Muscle cramps; reduced appetite	High blood pressure in genetically predisposed individuals
Potassium	(no formal recommen-dation)	Meats, milk, many fruits and vegetables, whole grains	Body water balance; nerve function	Muscular weakness, paralysis	Muscular weakness; cardiac arrest
Chloride	(no formal recommen-dation)	Same as for sodium	Plans a role in acid-base balance; formation of gastric juice	Muscle cramps; reduced appetite; poor growth	High blood pressure in genetically predisposed individuals
Trace Minerals					
Iron	Females: 15 mg Males: 10 mg	Meats, eggs, legumes, whole grains, green leafy vegetables	Component of hemoglobin, myoglobin, and enzymes	Iron deficiency, anemia, weakness, impaired immune function	Acute: shock, death Chronic: liver damage, cardiac failure
Iodine	150 µg	Marine fish and shellfish; dairy products; iodized salt; some breads	Component of thyroid hormones	Goiter (enlarged thyroid)	Iodide goiter

Continued

Table 18.2 continued

Mineral	RDA for Healthy Adults Ages 19–50	Major Dietary Sources	Major Functions	Signs of Severe, Prolonged Deficiency	Signs of Extreme Excess
Fluoride	1.5–4.0 mg[a]	Drinking water, tea, seafood	Maintenance of tooth (and maybe bone) structure	Higher frequency of tooth decay	Acute: GI distress; Chronic: mottling of teeth; skeletal deformation
Zinc	Females: 12 mg Males: 15 mg	Meats, seafood, whole grains	Component of enzymes	Growth failure; scaly dermatitis; reproductive failure; impaired immune function	Acute: nausea; vomiting; diarrhea Chronic: adversely affects copper metabolism, anemia, and immune function
Selenium	Females: 55 μg Males: 70 μg	Seafood, meat, whole grains	Component of enzyme; functions in close association with vitamin E	Muscle pain; maybe heart muscle deterioration	Nausea and vomiting; hair and nail loss
Copper	1.5–3 mg[a]	Seafood, nuts, legumes, organ meats	Component of enzymes	Anemia; bone and cardiovascular changes	Nausea; liver damage
Cobalt	(Required as vitamin B-12; no formal recommendation)	Animal products	Component of vitamin B-12	Not reported except as vitamin B-12 deficiency	With alcohol: heart failure
Chromium	50–200 μg[a]	Brewer's yeast, liver, seafood, meat, some vegetables	Involved in glucose and energy metabolism	Impaired glucose metabolism	Lung, kidney damage (occupational exposure only)
Manganese	2.0–5.0 mg[a]	Nuts, whole grains, vegetables and fruits, tea	Component of enzymes	Abnormal bone and cartilage	Central nervous system damage (occupational exposures)
Molybdenum	75–250 μg[a]	Legumes, cereals, some vegetables	Component of enzymes	Disorder in nitrogen excretion	Inhibition of enzymes; adversely affects copper metabolism

[a]Estimated safe and adequate daily dietary intake

From *Nutrition for Living* Fourth Edition, by Christian and Gregor. Copyright © 1994 Benjamin/Cummings Publishing Company, Menlo Park, CA. Reprinted by permission.

in summary

- The major minerals include calcium, phosphorus, magnesium, sulfur, sodium, potassium, and chloride. The trace elements include iron, iodine, fluoride, zinc, selenium, copper, cobalt, chromium, manganese, molybdenum, arsenic, nickel, and vanadium.
- Inadequate calcium and iron intake have been linked with osteoporosis and anemia, respectively. Those with a genetic predisposition for hypertension due to sodium retention benefit from a reduction in salt intake.

Carbohydrates

Carbohydrates and fats are the primary sources of energy in the average American diet (105). Carbohydrates suffer a bad reputation from those on diets, especially when you consider that you would have to eat over twice as much carbohydrate as fat to consume the same number of calories (4 kcal/gm versus 9 kcal/gm). Carbohydrates can be divided into two classes, those that can be digested and metabolized for energy (sugars and starches), and those that are undigestible (fiber). The sugars are found in jellies, jams, fruits, soft drinks, honey, syrups, and milk, while the starches are found in cereals, flour, potatoes, and other vegetables (141).

Sugars and Starches

Carbohydrate is a major energy source for all tissues and a crucial source for two: red blood cells and neurons. The red blood cells depend exclusively on anaerobic glycolysis for energy, and the nervous system functions well only on carbohydrate. These two tissues can consume 180 grams of glucose per day (39). Given this need it is no surprise that the plasma glucose concentration is maintained within narrow limits by hormonal control mechanisms (chapter 5). During strenuous exercise the muscle can use 180 grams of glucose in less than one hour. As a result of these needs one might expect that carbohydrate would make up a large fraction of our energy intake. Currently about 50% of energy intake is derived from carbohydrate (58a, 105), with the dietary goal being 55%–60% (144). While the goal is to increase carbohydrate intake, one of the *Dietary Guidelines for Americans* is to avoid too much sugar. The following suggestions were made relative to these guidelines (142):

- Use sugars in moderate amounts—sparingly if your calorie needs are low. Avoid excess snacking and brush and floss your teeth regularly.
- Read food labels. A food is likely to be high in sugars if its ingredient list shows one of the following first or second or if it shows several of them: table sugar (sucrose), brown sugar, raw sugar, glucose (dextrose), fructose, maltose, lactose, honey, syrup, corn sweetener, high-fructose corn syrup, molasses, fruit juice concentrate.

Dietary Fiber

Dietary fiber includes two insoluble forms, cellulose and hemicellulose, and three soluble forms, pectins, gums, and mucilages (36). Dietary fiber cannot be digested and metabolized, and consequently provides a sense of fullness (satiation) during a meal without the additional calories (45). This fact has been used by bakeries who lower the number of calories per slice of bread by adding cellulose from wood! Pectin and gum are used in food processing to thicken, stabilize, or emulsify the constituents of various food products (36).

Dietary fiber has long been linked to optimal health. Fiber acts as a hydrated sponge as it moves along the large intestine, making constipation less likely by reducing transit time (36, 45). Vegetarian diets high in soluble fiber have been linked to lower serum cholesterol due to the loss of more bile (cholesterol-containing) acids in the feces. However, the fact that vegetarian diets are also lower in the percent of calories from fat, which can also lower serum cholesterol, makes the interpretation of the data more complicated (45). While a high fiber diet reduces the incidence of diverticulosis, a condition in which outpouchings (diverticula) occur in the colon wall, the role of fiber in preventing colon cancer is still questionable (36, 45).

Given the broad role of dietary fiber in normal health, it is no surprise that the *Dietary Guidelines for Americans* recommends that Americans increase their intake of fiber (142). However, at this time no RDA exists for dietary fiber. According to *Dietary Guidelines for Americans*, to increase the intake of fiber and complex carbohydrates, we should eat on a daily basis:

- Three or more servings of various vegetables
- Two or more servings of various fruits
- Six or more servings of grain products (breads, cereals, pasta, and rice)

Fats

Dietary lipids include triglycerides, phospholipids, and **cholesterol.** If solid at room temperature, lipids are fats; if liquid, oils. Lipids contain 9 kcal/gm, and represent about 34% to 36% of the American diet, higher than the dietary goal of 30%, but lower than the 42% recorded in 1977 (37, 58a, 105, 144).

Fat not only provides fuel for energy, it is important in the absorption of fat-soluble vitamins, and for cell membrane structure, hormone synthesis (steroids), insulation, and protection of vital organs (36). Most fat is stored in adipose tissue, for subsequent release into the blood stream as free fatty acids (chapter 4). Because of fat's caloric density (9 kcal/gm), we are able to carry a large energy reserve, with little weight. In fact, the energy content of one pound of adipose tissue, 3,500 kcal, is sufficient to cover the cost of running a marathon. The other side of this coin is that because of this very high caloric density it takes a long time to decrease the mass of adipose tissue when on a diet.

The focus of attention in the medical community has been on the role of dietary fat in the development of atherosclerosis, a process in which the arterial wall becomes thickened, leading to a narrowing of the lumen of the artery. This is the underlying problem associated with coronary artery disease and stroke. While the specific cause is not known, it is believed that a variety of factors can damage the protective endothelial lining of the artery, allowing substances to build up and block the artery. The factors that can accelerate this process include elevated serum cholesterol and triglycerides, high blood pressure, and cigarette smoking (41). In the section on dietary goals, two of the recommendations dealt with this problem of atherosclerosis: a reduction in salt intake (see minerals), and a reduction in fat, saturated fat, and cholesterol. A reduction in each of the last three has been shown to reduce serum cholesterol, and with it, the risk of atherosclerosis (1a).

Usually the cholesterol concentration in the serum is divided into two classes on the basis of what type of **lipoprotein** is carrying the cholesterol. **Low-density lipoproteins (LDL)** carry more cholesterol than do the **high-density lipoproteins (HDL).** High levels of **LDL cholesterol** are directly related to cardiovascular risk, while high levels of **HDL cholesterol** offer protection from heart disease (1a). The concentration of HDL cholesterol is influenced by heredity, gender, exercise, and diet. Diets high in saturated fats increase LDL cholesterol. A reduction in the sources of saturated fats, including meats, animal fat, palm oil, coconut oil, hydrogenated shortenings, whole milk, cream, butter, ice cream, and cheese would reduce LDL cholesterol. Just substituting unsaturated fats for these saturated fats will lower serum cholesterol. Overall,

the consistent recommendation from the National Research Council (104) and the American Heart Association (1a) is to lower total fat consumption to less than 30% of total caloric intake. Dietary restriction of cholesterol has been shown to be effective in lowering serum cholesterol (1a); however, this effect is influenced by the percentage of saturated fat in the diet and the initial level of serum cholesterol (i.e., those with high serum cholesterol levels benefit the most) (46). Based on currently available evidence, it is reasonable and prudent to recommend a decrease in cholesterol in the diet to 300 mg/day or less (1a, 104). The following suggestions were provided as part of the *Dietary Guidelines for Americans* to have a diet low in fat, saturated fat, and cholesterol (142):

- Use fats and oils sparingly in cooking.
- Use small amounts of salad dressings and spreads, such as butter, margarine, and mayonnaise. One tablespoon of most of these spreads provides 10 to 11 grams of fat.
- Choose liquid vegetable oils most often because they are lower in saturated fat.
- Check labels on foods to see how much fat and saturated fat are in a serving.
- Trim fat from meat; take skin off poultry.
- Have cooked dry beans and peas instead of meat occasionally.
- Moderate the use of egg yolks and organ meats.
- Choose skim or low-fat milk and fat-free or low-fat yogurt and cheese most of the time.

Protein

Protein, at 4 kcal/gm, is not viewed as a primary energy source, as are fats and carbohydrates. Rather, it is important because it contains the nine essential amino acids, without which the body cannot synthesize all the proteins needed for tissues, enzymes, and hormones. The *quality* of protein in a diet is based on how well these essential amino acids are represented. In terms of quality, the best sources for protein are eggs, milk, and fish, with *good* sources being meat, poultry, cheese, and soybeans. *F*air sources of protein include grains, vegetables, seeds and nuts, and other legumes. Given that a meal contains a variety of foods, one food of higher quality protein tends to complement another of lower quality protein to result in an adequate intake of essential amino acids (36).

The adult RDA protein requirement of 0.8 gm/kg is easily met with diets that include a variety of the aforementioned foods. The protein requirement is also expressed as 10%–12% of total kcal ingested. Overall, most Americans meet either of these recommendations. The protein requirement for athletes is discussed in chapter 23.

in summary

- Carbohydrate is a primary source of energy in the American diet, and is divided into two classes: that which can be metabolized (sugars and starches) and dietary fiber.
- Two recommendations to improve health status in the American population are to increase the amount of complex carbohydrates to represent about 55%–60% of the calories, and to add more dietary fiber.
- Americans consume too much dietary fat, and the recommended change to reduce this total to no more than 30% is consistent with good health. Saturated fats should not represent more than 10% of the total calories.
- The protein requirement of 0.8 gm/kg can be met with low fat selections to minimize fat intake.

Meeting the Guidelines and Achieving the Goals

A good diet would allow an individual to achieve the RDA for protein, minerals, and vitamins, while emphasizing carbohydrates and minimizing fats. This can be accomplished by following one of the *Dietary Guidelines for Americans*: to eat a variety of foods. These guidelines (142) suggested that daily food selections should include:

- 3–5 servings of vegetables
- 2–4 servings of fruits
- 6–11 servings of breads, cereals, rice, and pasta
- 2–3 servings of milk, yogurt, and cheese
- 2–3 servings of meats, poultry, fish, dry beans and peas, eggs, and nuts

A variety of food group plans have been developed to help plan a diet consistent with these guidelines.

Food Group Plans

One of the best known plans, the Basic Four Food Group Plan, includes meat and meat substitutes, milk and milk products, fruits and vegetables, and grains (breads and cereals) as the food groups. Adults choose at least 2, 2, 4, and 4 servings per day from these respective groups. The emphasis is on eating a variety of items within each group in which **nutrient density** is relatively high. Nutrient density describes the nutrient content in 1,000 kcal of a food (105). Selecting foods of high nutrient density keeps the nutrients high and total kcals low. The quantity of each item within a food group in the Basic Four Food Group Plan is based on the quantity of a *specific nutrient* contained therein. For example, the items on the milk list have the calcium content in one cup of milk, and meat portion is based on protein content. Recently, the U.S. Department of Agriculture (140) introduced a new food group plan, the Food Guide Pyramid, to provide better guidance in making food selections consistent with the *Dietary Guidelines for Americans*.

Food Guide Pyramid

The Food Guide Pyramid, shown in figure 18.2, focuses on dietary fat, and how to make food selections to keep the intake of that nutrient below 30% of daily caloric intake. It also offers guidance related to the intake of sugars and salt. Table 18.3 shows some sample foods and serving sizes, as well as the recommended number of servings for three levels of caloric intake. The recommendation for a fat intake equal to 30% of caloric intake would allow 53, 73, and 93 grams of fat for the 1,600, 2,200, and 2,800 kcal intakes, respectively. It should be noted that only half of this total fat intake would be obtained if one selected the lowest fat choices in each food group (140).

Exchange System

Another method of planning a diet is the Exchange System. In this system the *caloric content and the percent of carbohydrate, fat, and protein* in each food is the focus of attention, rather than the nutrient density as in the Basic Four Food Group Plan or the Food Guide Pyramid. Foods in each group in the Exchange System are similar in these characteristics. Table 18.4 shows the breakdown for each of the six groups. This system is useful in weight control programs since the focus of attention is on calories. By knowing how many "exchanges" from each group are contained in the diet, the caloric content is known.

Evaluating the Diet

Independent of your dietary plan, the question arises as to how well you are achieving the guidelines. How do you analyze your diet? The first thing to do is to determine what you are eating, without fooling yourself. The use of the **twenty-four-hour recall** method relies on your ability to remember, from a specific time in one day, what you ate during the previous twenty-four hours. You have to judge the size of the portion you have eaten and make a judgment of whether or not that day was representative of what you normally eat. Other people use **food records,** in which a person records what is eaten throughout the day. It is recommended that a person obtain food records for three or four days per week to have a better estimate of usual dietary intake. Since the simple act of recording food intake may change our eating habits, one has to try and eat as normally as possible when recording food intake. It is important to remember that the RDA standards are to be met over the long run, and variations from those standards will exist from day to day (36).

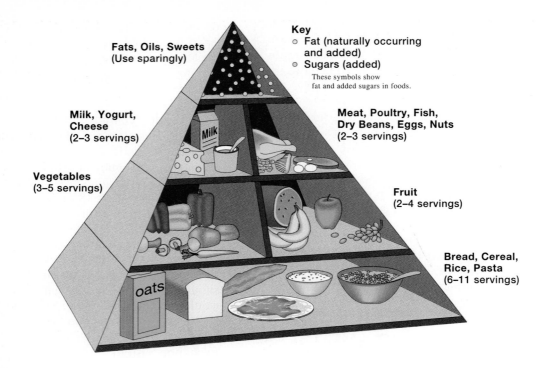

Key
○ Fat (naturally occurring and added)
◎ Sugars (added)
These symbols show fat and added sugars in foods.

Fats, Oils, Sweets
(Use sparingly)

Milk, Yogurt, Cheese
(2–3 servings)

Meat, Poultry, Fish, Dry Beans, Eggs, Nuts
(2–3 servings)

Vegetables
(3–5 servings)

Fruit
(2–4 servings)

Bread, Cereal, Rice, Pasta
(6–11 servings)

Figure 18.2

The U.S. Department of Agriculture introduced the food pyramid in 1992. The chart is a guideline to healthy eating. In contrast to former food group plans, the pyramid gives an instant idea of which foods should make up the bulk of the diet—whole grains, fruits, and vegetables.

Source: U.S. Department of Agriculture, 1992.

Table 18.3 Food Guide Pyramid: Food Groups, Sample Foods, and Daily Servings

Food Group	Sample Foods and Serving Size	Servings for 3 levels of daily caloric intake (kcal/day)		
		1,600	2,200	2,800
Breads	1 slice of bread 1 oz ready-to-eat cereal ½ cup of cooked cereal, rice, or pasta	6	9	11
Vegetable	1 cup of raw leafy vegetables ½ cup of other vegetables ¾ cup of vegetable juice	3	4	5
Fruit	1 medium apple ½ cup of chopped, cooked, or canned fruit ¾ cup of fruit juice	2	3	4
Milk	1 cup of milk or yogurt 1½ oz of natural cheese 2 oz of processed cheese	2–3	2–3	2–3
Meat	2–3 oz of cooked lean meat, poultry, or fish (½ cup cooked beans or 1 egg counts as 1 oz of lean meat)	2–3 servings equal to 5 oz of lean meat	2–3 servings equal to 6 oz of lean meat	2–3 servings equal to 7 oz of lean meat

Source: U.S. Department of Agriculture.

Table 18.4 The Six Exchange Groups

Group	Serving Size	Similar Foods	Carbohydrate (gm)	Protein (gm)	Fat (gm)	Energy (kcal)
Milk (skim)	1 cup	1 cup skim milk 1 cup yogurt from skim milk	12	8	Trace	90
Vegetable	½ cup	String beans Greens Carrots Beets	5	2	0	25
Fruit	1 serving	½ small banana 1 small apple ½ grapefruit ½ cup orange juice	15	0	0	60
Bread (starch)	1 slice	¾ cup ready-to-eat cereal ½ cup beans ⅓ cup corn 1 small potato	15	3	Trace	80
Meat (lean)	1 oz	1 oz chicken meat, w/o skin 1 oz fish ¼ cup canned tuna, or salmon 1 oz low-fat cheese (<5% butterfat)	0	7	3	55
Fat	1 tsp	1 tsp margarine 1 tsp oil 1 tbsp salad dressing 1 strip crisp bacon	0	0	5	45

The exchange lists are the basis of a meal planning system designed by a committee of the American Diabetes Association and The American Dietetic Association. While designed primarily for people with diabetes and others who must follow special diets, the exchange lists are based on principles of good nutrition that apply to everyone. Based on material from The American Diabetes Association and The American Dietetic Association, 1986.

in summary

- The Food Guide Pyramid provides guidance for meeting the nutritional requirements specified in the *Dietary Guidelines for Americans*.
- The Exchange System includes six groups organized for their composition of carbohydrate, fat, and protein, with special consideration for the caloric content. The six groups include milk, vegetable, fruit, bread, meat, and fat.

Body Composition

Obesity is a major problem in our society, being related to hypertension, elevated serum cholesterol, and adult onset diabetes (74). In addition, there is growing concern that as the incidence of childhood obesity increases, so will the pool of obese adults. In order to deal with this problem we must be able to monitor changes in body fatness throughout life and evaluate the effectiveness of diet and exercise in dealing with this problem. This section presents a brief overview of the different methods used in body composition analysis, and provides detailed explanations of the most common methods.

Methods of Measuring Body Composition

The Metropolitan Life Insurance Company's 1959 height/weight table (97) is one of the most common methods used to make judgments about whether or

Table 18.5 Desirable Weights for Men and Women, Twenty-Five Years of Age and Over

Height* Feet	Inches	Small Frame	Medium Frame	Large Frame
Men				
5	2	112–120	118–129	126–141
5	3	115–123	121–133	129–144
5	4	118–126	124–136	133–148
5	5	121–129	127–139	135–152
5	6	124–133	130–143	138–156
5	7	128–137	134–147	142–161
5	8	132–141	138–152	147–166
5	9	136–145	142–156	151–170
5	10	140–150	146–160	155–174
5	11	144–154	150–165	159–179
6	0	148–158	154–170	164–184
6	1	152–162	158–175	168–189
6	2	156–167	162–180	173–194
6	3	160–171	167–185	178–199
6	4	164–175	172–190	182–204

Height** Feet	Inches	Smale Frame	Medium Frame	Large Frame
Women				
4	10	92–98	96–107	104–119
4	11	94–101	98–110	106–122
5	0	96–104	101–113	109–125
5	1	99–107	104–116	112–128
5	2	102–110	107–119	115–131
5	3	105–113	110–122	118–134
5	4	108–116	113–126	121–138
5	5	111–119	116–130	125–142
5	6	114–123	120–135	129–146
5	7	118–127	124–139	133–150
5	8	122–131	128–143	137–154
5	9	126–135	132–147	141–158
5	10	130–140	136–151	145–163
5	11	134–144	140–155	149–168
6	0	138–148	144–159	153–173

Courtesy *Statistical Bulletin*, Metropolitan Insurance Company.
*With shoes with one-inch heels.
**With shoes with two-inch heels.

not a person is overweight (table 18.5). These tables are based on that company's policyholders, and the body weights associated with the lowest rate of mortality are listed by frame size. In 1983 an updated table was published that allowed more weight at each height. It has been suggested that the lower death rates at the higher weights in the 1983 table were a result of better treatment of coronary heart disease and diabetes, which allows heavier people to live longer; a reduction in cigarette smoking; and an increase in physical activity (41). The American Heart Association continues to recommend the 1959 table.

Independent of which table is used, there are some problems associated with their use (4):

- Persons seeking and receiving insurance are not representative of the general population.
- Some persons are represented more than once in the table, since policies (not people) were tabulated.
- Heights and weights were not measured in every case (some policyholders simply stated these).
- Body frame size was not measured.

In spite of these limitations, one of the most common indices of body composition is calculated from this table. In this procedure the midpoint in the weight range for a medium frame for a given height is used as a standard against which other body weights are compared. Dividing a person's weight by the midpoint in the weight range generates a relative weight (RW) or obesity index. A person with a body weight equal to the midpoint value would have an RW = 1.00. In contrast, if we look at the 1959 table (table 18.5), a man who is six feet tall and weighs 200 lbs, has an RW = 1.23 (200 lb ÷162 lb). A person who is 10% above normal (RW = 1.10) is classified as overweight, and if 20% above normal (RW = 1.20), is classified as obese. Our male subject at 23% above normal would be classified as obese.

Another measure of body composition that has been universally adopted is the Body Mass Index (BMI), which is the ratio of body weight (in kilograms) to height (in meters) squared: BMI = wt [kg] ÷ ht [m^2]. This index of body composition is easily calculated, and obesity guidelines related to percentile rankings (85th or 95th) or fixed values (27.8 for men and 27.3 for women) exist (90). However, concern has been expressed about recommendations in which the "healthy range" of BMI is listed as 19 to 25 for those 19 to 35 years of age, and 21 to 27 for those older than 35 years of age. Some feel that the upper value is too generous given that it is associated with a higher rate of morbidity and mortality (19, 152, 153).

One of the major problems associated with height/weight tables and the BMI is that there is no way to know if the person is heavily muscled or simply overfat. One of the earliest uses of body composition analysis showed that with height/weight tables "All American" football players weighing 200 lbs would have been found unfit for military service and would not have received life insurance (151). Clearly there is a need to distinguish overweight from overfat, and that will be the purpose of the next section of this chapter.

The most direct way to measure body composition is to do a chemical analysis of the whole body to determine the amount of water, fat, protein, and minerals. This is a common method used in nutritional studies on rats, but is useless in providing information for the average person. The following is a brief summary of techniques providing information about (a) the composition of the whole body and (b) the development or change in specific tissues of the body.

Isotope Dilution Total body water (TBW) is determined by the isotope dilution method. In this method a subject drinks an isotope of water (tritiated water—^3H_2O), deuterated water (^2H_2O), or ^{18}O-labeled water ($H_2{}^{18}O$) that is distributed throughout the body water. After three to four hours to allow for distribution of the isotope, a sample of body fluid (serum or saliva) is obtained and the concentration of the isotope is determined. The volume of TBW is obtained by calculating how much body water would be needed to achieve that concentration. A person with a large amount of body water will dilute the isotope to a greater extent. People with large TBW volumes possess more lean tissue and less fat tissue, so TBW can be used to determine body fatness (48, 118).

Photon Absorptiometry This method is used to determine the mineral content and density of bones. A beam of photons from iodine-125 is passed over a bone or bones, and the transmission of the photon beam through bone and soft tissue is obtained. There is a very strong positive relationship between the absorption of the photons and the mineral density of the bones (33, 90).

Potassium-40 Potassium is located primarily within the cells, along with a naturally occurring radioactive isotope of potassium: ^{40}K. The ^{40}K can be measured in a whole-body "counter," and is proportional to the mass of lean tissue (23).

Hydrostatic (Underwater) Weighing Water has a density of about 1 gm/ml, and body fat, with a density of about 0.900 gm/ml, will float in water. Lean tissue has a density of about 1.100 in adults and will sink in water. Whole body density provides information about the portion of the body that is lean and fat. Underwater weighing methods are commonly used to determine body density, and will be discussed in more detail (90).

Dual Energy X-ray Absorptiometry (DEXA) In this new technology a single X-ray source is used to determine whole-body and regional estimates of lean tissue, bone, mineral, and fat with a high degree of accuracy. The software required for this process continues to be refined and DEXA is expected to play a major role in the future of body composition analysis (45a, 90, 94a, 146a).

Near Infrared Interactance (NIR) This method is based on the absorption of light, reflectance, and near infrared spectroscopy (24). A fiber-optic probe is placed over the biceps and an infrared light beam is emitted. The light passes through subcutaneous fat and muscle and is reflected by bone back to the probe. Generally, there has been little interaction between scientists and the manufacturers in the development and validation of this type of device (90), and recent studies suggest that this technology has a way to go (26a, 95).

Radiography An X-ray of a limb allows one to measure the widths of fat, muscle, and bone, and has been used extensively in tracing the growth of these tissues over time (72). Fat-width measurements can also be used to estimate total body fat (52, 75).

Ultrasound Sound waves are transmitted through tissues and the echoes are received and analyzed. This technique has been used to measure the thickness of subcutaneous fat. Present technology allows for whole body scans and the determination of the volumes of various organs (24).

Nuclear Magnetic Resonance (NMR) In this method electromagnetic waves are transmitted through tissues. Select nuclei absorb and then release energy at a particular frequency (resonance). The resonant-frequency characteristics are related to the type of tissue. Computer analysis of the signal can provide detailed images, and the volumes of specific tissues can be calculated (24).

Total Body Electrical Conductivity (TOBEC) Body composition is analyzed by TOBEC on the basis that lean tissue and water conduct electricity better than does fat. In this method the subject lies in a large cylindrical coil while an electric current is injected into the coil. The electromagnetic field developed in the space enclosed by the cylindrical coil is affected by the subject's body composition (115, 122, 146).

Bioelectrical Impedance Analysis (BIA) The basis for BIA is similar to that of TOBEC, but uses a small portable instrument. An electrical current (50 µA usually set at a frequency of 50 kHz) is applied to an extremity and resistance to that current (due to the specific resistivity and volume of the conductor—the fat-free mass) is measured (90, 122, 146). Total body water is calculated, and the value can be used to estimate percent body fatness, as was mentioned for the isotope dilution procedure. BIA devices using multiple frequencies (5, 50, and 100 kHz) show promise of improved accuracy (90, 124, 146b). This technique may be an appropriate field method to use in place of or in addition to skinfolds in testing the elderly (55a).

Skinfold Thickness An estimate of total body fatness is made from a measure of subcutaneous fat. A number of skinfold measurements are obtained and the values used in equations to calculate body density (85, 90). Details on this technique will be presented in a later section.

Some of these procedures are expensive in terms of personnel and equipment (e.g., potassium-40, TOBEC, radiography, ultrasound, NMR, DEXA, TBW), and are not used on a routine basis for body composition analysis. BIA has gained greater acceptance in the past few years, due in part to a collaborative multiuniversity research project that showed it to be comparable to skinfold estimates of body fatness in men and women (90). The data from these techniques can be used alone or in combination to provide an assessment of body composition. A variety of models have been proposed for this purpose (65b, 90, 90a):

- Four-component model—this model uses information on mineral, water, protein, and fat to assess body composition. The careful measurement of each of these components allows one to account for variations in bone density (mineral) and total body water that might vary dramatically in certain populations (e.g., growing children, the elderly). These procedures would give one the best estimates of percent fat.

- Three-component model—in this model the body is divided into three components: (a) body water, protein + mineral, and fat, or (b) body water + protein, mineral, and fat. The three-component model also allows one to account for variations in either bone density or body water and improve estimates of body fatness.

- Two-component model—this, the oldest model, divides the body into two components, the fat mass and the fat-free mass. Although it is still the most commonly used approach to estimate percent fat, the assumptions underlying this model have been questioned. The limitations of the two-component model have been addressed using information collected with the multicomponent (3- and 4-component) models. The details will be provided in the following sections.

in summary

- A height/weight table and the body mass index (BMI) can indicate "overweight" relative to an average weight, but do not provide quantitative information about the composition of that weight in terms of fat-free mass and fat mass.

- Body composition can be measured in terms of total body water (isotope dilution, bioelectric impedance analysis), bone density (photon absorptiometry), lean tissue mass (potassium-40), density (underwater weighing), and thickness of various tissues (ultrasound, radiography, skinfolds).

- Body composition assessment can be based on 4-component (mineral, water, protein, and fat), 3-component (body water, protein + mineral, and fat, or body water + protein, mineral, and fat), or 2-component (fat-free mass and fat mass) models. The four component model is the most accurate.

Table 18.6 Equations for Estimating % Fat from Body Density Based on Age and Gender

Age, yrs.	Male C_1	Male C_2	Female C_1	Female C_2
1	572	536	569	533
1–2	564	526	565	526
3–4	553	514	558	520
5–6	543	503	553	514
7–8	538	497	543	503
9–10	530	489	535	495
11–12	523	481	525	484
13–14	507	464	512	469
15–16	503	459	507	464
Young adult	495	450	505	462

Note: C_1 and C_2 are the terms in percent fat equation to substitute for the Siri equation of percent fat = $\left[\dfrac{C_1}{D_b} - C_2 \right]$.

Reprinted, by permission, from T. G. Lohman, 1989, "Assessment of Body Composition in Children," in *Pediatric Exercise Science*, Vol. 1(1):22.

Two-Component System of Body Composition

Two approaches that are used extensively to estimate percent fat include the **underwater weighing** and skinfold methods. In both of these methods the investigator obtains an estimate of **whole body density,** and from this calculates the percentage of the body that is fat and the percentage that is fat-free. This is the two-component body composition system described by Behnke that is commonly used to describe changes in body composition (7). The conversion of whole body density values to fat and fat-free tissue components relies on "constants" used for each of those tissue components. Human fat tissue is believed to have a density of 0.900 gm/ml, and fat-free tissue a density of 1.100 gm/ml. Using these density values, Siri (130) derived an equation to calculate percent body fat from whole body density:

$$\% \text{ body fat} = \frac{495}{\text{Density}} - 450$$

This equation is correct only if the density values for fat tissue and fat-free tissue are 0.900 and 1.100 gm/ml, respectively. Investigators sensed that certain populations might have fat-free tissue densities different from that of 1.100 gm/ml when they observed high values for body fatness for children and the elderly, and extremely low values (<0% body fat) in professional football players (55a, 91, 156). Children have lower bone mineral contents, less potassium, and more water per unit fat-free mass, yielding a lower density for fat-free mass (91). Lohman (88) reports density values (gm/ml) of 1.080 at age six, 1.084 at age ten, and 1.097 for boys aged fifteen and one-half. The lower values in the prepubescent child would overestimate percent body fat by 5%. Based on data from the multicomponent models of body composition, Lohman (89a) recommends the values found in table 18.6 for Siri's equation when applied to children, youth, and young adults (see table 18.6).

In contrast to children who have density values below 1.100 for the fat-free mass, African Americans were shown to have a density of 1.113 gm/ml (121). The Siri equation would have to be modified as follows:

$$\% \text{ body fat} = \frac{437}{\text{Density}} - 393$$

While this may appear to be quite complicated, there is good reason to have the correct equation for a specific population. If judgments are to be made about the distribution of obesity in our society, it is important that estimates of body fatness be reasonably accurate. The following sections will discuss how whole-body density values are determined by underwater weighing and skinfold procedures.

Underwater Weighing

Density is equal to mass divided by volume ($D = M/V$). Since we already know body mass (body weight), we only have to determine body volume in order to calculate whole-body density (57). The underwater weighing method applies Archimedes' principle, which states that when an object is placed in water it is buoyed up by a counterforce equal to the water it displaces. The volume of water displaced (spilled over) would equal the *loss of weight* while the object is completely submerged. Some investigators determine body volume by measuring the actual volume of water displaced; others measure weight while the subject is underwater, and obtain body volume by subtracting the weight measured in water (M_W) from that measured in air (M_A), or ($M_A - M_W$). Both methods of determining volume are reproducible, but percent body fat values are

Figure 18.3
The underwater weighing technique illustrating two individuals with the same weight and height, but different body composition.

slightly but significantly (0.7%) lower with the volume displacement method (149). The weight of water displaced is converted to a volume by dividing by the density of the water (D_W) at the time of measurement.

$$D = \frac{M}{V} = \frac{M_A}{\dfrac{(M_A - M_W)}{D_W}}$$

This denominator must now be corrected for two other volumes: the volume of air in the lungs at the time of measurement [usually residual volume (V_R)], and the volume of gas in the gastrointestinal tract (V_{GI}). It is recommended that V_R be measured at the time that underwater weight is measured, but measurement on land with the subject in the same position is a suitable alternative (88). Residual volume can also be estimated with gender-specific regression equations, or by taking 24% (males) or 28% (females)

of vital capacity. However, the latter two procedures introduce measurement errors of 2%–3% fat for a given individual (102). V_{GI} can be quite variable, and while some investigators ignore this measure, others assume a 100 ml volume for all subjects (90).

The density equation can now be rewritten (30).

$$D = \frac{M}{V} = \frac{M_A}{\dfrac{(M_A - M_W)}{D_W} - V_R - V_{GI}}$$

Figure 18.3 shows the equipment used to measure underwater weight. Water temperature is measured to obtain the correct water density. The subject is weighed on land on a scale accurate to within 100 gms. The subject puts on a diver's belt with sufficient weight to prevent floating during the weighing procedure, and sits on the chair suspended from the precision scale. The scale can be read to 10 gms, and has major divisions of 50 gms. The subject sits on the chair with the water at chin level and as a maximal exhalation is just about completed, the subject bends over and pulls the head under. When a maximal expiration is achieved, the subject holds that position for about five to ten seconds while the investigator reads the scale. This procedure is repeated six to ten times until the values stabilize. The weight of the diver's belt and chair are subtracted from this weight to obtain the true value for M_W. If V_R were to be measured at the time underwater weight is measured, the subject would have to be breathing through a mouthpiece and valve assembly that could be activated at the correct time (113).

The following data were obtained on a white male, aged thirty-six: $M_A = 75.20$ kg, $M_W = 3.52$ kg, $V_R = 1.43$ liters, $D_W = 0.9944$ at 34° C, $V_{GI} = 0.1$ liters.

$$D = \frac{M}{V} = \frac{75.20}{\dfrac{(75.20 - 3.52)}{0.9944} - 1.43 - 0.1} = \frac{75.20}{70.55} = 1.066$$

This density value is now used in Siri's equation to calculate percent body fat.

$$\% \text{ body fat} = \frac{495}{\text{Density}} - 450$$

$$14.3 = \frac{495}{1.066} - 450$$

The underwater weighing procedure in which RV is measured (and not estimated) has been used as the "standard" against which other methods are compared. However, remember that due to the normal biological variability in the fat-free mass in a given population, the percent body fat value is estimated to be within about ±2.0% of the "true" value (90).

in summary

- In the two-component system of body composition analysis, the body is divided into fat-free and fat mass, with densities of 1.100 and 0.900, respectively. The estimate of the density of the fat-free mass must account for differences that exist in various populations (i.e., children and African Americans).
- Body density is equal to mass ÷ volume. Underwater weighing is used to determine body volume using the principle of Archimedes: when an object is placed in water it is buoyed up by a counterforce equal to the water it displaces. One can measure the actual volume of water displaced, or the loss of weight while underwater. The weight of water is divided by the density of water to yield body volume, which must then be corrected for the residual volume and the volume of gas in the GI tract.
- The percent body fat value has an error of about ±2.0% due to the normal biological variation of the fat-free mass.

Sum of Skinfolds

Underwater weighing, although a good way to obtain a measurement of body density, is time consuming and requires special equipment and personnel. Paralleling the development of the advanced technologies used in body composition analysis, scientists developed equations that predicted body density from a collection of skinfold measurements. The skinfold method relies on the observation that within any population a certain fraction of the total body fat lies just under the skin (subcutaneous fat), and if one could obtain a representative sample of that fat, overall body fatness (density) could be predicted. Generally, these prediction equations were developed with the underwater weighing method used as the standard. For example, a group of college males and females would have body density measured by underwater weighing, and a variety of skinfold measures would also be obtained. The investigator would then determine what collection of skinfolds would most accurately predict the body density determined by underwater weighing.

Investigators found that subcutaneous fat represents a variable fraction of total fat (20%–70%), depending on age, sex, overall fatness, and the measurement technique used. At a specific body fatness women have less subcutaneous fat than men, and older subjects of the same sex have less than younger subjects (85). Given that these variables could influence an estimate of body density, it is no surprise that of the more than one hundred equations developed, most were found to be "population specific" and could not be used for groups of different ages or sex. This obviously creates problems for exercise leaders in adult fitness programs or elementary or high school physical education teachers when they try to find the equation that works best for their particular group. Fortunately, a good deal of progress has been made to reduce these problems.

Jackson and Pollock (68) and Jackson, Pollock, and Ward (70) developed "generalized equations" for men and women, that is, equations that could be used across various age groups. In addition, these equations have been validated for athletic and nonathletic populations, including postpubescent athletes (88, 128, 129). In these equations, specific skinfold measurements are obtained and the values are used along with age to calculate body density. Here are two such equations, one for men and one for women, which can be used to predict body density (69). The body density value obtained is used in the Siri equation presented earlier to calculate % body fat.

Men
$$\text{Density} = 1.1125025 - 0.0013125 \, (X_1) + 0.0000055 \, (X_1)^2 - 0.0002440 \, (X_2)$$

Where X_1 = sum of chest, triceps, subscapular skinfolds, and X_2 = age in years.

Women
$$\text{Density} = 1.089733 - 0.0009245 \, (X_1) + 0.0000025 \, (X_1)^2 - 0.0000979 \, (X_2)$$

Where X_1 = sum of triceps, suprailium, and abdominal skinfolds, and X_2 = age in years.

Jackson and Pollock (69) simplified this procedure by providing tabulated % body fatness values for different skinfold thicknesses across age. All that is needed is the sum of skinfolds in order to obtain a % body fatness value. Appendixes H and I show the % body fat tables for men and women, respectively, using the sum of three skinfolds. For example, a woman, aged twenty-five, with a sum of skinfolds equal to 50 mm has a % body fat equal to 22.9% (look to the right of the sum of skinfold column where 48–52 is shown, over to the second column—ages 23–27). Estimates of % body fatness from skinfold measures has an error of about ±3.7% (86). Recently, concern has been expressed about the need to cross-validate the skinfold equations against the multicomponent models and to clarify the effects that age, gender, ethnicity, and fitness have on the various components of body composition, for example, the density of the fat-free mass (55a, 90).

The use of skinfold measurements was extended to children in the schools for early identification of obesity. The American Alliance for Health, Physical Education, Recreation, and Dance (3, 89) developed a health-related fitness test to evaluate cardiorespiratory function, muscular strength, low back function, and body fatness. The body fatness assessment relies on a triceps and subscapular or calf skinfold(s), and percentile norms are provided. When this test was developed the skinfold values could not be converted to percent body fatness values because the assumption that the fat-free mass had a density of 1.100 gm/cc was known to be false. However, based on recent research with young populations using the four-component model (134a), appropriate equations are available to convert skinfolds to body fat for young African American and white girls and boys (90) (see table 18.7).

Body Fatness for Health and Fitness

The previous sections showed how to determine body density by underwater weighing and skinfold procedures. This information on body density is converted to % body fat and can be used to make judgments about one's status relative to health and fitness. Lohman (86) recommends a range of 10%–20% as an optimal health and fitness goal for males. He indicates that this range allows for individual differences in physical activity and preferences, and is associated with little or no health risk due to diseases associated with fatness. Values above 20% increase the risks of diabetes, heart disease, and hypertension. Values of 20%–25% are considered moderately high, 25%–31% as high, and >31% as very high. Females are generally about 3% fatter than males prior to puberty and 11% fatter after puberty. The optimal range of body fat for adult females is 15%–25%, with 25%–30% listed as moderately high, 30%–35% as high, and >35% as very high (86).

Now that we know how to obtain a % body fatness measure, and what the optimal % body fat values are, how can we determine what the optimal body

Table 18.7 Prediction Equations of Percent Fat From Triceps and Calf and From Triceps and Subscapular Skinfolds in Children and Youth for Males and Females

Triceps and calf skinfolds
Males, all ages: % Fat = 0.735 $\sum$SF + 1.0
Females, all ages: % Fat = 0.610 $\sum$SF + 5.0
Triceps and subscapular skinfolds (>35 mm)
Males: % Fat = 0.783 $\sum$SF + I
Females: % Fat = 0.546 $\sum$SF + 9.7
Triceps and subscapular skinfolds (<35 mm)[a]
Males: % Fat = 1.21 ($\sum$SF) – 0.008 ($\sum$SF)^2 + I
Females: % Fat = 1.33 ($\sum$SF) – 0.013 ($\sum$SF)^2 + 2.5 (2.0 African Americans, 3.0 whites)
I = Intercept varies with maturation level and racial group for males as follows:

Age	African Americans	Whites
Prepubescent	–3.5	–1.7
Pubescent	–5.2	–3.4
Postpubescent	–6.8	–5.5
Adult	–6.8	–5.5

[a]Thus for a white pubescent male with a triceps of 15 and a subscapular of 12, the % fat would be: % Fat = 1.21 (27) – 0.008 (27)^2 – 3.4 = 23.4%
Note. Calculations were derived using Slaughter et al. (1988) equation. Reprinted, by permission, from T. G. Lohman, 1992, *Advances in Body Composition Assessment*, (Champaign, IL: Human Kinetics Publishers), 74. Calculations were derived using Slaughter et al. (1988).

weight range is? In the following example, a female college student has 30% body fat and weighs 142 lbs. Her optimal % fat range is 15%–25%.

Step 1. Calculate fat-free weight:
100% – 30% fat = 70% fat free
70% × 142 lb = 99.4 lb fat-free weight

Step 2. Optimal weight = $\dfrac{\text{fat-free weight}}{(1 - \text{optimal \% fat})}$, with optimal % fat expressed as a fraction:

For 15% = $\dfrac{99.4 \text{ lb}}{(1 - .15)}$ = 117 lb;

for 25% = $\dfrac{99.4 \text{ lb}}{(1 - .25)}$ = 132.5 lb

Her optimal weight range is 117–133 lb

Lohman (86) also provides values for % body fat that are below the optimal range: for boys, 6% to 10% is classified as low and <6% as very low; comparable values for girls are 12% to 15% and <12%, respectively. There is a great pressure in our society to be thin, and this can be carried to an extreme. A far too common problem in our high schools and colleges is an eating disorder known as **anorexia nervosa,** in which young females have an exaggerated fear of getting fat. This fear leads to food restriction and increased exercise in an attempt to stay thin, when they are, in fact, already thin (51). **Bulimia nervosa** is an eating disorder in which large quantities of food are taken in (binging), only to be followed by self-induced vomiting or the use of laxatives to rid the body of the food that was eaten (purging). While anorexia nervosa is characterized by the cessation of the menstrual cycle and the development of an emaciated state, the majority of the bingers/purgers are in the normal weight range (36).

It is clear that to stay in the optimal % body fat range an individual must balance the dietary consumption of calories with energy expenditure. We will now consider that topic.

in summary

- Subcutaneous fat can be "sampled" as skinfold thicknesses, and a sum of skinfolds can be converted to a percent body fat with formulas derived from the relationship of the sum of skinfolds to a body composition standard based on a 2-, 3-, or 4-component model.
- The recommended body fatness for males is 10%–20%, and for females is 15%–25%. There is concern about obesity and anorexia for those above and below these values, respectively.

Obesity and Weight Control

In chapter 14 we discussed the major risk factors associated with degenerative diseases. While high blood pressure, cigarette smoking, elevated serum cholesterol, and inactivity are the primary risk factors (114), more and more evidence points to obesity as being a separate and independent risk factor for CHD, and one directly tied to two of the above primary risk factors. Two separate epidemiological studies found that increases in relative weight or body mass index were related to an increase in the risk of heart disease (74, 116). Data from the Framingham Heart Study showed that relative weight was positively related to high serum triglycerides, total cholesterol (with lower HDL), and uric acid, elevated blood pressure, and a greater degree of glucose intolerance (74). The following is a summary of the diseases that are believed to be caused by or associated with obesity (117).

Causal

- Diseases or conditions in which obesity is a *primary contributing factor*: adult-onset diabetes, menstrual abnormalities, reproductive problems, heart size and function, arthritis, gout, and hypertension.
- Disease or condition in which obesity is a *secondary contributing factor*: endometrial carcinoma.

Association

- Diseases or conditions that are correlated with obesity, but not caused by obesity: atherosclerotic disease, gallbladder disease, and death.

As mentioned earlier, in spite of this information, the 1983 height/weight table of the Metropolitan Life Insurance Company listed higher weights at each height as being associated with lower death rates. In response, a twenty-six-year follow-up study of participants in the Framingham Heart Study recommended against this revision of the height/weight table with data indicating that higher relative weight was associated with increases in cardiovascular diseases (CVD) and death from CVD (67). The reason for the confusion was that the death rate was actually decreasing while the relative weight was increasing. The decrease in the death rate was believed to be due to decreases in cigarette smoking and improved health care and not the fact that people were fatter (47). It has been suggested that the better treatments available for those with diabetes and heart disease allows them to live longer at the higher body weights. It is a case of where the *average* body weight of a group is not the *optimal* weight for low risk of disease. In fact, Kannel and Gordon have stated that ". . . if everyone were at optimal weight we would have 25% less coronary heart disease and 35% less congestive heart failure and brain infarctions" (74).

Obesity

Obesity is defined as a high percentage of body fat, usually >25% for men and >32% for women. This corresponds to BMI values of 27.8 for men and 27.3 for women (90). Using these values it is estimated that 19 million women and 15 million men in the United States are obese (81). However, all obesity is not the same. Recent studies suggest that not only is the relative body fatness related to an increased risk of CVD, but the distribution of that fatness must also be considered. Individuals with a large waist circumference compared to hip circumference have a higher risk of CVD and sudden death (132, 133). These data suggest that in addition to skinfold or underwater weighing estimates of body density, measurements of waist and hip circumferences should also be obtained (82, 83). Ratios of waist to hip circumference >0.95 for men and >0.8 for women are associated with the CVD risk factors of insulin resistance, high cholesterol, and hypertension, and such individuals are treated even if they are only borderline obese (10, 18, 34, 132).

In addition to fat tissue distribution, there is a need to determine whether the obesity is due to an increase in the amount of fat in each fat cell (hypertrophic obesity), or to an increase in the number of fat cells (hyperplastic obesity), or both (9, 11, 12). In moderate obesity where the mass of adipose tissue is less than 30 kg, the increase in fat cell size appears to be the primary means of storing the additional fat. Beyond that, the cell number is the variable most strongly related to the mass of adipose tissue (12, 65a). This is shown in figure 18.4 where cell size increases up to about 30-kg body fat,

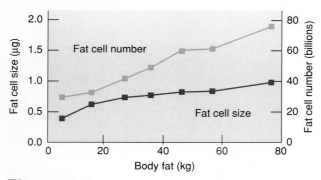

Figure 18.4

Relationship of fat cell size and fat cell number to total kilograms of body fat. Fat cell size is given in µg of fat, and fat cell number in billions of cells. The increase in body fatness beyond about 30 kg of fat is directly related to an increasing fat cell number; fat cell size remains relatively constant.

but does not significantly change thereafter. In contrast, fat cell number is strongly related to the mass of adipose tissue (131, 134).

There are about 25 billion fat cells in a normal-weight individual versus 60–80 billion in the extremely obese (12, 65a, 134). When a person undergoes dietary restriction, the size of the fat cells decreases but the number does not (12, 65a). This high fat cell number is believed to be related to the difficulty obese patients have in maintaining body weight once it has been lost (80). For example, a study was conducted to determine the pattern of weight loss, maintenance, and gain of groups classified as having obesity that is hyperplastic, hypertrophic, or both. Those with hyperplastic obesity or combined hyperplastic and hypertrophic obesity lost weight quickly, kept it off for only a short period of time, and regained it at a high rate. At this point we have seen that dieting does not change fat cell number, and that those who possess a high number of fat cells have difficulty maintaining a reduced body weight. The next question to consider is, when does the fat cell number increase?

In a longitudinal study of children during the first eighteen months of life, the fat cell number did not increase during the first twelve months, the increase in cell size being entirely responsible for the increase in body fat. In contrast, the gain in body fat from twelve to eighteen months was due entirely to an increase in fat cell number with cell size remaining stable (60). When these data were plotted along with data from other studies, the results indicated that cell number increases throughout growth (60, 65a). Given that physical activity and dietary intervention in grossly obese young children (eight years old) can slow the rate of growth in fat cell number, and that the fat cell number is tied to the inability of obese children to lose their obesity as adults, the emphasis on treatment during childhood is obvious (61, 78). Unfortunately, in

spite of our understanding of the problem, the prevalence of pediatric obesity has increased by 54% among six- to eleven-year-olds and by 39% among twelve- to seventeen-year-olds over the past fifteen to twenty years (58, 79). What causes obesity?

There is clearly no single cause of obesity. Obesity is related to both genetic and environmental variables. In 1965 Mayer (92) commented on the numerous studies showing that 70%–80% of obese children had at least one obese parent, but concluded that it was difficult to interpret those data given the way cultural background interacts with genetics. In effect, the need to do hard physical work in some countries, or extreme social pressure against obesity (discussed later), might not allow a genetic predisposition to express itself. Garn and Clark (53) found a strong relationship between parental fatness and the fatness of children. They identified three categories of fatness on the basis of triceps skinfold: lean = <15th percentile; medium = 15th–85th percentile, and obese = >85th percentile. The triceps skinfold thickness was related to parental fatness, being below average for the lean-dad/lean-mom pair and above average for the obese-dad/obese-mom pair. While this might imply that a genetic link exists, when the investigators compared husbands to wives (usually no genetic tie), the relationship was similar to that for their children, suggesting either that there was a tendency of like to mate like, or that communal living exerts a major influence.

A slightly different approach to this question was taken when the body mass index of biological and adoptive parents were compared to the values of the adopted child, as an adult. On the basis of a health questionnaire they were classified as thin (≤4th percentile), median (50th percentile), overweight (92nd–96th percentile), and obese (>96th percentile). A stronger relationship existed between the BMI of the adoptee and that of the biological parent (137). However, a subsequent review of this work pointed out that while the results were consistent with a genetic effect, it was not a very strong one (15). Other observations support the importance of the environment as a cause of obesity. In American women, obesity is inversely related to socioeconomic class: 30% for lower, 18% for middle, and 5% for the upper class (56). Further, women and adolescent girls have been shown to suffer the most direct discrimination because of this obesity (148). Clearly, while we may possess a genetic predisposition for obesity, there are a variety of social factors that influence its appearance. Is there any way to determine the importance of each?

Bouchard (15) and colleagues have determined, on the basis of an analysis of the relationships between and among nine types of relatives (spouses, parent-child, siblings, uncle-nephew etc.), that 25% of body fat and fat mass is tied to genetic factors, and 30% is due to cultural transmission. What is interesting is the components of energy expenditure that are influenced by genetic factors: (a) the amount of spontaneous physical activity, (b) resting metabolic rate, (c) thermic effect of food, and (d) relative rate of carbohydrate and fat oxidation. Further, when challenged with an excess of calories due to overeating, there is a genetic component related to the amount of weight gained, and the proportion of that weight that is stored as fat or lean tissue. Given that information, it should be no surprise that physicians and scientists who work in this area believe that genetic factors are the most important causes of obesity (20). However, as we will see, there is more to the story.

in summary

- If everyone were at optimal weight there would be a 25% reduction in CHD, and a 35% reduction in congestive heart failure and stroke.
- Obesity associated with fat mass in excess of 30 kg is due primarily to an increase in fat cell number, with fat cell hypertrophy being related to smaller degrees of obesity. Those with hyperplasia have a more difficult time losing weight and keeping it off.
- Genetic factors account for about 25% of the transmissible variance for fat mass and percent body fat; culture accounts for 30%.

Set Point and Obesity

Obese individuals, as previously mentioned, have a great deal of difficulty maintaining a reduced weight. In fact, the tendency of a person to return to a certain weight suggests that there is a biological set point for body weight much like the set points for any negative feedback biological control system. While the hypothalamus contains centers associated with satiety and feeding behavior, we must remember that the *body weight set point is a concept, rather than a reality* (14). Figure 18.5 shows a physiological model of a body weight set point in which biological signals with regard to blood glucose (glucostatic signal), lipid stores (lipostatic signal), or weight on feet (ponderostatic signal) provide input to the hypothalamus (14). If the collective signals indicate low energy stores, food intake is stimulated until the source of the signal is diminished and the energy stores now equal the set point. Like any biological control system, if the set point were to be increased, body weight would increase to meet this new value. Exercise can modify the signals going to the hypothalamus, and the type of diet can also influence feeding behavior.

In contrast to this physiological model, Booth's cognitive set-point model (14) deals with the role the environment (culture, socioeconomic class, etc.) has on body weight. Figure 18.6 shows that relative to a personally selected "ideal" body weight set point, we

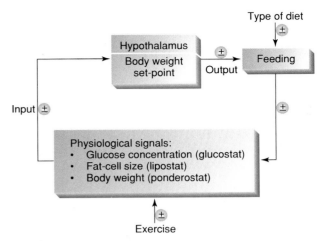

Figure 18.5

Physiological set point for control of body weight by altering feeding behavior showing the glucostatic (blood glucose), lipostatic (adipose tissue), and ponderostatic (weight) input to the hypothalamus. The signals from these latter mechanisms are compared against a "set point," and an appropriate increase or decrease in feeding behavior occurs. In this model, exercise can modify the input, and the type of diet can modify feeding behavior.

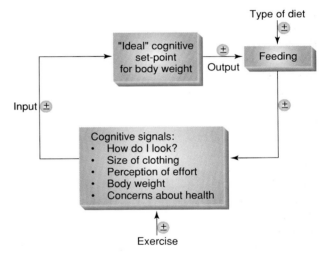

Figure 18.6

Cognitive set point for control of body weight by altering feeding behavior. A person's perception of "ideal" body weight is balanced against signals about how one looks, body weight, clothing, size, and so on. Exercise can modify the input, and the type of diet can modify feeding behavior.

are constantly receiving a variety of cognitive signals about how we look, body weight, clothing size, perception of effort, and concerns about health. A mismatch between the "ideal" set point and these perceptions leads to appropriate eating behavior. Exercise can modify the signals, and the type of diet can influence the feeding behavior. This set-point model is closely related to the behavior modification approach to diet, exercise, and weight control.

in summary

- Investigators have proposed a set-point theory to explain obesity given the tendency for people who diet to return to their former weight. Theories based on weight sensors (ponderostatic), the blood glucose concentration (glucostatic), and the mass of lipid (lipostatic) have been proposed.
- A behavioral set-point theory has been proposed that relies on the person making appropriate activity and dietary judgments when body weight, size, or shape does not match up with that person's ideal.

Diet, Exercise, and Weight Control

The Framingham Heart Study showed that body weight increases as we age. A reasonable question to ask is whether this gain in weight was due to an increase in caloric intake. Interestingly, caloric intake decreased over the same age span (17). We are forced to conclude that energy expenditure decreased faster than the decrease in caloric intake, and as a result, weight gain occurred. This weight gain problem can be corrected by understanding and dealing with one or both sides of the energy balance equation. We will deal with the energy balance equation first, and then discuss how modifications in energy intake can affect weight loss. Finally, we will explore the variables on the energy expenditure side of the equation.

Energy and Nutrient Balance

Weight gain occurs when there is a chronic increase in caloric intake, compared to energy expenditure. A net gain of about 3,500 kcal is needed to add 1 lb (454 grams) of adipose tissue. We are all familiar with the energy balance equation:

> Change in energy stores = energy intake – energy expenditure.

What is implied by this equation is that an excess energy intake of 250 kcal/d will cause body weight to increase one pound in 14 days (250 kcal/d × 14 d = 3500 kcal = 1 pound). At the end of one year the person will have gained about 24 pounds. As reasonable as this equation may appear, we know that a weight gain of that magnitude will not occur. The above equation is a "static" energy balance equation that does not consider the effect that the weight gain will have on energy expenditure (137b).

The energy balance equation can be expressed in a manner to account for the dynamic nature of energy balance in biological systems:

Rate of change of = rate of change of – rate of change of
energy stores   energy intake   energy expenditure

When body weight increases as a result of a chronically elevated energy intake, there is a compensatory increase in the amount of energy used at rest, as well as during activity when body weight is carried about. At some point then, the additional 250 kcal/d of energy intake will be balanced by a higher rate of energy expenditure brought about by the higher body weight. Body weight will stabilize at a new and higher value, but it will be more like 3.5 pounds, rather than 24 pounds higher (137b).

in summary

- The dynamic energy balance equation correctly expresses the dynamic nature of changes in energy intake and body weight. An increase in energy intake leads to an increase in body weight; in turn, energy expenditure increases to eventually match the higher energy intake. Body weight is now stable at a new and higher value.

Nutrient Balance

Investigators have taken this issue of energy balance one step further in an attempt to understand the causes of obesity. The dynamic energy balance equation can be subdivided into its components, representing the three major nutrients to generate nutrient-balance equations:

Rate of change of = rate of change of – rate of change of
protein stores   protein intake   protein oxidation

Rate of change of = rate of change of – rate of change of
carbohydrate   carbohydrate   carbohydrate
stores   intake   oxidation

Rate of change = rate of change of – rate of change of
of fat stores   of fat intake   fat oxidation

If a person maintains balance for each of these nutrients, that is, what is taken in, is expended, then energy balance is achieved. Nutrient balance is not a problem for protein and carbohydrate. The daily protein intake is used to maintain existing tissue protein, hormones, and enzymes. If more is taken in than is needed, the "extra" is oxidized for metabolic needs, and fat mass is not increased. The same is true for carbohydrates. Ingested carbohydrates are used to fill liver and muscle glycogen stores; the excess is oxidized and *is not* converted to fat (1, 12a, 64a). Carbohydrate intake promotes its own oxidization. This is a relatively new idea that has major ramifications for our understanding of nutrient and energy balance. The evidence seems to be quite convincing that *de novo* lipogenesis from carbohydrates (the making of new lipids from other nutrients) is of only minor consequence in humans. Simply, carbohydrates are either stored as carbohydrates or oxidized; they do not add <u>directly</u> to adipose tissue mass. This leaves fat.

In contrast to carbohydrate and protein, fat intake is not automatically balanced by fat oxidation. When "extra" fat is added to the diet, the same amount of carbohydrate, fat, and protein are oxidized as before; the extra fat is stored in adipose tissue. Fat intake *does not* promote its own oxidation. Fat oxidation is determined primarily by the difference between total energy expenditure and the amount of energy ingested in the form of carbohydrate and protein. Consequently, if one wishes to keep the size of the adipose tissue stores constant (i.e., maintain body weight), then one should not eat more fat than one can oxidize (48a, 48b, 48c, 71a, 71b, 137b). One last point. Alcohol intake is balanced by its own oxidation, but in the process, it suppresses fat oxidation. In this sense, the calories from alcohol should be included with that provided by fat (48c).

In chapter 4 you were introduced to the concept of the respiratory quotient (RQ = $\dot{V}CO_2/\dot{V}O_2$) as an indicator of the fuel oxidized during exercise. An RQ of 1.0 indicates that 100% of the energy is derived from carbohydrates and an RQ of 0.7 indicates that 100% of the energy comes from fat. An RQ of 0.85 indicates that a 50%/50% mixture of carbohydrate and fat was used. This RQ concept has been extended to the foods we ingest, and it is called the Food Quotient or FQ. The FQ is defined as the ratio of the CO_2 produced to the O_2 consumed during the oxidation of a representative sample of the diet (48a). The reason for describing this is that the FQ concept can be used with the RQ concept to determine if an individual is in nutrient balance (71a, 71b). Figure 18.7 presents this concept, and the following comments summarize its content:

- When RQ = FQ, the person is in nutrient and energy balance; the RQ/FQ ratio is 1.0.
- When RQ > FQ, the person is not oxidizing as much fat as was consumed (positive energy balance), and some fat has been stored in adipose tissue; the RQ/FQ ratio is >1.0.
- When RQ < FQ, the person used more fat than was consumed (negative energy balance), and some of the fat stores were used; the RQ/FQ ratio is <1.0.

This concept is helpful in discussing weight control, because one could improve nutrient and energy balance with regard to fat by either reducing the amount of fat in the diet (increasing the FQ), or doing exercise to use more fat (decreasing the RQ). We will now discuss both of these options.

Figure 18.7

Relationship between respiratory quotient (RQ)-to-food quotient (FQ) ratio and energy balance in humans. Each point represents values for a given subject measured over a 24-hr period.

(From E. Jéquier. 1992. Calorie balance versus nutrient balance. In *Energy Metabolism: Tissue Determinants and Cellular Corollaries*, eds. J. M. Kinney and H. N. Tucker, p. 131 New York: Raven.)

in summary

- Nutrient balance exits for both protein and carbohydrate. Excess intake is oxidized and is not converted to fat.
- Excess fat intake does not drive its own oxidation; the excess is stored in adipose tissue. Achieving fat balance is an important part of weight control.
- The ratio of the Food Quotient (FQ) to the Respiratory Quotient (RQ) provides good information about the degree to which an individual is in nutrient balance.

Diet and Weight Control

A good diet provides the necessary nutrients and calories to provide for tissue growth and regeneration, and to meet the daily energy requirements of work and play. In our society we are fortunate to have a wide variety of foods to meet these needs. However, we tend to consume more than the recommended amount of fat, which is believed to be related to our country's obesity problem. The focus on dietary fat is two-fold:

- fat grams contain more than twice the number of calories as carbohydrate and can contribute to a positive energy balance, and
- it is difficult to achieve nutrient balance for fat when it represents a large fraction of caloric intake.

The hypothesis that the FQ of the diet is an important aspect of weight control revolves around the factors driving energy intake. There is a mandatory need for carbohydrate oxidation by the nervous system, and we are driven to eat what is used (48b, 65). If we eat a high-fat diet, we will take in a considerable amount of fat while consuming the necessary carbohydrates to refill the carbohydrate stores. This fat is stored and body weight will increase. As mentioned earlier, as body weight increases daily energy expenditure increases until an energy balance is achieved at a new and higher body weight. The fat-balance concept is consistent with this. Flatt (48b) proposes that the increase in adipose tissue mass that accompanies weight gain increases the mobilization of free fatty acids, shifting the RQ to a lower value, and bringing it into balance with the FQ. In this sense, the elevation of body weight and fat mass due to a high fat/calorie diet is a compensatory mechanism that results in weight maintenance.

However, while we focus on the FQ/RQ concept, we should not forget that calories count in any weight-loss or weight-maintenance program. For example, studies in which subjects were switched from a high-fat to a low-fat diet, *while maintaining a constant caloric intake*, showed no change in energy expenditure or body weight (65, 84, 117e). In addition, in conditions in which a negative caloric balance was imposed to achieve weight loss, the composition of the diet (high-fat vs. low-fat) did not matter (64b). In this sense, one should not get carried away with the high carbohydrate diet and consume calories in excess of what is needed (48c). Given these facts, why should diet composition matter in terms of weight control and obesity?

Quite simply, diets with a high fat-to-carbohydrate ratio are associated with obesity (98). When subjects are given free access to food, more calories are consumed when one eats a high-fat diet than when one eats a high-carbohydrate diet (13a, 137d). The high-carbohydrate content may contribute to satiety better than the high-fat diet, resulting in an earlier termination of eating (117b). The nutrient balance (RQ = FQ) concept helps focus our attention on the need for a high-carbohydrate/low-fat diet to achieve and maintain a healthy level of body fatness. This diet is also consistent with what is needed to have normal cholesterol levels and sufficient carbohydrate for physical performance (see chapter 23). One of the *Dietary Guidelines for Americans* was to maintain healthy weight. The recommendations to avoid overeating included: eat smaller portions and limit second helpings. Further, to lose weight the following suggestions were made:

- Eat a variety of foods that are low in calories and high in nutrients.
- Eat more fruits, vegetables, and breads and cereals—without fats or sugars added in preparation and at the table.

- Eat less fat, and fatty foods.
- Eat less sugar and sweets.
- Drink little or no alcoholic beverages.
- Be more physically active to increase energy expenditure.

One last point before leaving this topic. As we mentioned earlier in the chapter, data on energy intake is assessed by twenty-four-hour recall or food records. However, one has to be cautious when interpreting these data as part of a weight-loss program. Research suggests that these methods may result in a considerable underestimation of caloric intake, especially in obese individuals (13, 41a, 84a, 96, 139). This, of course, would create a misdirection in looking for the cause of the obesity problem. It should be no surprise then that careful energy balance studies are done in highly controlled laboratory situations.

in summary

- Diets with a high fat-to-carbohydrate ratio are linked to obesity. Nutrient balance for fat can be most easily achieved with a low-fat diet (high FQ).
- Calories do count, and must be considered in any diet aimed at achieving or maintaining a weight loss goal.

Energy Expenditure and Weight Control

The other side of the energy balance equation involves the expenditure of energy and includes the basal metabolic rate, thermogenesis (shivering and nonshivering), and exercise. We will examine each of these relative to its role in energy balance.

Basal Metabolic Rate

Basal metabolic rate (BMR) is the rate of energy expenditure measured under standardized conditions (i.e., immediately after rising, twelve to eighteen hours after a meal, in a supine position in a thermoneutral environment). Because of the difficulty of achieving these conditions during routine measurements, investigators have measured **resting metabolic rate (RMR)** instead. In this latter procedure, the subject simply reports to the lab about four hours after eating a light meal, and after a period of time (thirty to sixty minutes) the metabolic rate is measured (99). Given the low level of oxygen uptake measured for BMR or RMR (200–400 ml $\cdot$ min^{-1}), a variation of only ±20 to 40 ml $\cdot$ min^{-1} represents a potential $\pm10\%$ error. In the following discussion both BMR and RMR will be discussed interchangeably, except where a specific contrast must be made for clarification.

The BMR is important in the energy balance equation because it represents 60% to 75% of total energy expenditure in the average sedentary person (111). The BMR is proportional to the fat-free mass, and after age twenty it decreases approximately 2% and 3% per decade in women and men, respectively. Women have a significantly lower BMR at all ages, due primarily to their lower fat-free mass (38, 43, 110, 150). Consistent with this, when RMR is expressed per unit of fat-free mass, there is no gender difference. At any body weight the RMR decreases about 0.01 kcal/min for each 1% increase in body fatness (110). While this may appear to be insignificant, this small difference can become meaningful in the progressive increase in weight gain over time. For example, a 5% difference in body fatness at the same body weight results in a difference of 0.05 kcal · min^{-1}, or 3 kcal · hr^{-1}, which is equal to 72 kcal · d^{-1}. It must be emphasized that percent body fat makes only a small contribution to the BMR. This was confirmed in a recent study examining the relationship of body composition to BMR; fat mass did not improve the prediction of BMR based on the fat-free mass alone (38).

As mentioned earlier, part of the variation in BMR is due to a genetic predisposition to be higher or lower (15). The range (±3 SD) in normal BMR values is about ±21% from the average value, and such variation helps to explain the observation that some have an easier time at maintaining body weight than others. If an average adult male has a BMR of 1,500 kcal · d^{-1}, those at +3 SD can take in an additional 300 kcal · d^{-1} (21% of 1,500 kcal) to maintain weight, while others at the low end of the range (−3 SD) would have to take in 300 fewer kcals (43, 54).

The fat-free mass is not the only factor influencing the BMR. In 1919 Benedict et al. (8) showed that prolonged dieting (reduction from about 3,100 kcal to 1,950 kcal) was associated with a 20% decrease in the BMR expressed per kilogram of body weight. This observation was confirmed in the famous Minnesota Starvation Experiment (77), and is shown in figure 18.8. In this figure the BMR is expressed as a percent of the value measured before the period of semi-starvation. The percent decrease in BMR is larger "per man" because of the loss of lean tissue (as well as fat tissue); however, when the value is expressed per kilogram of body weight or per unit of surface area (m^2), the BMR is still shown to be reduced. A decrease in the concentration of one of the thyroid hormones (T$_3$) and a reduced level of sympathetic nervous system activity have been implicated in this lower BMR due to caloric restriction (16). What these data mean is that during a period of low caloric intake the energy production of the tissues decreases in an attempt to adapt to the lower caloric intake and reduce the rate of weight loss. This is an appropriate adaptation in periods of semi-starvation, but is counterproductive in weight reduction programs. This information bears heavily on the use of low-calorie diets as a primary means of weight reduction (42, 50, 145, 147).

Figure 18.8
Decrease in basal metabolic rate during twenty-four weeks of semi-starvation.

The BMR is also responsive to periods of overfeeding. In the dieting experiment of Benedict et al. (8), mentioned earlier, when the subjects were allowed a day of free eating, the BMR was elevated on the following day. Further, in long-term (fourteen to twenty days) overfeeding to cause obesity, increases in resting and basal metabolic rates have been recorded. In essence, during the dynamic phase of weight gain (going from a lower to a higher weight) more calories are required per kg of body weight to maintain the weight gain than to maintain normal body weight (54, 127). This increased heat production due to an excess caloric intake, called **thermogenesis,** will be discussed in the next section. However, before leaving this discussion of the BMR, we need to mention the effect of exercise.

There is no doubt that the resting metabolic rate is elevated following exercise. The questions relate to how much and how long it is elevated, and to what extent it contributes to total daily energy expenditure (21, 112). A recent review of this topic indicates that controversies still exist even though the questions have been studied for over ninety years (99). At the heart of the matter is the measure of the metabolic rate that is taken as the baseline in these experiments. Should it be the BMR? The RMR? Molé (99) suggests that we need to create a new measurement called the Standard Metabolic Rate that would take into consideration the day-to-day fluctuations in normal physical activity, dietary intake, added exercise, and body composition. In support of these concerns it has been shown that trained subjects had a higher RMR than untrained subjects only when they did heavy exercise and consumed sufficient calories to maintain energy balance (28a). This suggests that the higher RMR in trained individuals is not due to chronic adaptations associated with training, but more to the higher energy flux associated with the training and diet. This is consistent with other studies showing that the RMR, expressed per kg of fat-free mass, is similar for trained and untrained individuals, and that resistance and endurance training do not affect the value (25, 26). Aside from helping to maintain or increase the lean body mass and the RMR, exercise training may favorably impact nutrient balance. Two studies, using strength training, showed a significant decrease in the 24-hr (139b) and sleeping (144a) metabolic rate RQ values, signifying an increased use of fat. This is consistent with achieving nutrient balance and energy balance over time (159).

in summary

- The BMR represents the largest fraction of total energy expenditure in sedentary persons. The BMR decreases with age, and women have lower BMR values than men.
- The fat-free mass is related to both the gender difference and to the decline in BMR with age. A reduction in caloric intake by dieting or fasting can reduce the BMR, while physical activity is important in maintaining it.

Thermogenesis

Core temperature is maintained at about 37° C by balancing heat production with heat loss. Under thermoneutral conditions the BMR (RMR) provides the necessary heat, but under cold environmental conditions the process of shivering is actuated, and 100% of the energy required for involuntary muscle contraction appears as heat to maintain core temperature. In addition, some animals (including newborn humans) produce heat by a process called nonshivering thermogenesis, involving brown adipose tissue. This type of adipose tissue is rich in mitochondria and increases heat production in response to norepinephrine (NE). Thyroid hormones, especially T_3, may either directly affect this process, or act in its permissive manner to facilitate the action of NE (16, 17, 71). Heat production is increased by uncoupling oxidative phosphorylation; that is, oxygen is used without ATP formation, so the energy contained in NADH and FADH appears directly as heat. Those individuals with large quantities of brown adipose tissue have a greater capacity to "throw off" calories in the form of heat rather than store them in adipose tissue. It has been hypothesized that variations in brown adipose tissue might be related to the ease or difficulty with which one gains weight.

Thermogenesis involves more than brown adipose tissue. The heat generated due to the food we consume accounts for about 10%–15% of our total daily energy expenditure; this is called the *thermic effect of feeding* (17, 111). Generally, this is determined by having a subject ingest a test meal (700 to 1,000 kcal), and the elevation in the metabolic rate is measured following the meal. This portion of our daily energy expenditure is influenced by genetic factors (15, 111), is

lower in obese than lean individuals (73, 123), and is influenced by the level of spontaneous activity and the degree of insulin resistance (137c). However, because it represents such a small part of the overall daily energy expenditure, it is not a good predictor of subsequent obesity.

In individuals who have been on a diet (underfeeding), just one day of overfeeding leads to an increase in the next day's BMR. The BMR then quickly returns to the level consistent with the low-caloric intake specified in the diet (8). It is as if the body is throwing off extra heat to maintain body weight during this period of relative overfeeding. This phenomenon has also been observed in the chronic overfeeding of human subjects. In Garrow's (55) and Danforth's (40) reviews of these overfeeding studies, the subjects showed an unexplained heat production associated with chronic excess caloric intakes. The elevations of the BMR have been explained on the basis of an increase in the mass of brown adipose tissue (mentioned earlier), and the involvement of other **energy wasteful systems.** These latter systems include a change in the Na^+/K^+ pump activity, or "futile cycles" in which the equivalent of one ATP is lost in each turn of the cycle (16, 17). An example of a futile cycle is when an ATP is used to convert fructose-6-phosphate to fructose-1,6-diphosphate, which, in the next step, is converted back to fructose-6-phosphate. In situations where heat, but no ATP, is produced, the resting oxygen consumption would have to be higher to maintain the normal ATP-consuming systems. Whatever the mechanism by which this dietary thermogenesis is induced, via brown fat or by futile cycles, it must be made clear that, like the BMR, there are marked differences in how individuals respond to an increased dietary intake. Clearly, those who have a normally high BMR and are very responsive to a large caloric excess would have an easier time staying at normal weight than those who do not.

in summary

- Thermogenesis (heat generation) is associated with the ingestion of meals (thermic effect of feeding), brown adipose tissue, and "futile cycles."
- The thermic effect of feeding represents a small part of total energy expenditure and is not predictive of obesity.

Physical Activity and Exercise

Physical activity constitutes the most variable part of the energy expenditure side of the energy balance equation, being 5% to 40% of the daily energy expenditure (32, 111). There are those who have sedentary jobs and who do little physical activity during their leisure time. Others may have strenuous jobs, or expend 300–1,000 kcal during their leisure time every day or two. Just how important is physical activity in

Figure 18.9

Relationship between body fatness and nonbasal energy expenditure is highly significant (P < 0.01) for females $r = -0.83$. for males $r = -0.55$.

Figure 18.10

Pattern of caloric intake for rats versus the durations of exercise. When rats do little or no exercise, caloric intake exceeds what is needed and body weight increases (see top-left part of figure). However, over a broad range of physical activity, caloric intake increases proportional to the activity, and body weight (top line) remains constant.

weight control? Epidemiological evidence suggests an inverse association between physical activity and body weight, with body fat being more favorably distributed in those who are physically active (41b). A recent study examined the relationship of body fatness to the different components of energy expenditure. Figure 18.9 shows that body fatness was inversely related to "nonbasal" (primarily that associated with physical activity) energy expenditure. In this sense, the level of physical activity is a permissive factor for obesity (117a, 120a).

Appetite The classic animal study describing the role of exercise on appetite was conducted by Mayer and colleagues (93). Figure 18.10 shows that when female rats exercised for twenty to sixty minutes per day (sedentary range) the caloric intake actually decreased slightly and the animals lost weight. Over the durations of one to six hours of activity the caloric intake increased proportionately and body weight was maintained, but at a level below that of the sedentary rat. Durations in excess of six hours were associated with a relative decrease in caloric intake and body weight (exhaustion). Twenty-five years after this study, Katch et al. (76) showed that in male rats accomplishing the same amount of work, those exercising at the higher intensity had a greater depression in appetite and weight gain than those at the lower intensity, with both groups being lower than the sedentary animals. In contrast, female rats tend to respond to increasing exercise intensity with an increase in appetite (108).

Mayer and colleagues (94) also studied the relationship of exercise to caloric intake on mill workers in West Bengal, India. Figure 18.11 shows a pattern of response similar to Mayer et al.'s (93) study on rats. In the activity classifications from light to very heavy work, caloric intake increased proportionally so that

body weight was not different among the various groups. However, in the sedentary classification, caloric intake was as high as for the very heavy work classification, and body weight was higher than the other groups. This suggests that a minimal level of exercise is needed to help regulate appetite. This study has been cited over the years as a primary supporting piece of evidence showing exercise to be important in the regulation of appetite. However, in 1978 Garrow (54) questioned the analysis of the data at the sedentary end of the scale where the group called "Clerks I" had a body weight similar to the more active groups, *but consumed about 400 kcal/day more* than those in the light work category. This analysis of the data would support a conclusion opposite that of Mayer et al. (94).

It should be clear that there would have to be some proportional increase in appetite as subjects increased physical activity, otherwise an athlete would gradually waste away during the course of a competitive season! However, when an exercise program is introduced to obese and/or sedentary individuals, appetite does not appear to increase. In Wilmore's (157) and Titchenal's (138) reviews of such exercise intervention studies, appetite did not increase in proportion to energy expenditure, suggesting a net loss of appetite. In summary, in male animals exercise decreases appetite in proportion to exercise intensity, while in female animals exercise stimulates appetite. Generally, in humans, caloric intake is regulated in proportion to energy expenditure over a broad range of exercise intensities and durations to help maintain body weight, but when exercise is introduced to a formerly sedentary population, a net decrease in appetite results.

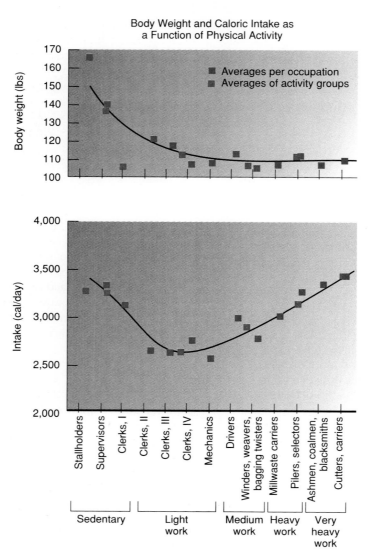

Body Weight and Caloric Intake as
a Function of Physical Activity

■ Averages per occupation
■ Averages of activity groups

Figure 18.11

Pattern of caloric intake versus occupational activity in humans. For occupations ranging from light work to very heavy work, there is a balance between caloric intake and physical activity such that body weight remains constant. For sedentary occupations, caloric intake (see left side of lower figure) exceeds needs and body weight is higher than expected (see left side of top figure).

Body Composition While exercise may help regulate appetite to maintain body weight, exercise has an independent effect on the composition of that weight. This has been shown in both animal as well as human studies. In general, male rats that participate in regular exercise have lower body weights, less lean body mass, and very little body fat compared to their sedentary control litter mates. In contrast, female rats tend to respond to exercise training with an increase in appetite such that they are as heavy as the sedentary group, with a lower fat weight and a higher lean weight (106). Oscai et al. (107) have shown that, in addition to these general changes in body composition due to exercise, exercise or food restriction in rats results in fewer and smaller fat cells. This observation is

supported by Hager et al.'s (60) finding that in a group of eight-year-old obese girls a diet/activity program was instrumental in reducing the rate of gain in fat cell number.

The advantage of using exercise compared to caloric restriction alone in weight-loss programs is that the composition of the weight that is lost is more fat tissue than lean tissue. In both animal (107) as well as human (28, 31, 44) studies using dietary restriction alone, lean body mass loss can equal 30%–40% of the weight loss. Exercise plus diet results in less lean body mass loss and a proportionately greater fat loss (107). In addition, the preferential mobilization of fat from visceral adipose tissue results in an improved body fat distribution and risk factor profile (117d, 147a).

However, it must be remembered that body composition changes take place slowly in human exercise studies, and the magnitude of the change is small. Wilmore's summary (156) of exercise and body composition studies showed the average decrease in percent body fat to be only 1.6% with fitness programs ranging in duration from 6 to 104 weeks.

in summary

- Humans increase appetite over a broad range of energy expenditure to maintain body weight; however, formerly sedentary individuals show a net loss of appetite when they undertake an exercise program.
- When weight loss occurs with an exercise and diet program, less lean body mass is lost than when the same weight loss is achieved by diet alone.

Weight Loss vs. Weight Maintenance One point that needs to be stated at the outset is that exercise is not required to achieve weight loss. All that is necessary is a caloric deficit, the magnitude of which is easily controlled by diet (64b). However, as mentioned above, the use of exercise as a part of a weight-loss program might serve to maintain a higher lean body mass and RMR, and result in an optimal body fatness at a higher body weight.

Although exercise might not be an essential ingredient in a weight-loss program, it is in a weight-maintenance program (134b). A major, unresolved question is how much? That said, some of the general exercise recommendations for health and fitness presented in chapter 16 would be considered reasonable for weight-maintenance programs. The primary factor involved in energy expenditure is the total work accomplished, so low-intensity, long-duration exercise is as good as high-intensity, short-duration exercise in expending calories. For the sedentary, overweight person, low intensity exercise is the proper choice since it can be done for longer periods of time in each exercise session, can be done each day, and is effective in conserving the fat-free mass (5). This is consistent with the Exercise Lite program presented in chapter 16.

Further, at low intensities (e.g., 25% $\dot{V}O_2$ max) free fatty acids are mobilized from the periphery to provide the majority of the fuel used, and help with maintaining fat-balance (117c). This does not mean that "fat-burning" is restricted to low-intensity activities. Individuals interested in more vigorous activity (~65% $\dot{V}O_2$ max) that can increase $\dot{V}O_2$ max can also reap the benefits of high rates of calorie and fat use (117c). Finally, even though carbohydrate makes up a large fraction of the energy supply during high intensity (~85% $\dot{V}O_2$ max) exercise (117c), training programs

using intermittent high-intensity exercise have been shown to cause a greater reduction in skinfold thickness than that conducted at the target heart rate range (139a). It is clear that virtually any form of exercise contributes to fat loss and the maintenance of body weight. The important thing is to just do it.

in summary

- Light-to-moderate exercise is an appropriate choice for most Americans to achieve health-related and weight-loss goals. Plasma free fatty acids make up a large fraction of the energy supply for that level of physical activity.
- Moderate exercise promotes the expenditure of large amounts of fat and calories, consistent with achieving weight-loss and fitness goals.
- Vigorous activity is effective in expending calories and achieving performance and fat-loss goals.

For weight-loss considerations, the caloric cost of an activity should be listed as the *net* cost (that above resting) since the *gross* cost of the activity includes energy already associated with resting metabolism. Table 18.8 shows the *net* energy cost per kg for walking and running 1 mile. In chapter 6 the net cost per m · min^{-1} of horizontal travel was 0.1 ml · kg^{-1} · min^{-1} for walking (up to about 3.75 mph), and 0.2 ml · kg^{-1} · min^{-1} for jogging or running. This translates to about 0.77 kcal per kg per mile for walking (0.1 ml · kg^{-1} · m^{-1} times 1,609 m · mile^{-1} times .0048 kcal per ml O_2), and 1.53 kcal per kg per mile for jogging or running. If a 60-kg person wished to expend 250 kcal by walking, a distance of 5.4 miles would have to be covered (250 kcal = [60 kg × 0.77 kcal · kg^{-1} · mile^{-1}]); the distance would be only 2.7 miles if jogged. If the person walks at relatively high walking speeds, the caloric cost is higher than for the slower walking speeds, and a shorter distance would have to be walked to expend the same number of calories. As mentioned earlier, since it is the total amount of work that is important in weight loss, the total distance walked or jogged does not have to be done at any one time.

In selecting activities to achieve weight-loss goals, one must be careful not to overestimate the energy expenditure. If a table of values of the caloric cost of activities lists climbing stairs as requiring 15 kcal · min^{-1}, one must realize that this is an impossible goal to achieve aerobically for those with a maximal oxygen uptake less than 3 liters · min^{-1}. Further, while an average value may be stated in such tables, some activities (e.g., swimming) have extreme variations in the energy required for the task. To deal realistically with this problem, Sharkey (125) provides a means of estimating the caloric expenditure associated with exercise for people of different fitness levels. If a person has a $\dot{V}O_2$

Table 18.8 Net Caloric Cost Per Mile for Walking, Jogging, and Running

Walking

Mph	2	2.5	3	3.5	4	4.5	5
Meters/min	54	67	80	94	107	121	134
Net cost kcal · kg⁻¹ · mile⁻¹	.77	.77	.77	.77	.96	1.15	1.38

$Net\ cost\ kcal \cdot kg^{-1} \cdot mile^{-1}$

Jogging/Running

Mph	3	4	5	6	7	8	9
Meters/min	80	107	134	160	188	215	241
Net cost kcal · kg⁻¹ · mile⁻¹	1.53	1.53	1.53	1.53	1.53	1.53	1.53

Note: Multiply by body weight in kilograms to obtain the number of kilocalories used per mile.

From E. T. Howley and B. D. Franks, *Health/Fitness Instructor's Handbook*, 2d ed. Copyright © 1992 Human Kinetics Publishers, Inc., Champaign IL. Used by permission.

Table 18.9 Estimated Net Energy Expenditure at 70% of $\dot{V}O_2$ Max During 1 Hour of Activity

$\dot{V}O_2$Max (METs) (kcal · kg⁻¹ · hr⁻¹)	Net Energy Expenditure at 70% $\dot{V}O_2$ Max (kcal · kg⁻¹ · min⁻¹)	Body Weight (kg) 50	70 (kcal · hr⁻¹)	90
20	13.0	650	910	1,170
18	11.6	580	812	1,044
16	10.2	510	714	918
14	8.8	440	616	792
10	6.0	300	420	540
8	4.6	230	322	414
6	3.2	160	224	287

From E. T. Howley and B. D. Franks, *Health/Fitness Instructor's Handbook*, 2d ed. Copyright © 1992 Human Kinetics Publishers, Inc., Champaign IL. Used by permission.

max equal to 10 METs, then the appropriate range of exercise intensities to be in the THR zone would be 6–8 METs (60%–80% $\dot{V}O_2$ max). Since 1 MET is 1 kcal · kg⁻¹ · hr⁻¹ (in addition to 3.5 ml · kg⁻¹ · min⁻¹), this subject would be working in the range of 6–8 kcal · kg⁻¹ · hr⁻¹. If the person weighs 70 kg and exercises for thirty minutes at 7 kcal · kg⁻¹ · hr⁻¹, the person would expend a total of 245 kcal (70 kg × 7 kcal · kg⁻¹ · hr⁻¹ × 0.5 hr). The net caloric expenditure would be about 210 kcal. Table 18.9 summarizes the estimated energy expenditure associated with exercise training for those with different $\dot{V}O_2$ max values (66). It should be clear that as the person loses weight the number of kcal used per fixed workout decreases, along with a decrease in the BMR. The combined effect of these two elements on the expenditure side of the weight-balance equation is that there will be a slowing of the rate of weight loss over time.

in summary

- Participation in regular physical activity achieves a wide variety of health-related goals (e.g., increased cardiorespiratory fitness, HDL-cholesterol, and fibrinolysis), and increases the chance that energy balance will be achieved.

study questions

1. Summarize the *Dietary Goals for the* U.S. and contrast them with the current dietary intake.
2. What is the difference between an RDA standard and a Daily Value?
3. Is there any risk in taking fat-soluble vitamins in large quantities? Explain.
4. Which two minerals are believed to be inadequate in women's diets?
5. Relative to coronary heart disease, why is there a major focus on dietary fat?
6. Compared to the Food Guide Pyramid, what is the rationale for including foods in specific groupings in the Exchange System?
7. Using a height/weight table, how fat is a football player who is 74 inches tall and weighs 235 lb?
8. Identify and describe the following methods of measuring body composition: isotope dilution, potassium-40, ultrasound, bioelectrical impedance analysis, dual energy x-ray absorptiometry, skinfold thickness, and underwater weighing.
9. Contrast the four-component with the two-component models of body composition assessment.
10. What is the principle of underwater weighing? Why should a different body density equation be used for children, in contrast to adults?
11. Given: a twenty-year-old college male, 180 lb, 28% fat. What is his target body weight to achieve 17% fat?

12. In terms of the resistance to weight reduction, contrast obesity due to hypertrophy with obesity due to hyperplasia of fat cells.
13. Is obesity more related to genetics or the environment?
14. If a person consumes 120 kcal per day in excess of need, what weight gain does the static energy balance equation predict compared to the dynamic energy balance equation?
15. What does nutrient balance mean and how is the ratio of the RQ to FQ used to determine nutrient balance?
16. Contrast a physiological set point with a behavioral set point related to obesity.
17. What happens to the BMR when a person goes on a low-calorie diet?
18. What recommendations would you give about the use of diet alone versus a combination of diet and exercise?
19. What is thermogenesis and how might it be related to a weight gain?
20. What is the effect of exercise on appetite and body composition?
21. What exercise recommendation is appropriate for someone who is sedentary and overweight, and is consistent with achieving caloric-expenditure and fat-loss goals?

suggested readings

Guthrie, H. A., and M. F. Picciano. 1995. *Human Nutrition*. St. Louis: Mosby.

Lohman, T. G. 1992. *Advances in Body Composition Assessment*. Champaign, IL: Human Kinetics.

references

1. Acheson, K. J. 1987. Carbohydrate metabolism and de novo lipogenesis in human obesity. *American Journal of Clinical Nutrition* 45:78–85.

1a. AHA Committee Report. 1982. Rationale of the diet-heart statement of the American Heart Association. *Nutrition Today* (Sept./Oct.):16–20, (Nov./Dec.):15–19.

2. Aloia, J. R. 1981. Exercise and skeletal health. *Journal of the American Geriatrics Society* 29:104–7.

3. American Alliance for Health, Physical Education, Recreation, and Dance. 1988. *Physical Best*. Reston, VA: Author.

4. Andres, R. 1985. Mortality and obesity: The rationale for age-specific height-weight tables. In *Principles of Geriatric Medicine*, eds. E. L. Bierman and W. R. Hazzard, chap. 29, 311–18. New York: McGraw-Hill.

5. Ballor, D. L., J. P. McCarthy, and E. J. Wilterdink. 1990. Exercise intensity does not affect the composition of diet- and exercise-induced body mass loss. *American Journal of Clinical Nutrition* 51:142–46.

6. Barnard, D. L. et al. 1969. Changes in body composition produced by prolonged total starvation and refeeding. *Metabolism* 18:564–69.

7. Behnke, A. R., B. G. Feen, and W. C. Welham. 1942. The specific gravity of healthy men: Body weight ÷ volume as an index of obesity. *Journal of the American Medical Association* 118:495–98.

8. Benedict, F. G. et al. 1919. *Human Vitality and Efficiency Under Prolonged Restricted Diet*. Washington, D.C.: The Carnegie Institution of Washington.

9. Björntrop, P. 1978. The fat cell: A clinical view. In *Recent Advances in Obesity Research*: II., ed. George Bray, 153–68. Westport, CN: Technomic.

10. ———. 1985. Regional patterns of fat distribution. *Annals of Internal Medicine* 103:994–95.

11. Björntrop, P. et al. 1971. Adipose tissue fat cell size and number in relation to metabolism in randomly selected middle-aged men and women. *Metabolism* 20:927–35.

12. Björntrop, P., and L. Sjöström. 1971. Number and size of adipose tissue fat cells in relation to metabolism in human obesity. *Metabolism* 20:703–13.

12a. ———. 1978. Carbohydrate storage in man: Speculations and some quantitative considerations. *Metabolism Clinical Experimental* 27:1853–65.

13. Black, A. E. et al. 1991. Critical evaluation of energy intake data using fundamental principles of energy physiology: 2. Evaluating the results of published surveys. *European Journal of Clinical Nutrition* 45:583–99.

13a. Blundell, J. E. et al. 1993. Dietary fat and the control of energy intake: Evaluating the effects of fat on meal size and postmeal satiety. *American Journal of Clinical Nutrition* (Suppl. 57):772S–778S.

14. Booth, D. A. 1980. Acquired behavior controlling energy intake and output. In *Obesity*, ed. A. J. Stunkard, 101–43. Philadelphia: W. B. Saunders.

15. Bouchard, C. 1991. Heredity and the path to overweight and obesity. *Medicine and Science in Sports and Exercise* 23:285–91.

16. Bray, G. A. 1969. Effect of caloric restriction on energy expenditure in obese patients. *The Lancet* 2:397–98.

17. ———. 1983. The energetics of obesity. *Medicine and Science in Sports and Exercise* 15:32–40.

18. ———. 1992. Pathophysiology of obesity. *American Journal of Clinical Nutrition* 55:488S–494S.

19. Bray, G. A., and R. L. Atkinson. 1992. New weight guidelines for Americans. *American Journal of Clinical Nutrition* 55:481–82.

20. Bray, G. A., B. York, and J. Delany. 1992. A survey of the opinions of obesity experts on the causes and treatment of obesity. *American Journal for Clinical Nutrition* 55:151S–154S.

21. Brehm, B. A. 1988. Elevation of metabolic rate following exercise implications for weight loss. *Sports Medicine* 6:72–78.

22. Brewer, V. 1983. Role of exercise in prevention of involutional bone loss. *Medicine and Science in Sports and Exercise* 15:445–49.

23. Brodie, D. A. 1988. Techniques of measurement of body composition Part I. *Sports Medicine* 5:11–40.

24. ———. 1988. Techniques of measurement of body composition Part II. *Sports Medicine* 5:74–98.

25. Broeder, C. E., K. A. Burrhus, L. S. Svanevik, and J. H. Wilmore. 1992. The effects of aerobic fitness on resting metabolic rate. *American Journal of Clinical Nutrition* 55:795–801.

26. ———. 1992. The effects of either high-intensity resistance or endurance training on resting metabolic rate. *American Journal of Clinical Nutrition* 55:802–10.

26a. Brooke-Wavell, K. et al. 1995. Evaluation of near infra-red interactance for assessment of subcutaneous and total body fat. *European Journal of Clinical Nutrition* 49:57–65.

27. Brownell, K. D., and A. J. Stunkard. 1980. Behavioral treatment for obese children and adolescents. In *Obesity*, ed. A. J. Stunkard, 415–37. Philadelphia: W. B. Saunders.

28. Brozek, J. et al. 1963. Densitometric analysis of body composition: Revision of some quantitative assumptions. *Annals of New York Academy of Science* 110:113–40.

28a. Bullough, R. C. 1995. Interaction of acute changes in exercise energy expenditure and energy intake on resting metabolic rate. *American Journal of Clinical Nutrition* 61:473–81.

29. Bunt, J. C. 1986. Hormonal alterations due to exercise. *Sports Medicine* 3:331–45.

30. Buskirk, E. R. 1961. Underwater weighing and body density: A review of procedures. In *Techniques for Measuring Body Composition*, eds. J. Brozek and A. Henschel. Washington, D.C.: National Academy of Sciences—National Research Council.

31. Buskirk, E. R. et al. 1963. Energy balance of obese patients during weight reduction: Influence of diet restriction and exercise. *Annals of New York Academy of Science* 110 (part II):918–40.

32. Calles-Escandón, J., and E. S. Horton. 1992. The thermogenic role of exercise in the treatment of morbid obesity: A critical evaluation. *American Journal of Clinical Nutrition* 55:533S–537S.

33. Cameron, J. R., and J. Sorenson. 1963. Measurement of bone mineral in-vivo: An improved method. *Science* 142:230–32.

34. Campaigne, B. N. 1990. Body fat distribution in females: Metabolic consequences and implications for weight loss. *Medicine and Science in Sports and Exercise* 22:291–97.

35. Cann, C. E. et al. 1984. Decreased spinal mineral content in amenorrheic women. *Journal of the American Medical Association* 251:626–29.

36. Christian, J. L., and J. L. Greger. 1994. *Nutrition for Living*. Redwood City, CA.: Benjamin/Cummings.

37. Coniglio, J. G. 1984. Fat. In *Nutrition Reviews' Present Knowledge in Nutrition*, 5th ed., chap. 7, 79–89. Washington, D.C.: The Nutrition Foundation.

38. Cunningham, J. J. 1991. Body composition as a determinant of energy expenditure: A synthetic review and a proposed general prediction equation. *American Journal of Clinical Nutrition* 54:963–69.

39. Dahlquist, A. 1984. Carbohydrates. In *Nutrition Reviews' Present Knowledge in Nutrition*, 5th ed., chap. 9, 116–30. Washington, D.C.: The Nutrition Foundation.

40. Danforth, E. et al. 1978. Undernutrition contrasted to overnutrition. In *Recent Advances in Obesity Research*: II, ed. G. Bray, 229–36. Westport, CN: Technomic.

41. DeBakey, M. E. et al. 1984. *The Living Heart Diet*. New York: Raven Press.

41a. de Vries, J. et al. 1994. Underestimation of energy intake by 3-d records compared with energy intake to maintain body weight in 269 nonobese adults. *American Journal of Clinical Nutrition* 60:855–60.

41b. di Pietro, L. 1995. Physical activity, body weight, and adiposity: An epidemiologic perspective. In *Exercise and Sport Sciences Reviews*, vol. 23, ed. J. O. Holloszy, 275–303. Baltimore: Williams & Wilkins.

42. Donnelly, J. E., J. Jakicic, and S. Gunderson. 1991. Diet and body composition: Effect of very low calorie diets and exercise. *Sports Medicine* 12:237–49.

43. DuBois, E. F. 1968. Basal energy, metabolism at various ages: Man. In *Metabolism*, eds. P. L. Altman and D. S. Dittmer, 345. Bethesda, MD: Federation of American Societies for Experimental Biology.

44. Durnin, J. V. G. A. 1978. Possible interaction between physical activity, body composition, and obesity in man. In *Recent Advances in Obesity Research*: II, ed. G. Bray, 237–41. Westport, CN: Technomic.

45. Eastwood, M. 1984. Dietary fiber. In *Nutrition Reviews' Present Knowledge in Nutrition*, 5th ed., chap. 12, 156–75. Washington, D.C.: The Nutrition Foundation.

45a. Ellis, K. J. et al. 1994. Accuracy of dual-energy x-ray absorptiometry for body-composition measurements in children. *American Journal of Clinical Nutrition* 60:660–65.

46. Ernst, N. D., and R. I. Levy. 1984. Diet and cardiovascular disease. In *Nutrition Reviews' Present Knowledge in Nutrition*, 5th ed., chap. 50, 724–39. Washington, D.C.: The Nutrition Foundation.

47. Feinleib, M. 1985. Epidemiology of obesity in relation to health hazards. *Annals of Internal Medicine* 103:1019–24.

48. Finberg, L. 1985. Clinical assessment of total body water. In *Body-Composition Assessments in Youth and Adults*, ed. A. F. Roche, 22–23. Columbus, OH: Ross Laboratories.

48a. Flatt, J. P. 1988. Importance of nutrient balance in body weight regulation. *Diabetes/Metabolism Reviews* 4:571–81.

48b. Flatt, J. P. 1993. Dietary fat, carbohydrate balance, and weight maintenance. *Annals of New York Academy of Science* 683:122–40.

48c. Flatt, J. P. 1995. Use and storage of carbohydrate and fat. *American Journal of Clinical Nutrition* (Suppl. 61):952S–959S.

49. Foreyt, J. P., and G. K. Goodrick. 1991. Factors common to successful therapy for the obese patient. *Medicine and Science in Sports and Exercise* 23:292–97.

50. Foster, G. D. et al. 1990. Controlled trial of the metabolic effects of a very-low-calorie diet: Short- and long-term effects. *American Journal of Clinical Nutrition* 51:167–72.

51. Garfinkle, P. E., and D. M. Garner. 1982. *Anorexia Nervosa*. New York: Brunner/Mazel.

52. Garn, S. M. 1961. Radiographic analysis of body composition. In *Techniques for Measuring Body Composition*, eds. J. Brozek and H. Henschel, 36–58. Washington, D.C.: National Academy of Sciences—National Research Council.

53. Garn, S., and D. C. Clark. 1976. Trends in fatness and the origins of obesity. *Pediatrics* 57:443–56.

54. Garrow, J. S. 1978. *Energy Balance and Obesity in Man*. New York: Elsevier North-Holland.

55. Garrow, J. S. 1978. The regulation of energy expenditure in man. In *Recent Advances in Obesity Research*: II, ed. G. Bray, 200–210. Westport, CN: Technomic.

55a. Going, S., D. Williams, and T. Lohman. 1995. Aging and body composition: Biological changes and methodological issues. In *Exercise and Sport Sciences Reviews* vol. 23, ed. J. O. Holloszy, 411–58. Baltimore: Williams & Wilkins.

56. Goldblatt, P. B., M. E. Moore, and A. J. Stunkard. 1965. Social factors in obesity. *Journal of the American Medical Association* 192:1039–44.

57. Goldman, R. F., and E. R. Buskirk. 1961. Body volume measurement by underwater weighing: Description of a method. In *Techniques for Measuring Body Composition*, eds. J. Brozek and A. Henschel, 78–89. Washington, D.C.: National Academy of Sciences—National Research Council.

58. Gortmaker, J. L. et al. 1987. Increasing pediatric obesity in the United States. *American Journal of Diseases of Children* 141:535–40.

58a. Guthrie, H. A., and M. F. Picciano. 1995. *Human Nutrition*. St. Louis: Mosby.

59. Guyton, A. G. 1981. *Textbook of Medical Physiology*. 6th ed. Philadelphia: W. B. Saunders.

60. ———. 1977. Body fat and adipose tissue cellularity in infants: A longitudinal study. *Metabolism* 26:607–14.

61. Hager, A., L. Sjöström, and B. Arvidsson. 1978. Adipose tissue cellularity in obese school girls before and after dietary treatment. *American Journal of Clinical Nutrition* 31:68–75.

62. Hallberg, L. 1984. Iron. In *Nutrition Reviews' Present Knowledge in Nutrition*. 5th ed., chap. 32, 459–78. Washington, D.C.: The Nutrition Foundation.

63. Heaney, R. P. 1987. The role of calcium in prevention and treatment of osteoporosis. *The Physician and Sportsmedicine* 15(11):83–88.

64. Heinrich, C. H. et al. 1990. Bone mineral content of cyclically menstruating female resistance and endurance trained athletes. *Medicine and Science in Sports and Exercise* 22:558.

64a. Hellerstein, M. K. et al. 1991. Measurement of de novo hepatic lipogenesis in humans using stable isotopes. *The American Society for Clinical Investigation, Inc.* 87:1841–52.

64b. Hill, J. O. et al. 1993. Obesity treatment: Can diet composition play a role? *American College of Physicians* 119:694–97.

65. Hirsch, J. 1995. Role and benefits of carbohydrate in the diet: Key issues for future dietary guidelines. *American Journal of Clinical Nutrition* (Suppl. 61):996S–1000S.

65a. Hirsch, J., and J. L. Knittle. 1970. Cellularity of obese and nonobese human adipose tissue. *Federation Proceedings* 29:1516–21.

65b. Houtkooper, L. B., and S. B. Going. 1994. Body composition: How should it be measured? Does it affect performance? *Sports Science Exchange* vol. 7, no. 5. Barrington, IL: Gatorade Sports Science Institute.

66. Howley, E. T., and B. Don Franks. 1992. *Health/Fitness Instructor's Handbook*. 2d ed. Champaign, IL: Human Kinetics.

67. Hubert, H. B. et al. 1983. Obesity as an independent risk factor for cardiovascular disease: A 26-year follow-up of participants in the Framingham Heart Study. *Circulation* 67:968–77.

68. Jackson, A. S., and M. L. Pollock. 1978. Generalized equations for predicting body density of men. *British Journal of Nutrition* 40:497–504.

69. Jackson, A. S., and M. L. Pollock. 1985. Practical assessment of body composition. *The Physician and Sportsmedicine* 13:76–90.

70. Jackson, A. S., M. L. Pollock, and A. Ward. 1980. Generalized equations for predicting body density of women. *Medicine and Science in Sports and Exercise* 12:175–82.

71. James, W. P. T., and P. Trayhurn. 1981. Thermogenesis and obesity. *British Medical Bulletin* 37:43–48.

71a. Jéquier, E. 1992. Calorie balance versus nutrient balance. In *Energy Metabolism: Tissue Determinants and Cellular Corollaries*, eds. J. M. Kinney and H. N. Tucker, 123–37. New York: Raven.

71b. ———. 1993. Body weight regulation in humans: The importance of nutrient balance. *News in Physiological Sciences* 8:273–76.

72. Johnston, F. E., and R. Malina. 1966. Age changes in the composition of the upper arm in Philadelphia children. *Human Biology* 38:1–21.

73. Jung, R. T. et al. 1979. Reduced thermogenesis in obesity. *Nature* (London) 279:322–23.

74. Kannel, W. B., and T. Gordon. 1979. Physiological and medical concomitants of obesity: The Framingham study. In *Obesity in America*, 125–43. U.S. Department of Health, Education, and Welfare. NIH Publication No. 79-359.

75. Katch, F. I. 1985. Assessment of lean body tissues by radiography and bioelectrical impedance. In *Body-Composition Assessment in Youths and Adults*, ed. A. F. Roche, 46–51. Columbus, OH: Ross Laboratories.

76. Katch, V. L., R. Martin, and J. Martin. 1979. Effects of exercise intensity on food consumption in the male rat. *American Journal of Clinical Nutrition* 32:1401–7.

77. Keys, A. et al. 1950. *The Biology of Human Starvation*, vol. I. Minneapolis: The University of Minnesota Press.

78. Knittle, J. L. 1972. Obesity in childhood: A problem in adipose tissue cellular development. *Journal of Pediatrics* 81:1048–59.

79. Kolata, G. 1986. Obese children: A growing problem. *Science* 233:20–21.

80. Krotkiewski, M. et al. 1977. Adipose tissue cellularity in relation to prognosis for weight reduction. *International Journal of Obesity* 1:395–416.

81. Kuczmarski, R. J. 1992. Prevalence of overweight and weight gain in the United States. *American Journal of Clinical Nutrition* 55:495S–502S.

82. Lapidus, L. et al. 1984. Distribution of adipose tissue and risk of cardiovascular disease and death: A 12-year follow-up of participants in the population study of women in Gothenburg, Sweden. *British Medical Journal* 289:1257–61.

83. Larsson, B. et al. 1984. Abdominal adipose tissue distribution, obesity, and risk of cardiovascular disease and death: 13-year follow-up of participants in the study of men born in 1913. *British Medical Journal* 288:1401–4.

84. Leibel, R. L. et al. 1992. Energy intake required to maintain body weight is not affected by wide variation in diet composition. *American Journal of Clinical Nutrition* 55:350–55.

84a. Lightman, S. W. et al. 1992. Discrepancy between self-reported and actual caloric intake and exercise in obese subjects. *The New England Journal of Medicine* 327:1893–98.

85. Lohman, T. G. 1981. Skinfolds and body density and their relation to body fatness: A review. *Human Biology* 53:181–225.

86. ———. 1982. Body composition methodology in sports medicine. *The Physician and Sportsmedicine* 10(12):47–58.

87. ———. 1985. Research relating to assessment of skeletal status. In *Body-Composition Assessments in Youth and Adults*, ed. A. F. Roche, 38–41. Columbus, OH: Ross Laboratories.

88. ———. 1986. Applicability of body composition techniques and constants for children and youths. In *Exercise and Sport Sciences Reviews*, vol. 14, ed. K. B. Pandolf, chap. 11, 325–57. New York: Macmillan.

89. ———. 1987. The use of skinfold to estimate body fatness in children and youth. *Journal of the Alliance for Health, Physical Education, Recreation and Dance* 58 (Nov.–Dec.): 98–102.

89a. ———. 1989. Assessment of body composition in children. *Pediatric Exercise Science* 1:19–30.

90. ———. 1992. *Advances in Body Composition Assessment*. Champaign, IL: Human Kinetics.

90a. Lohman, T. G., and S. B. Going. 1993. Multicomponent models in body composition research: opportunities and pitfalls. In *Human Body Composition*, eds. K. J. Ellis and J. D. Eastman, 53–58. New York: Plenum Press.

91. Lohman, T. G. et al. 1984. Bone mineral measurements and their relation to body density in children, youth and adults. *Human Biology* 56:667–79.

92. Mayer, J. 1965. Genetic factors in human obesity. *Annals of New York Academy of Science* 131:412–21.

93. Mayer, J. et al. 1954. Exercise, food intake, and body weight in normal rats and genetically obese mice. *American Journal of Physiology* 177:544–48.

94. Mayer, J., P. Roy, and K. P. Mitra. 1956. Relation between caloric intake, body weight and physical work: Studies in an industrial male population in West Bengal. *American Journal of Clinical Nutrition* 4:169–75.

94a. Mazess, R. B. et al. 1990. Dual-energy x-ray absorptiometry for total-body and regional bone-mineral and soft-tissue composition. *American Journal of Clinical Nutrition* 51:1106–12.

95. McLean, K. P., and J. S. Skinner. 1992. Validity of Futrex-5000 for body composition determination. *Medicine and Science in Sports and Exercise* 24:253–58.

96. Mertz, W. et al. 1991. What are people really eating? The relation between energy intake derived from estimated diet records and intake determined to maintain body weight. *American Journal of Clinical Nutrition* 54:291–95.

97. Metropolitan Life Insurance Company. 1959. New weight standards for men and women. *Statistical Bulletin Metropolitan Life Insurance Company* 40:1–4.

98. Miller, W. C. 1991. Diet composition, energy intake, and nutritional status in relation to obesity in men and women. *Medicine and Science in Sports and Exercise* 23:280–84.

99. Molé, P. A. 1990. Impact of energy intake and exercise on resting metabolic rate. *Sports Medicine* 10:72–87.

100. Montoye, H. J. et al. 1980. Bone mineral in senior tennis players. *Scandanavian Journal of Sport Science* 2:26–32.

101. Moore, R., and E. R. Buskirk. 1974. Exercise and body fluids. In *Science and Medicine of Exercise and Sport*, 2d ed., eds. W. R. Johnson and E. R. Buskirk. New York: Harper & Row.

102. Morrow, J. R. et al. 1986. Accuracy of measured and predicted residual lung volume on body density measurement. *Medicine and Science in Sports and Exercise* 18:647–52.

103. Nachtigall, L. E. et al. 1979. Estrogen replacement therapy I: A 10-year prospective study in the relationship to osteoporosis. *Obstetrics and Gynecology* 53:277–81.

104. National Research Council. 1989. *Diet and Health*. Washington, D.C.: National Academy Press.

105. National Research Council, National Academy of Sciences. 1989. *Recommended Dietary Allowances*. Washington, D.C.: National Academy Press.

106. Oscai, L. B. 1973. The role of exercise in weight control. In *Exercise and Sport Sciences Reviews*, vol. 1, ed. J. H. Wilmore, 103–20. New York: Academic Press.

107. Oscai, L. B. et al. 1972. Effects of exercise and food restriction on adipose tissue cellularity. *Journal of Lipid Research* 13:588–92.

108. Oscai, L. B., P. A. Mole, and J. O. Holloszy. 1971. Effects of exercise on cardiac weight and mitochondria in male and female rats. *American Journal of Physiology* 220:1944–48.

109. Oyster, N., M. Morton, and S. Linnell. 1984. Physical activity and osteoporosis in post-menopausal women. *Medicine and Science in Sports and Exercise* 16:44–55.

110. Passmore, R. 1968. Energy metabolism at various weights: Man. Part II. Resing: Adults. In *Metabolism*, eds. P. L. Altman and D. S. Dittmer, 344–45. Bethesda, MD: Federation of American Societies for Experimental Biology.

111. Poehlman, E. T. 1989. A review: Exercise and its influence on resting energy metabolism in man. *Medicine and Science in Sports and Exercise* 21:515–25.

112. Poehlman, E. T., C. L. Melby, and M. I. Goran. 1991. The impact of exercise and diet restriction on daily energy expenditure. *Sports Medicine* 11:78–101.

113. Pollock, M. L., and J. H. Wilmore. 1990. *Exercise in Health and Disease* 2d ed. Philadelphia: W. B. Saunders.

114. Pooling Project Research Group. 1978. Relationship of blood pressure, serum cholesterol, smoking habit, relative weight and ECG abnormalities to incidence of major coronary events: Final report of the pooling project. *Journal of Chronic Diseases* 31:201–306.

115. Presta, E. et al. 1987. Body composition in adolescents: Estimation by total body electrical conductivity. *Journal of Applied Physiology* 63:937–41.

116. Rabkin, S. W., F. A. L. Mathewson, and Ping-hwa Hsu. 1977. Relation of body weight to development of ischemic heart disease in a cohort of young North American men after a 26-year observation period: The Manitoba study. *The American Journal of Cardiology* 39:452–58.

117. Rimm, A. A., and P. L. White. 1979. Obesity: Its risks and hazards. In *Obesity in America*, U.S. Department of Health, Education and Welfare. NIH Publication No. 79-359.

117a. Rising, R. et al. 1994. Determinants of total daily energy expenditure: Variability in physical activity. *American Journal of Clinical Nutrition* 59:800–804.

117b. Rolls, B. J. 1995. Carbohydrates, fats, and satiety. *American Journal of Clinical Nutrition* (Suppl. 61):960S–7S.

117c. Romijn, J. A. et al. 1993. Regulation of endogenous fat and carbohydrate metabolism in relation to exercise intensity and duration. *American Journal of Physiology* 265:E380–E391.

117d. Ross, R., and J. Rissanen. 1994. Mobilization of visceral and subcutaneous adipose tissue in response to energy restriction and exercise. *American Journal of Clinical Nutrition* 60:695–703.

117e. Roust, L. R., K. D. Hammel, and M. D. Jensen. 1994. Effects of isoenergetic, low-fat diets on energy metabolism in lean and obese women. *American Journal of Clinical Nutrition* 60:470–75.

118. Schoeller, D. A. et al. 1985. Measurement of total body water: Isotope dilution techniques. In *Body-Composition Assessment in Youths and Adults*, ed. A. F. Roche, 24–29. Columbus, OH: Ross Laboratories.

119. Schoutens, A., E. Laurent, and J. R. Poortmans. 1989. Effects of inactivity and exercise on bone. *Sports Medicine* 7:71–81.

120. Schuette, S. A., and H. M. Linkswiler. 1984. Calcium. In *Nutrition Reviews' Present Knowledge in Nutrition*, 5th ed., chap. 28, 400–412. Washington, D.C.: The Nutrition Foundation.

120a. Schulz, L. O, and D. A. Schoeller. 1994. A compilation of total daily energy expenditures and body weights in healthy adults. *American Journal of Clinical Nutrition* 60:676–81.

121. Schutte, J. E. et al. 1984. Density of lean body mass is greater in blacks than in whites. *Journal of Applied Physiology: Respiratory, Environmental, and Exercise Physiology* 56:1647–49.

122. Segal, K. R. et al. 1985. Estimation of human body composition by electrical impedance methods: A comparative study. *Journal of Applied Physiology* 58:1565–71.

123. Segal, K. R. et al. 1990. Comparison of thermic effects of constant and relative caloric loads in lean and obese men. *American Journal of Clinical Nutrition* 51:14–21.

124. Segal, K. R. et al. 1991. Estimation of extracellular and total body water by multiple-frequency bioelectrical-impedance measurement. *American Journal of Clinical Nutrition* 54:26–29.

125. Sharkey, B. 1984. *The Physiology of Fitness*. 2d ed. Champaign, IL: Human Kinetics.

126. Sheppard, L., A. R. Kristal, and L. H. Kushi. 1991. Weight loss in women participating in a randomized trail of low-fat diets. *American Journal of Clinical Nutrition* 54:821–28.

127. Sims, E. A. H. et al. 1973. Endocrine and metabolic effects of experimental obesity in man. *Recent Progress in Hormonal Research* 29:457–87.

128. Sinning, W. E. et al. 1985. Validity of "generalized" equations for body composition analysis in male athletes. *Medicine and Science in Sports and Exercise* 17:124–30.

129. Sinning, W. E., and J. R. Wilson. 1984. Validity of "generalized" equations for body composition analysis in women athletes. *Research Quarterly for Exercise Sport* 55:153–60.

130. Siri, W. E. 1961. Body composition from fluid spaces and density: Analysis of methods. In *Techniques for Measuring Body Composition*, eds. J. Brozek and A. Henschel, 223–44. Washington, D.C.: National Academy of Sciences—National Research Council.

131. ———. 1980. Fat cells and body weight. In *Obesity*, ed. A. J. Stunkard, 72–100. Philadelphia: W. B. Saunders.

132. Sjöström, L. V. 1992. Morbidity of severely obese subjects. *American Journal of Clinical Nutrition* 55:508S–515S.

133. ———. 1992. Mortality of severely obese subjects. *American Journal of Clinical Nutrition* 55:516S–523S.

134. Sjöström, L., and P. Björntrop. 1974. Body composition and adipose tissue cellularity in human obesity. *Acta Media Scandinavica* 195:201–11.

134a. Slaughter, M. H. et al. 1988. Skinfold equations for estimation of body fatness in children and youth. *Human Biology* 60:709–23.

134b. Stefanick, M. L. 1993. Exercise and weight control. *Exercise and Sport Sciences Reviews* vol. 21, ed. J. O. Holloszy, 363–96. Baltimore: Williams & Wilkins.

135. Stuart, R. B., and B. Davis. 1972. *Slim Chance in a Fat World*. Champaign, IL: Research Press.

136. Stunkard, A. J. 1979. Obesity and the social environment: Current status, future prospects. In *Obesity in America*, 206–40. U.S. Department of Health, Education, and Welfare. NIH Publication No. 79-359.

137. Stunkard, A. J. et al. 1986. An adoption study of human obesity. *The New England Journal of Medicine* 314:193–98.

137a. Swan, P. D., and E. T. Howley. 1994. Substrate utilization during prolonged exercise in obese women differing in body fat distribution. *International Journal of Obesity* 18:263–68.

137b. Swinburn, B., and E. Ravussin. 1993. Energy balance or fat balance? *American Journal of Clinical Nutrition* (Suppl. 57):766S–771S.

137c. Tataranni, P. et al. 1995. Thermic effect of food in humans: Methods and results from use of a respiratory chamber. *American Journal of Clinical Nutrition* 61:1013–19.

137d. Thomas, C. D. et al. 1992. Nutrient balance and energy expenditure during ad libitum feeding of high-fat and high-carbohydrate diets in humans. *American Journal of Clinical Nutrition* 55:934–42.

138. Titchenal, C. A. 1988. Exercise and food intake: What is the relationship? *Sports Medicine* 6:135–45.

139. Tremblay, A. et al. 1991. Energy requirements of a postobese man reporting a low energy intake at weight maintenance. *American Journal of Clinical Nutrition* 54:506–8.

139a. Tremblay, A., J-A Simoneau, and C. Bouchard. 1994. Impact of exercise intensity on body fatness and skeletal muscle metabolism. *Metabolism* 43:814–18.

139b. Treuth, M. S. et al. 1995. Energy expenditure and substrate utilization in older women after strength training: 24-h calorimeter results. *Journal of Applied Physiology* 78:2140–46.

140. U.S. Department of Agriculture. 1992. USDA's *Food Guide Pyramid*. Washington, D.C.: Author.

141. U.S. Department of Agriculture. 1980. *Nutrition and Your Health: Dietary Guidelines for Americans*. Washington, D.C.

142. U.S. Department of Agriculture and U.S. Department of Health and Human Services. 1990. *Nutrition and Your Health: Dietary Guidelines for Americans*. 3d ed. Washington, D.C.

143. U.S. Senate Select Committee on Nutrition and Human Needs. 1977. *Dietary Goals for the U.S.— Supplemental Views*. Washington, D.C.: U.S. Government Printing Office.

144. U.S. Senate Select Committee on Nutrition and Human Needs. 1977. *Eating in America: Dietary Goals for the* U.S. Cambridge, MA: The MIT Press.

144a. Van Etten, L. M. L. A., K. R. Westerterp, and F. T. J. Verstappen. 1995. Effect of weight-training on energy expenditure and substrate utilization during sleep. *Medicine and Science in Sports and Exercise* 27:188–93.

145. Van Itallie, T. B. 1979. Conservative approaches to treatment. In *Obesity in America*, ed. G. Bray. Department of Health, Education, and Welfare. NIH Publication No. 79-359.

146. Van Itallie, T. B. et al. 1985. Clinical assessment of body fat content in adults: Potential role of electrical impedance methods: In *Body-Composition Assessments in Youth and Adults*, ed. A. F. Roche, 5–8. Columbus, OH: Ross Laboratories.

146a. Van Loan, M. D., et al. 1995. Evaluation of body composition by dual energy x-ray absorptiometry and two different software packages. *Medicine and Science in Sports and Exercise* 27:587–91.

146b. Van Marken Lichtenbelt, W. D. et al. 1994. Validation of bioelectrical-impedance measurements as a method to estimate body-water compartments. *American Journal of Clinical Nutrition* 60:159–66.

147. Vasselli, J. R., M. P. Cleary, and T. B. Van Itallie. 1984. Obesity. In *Nutrition Reviews' Present Knowledge in Nutrition*. 5th ed., chap. 4, 35–36. Washington, D.C.: The Nutrition Foundation.

147a. Wabitsch, M. et al. 1994. Body-fat distribution and changes in the atherogenic risk-factor profile in obese adolescent girls during weight reduction. *American Journal of Clinical Nutrition* 60:54–60.

148. Wadden, T. A., and A. J. Stunkard. 1985. Social and psychological consequences of obesity. *Annals of Internal Medicine* 103:1062–67.

149. Ward, A. et al. 1978. A comparison of body fat determined by underwater weighing and volume displacement. *American Journal of Physiology* 234:E94–E96.

150. Weinsier, R. L., Y. Schutz, and D. Bracco. 1992. Reexamination of the relationship of resting metabolic rate to fat-free mass and to the metabolically active components of fat-free mass in humans. *American Journal of Clinical Nutrition* 55:790–94.

151. Welham, W. C., and A. R. Behnke. 1942. The specific gravity of healthy men. *Journal of the American Medicine Association* 118:498–501.

152. Willett, W. C., M. Stampfer, J. Manson, and T. Van Itallie. 1991. New weight guidelines for Americans: Justified or injudicious. *American Journal of Clinical Nutrition* 53:1102–3.

153. Willett, W. C., M. Stampfer, J. Manson, and T. Van Itallie. 1992. Reply to G. A. Bray and R. L. Atlinson. *American Journal of Clinical Nutrition* 55:482–83.

154. Williams, M. H. 1985. *Nutritional Aspects of Human Physical and Athletic Performance*. 2d ed. Springfield, IL: Charles C Thomas.

155. Williams, R. L., and J. D. Long. 1983. *Toward a Self-Managed Lifestyle*, 3d ed. Boston, MA: Houghton Mifflin.

156. Wilmore, J. H. 1983. Body composition in sport and exercise: Directions for future research. *Medicine and Science in Sports and Exercise* 15:21–31.

157. ———. 1983. The 1983 C. H. McCloy Research Lecture. Appetite and body composition consequent to physical activity. *Research Quarterly for Exercise and Sport* 54:415–25.

158. Wing, R. R. 1992. Behavioral treatment of severe obesity. *American Journal of Clinical Nutrition* 55:545S–551S.

159. Zurlo, F. et al. 1990. Low ratio of fat to carbohydrate oxidation as predictor of weight gain: Study of 24-h RQ. *American Journal of Physiology* 259:E650–E657.

SECTION III

Physiology of
Performance

Factors Affecting Performance

objectives

By studying this chapter, you should be able to do the following:

1. Identify factors affecting maximal performance.
2. Provide evidence for and against the central nervous system being a site of fatigue.
3. Identify potential neural factors in the periphery that may be linked to fatigue.
4. Explain the role of cross-bridge cycling in fatigue.
5. Summarize the evidence on the order of recruitment of muscle fibers with increasing intensities of activity, and the type of metabolism upon which each is dependent.
6. Describe the factors limiting performance in all-out activities lasting less than ten seconds.
7. Describe the factors limiting performance in all-out activities lasting 10–180 seconds.
8. Discuss the subtle changes in the factors affecting optimal performance as the duration of a maximal performance increases from three minutes to four hours.

outline

Sites of Fatigue   362
   Central Fatigue   362
   Peripheral Fatigue   363
Factors Limiting All–Out Anaerobic Performances   365
   Ultra Short-Term Performances (Less than Ten Seconds)   366

Short-Term Performances (10 to 180 Seconds)   366
Factors Limiting All–Out Aerobic Performances   367
   Moderate-Length Performances (Three to Twenty Minutes)   367

Intermediate-Length Performances (Twenty-One to Sixty Minutes)   367
Long-Term Performances (One to Four Hours)   368
Athlete as Machine   369

n the last few chapters we have focused on proper exercise and nutrition for health and fitness. The emphasis was on *moderation* in both in order to reduce the risk factors associated with a variety of diseases. We must now change that focus in order to discuss the factors limiting physical performance.

Performance goals require much more time, effort, and risk of injury than fitness goals. What are the requirements for optimal performance? In order to answer this question we must ask another: What kind of performance? It is clear that the requirements for the best performance in the 400-meter run are different from those associated with the marathon. Figure 19.1 shows a diagram of factors influencing performance (5). Every performance requires a certain amount of strength, as well as the "skill" to apply that strength in the best way. Further, energy must be supplied in the manner needed or performance will suffer. Different activities require differing amounts of energy from aerobic and anaerobic processes. Both the environment (altitude and heat) and diet (carbohydrate and water intake) play a role in endurance performance. Lastly, best performances require a psychological commitment to "go for the gold." The purpose of this chapter is to expand on this diagram and discuss the factors limiting performance in a variety of activities, which will point the way to the remaining chapters. However, before we discuss these factors, we will summarize the potential sites of fatigue that would clearly affect performance.

Sites of Fatigue

Fatigue is simply defined as an inability to maintain a power output or force during repeated muscle contractions (10). As the two examples of the 400-meter run and the marathon suggest, the causes of fatigue vary, and are usually specific to the type of physical activity. Figure 19.2 provides a summary of potential sites of fatigue (10). The discussion of mechanisms starts at the brain, where a variety of factors can influence the "will to win," and continues to the cross-bridges of the muscles themselves. There is evidence to support most of the sites listed in figure 19.2 as "weak links" in the development of muscle tension needed for optimal performance. However, there is far from perfect agreement among scientists about the exact causes of fatigue. The reasons for this include: (a) the fiber type and training state of the subject, (b) whether the muscle was stimulated voluntarily or electrically, (c) the use of both amphibian and mammalian muscle preparations, with some isolated from the body, and (d) the intensity and duration of the exercise, and whether it was continuous or intermittent activity (15, 16). Within the scope of these limitations, we will now provide a summary of the evidence about each weak link, and then apply the information to specific types of performances.

Central Fatigue

The central nervous system (CNS) would be implicated in fatigue if there were (a) a reduction in the number of functioning motor units involved in the activity or (b) a reduction in motor unit firing frequency (8). There is evidence both for and against the concept of "central fatigue"; that is, that fatigue originates in the CNS.

Merton's classic experiments showed no difference in tension development when a *voluntary* contraction was compared to an *electrically induced* maximal contraction. When the muscle was fatigued

Figure 19.1

Factors affecting performance.

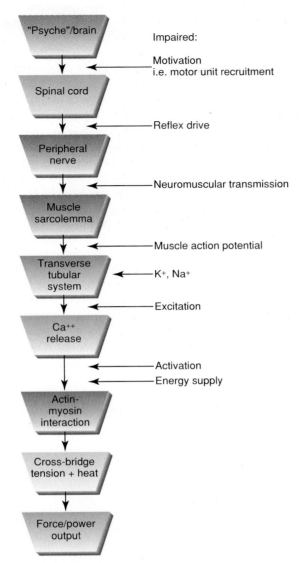

Possible Fatigue Mechanisms

"Psyche"/brain

Impaired:

Motivation
i.e. motor unit recruitment

Spinal cord

Reflex drive

Peripheral
nerve

Neuromuscular transmission

Muscle
sarcolemma

Muscle action potential

Transverse
tubular
system

K^+, Na^+

Excitation

Ca^{++}
release

Activation
Energy supply

Actin-
myosin
interaction

Cross-bridge
tension + heat

Force/power
output

Figure 19.2
Possible sites of fatigue.

by voluntary contractions, electrical stimulation could not restore tension (14). This suggested that the CNS was not limiting performance, and that the "periphery" was the site of fatigue.

In contrast, the early work of Ikai and Steinhaus (11) showed that a simple shout during exertion could increase what was formerly believed to be "maximal" strength. Later work showed that electrical stimulation of a muscle fatigued by voluntary contractions resulted in an increase in tension development (12). These studies suggest that the upper limit of voluntary strength is "psychologically" set, given that certain motivational or arousal factors are needed to achieve a physiological limit (12). In agreement with these results (that the CNS can limit performance) are two studies by Asmussen and Mazin (3, 4). Their subjects lifted weights thirty times a minute, causing fatigue in two to three minutes. Following a

two-minute pause, the lifting continued. These investigators showed that when either a physical diversion, consisting of the contraction of nonfatigued muscles, or mental diversion, consisting of doing mental arithmetic, was used between fatiguing bouts of exercise, work output was greater than when nothing was done during the pause. They also found that if a person did a series of muscle contractions to the point of fatigue with the eyes closed, simply opening the eyes restored tension (3). These studies suggest that alterations in central nervous system "arousal" can facilitate motor unit recruitment to increase strength, and alter the state of fatigue.

Peripheral Fatigue

While there is evidence both for and against the CNS being a site of fatigue, the vast majority of evidence points to the periphery, where neural, mechanical, or energetic events can hamper tension development (8a, 19).

Neural Factors

Fatigue due to neural factors could be associated with failure at the neuromuscular junction, the sarcolemma, the transverse tubules (t-tubule), or the sarcoplasmic reticulum (SR) that is involved in calcium (Ca^{++}) storage, release, and reuptake.

Neuromuscular Junction The action potential appears to reach the neuromuscular junction even when fatigue occurs (14). In addition, evidence based on simultaneous measurements of electrical activity at the neuromuscular junction and in the individual muscle fibers suggests that the neuromuscular junction is not the site of fatigue (7).

Sarcolemma and Transverse Tubules It has been hypothesized that the sarcolemma might be the site of fatigue due to its inability to maintain Na^+ and K^+ concentrations during repeated stimulation. When the Na^+/K^+ pump cannot keep up, K^+ accumulates outside the membrane and decreases inside the cell. This results in a depolarization of the cell and a reduction in action potential amplitude. The gradual depolarization of the sarcolemma could result in altered t-tubule function, including a block of the t-tubule action potential. If the latter occurs, Ca^{++} would not be released from the SR and muscle contraction would be blocked (1). However, the most recent evidence indicates that the typical reduction in the size of the action potential amplitude has little effect on force output by the muscle. In addition, the lower frequency of action potential firing with repeated stimulation of muscle seems to protect the muscle from further fatigue (rather than cause fatigue) by shifting the activation to a lower more optimal rate of firing (8a). This does not mean that the t-tubule is not involved in the fatigue process. Under certain stimulation conditions an action potential block can occur in the t-tubule, leading to a reduction in Ca^{++} release from the SR (8a, 19). As a result, myosin cross-bridge activation would be adversely affected.

Free Radical Production During Exercise May Contribute to Muscle Fatigue

Free radicals are highly reactive molecules that contain an unpaired electron in their outer orbital. Recall that free radicals are produced as a by-product of aerobic metabolism (chapter 3). Therefore, exercise results in an increased rate of free radical production in muscle and oxidative tissue damage may result. Further, recent evidence has shown that free radical production can promote muscle fatigue (6a, 14a). The mechanism of how free radicals produce muscle fatigue remains unknown. Some investigators have argued that free radical production during heavy or prolonged exercise may result in damage to the sarcoplasmic reticulum resulting in reduced calcium release during depolarization of the muscle. Although this is an attractive hypothesis, more research is required to confirm or deny this postulate. Because free radicals may contribute to fatigue some investigators have proposed that the use of antioxidant vitamins (e.g., vitamin C and E) may decrease the rate of free-radical mediated fatigue during exercise. This issue is discussed in chapter 25.

in summary

- Increases in CNS arousal facilitate motor unit recruitment to increase strength and alter the state of fatigue.
- The ability of the muscle membrane to conduct an action potential may be related to fatigue in activities demanding a high frequency of stimulation.
- Repeated stimulation of the sarcolemma can result in a reduction in the size and frequency of action potentials, however, shifts in the optimal frequency needed for muscle activation preserves force output.
- Under certain conditions an action potential block can occur in the t-tubule to result in reduction in Ca^{++} release from the SR.

Mechanical Factors

The primary mechanical factor that may be related to fatigue is cross-bridge "cycling." The action of the cross-bridge depends on (a) the functional arrangement of actin and myosin, (b) Ca^{++} being available to bind with troponin to allow the cross-bridge to bind with the active site on actin, and (c) ATP, which is needed for both the activation of the cross-bridge to cause movement, and the dissociation of the cross-bridge from actin. Exercise, especially eccentric exercise, can cause a physical disruption of the sarcomere, and reduce the capacity of the muscle to produce tension (2). A high H^+ concentration, due to a high rate of lactate formation, may contribute to fatigue in a variety of ways (8a, 9, 15, 16):

- reduce the force per cross bridge,
- reduce the force generated at a given Ca^{++} concentration (related to H^+ ion interference with Ca^{++} binding to troponin), and
- inhibit SR Ca^{++} release.

One sign of fatigue in isometric contractions is a longer "relaxation time"—the time from peak tension development to baseline tension. This longer relaxation time could be due to a slower cycling of the cross-bridge due to Ca^{++} not being pumped back to the sarcoplasmic reticulum fast enough, and/or inadequate ATP, which is needed for dissociation of the cross-bridge as well as for Ca^{++} pumping (13, 15, 16). It is this last factor, the availability of ATP, that has received the greatest attention.

in summary

- The cross-bridge's ability to "cycle" is important in continued tension development. Fatigue may be related to the effect of a high H^+ concentration on the ability of troponin to bind to Ca^{++}, the inability of the sarcoplasmic reticulum to take up Ca^{++}, or the lack of ATP needed to dissociate the cross-bridge from actin.

Energetics of Contraction

Fatigue can be viewed as the result of a simple imbalance between the ATP requirements of a muscle, and its ATP-generating capacity (16). As described in chapter 3, when exercise begins and the need for ATP accelerates, a series of ATP-generating reactions occur to replenish the ATP. As the cross-bridges use ATP and generate ADP, phosphocreatine provides for the immediate resynthesis of the ATP (PC + ADP $\rightarrow$ ATP + C). As the phosphocreatine becomes depleted, ADP begins to accumulate and the myokinase reaction occurs to generate ATP (ADP + ADP $\rightarrow$ ATP + AMP). The accumulation of all these products stimulates glycolysis to generate additional ATP, which may result in a H^+ accumulation (6). However, as ATP demand continues to exceed supply, a variety of reactions occur in the cell that limit work and protect the cell from damage. Remember that ATP is needed to pump ions and maintain cell structure. In this sense, fatigue serves a protective function. What are the signals to the muscle cell that energy utilization must slow down? When ATP generating mechanisms cannot keep up with ATP use, inorganic phosphate (P_i) begins to accumulate in the cell (P_i and ADP are not being converted to ATP). An increase in P_i in the muscle has been shown to inhibit maximal force, and the higher the P_i concentration, the lower the force measured during recovery from fatigue. The P_i seems to act directly on the cross-bridges to reduce its binding to actin (8a). What is interesting is that the cell does not run out of ATP, even in cases of extreme fatigue. Typically, the ATP concentration falls to approximately 70% of its pre-exercise level. The factors that cause fatigue reduce the rate of ATP utilization faster than ATP generation so that ATP concentration is maintained. This is believed to be a protective function aimed at minimizing changes in cellular homeostasis with continued stimulation.

in summary

- Fatigue is directly associated with a mismatch between the rate at which the muscle uses ATP and the rate at which ATP can be supplied.
- Cellular fatigue mechanisms slow down the rate of ATP utilization faster than the rate of ATP generation to preserve the ATP concentration and cellular homeostasis.

In chapter 8 we linked the different methods of ATP production to the different muscle fiber types that are recruited during activity. We will briefly summarize this information as it relates to our discussion of fatigue. Figure 19.3 shows the pattern of recruitment of muscle fiber types with increasing intensities of exercise. Up to about 40% of $\dot{V}O_2$ max, the Type I slow-twitch oxidative muscle fiber is recruited to provide tension development (17). This fiber type is dependent on a continuous supply of blood to provide the oxygen needed for the generation of ATP from carbohydrates and fats. Any factor limiting the oxygen supply to this fiber type (e.g., altitude, dehydration, blood loss, or anemia) would cause a reduction in tension development in these fibers and necessitate the recruitment of Type IIa fibers to generate tension.

Type IIa fast-twitch, fatigue-resistant muscle fibers are recruited between 40%–75% $\dot{V}O_2$ max (17). These fast-twitch fibers are rich in mitochondria, as are the Type I fibers, making them dependent on oxygen delivery for tension development. They also have a great capacity to produce ATP via anaerobic glycolysis. The mitochondrial content of Type IIa fibers is sensitive to endurance training, so that with detraining more of the ATP supply would be provided by glycolysis, leading to

Figure 19.3
Order of muscle fiber type recruitment in exercise of increasing intensity.

From Kent B. Pandolf, "Influence of Exercise and Training in Motor Unit Activation" in Kent B. Pandolf, Ed., *Exercise and Sport Sciences Reviews*, Vol. 15. Copyright © 1987 McGraw-Hill, Inc., New York. Reprinted by permission.

lactate production (see chapter 13). If oxygen delivery to this fiber type is decreased, or the ability of the fiber to use oxygen is decreased (due to low mitochondrial number), tension development will fall, requiring Type IIb fiber recruitment to maintain tension.

Type IIb is the fast-twitch muscle fiber with a low mitochondrial content. This fiber can generate great tension via anaerobic sources of energy, but fatigues quickly. It is recruited at about 75% $\dot{V}O_2$ max, making heavy exercise dependent upon its ability to develop tension (17).

in summary

- Muscle fibers are recruited in the following order with increasing intensities of exercise: Type I → Type IIa → Type IIb.
- The progression moves from the most to the least oxidative muscle fiber type. Intense exercise (>75% $\dot{V}O_2$ max) demands that Type IIb fibers be recruited, resulting in an increase in lactate production.

Factors Limiting All–Out Anaerobic Performances

As the intensity of exercise increases, the recruitment of muscle fibers progresses from Type I → Type IIa → Type IIb. This means that the ATP supply needed for tension development becomes more and more dependent upon anaerobic metabolism (17). In this way, fatigue is specific to the type of task undertaken. If a task

Figure 19.4
Factors affecting fatigue in ultra short-term events.

requires only Type I fiber recruitment, then the factors limiting performance will be very different from those associated with tasks requiring Type IIb fibers. With this review and summary in mind, let's now examine the factors limiting performance.

Ultra Short–Term Performances (Less than Ten Seconds)

The events that fit into this category include the shot put, high jump, long jump, and 50–100-meter sprints. These events require that tremendous amounts of energy be produced in a short period of time (high-power events), and Type II muscle fibers must be recruited. Figure 19.4 shows that maximal performance is limited by the fiber type distribution (Type I versus Type II) and by the number of muscle fibers recruited, which is influenced by the level of motivation (11). Optimal performance is also affected by skill and technique, which are dependent on practice. It should be no surprise that the anaerobic sources of ATP—the ATP-PC system and glycolysis—provide the energy. Chapter 20 provides tests for anaerobic power and chapter 21 provides a detailed list of the activities dependent upon such power. There is evidence that ingestion of creatine can influence performance in high-power exercise; see chapter 25 for details.

in summary

- In events lasting less than ten seconds, optimal performance is dependent on the recruitment of appropriate Type II fibers to generate the great forces that are needed.
- Motivation or arousal is required, as well as the skill needed to direct the force.
- The primary energy sources are anaerobic, with the focus on phosphocreatine.

Figure 19.5
Factors affecting fatigue in short-term events.

Short–Term Performances (10 to 180 Seconds)

Maximal performances in the ten to sixty second range are still predominantly (>70%) anaerobic, using the high force, fast-twitch fiber, but when a maximal performance is extended to three minutes, about 60% of the energy comes from the slower aerobic, ATP-generating processes. As a result of this transition from anaerobic to aerobic energy production, maximal running speed decreases as the length of the race increases. Given that the ATP-PC system can supply ATP for only several seconds, the vast majority of the ATP will be derived from anaerobic glycolysis (see chapter 3). Figure 19.5 shows that this will cause an accumulation of H$^+$ in muscle as well as blood. The elevated H$^+$ concentration may actually interfere with the continued production of ATP via glycolysis, or the contractile machinery itself, by interfering with troponin's ability to bind with Ca^{++}. However, it must be added that following exhausting exercise muscle tension recovers *before* the H+ concentration does, indicating the complex nature of the fatigue process (9, 15, 16, 18). In an effort to slow H+ accumulation, some athletes have attempted to ingest buffers prior to a race. This procedure is discussed in detail in chapter 25, which deals with ergogenic aids and performance.

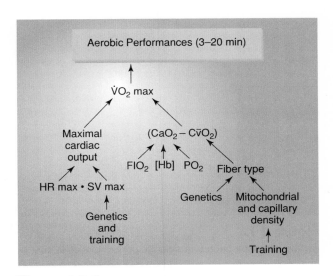

Figure 19.6
Factors affecting fatigue in aerobic performances lasting three to twenty minutes.

in summary

- In short-term performances lasting 10–180 seconds, there is a shift from 70% of the energy supplied anaerobically at ten seconds to 60% being supplied aerobically at 180 seconds.
- Anaerobic glycolysis provides a substantial portion of the energy, resulting in elevated lactate levels.

Factors Limiting All-Out Aerobic Performances

As the duration of an all-out performance increases, more demand is placed on the aerobic sources of energy. In addition, environmental factors such as heat and humidity, and dietary factors such as water and carbohydrate ingestion play a role in fatigue.

Moderate-Length Performances (Three to Twenty Minutes)

While 60% of ATP production is derived from aerobic processes in a three-minute maximal effort, the value jumps to 90% in a twenty-minute all-out performance. Given this dependence on oxidative energy production, the factors limiting performance include both the cardiovascular system, which delivers oxygen-rich blood to the muscles, and the mitochondrial content of the muscles involved in the activity. Since speed is a prerequisite in races lasting less than twenty minutes, Type IIa fibers, which are rich in mitochondria, are involved in supplying the ATP aerobically. Races lasting less than twenty minutes are run at 90%–100% of maximal aerobic power, so the athlete with the highest $\dot{V}O_2$ max has a distinct advantage. However, due to the fact that Type IIb fibers are also recruited, high levels of blood lactic acid are also experienced, and H+ accumulation would affect tension development as previously described (9, 15, 16, 18). Figure 19.6 summarizes the factors affecting performances requiring a high maximal oxygen uptake. The maximal

stroke volume is the crucial key to a high cardiac output (see chapter 13), and is influenced by both genetics and training. The arterial oxygen content (CaO_2) is influenced by the arterial hemoglobin content [Hb], the fraction of inspired oxygen (FIO_2), and PO_2 of the inspired air. Chapter 24 discusses the effect of altitude (low PO_2) on $\dot{V}O_2$ max, and chapter 25 discusses the use of blood doping (to raise the [Hb]) and oxygen breathing on aerobic performance. Training programs are discussed in chapter 21.

in summary

- In moderate-length performances lasting three to twenty minutes, aerobic metabolism provides 60%–90% of the ATP, respectively.
- These activities require an energy expenditure near $\dot{V}O_2$ max, with Type II fibers being recruited.
- Any factor interfering with oxygen delivery (e.g., altitude or anemia) would decrease performance since it is so dependent on aerobic energy production. High levels of lactate accompany these types of activities.

Intermediate-Length Performances (Twenty-One to Sixty Minutes)

In all-out performances lasting twenty-one to sixty minutes, the athlete will generally work at <90% $\dot{V}O_2$ max. A high $\dot{V}O_2$ max is certainly a prerequisite for success, but now other factors come into play. For example, an

Figure 19.7
Factors affecting fatigue in aerobic performances lasting twenty-one to sixty minutes.

individual who is an "economical" runner can move at a slightly higher speed for the same amount of oxygen compared to a runner who is not economical. Differences in running economy are due to biomechanical and/or bioenergetic factors. In this case measurements of both $\dot{V}O_2$ max and running economy would be needed to predict performance (see chapter 20). However, there is another variable that must be considered. Since races of this duration are not run at $\dot{V}O_2$ max, a person who can run at a high percentage of $\dot{V}O_2$ max would have an advantage. The ability to run at a high percentage of $\dot{V}O_2$ max is related to the concentration of lactate in the blood, and one of the best predictors of race pace is the lactate threshold. Interestingly, a high percentage of Type I muscle fibers is associated with both a greater lactate threshold and a higher mechanical efficiency (7a). The procedures to follow in estimating the maximal running speed for long distance races are presented in chapter 20. Factors limiting performance in runs of twenty-one to sixty minutes are summarized in figure 19.7. Please note that we must now consider the environmental factors of heat and humidity, as well as the state of hydration of the runner. The heat load will require that a portion of the cardiac output be directed to the skin, pushing the cardiovascular system closer to maximum at any running speed. See chapters 23 and 24 for information on how to deal with dehydration and environmental heat loads.

in summary
- Intermediate-length activities lasting twenty-one to sixty minutes are usually conducted at less than 90% $\dot{V}O_2$ max, and are predominantly aerobic.
- Given the length of the activity, environmental factors such as heat, humidity, and the state of hydration of the subject play a role in the outcome.

Long-Term Performances (One to Four Hours)

Performances of one to four hours are clearly aerobic performances involving little anaerobic energy production. Using the shorter aerobic performances (<sixty minutes) as a lead in, the longer the performance the greater the chance that environmental factors will play a role in the outcome. In addition, for performances greater than one hour the ability of the muscle and liver carbohydrate stores to supply glucose may be exceeded. As pointed out in chapter 4, fatty acids provide more fuel for oxidative metabolism the longer the race. However, it is clear that muscle fibers must have carbohydrate available, or muscle tension and performance will decline. Chapter 23 provides information about the optimal dietary strategies for performance in long-term events, including the consumption of fluids and carbohydrates during the run. Figure 19.8 summarizes the factors limiting performance in long-distance events.

in summary
- In long-term performances of one to four hours duration, environmental factors play a more important role as the muscle and liver glycogen stores try to keep up with the rate at which carbohydrate is used.
- Diet, fluid ingestion, and the ability of the athlete to deal with heat and humidity all influence the final outcome.

In conclusion, the factors limiting performance are specific to the type of performance. Short-term explosive performances are dependent on Type IIb fibers that can generate great power through anaerobic processes. In contrast, longer duration aerobic events

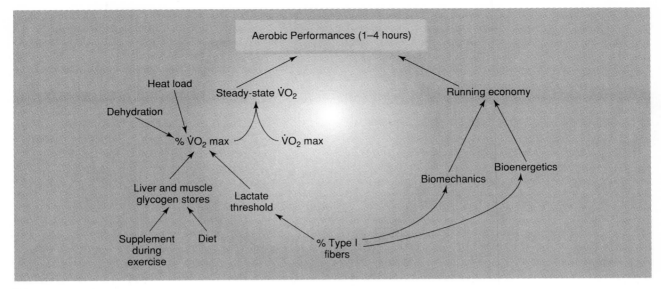

Figure 19.8
Factors affecting fatigue in aerobic performances lasting one to four hours.

require a cardiovascular system that can deliver oxygen at a high rate to muscle fibers with many mitochondria. It is clear that the testing and training of athletes must focus on the factors limiting performance for the specific event. For example, dietary carbohydrate and fluid ingestion are more crucial for the long distance runner than the high jumper. The following chapters will explore how to appropriately test, train, and feed athletes for optimal performance.

Athlete as Machine

One question we might keep in mind as we explore the details of how to improve performance is whether we might exceed what are regarded as reasonable and ethical boundaries for scientists, and treat the elite athlete as a machine rather than as a person. Are elite athletes being treated like racing cars in which engineers and mechanics (scientists and coaches) try to spot weaknesses that compromise performance, and then recommend solutions? Some may say yes, and indicate the worthiness of such an enterprise. Others may suggest that this has the potential to be dehumanizing if the athlete is reduced to no more than a

collection of working parts that are evaluated by a variety of specialists. Much would appear to depend on the goal of the research. If we are trying to understand how we function, and we develop healthy and safe methods that allow us to overcome personal limitations, we would appear to be on the right track. In contrast, if we *use* an athlete as a tool, that would be a different story. We are all familiar with the use of athletes by some countries to advance a particular political doctrine, and the complicity of scientists who were recruited to make athletes run faster and longer, and jump higher. Fortunately, universities, hospitals, and research centers have Institutional Review Boards (IRBs) to approve research proposals so that the rights of the subject are protected. This process also forces the investigator to provide a strong rationale showing that the risk to the subject (however small) is worth the benefits that might occur. Consistent with this, research journals require authors to follow IRB guidelines if they wish their work to be considered for publication. In this way we can move forward in our understanding of the physiological mechanisms underlying fatigue, while protecting the rights of the subject.

study questions

1. List the factors influencing performance.
2. Is the limiting factor for strength development located in the CNS or out in the periphery? Support your position.
3. Tracing the path the action potential takes from the time it leaves the motor end plate, where might the "weak link" be in the mechanisms coupling excitation to contraction?
4. When fatigue occurs there is still ATP present in the cell. What is the explanation for this?
5. Describe the pattern of recruitment of muscle fiber types during activities of progressively greater intensity, and explain them.
6. As the duration of a maximal effort increases from less than ten seconds to 10–180 seconds, what factor becomes limiting in terms of energy production?

7. Draw a diagram of the factors limiting maximal running performances of 1,500 m to 5 km.

8. While a high $\dot{V}O_2$ max is essential to world class performance, what role does running economy play in a winning performance?

9. Given that lactate accumulation will adversely affect endurance performance, what test might be an indicator of maximal sustained running (swimming, cycling) speed?

10. What is the role of environmental factors, such as altitude and heat, in very long-distance performances of one to four hours duration?

suggested readings

Jones, N. L., N. McCarney, and A. J. McComas, eds. 1986. *Human Muscle Power*. Champaign, IL: Human Kinetics.

Komi, P. V., ed. 1992. *Strength and Power in Sport*. London: Blackwell Scientific Publishers.

Porter, Ruth, ed. 1981. *Human Muscle Fatigue: Physiological Mechanisms*. London: Pitman Medical.

Simonson, E. 1971. *Physiology of Work Capacity and Fatigue*. Springfield, IL: Charles C. Thomas.

references

1. Allen, D. G., H. Westerblad, J. A. Lee, and J. Lannergren. 1992. Role of excitation-contraction coupling in muscle fatigue. *Sports Medicine* 13:116–26.

2. Appell, H. J., J. M. C. Soares, and J. A. R. Duarte. 1992. Exercise, muscle damage, and fatigue. *Sports Medicine* 13:108–15.

3. ———. 1978. A central nervous component in local muscle fatigue. *European Journal of Applied Physiology* 38:9–15.

4. Asmussen, E., and B. Mazin. 1978. Recuperation after muscular fatigue by "diverting activities." *European Journal of Applied Physiology* 38:1–7.

5. Åstrand, P. O., and K. Rodahl. 1977. *Textbook of Work Physiology*. 2d ed. New York: McGraw-Hill.

6. Banister, E. W., and B. J. C. Cameron. 1990. Exercise-induced hyperammonemia: Peripheral and central effects. *International Journal of Sports Medicine* 11:S129–S142.

6a. Barclay, J., and M. Hansel. 1991. Free radicals may contribute to skeletal muscle fatigue. *Canadian Journal of Physiology and Pharmacology* 69:279–84.

7. Bigland-Ritchie, B. 1981. EMG and fatigue of human voluntary and stimulated contractions. In *Human Muscle Fatigue: Physiological Mechanisms*, 130–56. London: Pitman Medical.

7a. Coyle, E. F. 1995. Integration of the physiological factors determining endurance performance. In *Exercise and Sport Sciences Reviews*, vol. 23, ed. J. O. Holloszy, 25–63. Baltimore: Williams & Wilkins.

8. Edwards, R. H. T. 1981. Human muscle function and fatigue. In *Human Muscle Fatigue: Physiological Mechanisms*, 1–18. London: Pitman Medical.

8a. Fitts, R. H. 1994. Cellular mechanisms of muscle fatigue. *Physiological Reviews* 74:49–94.

9. Fuchs, F., V. Reddy, and F. N. Briggs. 1970. The interaction of cations with the calcium-binding site of troponin. *Biochem. Biophys. Acta.* 221:407–9.

10. Gibson, H., and R. H. T. Edwards. 1985. Muscular exercise and fatigue. *Sports Medicine* 2:120–32.

11. Ikai, M., and A. H. Steinhaus. 1961. Some factors modifying the expression of human strength. *Journal of Applied Physiology* 16:157–63.

12. Ikai, M., and K. Yabe. 1969. Training effect of muscular endurance by means of voluntary and electrical stimulation. *European Journal of Applied Physiology* 28:55–60.

13. Jones, D. A. 1981. Muscle fatigue due to changes beyond the neuromuscular junction. In *Human Muscle Fatigue: Physiological Mechanisms*, 178–96. London: Pitman Medical.

14. Merton, P. A. 1954. Voluntary strength and fatigue. *Journal of Physiology* 123:553–64.

14a. Reid, M., K. Haack, K. Franchek, P. Valberg, L. Kobzik, and M. West. 1992. Reactive oxygen in skeletal muscle. I. Intracellular oxidant kinetics and fatigue in vitro. *Journal of Applied Physiology* 73:1797–1804.

15. Roberts, D., and D. J. Smith. 1989. Biochemical aspects of peripheral muscle fatigue—a review. *Sports Medicine* 7:125–38.

16. Sahlin, K. 1992. Metabolic factors in fatigue. *Sports Medicine* 13:99–107.

17. Sale, D. G. 1987. Influence of exercise and training on motor unit activation. In *Exercise and Sport Sciences Reviews*, vol. 15, ed. K. B. Pandolf, 95–151. New York: Macmillan.

18. Trevidi, B., and W. H. Danforth. 1966. Effect of pH on the kinetics of frog muscle phosphofructokinase. *Journal of Biological Chemistry* 241:4110–12.

19. Westerblad, H. et al. 1991. Cellular mechanisms of fatigue in skeletal muscle. *American Journal of Physiology* 261:C195–C209.

Work Tests to Evaluate Performance

objectives

By studying this chapter, you should be able to do the following:

1. Discuss the rationale for the determination of $\dot{V}O_2$ max in the evaluation of exercise performance in athletes competing in endurance events.
2. Explain the concept of "specificity of $\dot{V}O_2$ max."
3. State the rationale for the assessment of the lactate threshold in the endurance athlete.
4. Discuss the purpose and technique(s) involved in the measurement of exercise economy.
5. Provide an overview of how laboratory tests performed on the endurance athlete might be interpreted as an aid in predicting performance.
6. Describe several tests that are useful in assessing anaerobic power.
7. Discuss the techniques used to evaluate strength.

outline

Laboratory Assessment of Physical Performance 372

  Physiological Testing: Theory and Ethics 372

What the Athlete Gains by Physiological Testing 372

What Physiological Testing Will Not Do 373

Components of Effective Physiological Testing 373

Direct Testing of Maximal Aerobic Power 374

  Specificity of Testing 374

  Exercise Test Protocol 374

  Determination of Peak $\dot{V}O_2$ in Paraplegic Athletes 375

Laboratory Tests to Predict Endurance Performance 375

  Use of the Lactate Threshold to Evaluate Performance 375

  Measurement of Critical Power 377

Tests to Determine Exercise Economy 378

Estimating Success in Distance Running Using the Lactate Threshold and Running Economy 379

Determination of Anaerobic Power 380

  Tests of Ultra Short-Term Maximal Anaerobic Power 380

Tests of Short-Term Anaerobic Power 382

Evaluation of Muscular Strength 383

  Criteria for Selection of a Strength-Testing Method 384

  Isometric Measurement of Strength 384

  Isotonic Measurement of Strength 385

  Isokinetic Assessment of Strength 386

  Variable Resistance Measurement of Strength 386

critical power
dynamometer
isokinetic

Margaria power test
muscular strength
power tests

Quebec 10-second test
Sargent's jump-and-reach test
Wingate test

n general, there have been two principal approaches to the assessment of physical performance: (1) field tests of general physical fitness, which include a variety of measurements requiring basic performance demands and (2) laboratory assessments of physiological capacities such as maximal aerobic power ($\dot{V}O_2$ max), anaerobic power, and exercise economy (1, 33). It can be argued that physical fitness testing is important for an overall assessment of general conditioning, particularly in terms of evaluating student progress in a physical education conditioning class (1, 43). However, use of these test batteries does not provide the detailed physiological information needed to assess an athlete's current level of conditioning or potential weaknesses. Therefore, more specific laboratory tests are required to provide detailed physiological information relative to performance in specific athletic events. It is the purpose of this chapter to discuss laboratory tests designed to measure physical work capacity. Specifically, much of the chapter will center around laboratory tests to evaluate the maximum energy transfer capacities discussed in chapters 3 and 4.

Laboratory Assessment of Physical Performance

Physiological Testing: Theory and Ethics

Designing laboratory tests to assess physical performance requires an understanding of those factors that contribute to success in a particular sport or athletic event. In general, physical performance is determined by the individual's capacity for maximal energy output (i.e., maximal, aerobic, and anaerobic processes), muscular strength, coordination/economy of movement, and psychological factors (e.g., motivation and tactics) (1, 2, 23). Figure 20.1 illustrates a simple model of the components that interact to determine the quality of physical performance. Many types of athletic events require a combination of several of the above factors for an outstanding performance to occur. However, often one or more of these factors plays a dominating role in determining athletic success. In golf, there is little need for a high-energy output, but proper coordination is

Figure 20.1

Factors that contribute to physical performance. See text for details.

essential. Sprinting 100 meters requires not only good technique, but a high anaerobic power output as well. In distance running, cycling, or swimming, a high capacity for aerobic energy-yielding processes is essential for success. Again, laboratory evaluation of performance requires an understanding of those factors that are important for optimal performance in a particular athletic event. Thus, a test that stresses the same physiological systems required by a particular sport or athletic event would appear to be a valid means of assessing physical performance.

A key concern in the performance of "athletic" laboratory testing is maintaining respect for the athlete's human rights. In short, laboratory testing should be performed on athletes who are volunteers and have given written consent prior to testing. Prior to testing, the exercise scientist has the responsibility of informing the athlete about the purpose of the tests and the potential risks or discomfort associated with laboratory testing.

What the Athlete Gains by Physiological Testing

Laboratory measurement of physical performance can be expensive and time consuming. An obvious

Measurement of Peak Running Velocity to Predict Performance in Distance Running

The lactate threshold and critical power measurements have generally been used to predict performance in endurance events lasting longer than 20 minutes (e.g., 10 kilometer run). In an effort to develop a laboratory or field test to predict performance in endurance events less than 20 minutes (e.g., 5 kilometer run), researchers have developed a test called "peak running velocity" (26, 42a, 42b, 56a). The test is easy to administer and can be performed on a treadmill or track. For example, measurement of peak running velocity on a treadmill involves a short test of progressively increasing the treadmill speed every 30 seconds (0% grade) until volitional fatigue. Peak running velocity (meters · second^{-1}) is defined as the highest speed that can be maintained for >5 second duration (56a).

How well does peak running velocity predict performance? In a

Figure 20.5
Relationship between running peak velocity and finish time of a 5 kilometer (km) race. Data from reference 56a.

recent study, researchers demonstrated that peak running velocity was an excellent predictor of success in a 5 kilometer run (56a). This point is illustrated by the strong correlation between peak running velocity and 5 kilometer race time (see figure 20.5.). Surprisingly, similar findings have been reported for longer running events (e.g., 10–90 kilometer) as well (29a, 42b). Although additional research is required to fully investigate the application of this test to athletic performance, peak running velocity appears to be a promising laboratory or field test to predict endurance performance.

Figure 20.6
Concept of critical power.

of the lactate threshold, the usual procedure is to allow two independent researchers to visually inspect the graph and subjectively determine the point where there is a sudden increase in ventilation (figure 20.4). The point where ventilation increases rapidly is considered the ventilatory threshold and is used as an estimate of

the lactate threshold. Although some authors have criticized this technique for a lack of precision (51), it seems clear that this procedure is useful in predicting success in endurance events (50).

Measurement of Critical Power

Measurement of the maximal steady state power output is useful in predicting success in endurance events lasting 3–180 minutes in duration. Another laboratory measurement that can be used to predict performance in endurance events is **critical power.** The concept of critical power is based upon the notion that athletes can maintain a specific submaximal power output without fatigue (24a, 26, 29a). Figure 20.6 illustrates the critical power concept for running performance. In this illustration, running speed is plotted on the "y" axis and the time that the athlete can run at this speed prior to exhaustion is plotted on the "x" axis. Critical power is defined as the running speed (i.e., power output) at which the running speed/time curve reaches a plateau. Therefore, in theory, the critical power is considered the power output that can be maintained indefinitely. In practice, however, this is not the case. In fact, most athletes fatigue within 30–60 minutes when exercising at their critical power (24a).

Critical power can be determined in the laboratory by having subjects perform a series of five to seven timed exercise trials to exhaustion. This is generally accomplished over several days of testing. The results are graphed and critical power is determined by subjective assessment of the point where the power/time curve begins to plateau or by using a mathematical technique (see references 24a and 29a for details). Although figure 20.5 illustrates the critical power measurement for running, the same principle of measurement can be applied to other endurance sports (e.g., cycling, rowing, etc.) (24a, 25a).

How well does critical power predict performance? Several studies have shown that critical power is significantly correlated with performance in endurance events lasting 3–100 minutes (e.g., r = 0.67 – 0.85) (24a, 25a, 26, 29a). Therefore, critical power is a useful laboratory predictor of success in endurance sports.

Is critical power a better predictor of success in endurance events than other laboratory measures such as the lactate threshold or $\dot{V}O_2$ max? The answer remains controversial since many investigators report that $\dot{V}O_2$ max is the best single predictor of endurance performance success (12, 13, 21). However, in events lasting approximately 30 minutes, the lactate threshold, $\dot{V}O_2$ max, and critical power appear to be similar in their abilities to predict performance (29a). This is not surprising considering that critical power is dependent upon both $\dot{V}O_2$ max and the lactate threshold. Indeed, critical power is highly correlated to both $\dot{V}O_2$ max and the lactate threshold (29a, 40a). In other words, a subject with a high $\dot{V}O_2$ max and lactate threshold will also possess a high critical power.

in summary

- Common laboratory tests to predict endurance performance include measurement of the lactate threshold, critical power, and peak running velocity. All of these measurements have been proven useful in predicting performance in endurance events.
- The lactate threshold can be determined during an incremental exercise test using any one of several exercise modalities (e.g., treadmill, cycle ergometer, etc.). The lactate threshold represents an exercise intensity at which blood lactic acid levels begin to systematically increase.
- Critical power is defined as the running speed (i.e., power output) at which the running speed/time curve reaches a plateau.
- Peak running velocity (meters · second^{-1}) can be determined on a treadmill or track and is defined as the highest speed that can be maintained for >5 second duration.

Figure 20.7

An oxygen cost-of-running curve for two subjects. Note the higher $\dot{V}O_2$ cost of running at any given running speed for subject A when compared to subject B. See text for details.

Tests to Determine Exercise Economy

The topic of exercise economy was first introduced in chapter 6. The economy of a particular sport movement (e.g., running or cycling) has a major influence on the energy cost of the sport and consequently interacts with $\dot{V}O_2$ max in determining endurance performance (11, 16, 33, 40). For example, a runner who is uneconomical will expend a greater amount of energy to run at a given speed than an economical runner. With all other variables being equal, the more economical runner would likely defeat the less economical runner in head-to-head competition. Therefore, the measurement of exercise economy would seem appropriate when performing a battery of laboratory tests to evaluate an athlete's performance potential.

How is exercise economy evaluated? Conceptually, exercise economy is assessed by graphing energy expenditure during a particular activity (e.g., running, cycling, etc.) at several speeds. In general, the energy costs of running, cycling, or swimming can be determined using similar methods. Let's use running as an example to illustrate this procedure. The economy of running is quantified by measuring the steady-state oxygen cost of running on a horizontal treadmill at several speeds. The oxygen requirement of running is then graphed as a function of running speed (6, 25). Figure 20.7 illustrates the change in $\dot{V}O_2$ in two runners at a variety of running speeds. Notice that at any given speed, runner B requires less oxygen and therefore expends less energy than runner A (i.e., runner B is more economical than runner A). A marked difference in running economy between athletes can have an important impact on performance.

Estimating Success in Distance Running Using the Lactate Threshold and Running Economy

Over the past fifteen to twenty years, numerous investigators have attempted to apply laboratory tests to predict performance in a variety of sports (see reference 46 for examples). The sport that has received the most attention is distance running. Theoretically, prediction of potential performance in any endurance sport involves use of similar laboratory measurements ($\dot{V}O_2$ max, economy of movement, etc.). We will use distance running as an example of how a sport scientist or coach might use laboratory measurements to estimate an athlete's performance in a particular event. Let's begin our discussion with a brief overview of the physiological factors that contribute to distance running success. As previously mentioned, the best test for determining an endurance runner's potential is $\dot{V}O_2$ max. However, other factors modify the pace that can be maintained for races of different lengths. For example, anaerobic energy contributes significantly to the ability to maintain a specified pace during shorter distance runs (e.g., 1,500 meters) (8, 33). In longer runs (5,000 to 10,000 meters), running economy and the lactate threshold may play important roles in determining success (19, 50, 63). In order to predict endurance performance, we must determine the athlete's maximal race pace that can be maintained for a particular racing distance.

To illustrate how performance in distance running might be estimated, consider an example of predicting performance in a 10,000-meter race. We begin with an assessment of the athlete's running economy and then perform an incremental treadmill test to determine $\dot{V}O_2$ max and the lactate threshold. The test results for our runner are graphed in figure 20.8. How do we determine the maximal race pace from the laboratory data? Numerous studies have shown that a close relationship exists between the lactate or ventilatory threshold and the maximal pace that can be maintained during a 10,000-meter race (19, 50, 63). For instance, it appears that well-trained runners can run 10,000 meters at a pace that exceeds their lactate threshold by approximately 5 m · min^{-1} (25, 47). With this information and the data from figure 20.8, we can now predict a finish time for an athlete. First, we examine figure B to determine the $\dot{V}O_2$ at the lactate threshold. The lactate threshold occurred at a $\dot{V}O_2$ of 40 ml · kg^{-1} · min^{-1}, which corresponds to a running speed of 200 m · min^{-1} (part A of figure 20.8). Assuming that the athlete can exceed this speed by 5 m · min^{-1}, the projected average race pace for a 10,000-meter run would be 205 m · min^{-1}.

(a)

(b)

Figure 20.8
Incremental exercise test results for a hypothetical runner. These test results can be used to predict performance in an endurance race. See text for details.

Therefore, an estimate of the athlete's finish time could be obtained by dividing 10,000 meters by his predicted running speed (m · min^{-1}):

$$\text{Estimated finish time} = 10,000 \text{ m} \div 205 \text{ m} \cdot \text{min}^{-1}$$
$$= 48.78 \text{ min}$$

Although theoretical predictions of performance such as the example above can generally estimate performance with a reasonable degree of precision, a number of outside factors can influence racing performance. For example, motivation and race tactics play an important role in distance running success. Environmental conditions (heat/humidity, altitude, etc.) also influence an athlete's ultimate performance (see chapters 19 and 24).

in summary
- Prediction of success in an endurance event can be made by a laboratory assessment of the athlete's movement economy, $\dot{V}O_2$ max, and lactate threshold. These parameters can be used to determine the athlete's maximal race pace that can be maintained for a given racing distance and therefore performance can be predicted.

Figure 20.9
The percent contribution of the ATP-PC system, anaerobic glycolysis, and aerobic metabolism as a function of time during a maximal effort.

Determination of Anaerobic Power

For the assessment of anaerobic power, it is essential that the test employed use the muscle groups involved in the sport (i.e., specificity) and involve the energy pathways used in the performance of the event. Although several classification schemes have been proposed (3, 23a), tests to assess maximal anaerobic power can be generally classified into (1) ultra short-term tests designed to test the maximal capacity of the "ATP-PC system," and (2) short-term tests to evaluate the maximal capacity for anaerobic glycolysis (sometimes referred to as anaerobic endurance). Remember that events lasting less than ten seconds are considered to principally use the ATP-PC system to produce ATP, while events lasting thirty to sixty seconds utilize anaerobic glycolysis as the major bioenergetic pathway to synthesize ATP. This principle is illustrated in figure 20.9 and should be remembered when designing tests to evaluate an athlete's anaerobic power for a specific sport.

Tests of Ultra Short-Term Maximal Anaerobic Power

Several practical "field tests" have been developed to assess the maximal capacity of the ATP-PC system to produce ATP over a very short time period (e.g., one to ten seconds) (36). These tests are generally referred to as **power tests.** Recall from chapter 6 that power is defined as:

Power = (F × D) ÷ T

where F is the force generated, D is the distance over which the force is applied, and T is the time required to perform the work.

Margaria Power Test

One of the most commonly used power tests is the **Margaria power test** (36). This popular test requires the subject to run up a flight of steps as quickly as possible, and is conducted in the following manner. After several practice opportunities, the subject bounds up nine steps, taking three steps at a time. A timing "switch" mat starts a clock at step three and a second "switch" mat stops the clock at step nine which ends the test (see figure 20.10). The power output is calculated by multiplying the subject's body weight (i.e., the force) times the vertical distance traveled (usually 1–2 meters), and dividing by the time required to perform the test. Consider an example of an athlete (75 kg) who runs up six steps (vertical displacement = 2 meters) in 0.65 seconds. The power output is calculated as:

F = 75 kg
D = 2 m
T = 0.65 sec
power = (75 kg × 2 m) ÷ 0.65 sec
= 230.8 kgm · sec^{-1}

The Margaria power test has been shown to predict success in a 40-yard dash with a fair degree of accuracy (38). However, the absolute score or power output of the Margaria test needs to be interpreted with some caution. For example, if two athletes who differ in body weight perform a Margaria test in the same time, the heavier athlete will have a higher power output. This means that the larger athlete can generate a higher power output than the smaller athlete. However, in a weight-bearing activity like running the 100-meter dash, a higher Margaria score does not necessarily mean that the heavier athlete will complete the race in a faster time than the lighter athlete, because the heavier athlete must carry more body weight.

Jumping Power Tests

For many years, tests such as the standing long jump or **Sargent's jump-and-reach test** have been used as field tests to evaluate an individual's explosive anaerobic power. The standing long jump is the distance covered in a horizontal leap from a crouched position, while the Sargent's jump-and-reach test is the difference between the standing reach height and the maximum jump-and-touch height. Both tests probably fail to adequately assess an individual's maximal ATP-PC system capacity because of the brief duration of each test. Neither test is considered a good predictor of success in running a short dash (28).

Running Power Tests

The 40-yard dash has been a popular test to evaluate power output in football players for many years. The athlete generally performs two to three timed 40-yard dashes with full recovery between efforts. The fastest

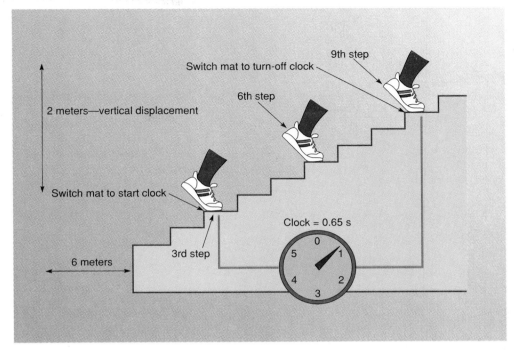

Figure 20.10

Illustration of the performance cf a Margaria power test. The subject begins with a running start and leaps three steps at a time up a stairs. The time required to leap up a total of six steps is recorded and the power output computed. See text for details.

Figure 20.11

Illustration of the use of a series of timed 40-yard dashes to determine the anaerobic fitness of football players. In this illustration, athlete A shows a small but constant decline in running speed with each additional dash. In contrast, athlete B shows a large systematic decline in speed across dash trials. Therefore, athlete A is considered to be in better condition than athlete B. See text for details.

time recorded is considered an indication of the individual's power output. Although a 40-yard dash is a rather specific test of power output for football players, there is little evidence that a 40-yard run in a straight line is a reliable predictor of an athlete's success at a particular position. Perhaps a shorter run (e.g., 10–20 yards), with several changes in direction, might provide a more specific test of power output in football players (38).

Recently, Stuart and colleagues (61) have proposed a fitness test for football players that is designed to evaluate the athlete's ability to perform repeated short bursts of power. The test is conducted in the following way. After a brief warm-up, the athlete performs a series of ten timed 40-yard dashes (maximum effort), with a twenty-five second recovery between dashes. The twenty-five second recovery period is designed to simulate the elapsed time between plays in a football game. The athletes' time for each 40-yard dash is graphed as a function of the trial number. This procedure is illustrated in figure 20.11 where line A represents data from a well-conditioned athlete and line B is data from a less fit athlete. Notice that both lines A and B have negative slopes (fatigue slope). This demonstrates that each of the two athletes is slowing down with each sequential 40-yard trial. Athletes who are highly conditioned will be able to maintain faster 40-yard dash times over the ten trials when compared to less conditioned athletes, and therefore will have a less negative fatigue slope. In an effort to establish a set of standards for this test, Stuart and coworkers have proposed that athletes be classified into one of four classifications on the basis of the maximal running velocity percentage that can be maintained over the final three 40-yard dash trials (see table 20.1). At

Table 20.1 Classification of Fitness Levels for Football Players on the Basis of a Series of 40-Yard Dash Times

Level	Category	Percentage of Maximal Velocity Maintained*
1	Superior	>90%
2	Good	85%–89%
3	Sub-par	80%–84%
4	Poor	<79%

*The "percentage of the maximal velocity maintained" is calculated by averaging the velocity of the last three trials and dividing by the average velocity over the first three trials. This ratio is then expressed as a percentage. See text for further details.

Table 20.2 The Resistance Setting for the Wingate Test Is Based on the Subject's Body Weight

Subject's Body Weight (kg)	Resistance Setting on the Flywheel (kg)
20–24.9	1.75
25–29.9	2.0
30–34.9	2.5
35–39.9	3.0
40–44.9	3.25
45–49.9	3.5
50–54.9	4.0
55–59.9	4.25
60–64.9	4.75
65–69.9	5.0
70–74.9	5.5
75–79.9	5.75
80–84.9	6.25
> 85	6.5

From B. Noble, *Physiology of Exercise and Sport*. Copyright © 1986. The C. V. Mosby Company, St. Louis MO. Reprinted by permission.

present, levels 1 and 2 are considered acceptable levels of fitness for football players of any position, while levels 3 and 4 are labeled as sub-par and poor fitness standards, respectively.

Cycling Power Tests

The **Quebec 10-second test** was developed in 1983 to assess ultra short-term anaerobic power in cyclists (59). The technical error of this test is small and the procedure is highly reliable (3). The test is performed on a friction-braked cycle ergometer that contains a photocell capable of measuring flywheel revolutions; the number of flywheel revolutions and resistance against the flywheel is electrically relayed to a microcomputer for analysis. The design of the test is simple. After a brief warm-up, the subject performs two all-out 10-second cycling trials separated by a rest period. The initial resistance on the cycle flywheel is determined by the subject's weight (about 0.09 kg per kg of body weight). Upon a verbal start command by the investigator, the subject begins pedaling at 80 rpm's and the load is rapidly adjusted within two to three seconds to the desired load. The subject then pedals as fast as possible for 10 seconds. Strong verbal encouragement is provided throughout the test. After a ten-minute rest period, a second test is performed and the results of the two tests averaged. The test results are reported in peak joules per kg of body weight and total joules per kg of body weight.

In addition to the evaluation of cyclists, the Quebec 10-second test has been used to test ultra short-term anaerobic power in nonathletes, runners, speed skaters, biathletes, and body builders. For complete details of these results see Bouchard et al. (3).

Tests of Short–Term Anaerobic Power

As illustrated in figure 20.9, the ATP-PC system for production of ATP during intense exercise is important for short bursts of exercise (one to ten seconds), whereas glycolysis becomes an important metabolic pathway for energy production in events lasting longer than fifteen seconds. In an effort to evaluate the maximal capacity for anaerobic glycolysis to produce ATP during exercise, several short-term anaerobic power tests have been developed. Like other performance tests, anaerobic power tests should involve the specific muscles used in a particular sport.

Cycling Anaerobic Power Tests

Researchers at the Wingate Institute in Israel have developed a thirty-second, maximal effort cycling test **(Wingate test)** designed to determine both peak anaerobic power and mean power output over the thirty-second test. This test has been shown to be highly reproducible (27) and offers an excellent means of evaluating anaerobic power output in cyclists. The test is administered in the following manner. The subject performs a short, two- to four-minute warm-up on the cycle ergometer at an exercise intensity sufficient to elevate heart rate to 150–160 beats $\cdot$ min^{-1}. After a three- to five-minute rest interval, the test begins with the subject pedaling the cycle ergometer as fast as possible without resistance on the flywheel. After the subject reaches full pedaling speed (e.g., two to three seconds), the test administrator quickly increases the flywheel resistance to a predetermined load. This predetermined load is an estimate (based on body weight) of a work load that would exceed the subject's $\dot{V}O_2$ max by 20%–60% (see table 20.2). The subject continues to pedal as rapidly as possible, and the pedal rate is recorded every five seconds during the test. The highest power output over the first few seconds is considered the peak power output and is indicative of the maximum rate of the ATP-PC system to produce ATP during this type of exercise. The decline in power output during the test is used as an index of anaerobic endurance and presumably represents the maximal capacity to produce ATP via a combination of the ATP-PC system and glycolysis. The decrease in power output is expressed as the percentage of peak power decline. The peak power output obtained during a Wingate test occurs near the beginning of the test, and the lowest power output is recorded during the last five seconds of the test. The difference in these two power outputs (i.e., highest power output minus lowest power output) is then divided by the peak power output and expressed as a percentage. For instance, if the peak power output was 600 watts and the lowest power output during the test was 200 watts, then the decline in power output would be computed as:

$$(600 - 200) \div 600 = .666 \times 100\% = 67\%$$

The 67% decline in power output means that the athlete decreases his or her peak power output by 67% over the thirty-second exercise period.

Since the introduction of the Wingate test in the early 1970s, a number of modifications to the original protocol have been proposed (17, 22, 27, 45, 54). Recently, an Australian team of sport scientists (22) have developed a new test for measurement of anaerobic power on a cycle ergometer that involves 60 seconds of maximal exercise and uses a variable resistance loading. The test design permits the measurement of both peak anaerobic power (i.e., peak ATP-PC system power) as well as mean (glycolytic) power output over the 60-second maximal exercise bout. The test is designed as follows. The subject performs a five-minute warm-up at a low work rate (e.g., 120 watts). After a two-minute recovery, the subject begins pedaling as fast as possible with no load against the cycle flywheel. When peak pedaling speed is obtained (i.e., three seconds), the investigator quickly increases the load on the flywheel to 0.095 kg resistance per kg of body weight. The subject continues to pedal as fast as possible at this load for 30 seconds; at the 30-second point, the load on the flywheel is reduced to 0.075 kg resistance per kg of body weight for the remainder of the test. The subject's power output during the test is continuously monitored electronically and work output is recorded as peak power output (joules per kg) and mean power output (joules per kg) during the entire test.

The rationale for the variable load is that while a high resistance is required to elicit maximal anaerobic power, such a resistance is too great for a supramaximal test of 60-second duration (22). By reducing the resistance midway through the test, the workload becomes more manageable, which enables the subject to complete a maximal effort test for the entire 60-second period. The advantage of this test over the Wingate test is that the variable resistance design permits the measurement of peak anaerobic power and

maximal anaerobic power over 60-second duration. This type of test would be useful for athletes who compete in events lasting between forty-five to sixty seconds. Note that while this test maximally taxes both the ATP-PC system and glycolysis, because of the test duration the aerobic system is also activated (see chapters 3 and 4). Therefore, while the energy required to perform 60 seconds of maximal exercise comes primarily (e.g., 70%) from anaerobic pathways, the aerobic energy contribution may reach 30%.

Running Anaerobic Power Tests

Maximal distance runs from 200 to 800 meters have been used to evaluate anaerobic power output in runners (55, 64). Because such factors as running technique and motivation influence the performance of these types of power tests, the development of appropriate norms has been difficult. Nevertheless, this type of test can be used effectively to determine improvement within individuals as a result of a training regimen.

Sport-Specific Tests

Ultra short-term and short-term sport specific anaerobic tests can be developed to meet the needs of team sports or individual athletic events. The tests could attempt to measure the peak power output in a few seconds or measure mean power output during a period of ten to sixty seconds depending upon the energy demands of the sport.

Tests could be developed for tennis, basketball, ice skating, swimming, and so on. In some cases, time or distance covered would be the dependent variable measured rather than a direct measurement of power output (3). This type of sport-specific test provides the coach and athlete with direct feedback relative to the athlete's present level of fitness; subsequent periodic testing can be used to evaluate the success of training programs.

in summary

- Anaerobic power tests are classified as:
  (a) ultra short-term tests to determine the maximal capacity of the ATP-PC system and (b) short-term tests to evaluate the maximal capacity for anaerobic glycolysis.
- Ultra short-term and short-term power tests should be sport-specific in an effort to provide the athlete and coach with feedback relative to the athlete's current fitness level.

Evaluation of Muscular Strength

Muscular strength is defined as the maximum force that can be generated by a muscle or muscle group (1). Measurement of muscular strength is a common practice in the evaluation of training programs for football players, shot putters, weight lifters, and other power athletes. Strength testing can be used to monitor training progress or monitor the rehabilitation of injuries (37). Muscular strength can be assessed by using one of four methods: (1) isometric testing, (2) isotonic testing, (3) isokinetic testing, and (4) variable resistance testing. Before we discuss these methods of strength measurement, let's consider some general guidelines for the selection of a strength testing method.

Criteria for Selection of a Strength-Testing Method

The criteria for selecting a method of strength testing includes the following factors (52): specificity, ease of data acquisition and analysis, cost, and safety. Given the importance of proper strength-test selection, a brief discussion of each of these factors is warranted.

Specificity of strength testing considers the muscles involved in the sport movement, the movement pattern and contraction type, and the velocity of the contraction. For example, the measurement of sport-specific strength should use the muscle groups involved in the activity. Further, the testing mode should simulate the type of contraction used in the sport (isometric vs. dynamic). If the contraction used in the sport is dynamic, further consideration should be given to whether the contraction is concentric or eccentric. A final level of specificity is the velocity of shortening. There is a degree of velocity specificity in strength training; speed and power athletes perform better on high velocity power tests compared to low (67). Therefore, there is a justification for attempting to make the velocity of test contractions similar to those used in the sport.

Factors such as convenience and time required for strength measurements are important considerations when measurements are made on a large number of athletes (29b). Presently, a number of companies market strength measurement devices that are interfaced with computer analysis packages. These devices greatly reduce the time required for strength measurement and analysis.

Much of the commerically available computerized equipment for strength measurement is expensive. The high cost of this equipment may prevent its purchase by physical therapy, exercise science, or athletic programs with small budgets. In these cases, the physical therapist, exercise scientist, or coach must choose the best available option within his/her budget.

A final concern for the selection of a strength testing method is the safety of the technique. Safety should be a key concern for any measurement of strength. Clearly, strength measurement techniques that put the athlete at high risk of injury should be avoided.

Figure 20.12
Use of the cable tensiometer to measure static force during a knee extension.

Isometric Measurement of Strength

Measurement of isometric strength requires a specifically constructed device that permits testing of the sport-specific muscle groups. These devices can be designed by the sports scientist or purchased commercially. The cable tensiometer is a tension-measuring device, and was one of the first techniques used to measure isometric force in a variety of muscle groups. Figure 20.12 illustrates the use of the cable tensiometer to measure leg strength during a knee extension. As the subject applies force over the cable, the cable tightens and the tensiometer pointer is deflected to indicate the amount of force applied during the movement.

The fact that the tensiometer is lightweight and portable makes it an attractive device for making strength measurements in the field. The cable tensiometer has been used in physical therapy to evaluate training progress to injured limbs. It has been argued that since the cable tensiometer can be applied to measure static strength at many different joint angles, this technique might be more effective in evaluating strength gains during therapeutic training than conventional weight-lifting tests (38).

Measurement of isometric strength is typically performed at several joint angles. Isometric testing at each joint angle usually consists of two or three trials of maximal contractions (contraction durations of approximately five seconds); the best of these trials is considered to be the measure of strength.

Advantages of isometric testing using computerized equipment include the fact that these tests are generally simple and safe to administer. Disadvantages include the high cost of some commercial devices and the fact that many sport activities involve dynamic movements. Further, because of strength differences over the full range of joint movement, isometric measurements must be made at numerous joint angles; this increases the amount of time required to perform a test.

Isotonic Measurement of Strength

The term *isotonic* means constant tension. This term is often applied to conventional weight-lifting exercise because the weight of the barbell or dumbbell remains constant as the weight is lifted over the range of movement. In a strict sense, application of the term *isotonic* to weightlifting can be criticized because the actual force or torque applied to the weight does not remain constant over the full range of movement. Acceleration and deceleration of the limbs during a weight-lifting movement often causes variation in the force applied. Nonetheless, because of the widespread usage in the literature, we will apply the term *isotonic* to conventional weight-lifting exercises. The most common measure of isotonic strength is the one-repetition maximum, but tests involving three to six repetitions have been employed.

The one-repetition maximum (1-RM) method of evaluating muscular strength involves the performance of a single, maximal lift. This refers to the maximal amount of weight that can be lifted during one complete dynamic repetition of a particular movement (e.g., bench press). To test the 1-RM for any given muscle group, the subject selects a beginning weight that is close to the anticipated 1-RM weight. If one repetition is completed, the weight is increased by a small increment and the trial repeated. This process is continued until the maximum lifting capacity is obtained. The highest weight moved during one repetition is considered the 1-RM. The 1-RM test can be performed using free weights (barbells) or an adjustable resistance exercise machine.

Because of safety concerns, some physical therapists and exercise scientists have recommended that an isotonic test consisting of three or six repetitions be substituted for the 1-RM test. The rationale is that the

Figure 20.13
Use of the typical hand-grip and back-lift dynamometer.

incidence of injury may be less with a weight that can be lifted a maximum of three or six times compared to the heavier weight that can be lifted during a 1-RM contraction.

In addition to the use of free weights or machines, maximal isotonic strength can be measured using dynamometers. A **dynamometer** is a device capable of measuring force. Hand-grip and back-lift dynamometers have been used to evaluate grip strength and back strength, respectively, for many years. Dynamometers operate in the following way. When force is applied to the dynamometer, a steel spring is compressed and moves a pointer along a scale. By calibrating the dynamometer with known weights, one can determine how much force is required to move the pointer a specified distance on the scale. Figure 20.13 illustrates the use of a hand-grip and back-lift dynamometer to assess grip and back strength.

The advantages of isotonic strength testing include low cost of equipment and the fact that force is dynamically applied, which may simulate sport specific movements. The disadvantage of isotonic testing using a 1-RM technique is the possibility of subject injury and it does not provide information concerning the force application over the full range of motion. This point will be discussed again in the next section.

Figure 20.14
Use of a commercially available computer-assisted isokinetic dynamometer to measure strength during a knee extension.

Photo courtesy of CYBEX, Inc.

Figure 20.15
Example of a "computer printout" from a computer-assisted isokinetic dynamometer during a maximal effort knee extension.

Isokinetic Assessment of Strength

Over the past several years, many commercial computer-assisted devices to assess dynamic muscular force have been developed. The most common type of computerized strength measurement device on the market is an isokinetic dynamometer, which provides variable resistance. The term **isokinetic** means moving at a constant rate of speed. A variable resistance isokinetic dynamometer is an electronic-mechanical instrument that maintains a constant speed of movement while varying the resistance during a particular movement. The resistance offered by the instrument is an accommodating resistance, which is designed to match the force generated by the muscle. A force transducer inside the instrument constantly monitors the muscular force generated at a constant speed and relays this information to a computer, which calculates the average force generated over each time period and joint angle during the movement. An example of this type of instrument is pictured in figure 20.14.

A typical computer printout of data obtained during a maximum effort leg extension on a computerized isokinetic dynamometer is illustrated in figure 20.15. This type of strength assessment provides a great deal more information than that supplied by a 1-RM test. The force curve pictured in figure 20.15 illustrates that the subject generates the smallest amount of force early in the movement pattern and the greatest amount of force during the middle portion of the movement. The 1-RM test provides only the final outcome, which is the maximum amount of weight lifted during this particular movement. That is, a 1-RM test does not provide information concerning the differences in force generation over the full range of movement. Therefore, a computer-assisted isokinetic instrument appears to offer advantages over the more traditional 1-RM test.

Variable Resistance Measurement of Strength

Several commercial companies market weight machines that vary the resistance (weight) during dynamic muscular contractions. The measurement of strength using a variable resistance device is similar in principle to isotonic tests using 1-RM or three to six repetitions with the exception that the variable resistance machine creates a variable resistance over the range of movement. This variable resistance is typically achieved via a "cam," which in theory is designed to vary the resistance according to physiological and mechanical factors that determine force generation by muscles over the normal range of movement.

Advantages of these devices is that most sport movement patterns are performed using variable forces and the design of these machines make adjustment of weight easy and therefore little time is required for measurement. A disadvantage of these machines is the high cost; this is compounded by the fact that several individual machines are often required to measure strength in different muscle groups.

in summary

- Muscular strength is defined as the maximum force that can be generated by a muscle or muscle group.
- Evaluation of muscular strength is useful in assessing training programs for athletes involved in power sports or events.
- Muscular strength can be evaluated using any one of the following techniques: (a) isometric, (b) isotonic, (c) isokinetic, or (d) variable resistance devices.

study questions

1. Discuss the rationale behind laboratory tests designed to assess physical performance in athletes. How do these tests differ from general physical fitness tests?

2. Define maximal oxygen uptake. Why might relative $\dot{V}O_2$ max be the single most important factor in predicting distance running success in a heterogeneous group of runners?

3. Discuss the concept of "specificity of testing" for the determination of $\dot{V}O_2$ max. Give a brief overview of the design of an incremental test to determine $\dot{V}O_2$ max. What criteria can be used to determine the validity of a $\dot{V}O_2$ max test?

4. Briefly, explain the technique employed to determine the lactate threshold and the ventilatory threshold.

5. Describe how the economy of running might be evaluated in the laboratory.

6. Discuss the theory and procedures involved in predicting success in distance running.

7. Explain how short-term maximal anaerobic power can be evaluated by field tests.

8. Describe how the Wingate test is used to assess medium-term anaerobic power.

9. Provide an overview of the 1-RM technique to evaluate muscular strength. Why might a computer-assisted dynamometer be superior to the 1-RM technique in assessing strength changes?

10. Discuss the advantages and disadvantages of each of the following types of strength measurement: (1) isometric, (2) isotonic, (3) isokinetic, and (4) variable resistance.

suggested readings

Green, S. 1995. Measurement of anaerobic work capacities in humans. *Sports Medicine* 19:32–42.

Hill, D. 1993. The critical power concept. A review. *Sports Medicine* 16:237–54.

MacDougall, J., H. Wenger, and H. Green. 1991. *Physiological Testing of the High Performance Athlete*. Champaign, IL: Human Kinetics.

Maud, P., and C. Foster (Eds.) 1995. *Physiological Assessment of Human Fitness*. Champaign, IL: Human Kinetics.

references

1. Åstrand, P. O., and K. Rodahl. 1986. *Textbook of Work Physiology*. New York: McGraw-Hill.

2. Beaver, W., K. Wasserman, and B. Whipp. 1986. A new method for detecting anaerobic threshold by gas exchange. *Journal of Applied Physiology* 60:2020–27.

3. Bouchard, C. et al. 1991. Testing anaerobic power and capacity. In *Physiological Testing of the High Performance Athlete*, eds. J. MacDougall, H. Wenger, and H. Green, 175–222. Champaign, IL: Human Kinetics.

4. Bouckaert, J., and J. Pannier. 1984. Specificity of $\dot{V}O_2$ max and blood lactate determinations in runners and cyclists. *International Archives of Physiology and Biochemistry* 93:30–31.

5. Bouckaert, J., J. Pannier, and J. Vrijens. 1983. Cardiorespiratory response to bicycle and rowing ergometer exercise in oarsmen. *European Journal of Applied Physiology* 51:51–59.

6. Bransford, D., and E. Howley. 1977. Oxygen cost of running in trained and untrained men and women. *Medicine and Science in Sports and Exercise* 9:41–44.

7. Buchfuhrer, M. et al. 1983. Optimizing the exercise protocol for cardiopulmonary assessment. *Journal of Applied Physiology* 55:1558–64.

8. Bulbulian, R., A. Wilcox, and B. Darabos. 1986. Anaerobic contribution to distance running performance of trained cross-country athletes. *Medicine and Science in Sports and Exercise* 18:107–13.

9. Burke, E. 1976. Validity of selected laboratory and field tests of physical working capacity. *Research Quarterly* 47:95–104.

10. Caiozzo, V. et al. 1982. A comparison of gas exchange indices used to detect the anaerobic threshold. *Journal of Applied Physiology* 53:1184–89.

11. Conley, D., and G. Krahenbuhl. 1980. Running economy and distance running performance of highly trained athletes. *Medicine and Science in Sports and Exercise* 12:357–60.

12. Costill, D. 1967. The relationship between selected physiological variables and distance running performance. *Journal of Sports Medicine and Physical Fitness* 7:61–66.

13. Costill, D. 1970. Metabolic responses to distance running. *Journal of Applied Physiology* 28:251–55.

14. Costill, D. 1979. *A Scientific Approach to Distance Running*. Los Altos: Track and Field News Press.

15. Costill, D., H. Thompson, and E. Roberts. 1973. Fractional utilization of the aerobic capacity during distance running. *Medicine and Science in Sports* 5:248–52.

16. Daniels, J., and N. Daniels. 1992. Running economy of elite male and elite female distance runners. *Medicine and Science in Sports and Exercise* 24:483–89.

17. Dotan R., and O. Bar-Or. 1983. Load optimization for the Wingate anaerobic test. *European Journal of Applied Physiology* 51:409–17.

18. Ebbeling, C. et al. 1991. Development of a single-stage submaximal treadmill walking test. *Medicine and Science in Sports and Exercise* 23:966–73.

19. Farrell, P. et al. 1979. Plasma lactate accumulation and distance running performance. *Medicine and Science in Sports* 11:338–44.

20. Foster, C. 1983. $\dot{V}O_2$ max and training indices as determinants of competitive running performance. *Journal of Sports Sciences* 1:13–27.

21. Foster, C., J. Daniels, and R. Yarbough. 1977. Physiological correlates of marathon running and performance. *Australian Journal of Sports Medicine* 9:58–61.

21a. Foster, C. et al. 1995. Blood lactate and respiratory measurement of the capacity for sustained exercise. In *Physiological Assessment of Human Fitness*, eds. P. Maud and C. Foster, 57–72. Champaign, IL: Human Kinetics.

22. Gastin, P. et al. 1991. Variable resistance loadings in anerobic power testing. *International Journal of Sports Medicine* 12:513–18.

23. Green, H. 1991. What do tests measure? In *Physiological Testing of the High Performance Athlete*, eds. J. MacDougall, H. Wenger, and H. Green. Champaign, IL: Human Kinetics.

23a. Green, S. 1995. Measurement of anaerobic work capacities in humans. *Sports Medicine* 19:32–42.

24. Hagan, R., M. Smith, and L. Gettman. 1981. Marathon performance in relation to maximal aerobic power and training indices. *Medicine and Science in Sports and Exercise* 13:185–89.

24a. Hill, D. 1993. The critical power concept. A review. *Sports Medicine* 16:237–54.

25. Hopkins, P., and S. Powers. 1982. Oxygen uptake during submaximal running in highly trained men and women. *American Corrective Therapy Journal* 36:130–32.

25a. Housh, D. et al. 1989. The accuracy of the critical power test for predicting time to exhaustion during cycle ergometry. *Ergonomics* 32:997–1004.

26. Hughson, R., C. Orok, and L. Staudt. 1984. A high-velocity treadmill running test to assess endurance running potential. *International Journal of Sports Medicine* 5:23–25.

27. Jacobs, I. 1980. The effects of thermal dehydration on performance of the Wingate anaerobic test. *International Journal of Sports Medicine* 1:21–24.

28. Katch, V. et al. 1977. Optimal test characteristics for maximal anaerobic work on the cycle ergometer. *Research Quarterly* 48:319–27.

29. Kenney, W., and J. Hodgson. 1985. Variables predictive of performance in elite middle-distance runners. *British Journal of Sports Medicine* 19:207–9.

29a. Kolbe, T. et al. 1995. The relationship between critical power and running performance. *Journal of Sports Sciences* 13:265–69.

29b. Kraemer, W., and A. Fry. 1995. In *Physiological Assessment of Human Fitness*, eds. P. Maud and C. Foster, 115–38. Champaign, IL: Human Kinetics.

30. LaFontaine, T., B. Londeree, and W. Spath. 1981. The maximal steady state versus selected running events. *Medicine and Science in Sports and Exercise* 13:190–92.

31. Lawler, J., S. Powers, and S. Dodd. 1987. A time saving incremental cycle ergometer protocol to determine peak oxygen consumption. *British Journal of Sports Medicine* 21:171–73.

32. Lehmann, M. et al. 1983. Correlations between laboratory testing and distance running performance in marathoners of similar ability. *International Journal of Sports Medicine* 4:226–30.

33. Londeree, B. 1986. The use of laboratory test results with long distance runners. *Sports Medicine* 3:201–13.

34. MacDougall, J., and H. Wenger. 1991. The purpose of physiological testing. In *Physiological Testing of the High Performance Athlete*, eds. J. MacDougall, H. Wenger, and H. Green. Champaign, IL: Human Kinetics.

35. Magel, J., and J. Faulker. 1967. Maximum oxygen uptake of college swimmers. *Journal of Applied Physiology* 22:929.

36. Margaria, R. 1966. Measurement of muscular power in man. *Journal of Applied Physiology* 21:1662.

37. Mayhew, T., and J. Rothstein. 1985. Measurement of muscle performance with instruments. In *Measurement of Muscle Performance with Instruments*, ed. J. Rothstein, 57–102. New York: Churchill Livingstone.

38. McArdle, W., F. Katch, and V. Katch. 1991. *Exercise Physiology: Energy, Nutrition, and Human Performance.* Philadelphia: Lea & Febiger.

39. McMiken, D., and J. Daniels. 1976. Aerobic requirements of maximal aerobic power in treadmill and track running. *Medicine and Science in Sports and Exercise* 8:14–17.

40. Morgan, D., and M. Craib. 1992. Physiological aspects of running economy. *Medicine and Science in Sports and Exercise* 24:456–61.

40a. Moritani, T. et al. 1981. Critical power as a measure of physical work capacity and anaerobic threshold. *Ergonomics* 24:339–50.

41. Murase, Y. et al. 1981. Longitudinal study of aerobic power in superior junior athletes. *Medicine and Science in Sports and Exercise* 13:180–84.

42. Mygind, E. et al. 1991. Evaluation of a specific test in cross-country skiing. *Journal of Sports Sciences* 9:249–57.

42a. Noakes, T. 1988. Implications of exercise testing for prediction of athletic performance: A contemporary perspective. *Medicine and Science in Sports and Exercise* 20:319–30.

42b. Noakes, T. et al. 1990. Peak treadmill running velocity during the max test predicts running performance. *Journal of Sports Sciences* 8:35–45.

43. Noble, B. 1986. *Physiology of Exercise and Sport.* St. Louis: C. V. Mosby.

44. Pannier, J., J. Vrijens, and C. Van Cauter. 1980. Cardiorespiratory response to treadmill and bicycle exercise in runners. *European Journal of Applied Physiology* 43:243–51.

45. Parry-Billings, M. et al. 1986. The measurement of anaerobic power and capacity: Studies on the Wingate anaerobic test. *Snipes* J9:48–58.

46. Peronnet, F., and G. Thibault. 1989. Mathematical analysis of running performance and world running records. *Journal of Applied Physiology* 67:453–65.

47. Pollock, M. 1977. Submaximal and maximal working capacity of elite distance runners: Cardiorespiratory aspects. *Annuals of the New York Academy of Sciences* 301:310–22.

48. Pollock, M., A. Jackson, and R. Pate. 1980. Discriminant analysis of physiological differences between good and elite runners. *Research Quarterly* 51:521–32.

49. Pollock, M. et al. 1976. A comparative analysis of four protocols for maximal treadmill stress testing. *American Heart Journal* 92:39–46.

50. Powers, S. et al. 1983. Ventilatory threshold, running economy, and distance running performance of trained athletes. *Research Quarterly for Exercise and Sport* 54:179–82.

51. Powers, S., S. Dodd, and R. Garner. 1984. Precision of ventilatory and gas exchange alterations as a predictor of the anaerobic threshold. *European Journal of Applied Physiology* 52:173–77.

52. Sale, D. 1991. Testing strength and power. In *Physiological Testing of the High Performance Athlete*, eds. J. MacDougall, H. Wenger, and H. Green, 21–106. Champaign, IL: Human Kinetics.

53. Sawka, M. et al. 1983. Determination of maximal aerobic power during upper body exercise. *Journal of Applied Physiology* 54:113–17.

54. Schenau, G. et al. 1991. Can cycle power output predict sprint running performance? *European Journal of Applied Physiology* 63:255–60.

55. Schnabel, A., and W. Kinderman. 1983. Assessment of anaerobic capacity in runners. *European Journal of Applied Physiology* 52:42–46.

56. Schwade, J., G. Blomquist, and W. Shapiro. 1977. A comparsion of the response to arm and leg work in patients with ischemic heart disease. *American Heart Journal* 94:203–8.

56a. Scott, B., and J. Houmard. 1994. Peak running velocity is highly related to distance running performance. *International Journal of Sports Medicine* 15:504–7.

57. Shaw, D. et al. 1974. Arm crank ergometer: A new method for the evaluation of coronary heart disease. *American Journal of Cardiology* 33:801–5.

58. Sherrill, D. et al. 1990. Using smoothing splines for detecting ventilatory thresholds. *Medicine and Science in Sports and Exercise* 22:684–89.

59. Simoneau, J. et al. 1983. Tests of anaerobic alactacid and lactacid capacities. *Canadian Journal of Applied Sports Sciences* 8:266–70.

60. Storer, T. et al. 1990. Accurate prediction of $\dot{V}O_2$ max in cycle ergometry. *Medicine and Science in Sports and Exercise* 22:704–12.

61. Stuart, M. K., S. Powers, and J. Nelson. Development of an anaerobic fitness test for football players. Unpublished observations.

62. Tanaka, K., and Y. Matsuura. 1984. Marathon performance, anaerobic threshold, and onset of blood lactate accumulation. *Journal of Applied Physiology* 57:640–43.

63. Tanaka, K. et al. 1983. Relationships of anaerobic threshold and onset of blood lactate accumulation with endurance performance. *European Journal of Applied Physiology* 52:51–56.

64. Taunton, J., H. Maron, and J. Wilkinson. 1981. Anaerobic performance in middle and long distance runners. *Canadian Journal of Applied Sports Sciences* 6:109–13.

65. Taylor, H., E. Buskirk, and A. Henschel. 1955. Maximal oxygen uptake as an objective measure of cardiorespiratory performance. *Journal of Applied Physiology* 8:73–80.

66. Thoden, J. 1991. Testing aerobic power. In *Physiological Testing of the High Performance Athlete*, eds. J. MacDougall, H. Wenger, and H. Green, 107–74. Champaign, IL: Human Kinetics.

67. Thorland, W. 1987. Strength and anaerobic response of elite young female sprint and distance runners. *Medicine and Science in Sports and Exercise* 19:56–61.

68. Walker, R., S. Powers, and M. Stuart. 1986. Peak oxygen uptake in arm ergometry: Effects of testing protocol. *British Journal of Sports Medicine* 20:25–26.

69. Wasserman, K. et al. 1973. Anaerobic threshold and respiratory gas exchange during exercise. *Journal of Applied Physiology* 35:236–43.

70. Weltman, A. et al. 1990. Reliability and validity of a continuous incremental treadmill protocol for the determination of lactate threshold, fixed blood lactate concentrations, and $\dot{V}O_2$ max. *International Journal of Sports Medicine* 11:26–32.

71. Williams, J., S. Powers, and S. Stuart. 1986. Hemoglobin desaturation in highly trained athletes during heavy exercise. *Medicine and Science in Sports and Exercise* 18:168–73.

72. Williams, L. 1978. Prediction of high-level rowing ability. *Journal of Sports Medicine and Physical Fitness* 18:11–15.

73. Wyndham, C. et al. 1969. Physiological requirements for world-class performances in distance running. *South African Medical Journal* 43:996–1002.

74. Zhang, Y. et al. 1991. Effect of exercise testing protocol on parameters of aerobic function. *Medicine and Science in Sports and Exercise* 23:625–30.

21

Training for Performance

objectives

By studying this chapter, you should be able to do the following:

1. Discuss the concept of designing a sport-specific training program based on an analysis of the energy systems utilized by the activity.
2. List and discuss the general principles of physical conditioning for improved sport performance.
3. Define the terms *overload*, *specificity*, and *reversibility*.
4. Outline the use of interval training and continuous training in the improvement of the maximal aerobic power in athletes.
5. Discuss the guidelines associated with planning a training program designed to improve the anaerobic power of athletes.
6. Outline the principles of training for the improvement of strength.
7. Discuss the role of gender differences in the development of strength.
8. List the factors that contribute to delayed onset muscle soreness.
9. Discuss the use of static and ballistic stretching to improve flexibility.
10. Outline the goals of: (1) off-season conditioning, (2) preseason conditioning, and (3) in-season conditioning.
11. List and discuss several common training errors.

outline

Training Principles   392
  Overload, Specificity, and Reversibility   392
  Influence of Gender, Initial Fitness Level, and Genetics   393
Components of a Training Session: Warm-Up, Workout, and Cool Down   394
Training to Improve Aerobic Power   394
  Interval Training   395
  Long, Slow Distance   396
  High-Intensity, Continuous Exercise   396
Injuries and Endurance Training   397

Training for Improved Anaerobic Power   397
  Training to Improve the ATP-PC System   397
  Training to Improve the Glycolytic System   398
Training to Improve Muscular Strength   398
  Progressive Resistance Exercise   398
  General Strength-Training Principles   398
  Free Weights versus Machines   399
  Combined Strength and Endurance Training Programs   399

Gender Differences in Response to Strength Training   400
Muscle Soreness   401
Training for Improved Flexibility   402
Year-Round Conditioning for Athletes   402
  Off-Season Conditioning   403
  Preseason Conditioning   403
  In-Season Conditioning   403
Common Training Mistakes   403

delayed onset muscle soreness
  (DOMS)
dynamic stretching
hyperplasia
hypertrophy

progressive resistance exercise (PRE)
proprioceptive neuromuscular
  facilitation (PNF)
repetition
rest interval

set
static stretching
tapering
variable resistance exercise
work interval

Traditionally, coaches and trainers have planned conditioning programs for their team by following regimens used by teams that have successful win-loss records. This type of reasoning is not sound, since win-loss records alone do not scientifically validate the specific conditioning program used by the successful team. In fact, the successful team might be victorious by virtue of having superior athletes and not as a result of an outstanding conditioning program. Without question the planning of an effective athletic conditioning program can best be achieved by the application of proven physiological training principles. Optimizing training programs for athletes is important, since failure to properly condition an athletic team results in a poor performance and often defeat. It is the purpose of this chapter to present an overview of how to apply scientific principles to the development of an athletic conditioning program.

Training Principles

The overall objective of a sport conditioning program is to improve performance by increasing the energy output during a particular movement (4, 53, 68). Recall that throughout this book (e.g., chapters 3, 4, and 20), emphasis has been placed on the fact that dissimilar sport activities utilize different metabolic pathways or "energy systems" to produce the ATP needed for movement. An understanding of exercise metabolism is important to the coach or trainer since the design of a conditioning program to optimize athletic performance requires knowledge of the principal energy systems utilized by the sport. Consider a few examples. The performance of a 60-meter dash uses the ATP-PC system almost exclusively to produce the needed ATP. In contrast, a marathon runner depends on aerobic metabolism to provide the needed energy to complete the race. However, most sport activities use multiple energy pathways. For instance, soccer uses a combination of metabolic pathways to provide the needed ATP. Knowledge of the relative anaerobic-aerobic contributions to ATP production during an activity is the cornerstone of planning a conditioning program. A well-designed conditioning program allocates the appropriate amount of aerobic and anaerobic conditioning time to match the energy demand of the sport. For instance, if an activity derives 40% of its ATP from anaerobic pathways and 60% from aerobic pathways (e.g., 1,500-meter run), the training program should be divided 40%/60% between anaerobic/aerobic training (4, 53). Table 21.1 contains a list of various sports and an estimation of their predominant energy systems. This information can be used by the coach or trainer to allocate the appropriate amount of time to training each energy system.

The above discussion does not necessarily imply that power athletes (e.g., sprinters) should not perform aerobic training. On the contrary, aerobic activity during the preseason to strengthen tendons and ligaments is generally recommended for all athletes. For a review of the effects of exercise training on the strength of tendons and ligaments, see reference 73.

Overload, Specificity, and Reversibility

The terms overload, specificity, and reversibility were introduced in chapters 13 and 15, and will be repeated here only briefly. Recall that an organ system (e.g., cardiovascular, skeletal muscle, etc.) increases its capacity in response to a training overload. That is, the training program must stress the system above the level to which it is accustomed. Conversely, when an athlete stops training, the training effect is quickly lost (reversibility). Studies have demonstrated that within two weeks after the cessation of training, significant reductions in $\dot{V}O_2$ max can occur (16, 17). A classic study of Saltin and colleagues (66) demonstrated that after twenty days of bed rest, a group of subjects showed a 25% reduction in $\dot{V}O_2$ max and maximal cardiac output. These rather dramatic decrements in working capacity as a result of inactivity clearly demonstrate the rapid reversibility of training.

The concept of specificity refers to not only the specific muscles involved in a particular movement, but to the energy systems that provide the ATP required to complete the movement under competitive conditions. Therefore, training programs need to deal with specificity by using not only those muscle groups engaged during competition, but also the energy systems that will be providing the ATP. For instance, "specific training" for a sprinter would involve running high-intensity dashes. Similarly, specific training for a

Table 21.1 The Predominant Energy Systems for Selected Sports

Sport/Activity	% ATP Contribution by Energy System		
	ATP–PC	Glycolysis	Aerobic
Baseball	80	15	5
Basketball	80	10	10
Field hockey	60	20	20
Football	90	10	—
Golf(swing)	100	—	—
Gymnastics	90	10	—
Ice hockey:			
Forwards/defense	80	20	—
Goalie	95	5	—
Rowing	20	30	50
Soccer:			
Goalie/wings/strikers	80	20	—
Halfbacks	60	20	20
Swimming:			
Diving	98	2	—
50 meters	95	5	—
100 meters	80	15	—
200 meters	30	65	5
400 meters	20	40	40
1,500 meters	10	20	70
Tennis	70	20	10
Track and field:			
100/200 meters	98	2	—
Field events	90	10	—
400 meters	40	55	5
800 meters	10	60	30
1,500 meters	5	35	60
5,000 meters	2	28	70
Marathon	—	2	98
Volleyball	90	10	—
Wrestling	45	55	—

From E. L. Fox and D. K. Mathews, *Interval Training: Conditioning for Sports and General Fitness.* Copyright © 1974 Saunders College Publishing, Orlando FL. Reprinted by permission of the author.

marathoner would involve long, slow-paced runs in which virtually all of the ATP needed by the working muscles would be derived from aerobic metabolism.

Influence of Gender, Initial Fitness Level, and Genetics

At one time, it was believed that conditioning programs for women had special requirements that differed from those used to train men. Today, however, much evidence exists to demonstrate that men and women respond to training programs in a similar fashion (8, 10, 46, 59, 60, 72). Therefore, the same general approach to physiological conditioning can be used in planning programs for men and women. This does not mean that men and women should perform identical exercise training sessions (e.g., same volume and intensity). Indeed, individual training programs, regardless of gender, should be designed appropriately to match the level of fitness and maturation of the athlete. Individual "exercise prescriptions" is an important concern in the design of training programs and will be discussed in further detail in the next several paragraphs.

It is a common observation that individuals differ greatly in the degree of improvement resulting from training programs. Many factors contribute to the observed individual variations in the training response. One of the most important influences is the athlete's beginning level of fitness. In general, the amount of training improvement is always greater in those individuals who are less conditioned at the beginning of the training program (67). It has been demonstrated that sedentary middle-aged men with heart disease may improve their $\dot{V}O_2$ max by as much as 50%, whereas the same training program in normal active adults improves $\dot{V}O_2$ max by only 10%–15% (44, 53). Similarly, conditioned athletes may improve their level of conditioning by only 3%–5% following an increase in training intensity. However, this 3%–5% improvement in the trained athlete may be the difference between winning an Olympic gold medal and failing to place in the event.

Additionally, it seems likely that genetics plays an important role in how an individual responds to a training program (4). For instance, an individual with a high genetic endowment for endurance sports is likely to respond differently to endurance training when compared to an individual with a markedly different genetic profile. It is for this reason, and the fact that athletes begin conditioning programs at different levels of fitness, that training programs should be individualized. It is unrealistic to expect each athlete on the team to perform the same amount of work or to exercise at the same work rate during training sessions.

Note that while training can greatly improve performance, there is no substitute for genetically inherited athletic talent if the individual is to compete at a world-class level. For example, there is a limit to how much training can improve aerobic power. Therefore, those individuals with a low genetic endowment for aerobic power cannot, under any training program, increase their $\dot{V}O_2$ max to world-class levels. Åstrand and Rodahl (4) have commented that if you want to become a world-class athlete you must choose your parents wisely.

in summary

- The general objective of sport conditioning is to improve performance by increasing the maximum energy output during a particular movement. A conditioning program should allocate the appropriate amount of training time to match the aerobic and anaerobic energy demands of the sport.
- Muscles respond to training as a result of a progressive overload. When an athlete stops training, there is a rapid decline in fitness due to detraining (reversibility).
- In general, men and women respond to conditioning in a similar fashion. The amount of training improvement is always greater in those individuals who are less conditioned at the onset of the training program.

Components of a Training Session: Warm-Up, Workout, and Cool Down

Every training session should consist of three components: (1) warm-up, (2) workout, and (3) cool down. This idea was first introduced in chapter 16 and will be

mentioned only briefly here. The warm-up prior to a training workout has several important objectives. First, warm-up exercises increase cardiac output and blood flow to the skeletal muscles to be used during the training session. Secondly, the warm-up activity results in an increase in muscle temperature, which elevates muscle enzyme activity (52). Finally, preliminary exercise affords the athlete an opportunity to perform stretching exercises. The duration of the warm-up may be from five to twenty minutes, depending on environmental conditions and the nature of the training activity (18, 81). Although limited data exist, it is commonly believed that a proper warm-up may reduce the possibility of muscle injury due to pulls or strains (7, 32, 61a, 63). Additional research is needed to definitively answer this question.

Immediately following the training session, a period of low intensity, "cool down" exercises should be performed. The principal objective of a cool down is to return "pooled" blood from the exercised skeletal muscles back to the central circulation. Similar to the warm-up, the length of the cool down may vary from ten to thirty minutes, depending on environmental conditions, the age and fitness level of the individual, and the nature of the training session.

in summary

- Every training session should consist of a warm-up period, workout session, and a cool down period.
- Although limited data exist, it is believed that a warm-up reduces the risk of muscle and/or tendon injury during exercise.

Training to Improve Aerobic Power

Recall from chapter 13 that endurance training improves $\dot{V}O_2$ max by increasing both maximal cardiac output and increasing the a-$\bar{v}$ O_2 difference (i.e., increasing the muscle's ability to extract O_2). Therefore, a training program designed to improve maximal aerobic power must overload the circulatory system and stress the oxidative capacities of skeletal muscles as well (4, 14, 18). As in all training regimens, specificity is critical. The athlete should stress the specific muscles to be used in his or her sport (78). In other words, runners should train by running, cyclists should train on the bicycle, swimmers should swim, and so forth.

There are three principal aerobic training methods used by athletes: (1) interval training, (2) long, slow distance (low-intensity), and (3) high-intensity, continuous exercise. Controversy exists as to which of these training methods results in the greatest improvement in $\dot{V}O_2$ max. Indeed, there does not appear to be a magic training formula for all athletes to

Table 21.2 Guidelines for Determining the Intensity or Work Rate During Interval Training for Running and Swimming Different Distances

Interval Training Distances (Yards) Running	Swimming	Work Rate for Each Interval
100	25	One to five seconds slower than best time
220	50	Three seconds slower than best time
440	100	One to four seconds faster than average 440-yard run or 100-yard swim times recorded during a mile run or 440-yard swim
880–1,320	165–320	Three to four seconds slower than the average 440-yard run or 100-yard swim times recorded during a mile run or 440-yard swim

From E. L. Fox and D. K. Mathews, *Interval Training: Conditioning for Sports and General Fitness*. Copyright © 1974 Saunders College Publishing, Orlando FL. Reprinted by permission of the author.

follow. However, there is evidence that it is training intensity and not duration that is the most important factor in improving $\dot{V}O_2$ max (9, 19, 24, 27, 35, 43, 61). Nonetheless, from a psychological standpoint, it would appear that a mixing of all three methods would provide the needed variety to prevent the athlete from becoming bored with a single and rather monotonous training program.

Note that improvement of $\dot{V}O_2$ max is only one variable related to endurance. Recall from chapter 20 that although a high $\dot{V}O_2$ max is important for success in endurance events, both movement economy and the lactate threshold are also important variables. Therefore, training to improve endurance performance should not only be geared toward the improvement of $\dot{V}O_2$ max, but should increase the lactate threshold and improve running economy. A brief discussion of various training methods used to improve endurance performance follows.

Interval Training

Interval training involves the performance of repeated exercise bouts, with brief recovery periods in between. The length and intensity of the work interval depends on what the athlete is trying to accomplish. For instance, a longer work interval requires a greater involvement of aerobic energy production, while a shorter, more intense interval provides greater participation of anaerobic metabolism. Therefore, interval training that is designed to improve $\dot{V}O_2$ max should generally utilize intervals > 60 sec to maximize the involvement of aerobic ATP production. Further, it is generally believed that high-intensity intervals are more effective in improving aerobic power, and perhaps the lactate threshold, than low-intensity intervals (28, 31, 48). These improvements may be due to the recruitment of fast-twitch (Types IIa and IIb) fibers during this type of high-intensity exercise.

One obvious advantage of interval training over continuous running is that this method of training provides a means of performing large amounts of high-intensity exercise in a short time. Further, this training method offers two ways of providing a training overload. For example, the interval training prescription can be modified to provide "overload" in terms of either increasing the total number of exercise intervals performed, or the intensity of the work interval. Adjustments to either of these factors allow the coach or athlete to alter the workout plan to accomplish specific training goals.

How does one design an interval workout? A complete discussion of the theory and rationale of designing an interval training program to improve athletic performance is beyond the scope of this chapter. For a detailed discussion of interval training, the reader is referred to Fox and Mathews (31). Additionally, table 21.2 provides some general guidelines for determining the intensity for running or swimming intervals.

In planning an interval training session, the following variables need to be considered: (1) length of the work interval, (2) intensity of the effort, (3) duration of the rest interval, (4) number of interval sets, and (5) the number of work repetitions. The length of the **work interval** refers to the distance to be covered during the work effort. In training to improve aerobic power, the work interval should generally last longer than sixty seconds. The intensity of the work effort during interval training can be monitored from a ten-second HR count upon completion of the interval (i.e., 10 sec HR count × 6 = HR per min). In general, exercise HRs should reach 85%–100% of the maximal HR during interval training. The time between work efforts is termed the **rest interval,** and consists of light activity such as walking. The length of the rest interval is generally expressed as a ratio of the duration of the work interval. For example, if the work interval for running 400 meters was seventy-five seconds, a rest interval of seventy-five seconds would result in a 1:1 ratio of work to rest. Generally, the rest interval should be at least as long as the work interval (4). In planning an interval training program for athletes who are not already highly trained, a work:rest ratio of 1:3 or 1:2 seems preferable. As a rule of thumb, the HR should drop to approximately 120 beats · min^{-1} near the end of the recovery interval (4).

A **set** is a specified number of work efforts performed as a unit. For instance, a set may consist of 8 × 400-meter runs with a prescribed rest interval between each run. The term **repetition** is the number of work efforts within one set. In the example just given, 8 × 400-meter run repetitions constituted one set. The number of repetitions and sets performed per workout depends on the purpose of the particular training session and the fitness levels of the athletes involved.

Long, Slow Distance

The use of long, slow distance (LSD) runs (or cycle rides, long swims, etc.) became a popular means of training for endurance events in the 1970s (13). In general, this method of training involves performing exercise at a low intensity (i.e., 57% $\dot{V}O_2$ max or approximately 70% of max HR) for durations that are generally greater in length than the normal competition distance. Although it seems reasonable that this type of training is a useful means of preparing an athlete to compete in long endurance competitions (marathon running), recent evidence suggests that short-term, high-intensity exercise is superior to long-term, low-intensity exercise in improving $\dot{V}O_2$ max (43, 44).

One of the historical reasons for researchers using training sessions of long duration is the common belief that improvements in endurance are proportional to the volume of training performed. Indeed, many coaches and athletes believe that improvements in athletic performance are directly related to how much work was performed during training, and that athletes can reach their potential only by doing long duration exercise bouts. Recent evidence by Costill and colleagues (15a) contradicts this belief. These workers demonstrated that athletes training 1.5 hours per day performed as well as athletes training 3 hours per day. In fact, the athletes that trained 3 hours per day performed poorer in some events than the group training 1.5 hours per day. This study illustrates the point that "more" is not always better in endurance training. Therefore, coaches and athletes should carefully consider the volume of training required to reach maximal benefits from long, slow-distance exercise.

High-Intensity, Continuous Exercise

Again, there is a growing volume of evidence to suggest that continuous high-intensity exercise is an outstanding means of improving $\dot{V}O_2$ max and the lactate threshold in athletes (19, 24, 27, 35, 43). Although the exercise intensity that promotes the greatest improvement in $\dot{V}O_2$ max may vary from athlete to athlete, it is believed that exercise intensities between 80%–90% $\dot{V}O_2$ max are optimal (see figure 21.1). Further, it seems

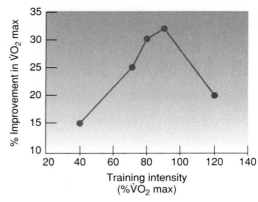

Figure 21.1

Relationship between training intensity and percent improvement in $\dot{V}O_2$ max. Data from references 24, 27, 28, and 43.

likely that a work rate that is equal to or slightly above the lactate threshold provides excellent improvement in maximum aerobic power and thus is a useful guideline for planning training programs (61).

Recall from chapter 20 that the lactate threshold can be determined in the laboratory during an incremental exercise test. Additionally, the lactate threshold can be estimated noninvasively using the ventilatory threshold (chapters 10 and 20). In the field, it is not practical to take repeated blood samples to determine the training speed that equals the lactate threshold during each training session, nor is it practical to continuously monitor ventilation during training. Therefore, the athlete needs a simple, noninvasive means of evaluating exercise intensity. Exercise heart rate appears to be the most practical means of evaluating exercise intensity during training. During the laboratory assessment of the lactate threshold or ventilatory threshold, it is standard practice to record heart rate stage-by-stage. The heart rate that corresponds to the metabolic rate at which the lactate threshold occurred can then be used by the athlete during training sessions as a guide to optimize training intensity. An alternative to direct laboratory testing to determine the lactate threshold is to have the athletes train at a fixed percentage of their maximal heart rates. Recently, Weltman and colleagues (79) have developed exercise prescription guidelines for male endurance runners. These authors suggest that if the lactate threshold is to be used as the exercise training intensity, then athletes should exercise at ≥ 90% heart rate max or 95% of heart rate reserve. Presently, it is unknown if these guidelines apply to women athletes or to athletes in sports other than distance running.

The objective during high-intensity, continuous training is to exercise at a heart rate near the lactate threshold for approximately twenty-five to fifty minutes, with the duration of the training session being dependent on the fitness level of the athlete. As the athlete improves, it may become necessary to repeat the laboratory testing and alter the training intensity accordingly.

in summary

- Historically, training to improve maximal aerobic power has used three methods: (1) interval training, (2) long, slow distance, and (3) high-intensity, continuous exercise.
- Although controversy exists as to which of the above training methods results in the greatest improvement in $\dot{V}O_2$ max, there is growing evidence that it is intensity and not duration that is the most important factor in improving $\dot{V}O_2$ max.

Injuries and Endurance Training

An important question associated with any type of endurance training is what type of training program presents the lowest risk of injury to the athlete. At present, a clear answer to this question is not available. However, a recent review of exercise-training-induced injuries suggests that the majority of training injuries are a result of overtraining (e.g., overuse injuries) (55). The overuse injury can come from either short-term, high-intensity exercise or long-term, low-intensity exercise (55). A common sense guideline to avoid overuse injuries is to avoid large increases in training volume or intensity. Perhaps the most useful rule of thumb guideline for increasing the training load is the "ten percent rule" (55). In short, the ten percent rule suggests that training intensity or duration should not be increased more than ten percent per week to avoid an overtraining injury. For example, a runner running 50 miles per week could increase his/her weekly distance to 55 miles (10% of 50 = 5) the following week.

In addition to overtraining, several other exercise-induced injury risk factors have been identified (55). Among these factors are musculotendonous imbalance of strength and/or flexibility, footwear problems (i.e., excessive wear), anatomical malalignment, poor running surface, and disease (e.g., arthritis, old fracture, etc.).

Note that gender is not an injury risk factor for endurance training (55). While some evidence exists that the female runner may sustain a higher incidence of overuse injuries than males of the same age, this may be due to cultural differences, the result of less running by teenage girls (56). Micheli (55) has suggested that many of the leg injuries in female runners appear to be the result of overtraining. This may be especially true for poorly conditioned women beginning training programs designed for well trained men.

in summary

- The majority of training injuries are a result of overtraining (e.g., overuse injuries) and can come from either short-term, high-intensity exercise or prolonged, low-intensity exercise.
- A useful rule of thumb guideline for increasing the training load is the "ten percent rule." The ten percent rule states that training intensity or duration should not be increased more than ten percent per week to avoid an overtraining injury.

Training for Improved Anaerobic Power

Athletic events lasting less than sixty seconds depend largely on anaerobic production of the necessary energy. In general, training to improve anaerobic power centers around the need to enhance either the ATP-PC system or anaerobic glycolysis (lactic acid system) (54). However, some activities require major contributions of both of the above anaerobic metabolic pathways to provide the necessary ATP for competition (see table 21.1). Again, it is critical that the training program use the specific muscle groups that are required by the athlete during competition.

Training to Improve the ATP–PC System

Sports such as football, weight lifting, and short dashes in track (100 meters) depend on the ATP-PC system to provide the bulk of the energy needed for competition. Therefore, optimal performance requires a training program that will maximize ATP production via the ATP-PC pathway.

Training to improve the ATP-PC system involves a special type of interval training. In order to maximally stress the ATP-PC metabolic pathway, short, high-intensity intervals (five to ten seconds duration) using the muscles utilized in competition are ideal. Because of the short durations of this type of interval, little lactic acid is produced and recovery is rapid. The rest interval may range between thirty to sixty seconds, depending on the fitness levels of the athletes. For example, a training program for football players might involve repeated 30-yard dashes (with several directional changes), with a thirty-second rest period between efforts. The number of repetitions per set would be determined by the athletes' fitness levels, environmental factors, and perhaps other considerations.

Training to Improve the Glycolytic System

After approximately ten seconds of a maximal effort, there is a growing dependence on energy production from anaerobic glycolysis (4, 29, 30). In order to improve the capacity of this energy pathway, the athlete must overload the "system" via short-term, high-intensity efforts. In general, high-intensity intervals of twenty to sixty seconds duration are useful in overloading this metabolic pathway.

This type of anaerobic training is both physically and psychologically demanding and thus requires a high commitment on the part of the athlete. Further, this type of training may drastically reduce muscle glycogen stores. It is for these reasons that athletes often alternate hard interval training days and light training sessions.

in summary

- Training to improve anaerobic power involves a special type of interval training. In general, the intervals are of short duration and consist of high-intensity exercise (near-maximal effort).

Training to Improve Muscular Strength

The goal of a strength-training program is to increase the maximum amount of force that can be generated by a particular muscle group. In general, any muscle that is regularly exercised at a high intensity (i.e., intensity near its maximum force generating capacity) will become stronger (42). Strength-training exercises can be classified into three categories: (1) isometric or static, (2) dynamic or isotonic (includes **variable resistance exercise**), and (3) isokinetic. Recall that isometric exercise is the application of force without joint movement, and that dynamic exercise involves force application with joint movement (chapters 8 and 20). Variable resistance exercise is the term used to describe exercise performed on machines such as Nautilus® equipment, which provide a variable amount of resistance during the course of an isotonic contraction. Isokinetic exercise is the exertion of force at a constant speed. Although isometric exercise has been shown to improve strength, either isotonic or isokinetic strength training are generally preferred in the preparation of athletes because isometric training does not increase strength over the full range of motion—only at the specific joint angle maintained during training (23, 30, 42, 81).

What physiological adaptations occur as a result of strength training? This issue was discussed in chapter 13 and will be addressed only briefly here. One of the obvious and perhaps most important physiological

changes that occurs following a strength-training program is the increase in muscle mass. Recall from chapter 8 that the amount of force that can be generated by a muscle group is proportional to the cross-sectional area of the muscle (47). Therefore, larger muscles exert greater force than smaller muscles. Many investigators believe that the increase in muscle size via resistance training is due to **hypertrophy** (an increase in muscle fiber diameter due to an increase in myofibrils) (1, 2, 14, 36–38, 72). However, Gonyea and associates argue that muscles also increase their size in response to strength training by **hyperplasia** (increase in the number of muscle fibers) (39–41, 57, 69, 71). Although this issue remains controversial, it appears that much of the increase in muscle size due to strength training occurs via hypertrophy (14, 36–38).

Of further interest is the recent finding that strength training may result in fast-fiber-type conversions in humans (72). Staron and colleagues (72) demonstrated that twenty weeks (two training sessions per week) of high-intensity strength training resulted in a conversion of Type IIb fibers to Type IIa in college age females. The physiological significance of this type of fiber conversion is unclear. However, these results reflect the dynamic nature of skeletal muscles to adapt to various workloads.

Strength training may also induce central nervous system changes, which can increase the number of motor units recruited, alter motor neuron firing rates, enhance motor unit synchronization during a particular movement pattern, and result in the removal of neural inhibition (58, 62). These four processes result in an improvement in the amount of muscular force generated and appear to occur within the few weeks after starting a strength-training program (58).

Progressive Resistance Exercise

The most common form of strength training is weight lifting using free weights or various types of weight machines (i.e., isotonic or isokinetic training). In order to improve strength, weight training must employ the overload principle by periodically increasing the amount of weight (resistance) used in a particular exercise. This method of strength training was first described in 1948 by DeLorme and Watkins (20) and is called **progressive resistance exercise (PRE).** Since this early work, numerous other systems of training to improve muscular strength have been proposed, but the concept of PRE is the basis for most weight-training programs.

General Strength-Training Principles

Muscles increase in strength by being forced to contract at tensions near their maximum. If muscles are not overloaded, then there is no improvement in strength. Perhaps the first application of the overload principle was applied by the famous Olympic wrestler, Milo of Crotona (500 B.C.). Milo incorporated overload in his training routine by carrying a bull calf on his back each day until the animal reached maturity. Since the days of Milo, athletes have applied the principle of overload to training by lifting heavy objects.

The perfect training regimen for optimum improvement of strength remains controversial. Indeed, there does not appear to be a magic formula for strength training that meets the needs of all individuals (23). This is not surprising given that subjects vary in their responses to training loads due to differences in fitness levels and trainability (50). Therefore, similar to endurance training, the exercise prescription for strength training must be tailored for the individual. However, a general guideline for a strength-training exercise prescription is as follows. The intensity is four to eight repetitions maximum (RM) and practiced in multiple sets of three or four (5, 6, 75). Clearly, strength gains are less when the number of repetitions are greater than fifteen. Rest days between strength workouts seem critical for optimal strength improvement (6, 75). Therefore, a training schedule of three to four days per week is recommended.

A common belief among coaches and athletes is that strength increases in direct proportion to the volume of weight training. Although there is a link between training intensity/volume and strength gains, the optimal training volume to improve strength is not known. It is likely that the optimal weight-training volume for maximal improvement of muscular strength varies among subjects of different ages and fitness levels. Further, it is clear that weight-training programs incorporating extremely high training volumes are not required for optimal strength gains (76).

Similar to other training methods, strength training should involve those muscles used in competition. Indeed, strength-training exercises should stress the muscles in the same movement pattern used during the athletic competition. For instance, a shot putter should perform exercises that strengthen the specific muscles of the arm, chest, back, and legs that are involved in "putting the shot."

A final concern in the design of strength-training programs for sport performance is that the speed of muscle shortening during training should be similar to those speeds used during the event. For example, many sports require a high velocity of movement. Several studies have shown that strength-training programs using high velocity movements in a sport specific movement pattern produce superior gains in strength/power-oriented sports (21, 26, 64). These findings reinforce the notion that specificity of training dictates specific adaptations to specific stresses (73).

Free Weights versus Machines

Over the past several years, much controversy has centered around the question of whether training with free weights (barbells) or various types of weight machines (Nautilus®, Universal®, etc.) produces the greatest strength gains in athletes. At present, a definitive answer to this question is not available. When comparing strength gains obtained on various types of weight machines, no differences exist between variable resistance machines and constant resistance machines (51). However, Stone et al. (75) argue that strength training using free weights is superior to training with many commercial weight machines (both constant and variable resistance) for the following reasons: (1) data exists to support the notion that free weights produce greater strength gains during short-term training periods than many types of weight machines (74, 77), (2) use of free weights provides movement versatility and allows a greater specificity of training than weight machines, and (3) training with free weights (unlike many weight machines) involves large muscle mass and multi-segment exercise, which forces the athlete to control both balance and stabilizing factors. This type of training is useful since most sports require the athlete to maintain balance and body stability during competition (75). Although free weights offer some advantages over commercial weight machines, disadvantages also exist. Possible disadvantages include potential for injury (dropping weights), extra people required for spotting, and the amount of time required to learn proper lifting technique. Table 21.3 summarizes some of the advantages and disadvantages of strength training using isometric, isotonic (free weights, Nautilus®, etc.), and isokinetic machines.

Combined Strength and Endurance Training Programs

Strength and endurance training are often done concurrently by athletes and fitness enthusiasts. Some investigators have argued that performing combined strength and endurance training programs may antagonize the strength gains achieved by weight training alone (25, 42, 65). For example, two studies have demonstrated that untrained subjects who perform a combination of endurance and strength training achieve lower strength gains compared to subjects performing weight training alone (25, 42). However, whether the combination of weight and endurance training impedes strength gains probably depends on several factors, including the training state of the subjects, the volume and frequency of training, and the way the two training methods are integrated (65). In this regard, Sale (65) has recently demonstrated that athletes who perform concurrent strength and endurance training programs on the same day show a reduction in strength gains compared to athletes performing strength training alone. In contrast, these authors reported that athletes who perform concurrent strength and

Table 21.3 Summary of Potential Advantages and Disadvantages of Weight-Training Programs Using Various Types of Equipment

Program	Equipment	Advantages	Disadvantages
Isometric	Variety of home-designed devices	Minimal cost; less time required	Not directly applicable to most sport activities; may become boring; progress is difficult to monitor
Isotonic	Free weights	Low cost; specialized exercises may be designed to simulate a particular sport movement; progress easy to monitor	Injury potential due to dropping weights; increase workout time due to time required to change weights
Isotonic	Commercial weight machines (i.e., Universal®)	Generally safe; progress easy to monitor; small amount of time required to change weight	Does not permit specialized exercise; high cost
Variable resistance	Commercial devices (e.g., Nautilus®)	Has a cam system that provides a variable resistance that changes to match the joint's ability to produce force over the range of motion; progress easy to monitor; safety	High cost; limited specialized exercises
Isokinetic	Commercial isokinetic devices (e.g., Cybex®)	Allows development of maximal resistance over full range of motion; exercises can be performed at a variety of speeds	High cost; limited specialized exercises

Modified from reference 8.

endurance training programs on separate days gain strength as rapidly as athletes performing strength training only. What is the explanation for these findings? A possible explanation is that same day endurance plus strength training may result in a reduced strength-training effort particularly when endurance training is performed first. Indeed, fatigue or anticipation may reduce the amount of effort that subjects apply to strength training when the two programs are performed on the same day. Therefore, although more research in this area is required, a current recommendation for the training of power athletes would be for the athlete to perform strength and endurance training programs on separate days.

Gender Differences in Response to Strength Training

It is well established that when absolute strength (i.e., total amount of force applied) is compared in untrained men and women, men are typically stronger. This difference is greatest in the upper body where men are approximately 50% stronger than women, whereas men are only 30% stronger than women in the lower body (59). This apparent sex difference in strength is eliminated when force production in men and women is compared on the basis of the cross-sectional area of muscle. Figure 21.2 illustrates this point. Notice that as the cross-sectional area of muscle increases (x-axis), the arm flexor strength (y-axis) increases in a linear fashion and is

Figure 21.2
Arm flexor strength of men and women graphed as a function of muscle cross-sectional area.

independent of sex. That is, human muscle can generate 3–4 kg of force per cm^2 of muscle cross-section regardless of whether the muscle belongs to a male or female (47).

An often-asked question is "Do women gain strength as rapidly as men when training with weights?" In an effort to answer this question, Wilmore (80) compared the strength change between a group of untrained men and women before and after ten weeks of isotonic weight training. The results revealed that no differences existed between sexes in the percent of strength gained during the training period (see figure 21.3). Similar findings have been reported in other studies, and demonstrate

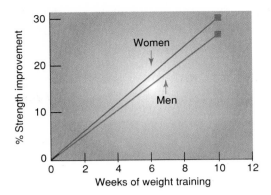

Figure 21.3
Strength changes in men and women as a result of a ten-week strength training program.

Figure 21.4
Proposed model for the occurrence of delayed muscular soreness.

that untrained men and women respond similarly to weight training (46, 60). However, the aforementioned studies are considered short-term training periods and may not reflect what occurs over long-term training. For instance, it is generally believed that men exhibit a greater degree of muscular hypertrophy than women as a result of long-term weight training. This gender difference in muscular hypertrophy appears to be related to the fact that men have twenty to thirty times higher blood levels of testosterone. For a review of strength training for female athletes, see reference 46.

Muscle Soreness

It is a common experience for novice weight trainers and sometimes even veteran strength athletes to notice a **delayed onset muscle soreness (DOMS)** that appears twenty-four to forty-eight hours after strenuous exercise. The search for an answer to the question of "What causes DOMS?" has extended over many years. A number of possible explanations have been proposed, including a buildup of lactic acid in muscle, muscle spasms, and torn muscle and connective tissue. Based on present evidence, it appears that DOMS is due to tissue injury caused by excessive mechanical force exerted upon muscle and connective tissue (3, 11, 33, 34, 70). Perhaps the strongest data to support this viewpoint comes from electron microscopy studies in which electron micrographs taken of muscles suffering from DOMS reveal microscopic tears in these muscle fibers (34).

How does DOMS occur and what is the physiological explanation for DOMS? A clear answer to this question is not currently available (for reviews, see references 3 and 12). However, Armstrong (3) has proposed that DOMS occurs in the following manner: (1) strenuous muscular contractions (especially eccentric contractions) result in structural damage in muscle and perhaps connective tissue as well, (2) calcium leaks out of the sarcoplasmic reticulum and

collects in the mitochondria, which inhibits oxidative phosphorylation (i.e., ATP production is halted), (3) the buildup of calcium also activates enzymes (proteases), which degrade cellular proteins including contractile proteins, (4) this breakdown of muscle proteins results in an inflammatory process, which includes an increase in prostaglandin and histamine production, and finally (5) the accumulation of histamines, potassium, prostaglandins, and edema surrounding muscle fibers stimulates free nerve endings (pain receptors), which results in the sensation of DOMS (see figure 21.4).

How does one avoid being a victim of DOMS following exercise? It appears that DOMS occurs most frequently following intense exercise using muscles that are unaccustomed to being worked (3). Further, eccentric exercise appears to cause greater suffering from DOMS than concentric work. Therefore, a general recommendation for the avoidance of DOMS is to begin an exercise training program gradually. That is, avoid intense exercise (particularly eccentric) during the first five to ten training sessions. This pattern of slow progression allows the exercised muscles to "adapt" to the exercise stress and therefore reduces the incidence or severity of DOMS.

in summary

- Improvement in muscular strength can be achieved via progressive overload by using either isometric, isotonic, or isokinetic exercise. Isotonic or isokinetic training seems preferable to isometric exercise in developing strength gains in athletes, since isometric strength gains occur only at the specific joint angles that are held during isometric training.
- Although untrained men exhibit greater absolute strength than untrained females, there does not appear to be gender differences in strength gains during a short-term weight-training program.
- Delayed onset muscle soreness (DOMS) is thought to occur due to microscopic tears in muscle fibers or connective tissue. This results in cellular degradation and an inflammatory response, which results in pain within twenty-four to forty-eight hours after strenuous exercise.

Training for Improved Flexibility

The ability to move joints through a full range of motion is important in many sports. Loss of flexibility can result in a reduction of movement efficiency and may increase the chance of injury in some sports (7). Therefore, many athletic trainers and coaches recommend regular stretching exercises to improve flexibility and thus reduce the chance of injury and perhaps optimize the efficiency of movement.

It should be noted however, that a high degree of flexibility in all joints may not be desirable in all sports. For instance, excessive flexibility is often indicative of proneness to injury in contact sports. For example, the shoulder joint is structurally weak when compared to the hip joint. This is because the glenoid fossa of the scapula (socket where the head of the humerus fits) is very shallow. Therefore, the main stability of the shoulder joint is provided by the surrounding musculature. Hence, an increase in shoulder muscle mass might reduce flexibility, but would lower the chance of shoulder injury in contact sports by increasing shoulder stability.

There are two general stretching techniques in use today: (1) **static stretching** (continuously holding a stretch position), and (2) **dynamic stretching** (sometimes referred to as *ballistic stretching* if movements are not controlled). Although both techniques result in an improvement in flexibility, static stretching is considered to be superior over dynamic stretching because: (1) there is less chance of injury (6), (2) static stretching causes less muscle spindle activity when compared to dynamic stretching, and (3) there is less

chance of muscle soreness. Stimulation of muscle spindles during dynamic stretching can produce a stretch reflex and therefore result in muscular contraction. This type of muscular contraction counteracts the desired lengthening of the muscle and may increase the chance of injury.

Research has shown that thirty minutes of static stretching exercises performed twice per week will improve flexibility within five weeks (22). It is recommended that the stretch position be held for ten seconds at the beginning of a flexibility program and increased up to sixty seconds after several training sessions. Each stretch position should be repeated three to five times, with the number increased up to ten repetitions. Overload is applied by increasing the range of motion during the stretch position and increasing the amount of time the stretch position is held.

Preceding a static stretch with an isometric contraction of the muscle group to be stretched is an effective means of improving muscle relaxation and may enhance the development of flexibility (7, 22, 81). This stretching technique is called **proprioceptive neuromuscular facilitation (PNF)**. The procedure generally requires two people and is performed as follows (49). A training partner moves the target limb passively through its range of motion; after reaching the end point of the range of motion, the target muscle is isometrically contracted (against the partner) for six to ten seconds. The target muscle then relaxes and is again stretched by the partner to a greater range of motion. The physiological rationale for the use of PNF stretching is that muscular relaxation follows an isometric contraction because the contraction stimulates Golgi tendon organs, which inhibit contraction during the subsequent stretching exercise.

in summary

- Improvement in joint mobility (flexibility) can be achieved via static or dynamic stretching, with static stretching being the preferred technique.

Year-Round Conditioning for Athletes

It is common for today's athletes to engage in year-round conditioning exercises. This is necessary to prevent gain of excessive body fat and prevent extreme physical detraining between competitive seasons. The training periods of athletes can be divided into three phases: (1) off-season training, (2) preseason training, and (3) in-season training. A brief description of each training period follows.

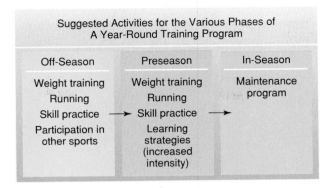

Suggested Activities for the Various Phases of A Year-Round Training Program		
Off-Season	Preseason	In-Season
Weight training	Weight training	Maintenance program
Running	Running	
Skill practice →	Skill practice →	
Participation in other sports	Learning strategies (increased intensity)	

Figure 21.5
Recommended activities for the various phases of year-round training.

Off-Season Conditioning

In general, the objectives of off-season conditioning programs are to: (1) prevent excessive fat weight gain, (2) maintain muscular strength or endurance, (3) maintain ligament and bone integrity, and (4) maintain a reasonable skill level in the athlete's specific sport. Obviously, the exact nature of the off-season conditioning program will vary from sport to sport. For example, a football player would spend considerably more time performing strength-training exercises than a distance runner. Conversely, the runner would incorporate more running into an off-season conditioning program than the football player. Hence, specific exercises should be selected on the basis of the sport's demands (30).

No matter what the sport, it is critical that an off-season conditioning program provide variety for the athlete. Further, off-season conditioning programs generally use a training regimen that is composed of low-intensity, high-volume work. This combination of low-intensity training and variety may prevent the occurrence of "overtraining syndromes" and the development of psychological staleness. Figure 21.5 contains a list of some recommended training activities for off-season conditioning.

Off-season conditioning allows the athletes to concentrate on fitness areas where they may be weak. Therefore, it is important that off-season programs be designed for the individual. For instance, a basketball player may lack leg strength and power and therefore have a limited vertical jump. An off-season conditioning program allows this athlete to engage in specific strength-training activities that will improve leg power and enhance vertical jumping capacity.

Preseason Conditioning

The principal objective of preseason conditioning (e.g., eight to twelve weeks prior to competition) is to increase to a maximum the capacities of the predominant energy systems used in a particular sport (30). In the transition from off-season conditioning to preseason conditioning there is a gradual shift from low-intensity, high-volume exercise to high-intensity, low-volume exercise. As in all phases of a training cycle, the program should be sport specific.

For a detailed preseason conditioning program for specific sports the reader is referred to Bowers and Fox (1992) in the suggested reading list. In general, the types of exercise performed during preseason conditioning are similar to those used during off-season conditioning (figure 21.5). The principal difference between off-season and preseason conditioning is the intensity of the conditioning effort. During preseason conditioning, the athlete applies a progressive overload by increasing the intensity of workouts, whereas off-season conditioning involves high-volume, low-intensity workouts.

In-Season Conditioning

The general goal of in-season conditioning for most sports is to maintain the fitness level achieved during the preseason training program. For instance, in a sport such as football, in which there is a relatively long competitive season, the athlete must be able to maintain strength and endurance during the entire season. A complicating factor in planning an in-season conditioning program for many team sports is that the season may not have a clear-cut ending. That is, at the end of the regular season, play-off games may extend the season an additional several weeks. Therefore, it is difficult in these types of sports to plan a climax in the conditioning program, and so there is the need for a maintenance training program.

In planning an in-season conditioning program, the goal is to design a program that is of sufficient volume and intensity to maintain strength and endurance during the entire playing season. Note that strength can be maintained during the competitive season by as little as one workout every seven to ten days (75). However, maintenance of cardiovascular fitness appears to require a minimum of two to three training days per week (45).

in summary
- Year-round conditioning programs for athletes include an off-season program, preseason program, and an in-season program.
- The general objectives of an off-season conditioning program are to prevent excessive fat weight gain, maintain muscular strength and endurance, maintain bone and ligament strength, and preserve a reasonable skill level in the athlete's specific sport.

Common Training Mistakes

Some of the most common training errors include: (1) overtraining, (2) undertraining, (3) using exercises and work-rate intensities that are not sport specific,

Overtraining and the Immune System

The human immune system is a complex array of cells and hormones charged with the responsibility of preventing infections and cancer. There is growing evidence that moderate levels of exercise training improve immune function and decrease the risk of infection (49a, 59a, 59b). However, it is now clear that heavy training regimens coupled with a lack of rest (i.e., overtraining) result in a weakened immune system and an increased risk of disease. The relationship between various levels of exercise training and the risk of infection is described by a "J"-shaped curve (see chapter 13, figure 13.13) (59b). Close inspection of figure 13.13 illustrates that movement from a sedentary life-style to an active life-style involving a moderate level of exercise training reduces the risk of infection. However, overtraining, due to a very high training intensity or volume, increases the risk of infection. Therefore, athletes should be able to recognize the symptoms of overtraining. When overtraining symptoms appear, the athlete must be prepared to reduce his/her training load to avoid a reduction in immune function.

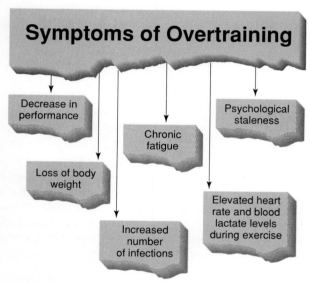

Figure 21.6

Common symptoms of overtraining.

symptoms of overtraining include: (1) elevated heart rate and blood lactate levels at a fixed submaximal work rate, (2) loss in body weight due to a reduction in appetite, (3) chronic fatigue, (4) psychological staleness, (5) multiple colds or sore throats, and/or (6) a decrease in performance (see figure 21.6). An overtrained athlete may exhibit one or all of these symptoms (7, 30, 34a, 46a, 81). Therefore, it is critical that the coach or trainer recognize the classic symptoms of overtraining and be prepared to reduce their athletes' work loads when overtraining symptoms appear. Recall that specific training programs should be planned for athletes when possible to compensate for individual differences in genetic potential and fitness levels. This is an important point to remember when planning training programs for athletic conditioning.

Another common mistake in the training of athletes is the failure to plan sport-specific training exercises. Often coaches or trainers fail to understand the importance of the law of specificity, and develop training exercises that do not enhance the energy capacities of the skeletal muscles used in competition. This error can be avoided by achieving a broad understanding of the training principles discussed earlier in this chapter.

Further, coaches, trainers, and athletes should plan and record training schedules designed to achieve specific fitness objectives at various times during the year. Failure to plan a training strategy may result in misuse of training time and ultimately result in inferior performance.

Finally, failure to reduce the intensity and volume of training prior to competition is also a common

(4) failure to plan long-term training schedules to achieve specific goals, and (5) failure to taper training prior to a competition. Let's discuss each of these training errors briefly.

Overtraining may be a more significant problem than undertraining for several reasons. First, overtraining (workouts that are too long or too strenuous) may result in injury or reduce the athlete's resistance to disease (see A Closer Look 21.1). Further, overtraining may result in a psychological staleness, which can be identified by a general lack of enthusiasm on the part of the athlete. The general training error. Achieving a peak athletic performance requires a healthy blend of proper nutrition, training, and rest. Failure to reduce the training volume and/or intensity prior to competition results in inadequate rest and compromises performance. Therefore, in an effort to achieve peak performance, athletes should reduce their training load for several days prior to competition; this practice is called **tapering.** The goal of tapering is to provide time for muscles to resynthesize glycogen to maximal levels and to allow muscles to heal from training-induced damage. While the optimum length of a taper period continues to be debated, a reduced training load of 3–21 days has been used successfully in both strength and endurance sports (15, 34b, 45, 46b, 52a). Indeed, runners and swimmers can reduce their training load by approximately 60% for up to 21 days without a reduction in performance (15, 34b, 46b).

in summary

- Common mistakes in training include undertraining, overtraining, performing nonspecific exercises during training sessions, failure to carefully schedule a long-term training plan, and failure to taper training prior to a competition.
- Symptoms of overtraining include: (1) elevated heart rate and blood lactate levels at a fixed submaximal work rate, (2) loss in body weight due to a reduction in appetite, (3) chronic fatigue, (4) psychological staleness, (5) increased number of infections, and/or (6) a decrease in performance.
- Tapering is the term applied to short-term reduction in training load prior to competition. Research has shown that tapering prior to a competition is useful in improving performance both in strength and endurance events.

study questions

1. Explain how knowledge of the energy systems used in a particular activity or sport might be useful in designing a sport-specific training program.
2. Provide an outline of the general principles of designing a training program for the following sports: (1) football, (2) soccer, (3) basketball, (4) volleyball, (5) distance running (5,000 meters), and (6) 200-meter dash (track).
3. Define the following terms as they relate to interval training: (1) work interval, (2) rest interval, (3) work-to-rest ratio, and (4) set.
4. How can interval training be used to improve both aerobic and anaerobic power?
5. List and discuss the three most common types of training programs used to improve $\dot{V}O_2$ max.
6. Discuss the practical and theoretical differences between an interval training program used to improve the ATP-PC system, and a program designed to improve the lactic acid system.
7. List the general principles of strength development.
8. Define the terms *isometric*, *isotonic*, and *isokinetic*.
9. Outline the model to explain delayed onset muscle soreness proposed by Armstrong.
10. Discuss the use of static and dynamic stretching to improve flexibility. Why is a high degree of flexibility not desired in all sports?
11. List and discuss the objectives of: (1) off-season conditioning, (2) preseason conditioning, and (3) in-season conditioning.
12. What are some of the more common errors made in the training of athletes?

suggested readings

Bowers, R., and E. Fox. 1992. *Sports Physiology.* Dubuque, IA: Wm. C. Brown.

Gibala, M. et al. 1994. The effect of tapering on strength performance in trained athletes. *International Journal of Sports Medicine* 15:492–97.

Komi, P. 1992. *Strength and Power in Sport.* London: Blackwell Scientific Publications.

Mazzeo, R. 1994. The influence of exercise and aging on immune function. *Medicine and Science in Sports and Exercise* 26:586–92.

Morrissey, M. et al. 1995. Resistance training modes: Specificity and effectiveness. *Medicine and Science in Sports and Exercise* 27:648–60.

Wilmore, J., and D. Costill. 1993. *Training for Sport and Activity.* Dubuque, IA: Wm. C. Brown.

references

1. Alway, S. 1990. Muscle cross sectional area and torque in resistance-trained subjects. *European Journal of Applied Physiology* 60:86–90.

2. ———. 1990. Twitch contractile adaptations are not dependent on the intensity of isometric exercise in human triceps surae. *European Journal of Applied Physiology* 60:346–52.

3. Armstrong, R. 1984. Mechanisms of exercise-induced delayed onset of muscular soreness: A brief review. *Medicine and Science in Sports and Exercise* 16:529–38.

4. Åstrand, P. O., and K. Rodahl. 1986. *Textbook of Work Physiology.* New York: McGraw-Hill.

5. Berger, R. A. 1962. Optimum repetitions for the development of strength. *Research Quarterly* 33:334–38.

6. ———. 1982. *Applied Exercise Physiology.* Philadelphia: Lea & Febiger.

7. Brooks, G. A., and T. Fahey. 1987. *Fundamentals of Human Performance.* New York: Macmillan.

8. Burke, E. 1977. Physiological similar effects of similar training programs in males and females. *Research Quarterly* 48:510–17.

9. Burke, E., and B. D. Franks. 1975. Changes in $\dot{V}O_2$ max resulting from bicycle training at different intensities holding total mechanical work constant. *Research Quarterly* 46:31–37.

10. Burke, E. J., ed. 1980. *Toward an Understanding of Human Performance.* Ithaca, NY: Mouvement Publications.

11. Clarkson, P. et al. 1986. Muscle soreness and serum creatine kinase activity following isometric, eccentric, and concentric exercise. *International Journal of Sports Medicine* 7:152–55.

12. Clarkson, P. et al. 1992. Muscle function after exercise-induced muscle damage and rapid adaptation. *Medicine and Science in Sports and Exercise* 24:512–20.

13. Costill, D. 1979. *A Scientific Approach to Distance Running.* Los Altos: Track and Field News.

14. Costill, D. et al. 1979. Adaptations in skeletal muscle following strength training. *Journal of Applied Physiology* 46:96–99.

15. Costill, D. et al. 1985. Effects of reduced training on muscular power in swimmers. *Physician and Sports Medicine* 13:94–101.

15a. Costill, D. et al. 1991. Adaptations to swimming training: Influence of training volume. *Medicine and Science in Sports and Exercise* 23:371–77.

16. Coyle, E. et al. 1984. Time course of loss of adaptations after stopping prolonged intense endurance training. *Journal of Applied Physiology* 57:1857–64.

17. Coyle, E. et al. 1985. Effects of detraining on responses to submaximal exercise. *Journal of Applied Physiology* 59:853–59.

18. Daniels, J., R. Fitts, and G. Sheehan. 1978. *Conditioning for Distance Running.* New York: John Wiley & Sons.

19. Davies, C. T. M., and A. Knibbs. 1971. The training stimulus: The effects of intensity, duration, and frequency of effort on maximum aerobic power output. *Int. Z. Angew* 20:299–305.

20. Delorme, T., and A. Watkins. 1948. Techniques of progressive resistance exercise. *Archives of Physical and Rehabilitative Medicine* 29:263–66.

21. Deschenes, M. 1989. Short review: Motor coding and motor unit recruitment pattern. *Journal of Applied Sport Science Research* 3:33–39.

22. DeVries, H. 1962. Evaluation of static stretching procedures for improvement of flexibility. *Research Quarterly* 33:222–29.

23. DiNubile, N. 1991. Strength training. *Clinics in Sports Medicine* 10:33–63.

24. Dudley, G., W. Abraham, and R. Terjung. 1982. Influence of exercise intensity and duration on biochemical adaptations in skeletal muscle. *Journal of Applied Physiology* 53:844–50.

25. Dudley, G., and R. Djamil. 1985. Incompatibility of strength and endurance training. *Journal of Applied Physiology* 59:1446–51.

26. Ewing, J. et al. 1990. Effects of velocity of isokinetic training on strength, power, and quadriceps muscle fiber characteristics. *European Journal of Applied Physiology* 61:159–62.

27. Fox, E. et al. 1973. Intensity and distance of interval training programs and changes in maximal aerobic power. *Medicine and Science in Sports* 5:18–22.

28. Fox, E. et al. 1975. Frequency and duration of interval training programs and changes in aerobic power. *Journal of Applied Physiology* 38:481–84.

29. Fox, E., S. Robinson, and D. Wiegman. 1969. Metabolic energy sources during continuous and interval running. *Journal of Applied Physiology* 27:174–78.

30. Fox, E. L. 1984. *Sports Physiology.* Philadelphia: W. B. Saunders.

31. Fox, E. L., and D. Mathews. 1974. *Interval Training: Conditioning for Sports and General Fitness.* Philadelphia: W. B. Saunders.

32. Franks, B. 1983. Physical warm-up. In *Ergogenic Aids in Sports,* ed. M. Williams. 340. Champaign, IL: Human Kinetics.

33. Friden, J., and R. Lieber. 1992. Structural and mechanical basis of exercise-induced injury. *Medicine and Science in Sports* 24:521–30.

34. Friden, J., M. Sjöström, and B. Ekblom. 1983. Myofibrillar damage following eccentric exercise in man. *International Journal of Sports Medicine* 4:170–76.

34a. Fry, R. et al. 1994. Psychological and immunological correlates of acute overtraining. *British Journal of Sports Medicine* 28:241–46.

34b. Gibala, M. et al. 1994. The effects of tapering on strength performance in trained athletes. *International Journal of Sports Medicine* 15:492–97.

35. Gibbons, E. et al. 1983. Effects of various training intensity levels on anaerobic threshold and aerobic capacity in females. *Journal of Sports Medicine and Physical Fitness* 23:315–18.

36. Goldberg, A. 1965. Muscle hypertrophy in hypophysectomized rats. *Physiologist* 8:175–78.

37. Gollnick, P. et al. 1981. Muscular enlargement and number of fibers in skeletal muscles of rats. *Journal of Applied Physiology* 50:936–43.

38. Gollnick, P. et al. 1983. Fiber number and size in overloaded chicken anterior latissimus dorsi muscle. *Journal of Applied Physiology* 54:1292–97.

39. Gonyea, W. 1980. The role of exercise in inducing skeletal muscle fiber splitting. *Journal of Applied Physiology* 48:421–26.

40. Gonyea, W. et al. 1986. Exercise induced increases in muscle fiber number. *European Journal of Applied Physiology* 55:137–41.

41. Gonyea, W., G. Ericson, and F. Bonde-Peterson. 1977. Skeletal muscle fiber splitting induced weight lifting exercise in cats. *Acta Physiologica Scandanavica* 99:105–9.

42. Hickson, R. 1980. Interference of strength development by simultaneously training for strength and endurance. *European Journal of Applied Physiology* 45:255–63.

43. Hickson, R., H. Bomze, and J. Holloszy. 1977. Linear increase in aerobic power induced by a strenuous program of endurance exercise. *Journal of Applied Physiology* 42:372–76.

44. Hickson, R. et al. 1981. Time course of the adaptive responses of aerobic power and heart rate to training. *Medicine and Science in Sports and Exercise* 13:17–20.

45. Hickson, R., and M. Rosenkoetter. 1981. Reduced training frequencies and maintenance of increased aerobic power. *Medicine and Science in Sports and Exercise* 13:13–16.

46. Holloway, J., and T. Baeche. 1990. Strength training for female athletes: A review of selected aspects. *Sports Medicine* 9:216–28.

46a. Hooper, S. 1995. Markers for monitoring overtraining and recovery. *Medicine and Science in Sports and Exercise* 27:106–12.

46b. Houmard, J. 1990. Reduced training maintains performance in distance runners. *International Journal of Sports Medicine* 11:46–51.

47. Ikai, M., and T. Fukunaga. 1968. Calculation of muscle strength per unit of cross-sectional area of a human muscle by means of ultrasonic measurements. *Int. Z. Angew. Physiol.* 26:26–31.

48. Knuttgen, H. et al. 1973. Physical conditioning through interval training with young male adults. *Medicine and Science in Sports* 5:220–26.

49. Liemohn, W., and G. Sharpe. 1992. Muscular strength and endurance, flexibility, and low-back function. In *Health/Fitness Instructor's Handbook*, eds. E. Howley and D. Frank, 179–96. Champaign, IL: Human Kinetics.

49a. MacKinnon, L. 1992. *Exercise and Immunology*. Champaign, IL: Human Kinetics.

50. Malina, R., and C. Bouchard. 1986. Sport and human genetics. *Proceedings of the 1984 Olympic Scientific Congress*, vol. 4. Champaign, IL: Human Kinetics.

51. Manning, R. et al. 1990. Constant vs. variable resistance knee extension training. *Medicine and Science in Sports and Exercise* 22:397–401.

52. Martin, B. et al. 1975. Effect of warm-up on metabolic responses to strenuous exercise. *Medicine and Science in Sports* 7:146–49.

52a. Martin, D. 1994. Effects of interval training and a taper on cycling performance and isokinetic leg strength. *International Journal of Sports Medicine* 15:485–91.

53. McArdle, W., F. Katch, and V. Katch. 1991. *Exercise Physiology: Energy, Nutrition, and Human Performance*. Philadelphia: Lea & Febiger.

54. Medbo, J., and S. Burgers. 1990. Effect of training on the anaerobic capacity. *Medicine and Science in Sports and Exercise* 22:501–7.

55. Micheli, L. 1988. Injuries and prolonged exercise. In *Prolonged Exercise*, eds. D. Lamb and R. Murray, 393–407. Indianapolis: Benchmark Press.

56. Micheli, L. et al. 1980. Etiological assessment of overuse stress fractures in athletes. *Nova Scotia Medical Bulletin* 43–47.

57. Mikesky, A. et al. 1991. Changes in muscle fiber size and composition in response to heavy-resistance exercise. *Medicine and Science in Sports and Exercise* 23:1042–49.

58. Moritani, T., and H. DeVries. 1979. Neural factors versus hypertrophy in the time course of muscle strength gain. *American Journal of Physical Medicine* 58:115–19.

59. Morrow, J., and W. Hosler. 1981. Strength comparisons in untrained men and trained women. *Medicine and Science in Sports and Exercise* 13:194–98.

59a. Nash, M. 1994. Exercise and immunology. *Medicine and Science in Sports and Exercise* 26:125–27.

59b. Nieman, D. 1994. Exercise, infection, and immunity. *International Journal of Sports Medicine* 15:S131–S141.

60. O'Shea, J., and J. Wegner. 1981. Power weight training in the female athlete. *Physician and Sports Medicine* 9:109–14.

61. Priest, J., and R. Hagan. 1987. The effects of maximum steady-state pace on running performance. *British Journal of Sports Medicine* 21:18–21.

61a. Rodenburg, J. et al. 1994. Warm-up, stretching and massage diminish harmful effects of eccentric exercise. *International Journal of Sports Medicine* 15:414–19.

62. Rube, N., and N. Secher. 1990. Effect of central factors on fatigue following two- and one-leg static exercise in man. *Acta Physiologica Scandanavica* 141:87–95.

63. Safran, M. et al. 1989. Warm-up and muscular injury prevention. *Sports Medicine* 4:239–49.

64. Sale, D. 1988. Neural adaptation to resistance training. *Medicine and Science in Sports and Exercise* 20 (Suppl.):S135–S145.

65. Sale, D. et al. 1990. Comparison of two regimens of concurrent strength and endurance training. *Medicine and Science in Sports and Exercise* 22:348–56.

66. Saltin, B. et al. 1968. Response to exercise after bed rest and after training. *Circulation* 38 (Suppl. 7):1–78.

67. Sharkey, B. 1970. Intensity and duration of training and the development of cardiorespiratory endurance. *Medicine and Science in Sports* 2:197–202.

68. ———. 1990. *Physiology of Fitness*. Champaign, IL: Human Kinetics.

69. Sjöström, M. et al. 1991. Evidence of fiber hyperplasia in human skeletal muscles from healthy young men? *European Journal of Applied Physiology* 62:301–4.

70. Smith, L. 1991. Acute inflammation: The underlying mechanism in delayed onset muscle soreness? *Medicine and Science in Sports and Exercise* 23:542–51.

71. Sola, O., D. Christensen, and A. Martin. 1973. Hypertrophy and hyperplasia of adult chicken anterior latissimus dorsi muscle following stretch with and without denervation. *Experimental Neurology* 41:76–100.

72. Staron, R. et al. 1989. Muscle hypertrophy and fast fiber type conversions in heavy resistance-trained women. *European Journal of Applied Physiology* 60:71–79.

73. Stone, M. 1990. Muscle conditioning and muscle injuries. *Medicine and Science in Sports and Exercise* 22:457–62.

74. Stone, M., R. Johnson, and D. R. Carter. 1979. A short-term comparison of two different methods of resistance training on leg strength and power. *Athletic Training* 14:158–60.

75. Stone, M., and H. O'Bryant. 1986. *Weight Training: A Scientific Approach.* Minneapolis: Burgess.

76. Trzaskoma, Z. et al. 1992. Investigation of an experimental weight-training programme. *Journal of Sports Sciences* 10:109–17.

77. Wathen, D. 1980. A comparison of the effects of selected isotonic and isokinetic exercises, modalities, and programs on the vertical jump in college football players. *National Strength Coaches Association Journal* 2:47–48.

78. Wells, C., and R. Pate. 1988. Training for performance of prolonged exercise. In *Prolonged Exercise*, eds. D. Lamb and R. Murray, 357–88. Indianapolis: Benchmark Press.

79. Weltman, A. et al. 1990. Percentages of maximal heart rate, heart rate reserve and VO_2 max for determining endurance training intensity for male runners. *International Journal of Sports Medicine* 11:218–22.

80. Wilmore, J. 1974. Alterations in strength, body composition, and anthrometric measurements consequent to a 10-week weight training program. *Medicine and Science in Sports* 6:133–39.

81. Wilmore, J., and D. Costill. 1993. *Training for Sport and Activity.* Dubuque, IA: Wm. C. Brown.

22

Training for the Female Athlete, Children, and Special Populations

objectives

By studying this chapter, you should be able to do the following:

1. Describe the incidence of amenorrhea in female athletes versus the general population.
2. List those factors thought to contribute to "athletic" amenorrhea.
3. Discuss the general recommendations for training during menstruation.
4. List the general guidelines for exercise during pregnancy.
5. Define the term "female athlete triad."
6. Discuss the possibility that chronic exercise presents a danger to: (1) the cardiopulmonary system or (2) the musculoskeletal system of children.
7. List those conditions in Type I diabetics that might limit their participation in a vigorous training program.
8. Explain the rationale for the selection of an insulin injection site for Type I diabetics prior to a training session.
9. List the precautions that should be taken by asthmatics during a training session.
10. Discuss the question "Does exercise promote seizures in epileptics?"

outline

Factors Important to Women Involved in Vigorous Training   410
    Exercise and Menstrual Disorders   410
    Training and Menstruation   411
    The Female Athlete and Eating Disorders   411
    Bone Mineral Disorders and the Female Athlete   412
    Training During Pregnancy   412

Sports Conditioning for Children   413
    Training and the Cardiopulmonary System   413
    Training and the Musculoskeletal System   414
Competitive Training for Diabetics   415
Training for Asthmatics   415

Epilepsy and Physical Training   416
    Does Exercise Promote Seizures?   416
    Risk of Injury Due to Seizures   416

amenorrhea

anorexia nervosa

articular cartilage

bulimia

dysmenorrhea

epilepsy

epiphyseal plate (growth plate)

ertainly the general physiological principles of exercise training to improve performance apply to anyone interested in improving athletic performance (see chapter 21). However, when planning competitive training programs for special populations, there are several specific issues that require individual consideration. For instance, there are special training concerns for both the female athlete and children. Also, there are specific guidelines for the training of diabetics, asthmatics, and epileptics. It is the purpose of this chapter to address each of these issues. Let's begin our discussion with the topic of exercise training for the female athlete.

Factors Important to Women Involved in Vigorous Training

Involvement of large numbers of women in competitive athletics has been a recent phenomenon. Over the past two decades, the number of women that are actively engaged in competitive athletics has increased exponentially. Unfortunately, many of the decisions regarding the participation of women in sports and exercise programs have been made on the basis of limited, or absent, physiological information. Research concerning women and exercise was scarce until recent years. Although many questions concerning the female athlete remain to be answered, current research indicates that there is no reason to limit the healthy female athlete from active participation in endurance or power sports (23). In fact, the general responses of females to exercise and training are essentially the same as those described for males (35) with the exception that exercise thermoregulation is moderately impaired in female athletes during the luteal phase of the menstrual cycle (37). The fact that men and women respond to exercise training in a similar manner is logical since the same cellular mechanisms that regulate most physiological and biochemical responses to exercise are the same for both sexes. However, there are several specific concerns related to female participation in vigorous training. In this section we will discuss four key issues related to the female athlete: (1) exercise and the menstrual cycle, (2) eating disorders, (3) bone mineral disorders, and (4) exercise during pregnancy.

Figure 22.1

The relationship between training distance and the incidence of amenorrhea. Notice that as the training distance increases, there is a direct increase in the incidence of amenorrhea.

Exercise and Menstrual Disorders

Over the past several years there have been increasing reports concerning the influence of intense exercise training on the length of the menstrual cycle (11, 12, 17, 19, 22, 33). Indeed, there are numerous reports in the literature of female athletes who experience "athletic" amenorrhea. The term **amenorrhea** refers to a cessation of menstruation, and is generally defined as less than four menses per year (31).

How common is athletic amenorrhea? It appears that the incidence of amenorrhea is higher in some activities than in others. For example, the occurrence of irregular menses is rather high in distance running and ballet dancing, while much lower incidences are reported for swimming and cycling (3, 31). Dale (11) reports that the incidence of amenorrhea in the general population is approximately 3 percent, while the incidence in distance runners is 24 percent.

What causes menstrual cycle dysfunction in athletes? The current belief is that the cause may vary between individual athletes and is probably due to multiple factors. Although some studies linked a low percentage of body fat with athletic amenorrhea (31), recent evidence does not fully support the notion that low body fat is the principal cause of amenorrhea (19, 43). Whatever the cause of amenorrhea in athletes, it appears to be related to the total amount of training (6, 17, 32). Figure 22.1 illustrates this point. As the weekly training distance increases, the incidence of athletic amenorrhea increases in proportion to the increase in training stress. This finding can be interpreted to mean that too much training either directly or indirectly influences the incidence of amenorrhea. There are at least two ways in which training might influence normal reproductive function. First, exercise alters blood concentrations of numerous hormones (26) which may result in a modification of feedback to the hypothalamus (chapter 5). This, in turn, may influence the release of female reproductive hormones and therefore modify the menstrual cycle (31). A second possibility is that high training mileage may result in increased psychological stress. Psychological stress may disrupt the menstrual cycle by increasing blood levels of catecholamines or endogenous opiates which play a role in regulating the reproductive system (31). For a review of the reproductive system and exercise in women see Loucks et al. (1992) in the suggested reading list.

Training and Menstruation

The consensus opinion among physicians is that there is little reason for the healthy female athlete to avoid training or competition during menses (23). Indeed, evidence exists that outstanding performances and world records have been established during all phases of the menstrual cycle (13). Therefore, it is not recommended that the female athlete alter her training or competitive schedule because of menses.

Dysmenorrhea (painful menstruation) is one of the greatest concerns of the female athlete. Several reports show that the incidence of dysmenorrhea is higher in athletic populations than nonathletic groups (23). The explanation for this observation is unknown. However, it is possible that prostaglandins (a type of naturally occurring fatty acid) are responsible for dysmenorrhea in both athletes and nonathletes. The release of prostaglandins begins just prior to the onset of menstrual flow, and may last for two to three days after menses begins. These prostaglandins cause the smooth muscle in the uterus to contract, which in turn causes ischemia (reduced blood flow) and pain (23).

Although athletes who experience dysmenorrhea can continue to train, this is often difficult since physical activity may increase the discomfort. Athletes who experience severe dysmenorrhea should see a physician for treatment. Hale (23) reports that athletes often experience a reduction in dysmenorrhea pain with the use of antiprostaglandin drugs. These drugs are considered safe and can be taken without interrupting training schedules.

The Female Athlete and Eating Disorders

The low social acceptance for individuals with a high percentage of body fat and an emphasis on having the "perfect" body have increased the incidence of eating

Figure 22.2
Warning signs for anorexia nervosa.

disorders. Two of the more common ones that affect young adults are anorexia nervosa and bulimia. Because of the relatively high occurrence of these eating disorders in female athletes, we discuss both the symptoms and health consequences of these abnormal eating behaviors.

Anorexia Nervosa

Anorexia nervosa is a common eating disorder that is unrelated to any specific physical disease. The end result of extreme anorexia nervosa is a state of starvation in which the individual becomes emaciated due to a refusal to eat. The psychological cause of anorexia nervosa is unclear, but it seems to be linked to an unfounded fear of fatness that may be related to family or societal pressures to be thin (44). The incidence of this eating disorder has grown in recent years. It appears that individuals with the highest probability of developing anorexia nervosa are upper-middle class young females who are extremely self critical. Currently, it is estimated that the incidence of anorexia nervosa is as high as one out of every 200 adolescent girls (1b, 4a).

The anorexic may use a variety of techniques to remain thin including starvation, exercise, and laxatives. The effects of anorexia include excessive weight loss, cessation of menstruation, and, in extreme cases, death. Since anorexia is a serious mental and physical disorder, medical treatment by a team of professionals (physician, psychologist, nutritionist) is necessary to correct the problem. Treatment may require years of psychological counseling and nutritional guidance. The first step in seeking professional treatment for anorexia nervosa is the recognition that a problem exists. Figure 22.2 illustrates the common symptoms of anorexia.

Warning signs for bulimia

- Noticeable weight loss
- Excessive concern about weight
- Bathroom visits after meals
- Depressive moods
- Strict dieting followed by eating binges
- Increasing criticism of one's body

Figure 22.3
Warning signs for bulimia.

Bulimia

Bulimia is overeating (called binge eating) followed by vomiting (called purging). The bulimic repeatedly ingests large quantities of food and then forces himself or herself to vomit in order to prevent weight gain. Bulimia may result in damage to the teeth and the esophagus due to vomiting of stomach acids. Like anorexia nervosa, bulimia is most common in female athletes, has a psychological origin, and requires professional treatment when diagnosed. Several authors indicate that the incidence of bulimia may be as low as 1 percent or as high as 20 percent among U.S. females aged 13–23 years (1b, 4a).

Most bulimics look normal and are of normal weight. Even when their bodies are slender, their abdomens may protrude due to being stretched by frequent eating binges. Common symptoms of bulimia are illustrated in figure 22.3.

Eating Disorders: A Final Comment

Eating disorders have become a major problem in female athletes. Some experts have estimated that as many as 50 percent of elite female athletes experience some type of eating disorder. The sports with the highest incidence of eating disorders are distance running, swimming, diving, figure skating, gymnastics, body building, and ballet. Although maintaining an optimal body composition for competition is important to achieve athletic success, eating disorders are not an appropriate means of weight loss. Therefore, trainers, athletes, and coaches need to recognize the warning signals of eating disorders and be prepared to assist the athlete in obtaining the appropriate help.

Bone Mineral Disorders and the Female Athlete

A growing concern for the female athlete is the loss of bone mineral content (osteoporosis). In general, there are two major causes of bone loss in the female athlete (14a, 14b):

1. estrogen deficiency due to amenorrhea and
2. inadequate calcium intake due to eating disorders.

Unfortunately, many female athletes suffer a bone loss due to both amenorrhea and the inadequate calcium intake associated with an eating disorder (14a, 14b). Although exercise training has been shown to reduce the rate of bone loss due to estrogen deficiency and low calcium intake, exercise cannot completely reverse this process (34a). Therefore, the only solution to the problem of bone mineral loss in the female athlete is to correct the estrogen deficiency and/or increase the calcium intake to normal levels. In both cases, a physician should be involved in prescribing the correct treatment for the individual athlete.

Training During Pregnancy

Chapter 17 provided a brief overview of what is currently known about exercising for fitness during pregnancy. While it is generally agreed that women who are physically fit prior to becoming pregnant may continue to perform moderate intensity (short duration) exercise during pregnancy (5, 9, 14, 27, 30, 34a, 39a), controversy exists concerning the wisdom of high-intensity training for pregnant women. Although controversial, some animal studies have demonstrated that long-duration exercise (more than thirty minutes) during pregnancy results in a reduction in both uterine blood flow and fetal weight at term (10, 20, 36, 41). For example, one study reported that placental diffusion capacity decreases as a direct function of both the duration and intensity of exercise during pregnancy (20). At present it is unclear if these results can be extrapolated to humans since pregnant women have performed maximal exercise with no apparent adverse effects on fetal or maternal outcome (8). However, because of the limited number of studies examining the effect of heavy exercise on the health of mother and baby, more research is needed before firm exercise guidelines can be established. Until a definitive answer to this question is available, Hale (23) has recommended that the pregnant female be discouraged from engaging in prolonged or high-intensity training. For those athletes wishing to maintain fitness during pregnancy, Hale recommends aquatic programs, since swimming or other forms of aquatic exercise allows cardiovascular training in a medium that offers the

A Closer Look 22.1

The Female Athlete Triad

It is generally accepted that the three most common health problems facing the young female athlete are:

1. amenorrhea,
2. eating disorders, and
3. bone mineral loss.

Collectively, these problems have been called the "female athlete triad" (45). Current evidence suggests that these problems are interrelated

and that one problem can potentially lead to another. For example, an eating disorder can lead to inadequate nutrient and calcium intake and eating disorders are known to promote amenorrhea. Long-term amenorrhea can result in low blood estrogen levels. The combination of inadequate calcium intake and low estrogen levels can result in a loss of bone mineral content.

At present, researchers do not completely understand the interrelationships between these three major problems facing the female athlete. The challenge for future research in this area is to develop a means of preventing the initiation of the female athlete triad and improving the treatment of each of these problems after they develop.

body support and accelerated heat transfer. Specific guidelines for exercise to maintain fitness during pregnancy were listed in chapter 17 (table 17.3).

in summary

- The incidence of amenorrhea in female athletes appears to be highest in distance runners and ballet dancers when compared to other sports. Although the cause of amenorrhea in female athletes is not clear, it appears likely that multiple factors (e.g., the amount of training and psychological stress) are involved.
- There appears to be little reason for female athletes to avoid training during menstruation unless they experience severe discomfort due to dysmenorrhea. Athletes who experience severe dysmenorrhea should see a physician for treatment.
- Some experts have estimated that as many as 50 percent of elite female athletes experience some type of eating disorder. Two of the more common eating disorders are anorexia nervosa and bulimia.
- The three most common health problems facing the young female athlete are amenorrhea, eating disorders, and bone mineral loss; collectively, these problems have been called the "female athlete triad."
- Short-term, low-intensity exercise does not appear to have negative consequences during pregnancy. However, data suggest that long-duration or high-intensity training should be avoided during pregnancy.

Sports Conditioning for Children

There are many unanswered questions related to the physiologic responses of the healthy child to various types of exercise. This is due to the limited number of investigators studying children and exercise, and because of ethical considerations in studying children. For instance, few investigators would puncture a child's artery, take a muscle biopsy, or expose a child to harsh environments (e.g., heat, cold, high altitudes) to satisfy scientific curiosity. Because of these ethical constraints, current knowledge concerning training for children is limited primarily to the cardiopulmonary system, with a growing body of information concerning the possibility of musculoskeletal injury as a result of specific types of sports training. The following discussion addresses some of the important issues concerning child participation in vigorous conditioning programs.

Training and the Cardiopulmonary System

As youth sports teams increase in popularity, one of the first questions asked is "Are the hearts of children strong enough for intensive sports conditioning?" In other words, is there a possibility of "overtraining" young athletes, with the end result being permanent damage to the cardiovascular system? The answer to this question is "no." Children involved in endurance sports such as running or swimming improve their maximal aerobic power comparable to adults and show no indices of damage to the cardiopulmonary system (15, 16, 24, 38a). Over the past several years, children have safely trained and completed marathon runs in less than four hours. If proper techniques of physical training are employed, with a progressive increase in cardiopulmonary stress, children appear to adapt to endurance training in a fashion similar to adults (15, 16, 34, 38a).

Training and the Musculoskeletal System

Organized vigorous training in some types of sports (e.g., swimming, basketball, volleyball, track and field) does not appear to adversely affect growth and development in children (34). This is true for both boys (16) and girls (2). In fact, moderate physical training has been shown to augment or optimize growth in children (1, 2, 15, 16). Therefore, many investigators have concluded that a certain amount of physical activity is necessary for normal growth and development (1, 2, 34). However, is there danger of overtraining? Can children perform heavy endurance training or strength training without long-term musculoskeletal problems? This issue remains controversial. There is evidence that the growing bones of a child are more susceptible to certain types of mechanical injury than those of the adult, primarily because of the presence of growth cartilage (34). Growth cartilage is present at the growth plate **(epiphyseal plate), articular cartilage** (cartilage at joints), and the sites of major muscle-tendon insertion in the child (34). The location of the growth plate, for the knee joint is illustrated in figure 22.4. The growth plate is the site of bone growth in long bones. The time at which bone growth ceases varies from bone to bone, but is generally complete by eighteen to twenty years of age (34). Upon completion of growth, growth plates ossify (harden with calcium) and disappear, and growth cartilage is replaced by a permanent "adult" cartilage.

Is there an optimal level of training for children, above which musculoskeletal injuries may occur? The apparent answer to this question is "yes." Clinical evidence suggests that excessive throwing in organized youth league baseball may result in injury to the elbow (Little League elbow) (34). This same problem is not observed in free-play situations (34). Indeed, new injury patterns are developing in children as the number of children participating in organized sports increases (1a). A recent statement from the American College of Sports Medicine indicated that up to 50 percent of all injuries sustained by children while playing organized sports could be avoided by attention to proper training techniques, safety procedures, and proper use of safety equipment (1a).

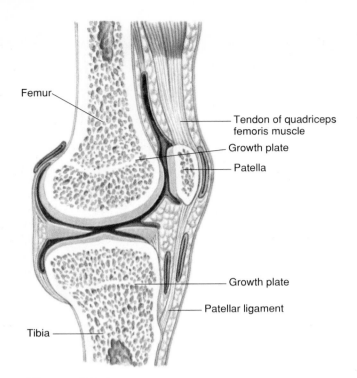

Figure 22.4
Location of the growth plate (epiphyseal plate) associated with the long bones in the leg.

A major concern for children participating in endurance training (e.g., running) or strength training (e.g., weight lifting) is that the constant microtrauma of repetitive training can cause premature closure of the growth plate and therefore retard normal long bone growth. Experimental literature on training and specific bone lengths indicates reduced bone lengths in rats and mice exposed to forced swimming and running (34). Corresponding data on humans do not exist. However, given the evidence available on the influence of physical activity on bone growth and development, it appears that the advice Steinhaus (39) offered over fifty years ago is sound. That is, the pressure effects of regular physical activity may stimulate bone growth to an optimal length, but excessive pressure (overtraining) can retard linear growth. The practical problem in dealing with young athletes is that it is difficult to define excessive pressure. In other words, how much training is optimal to bring about the desired physiological training responses without causing musculoskeletal problems? At present, a simple answer to this question is not available. There is an obvious need for detailed research in this area to produce guidelines for youth coaches and trainers in the development of conditioning programs for children engaged in competitive athletics.

in summary

- Although physical activity has been shown to optimize growth in children, questions remain as to the possibility of overtraining with resultant injuries to the musculoskeletal system. In particular, there is evidence that the growing bones of children are more susceptible to certain types of mechanical injury due to the presence of growth cartilage.

Competitive Training for Diabetics

As discussed in chapter 17, there is a beneficial effect of exercise on diabetes, and physicians often recommend regular exercise for diabetics as a part of their therapeutic regimen (i.e., to help maintain control of blood glucose levels) (18). We will limit our discussion to Type I diabetics since Type II diabetics are less likely to engage in training for performance purposes. Can Type I diabetics train vigorously and take part in competitive athletics? The answer to this question is a qualified yes. In long-term diabetic patients with microvascular complications (damage to small blood vessels) or neuropathy (nerve damage), exercise should be limited and extensive training is not generally recommended (34). However, in individuals who maintain good blood glucose control and are free from other medical complications, diabetes in itself should not limit the type of exercise or sporting event (40).

What precautions should the diabetic athlete take to allow safe participation in training programs? An overview of exercise training for fitness in diabetic populations was presented in chapter 17 and will be reviewed here only briefly. The key to safe participation in sport conditioning for the diabetic athlete is to learn to avoid hypoglycemic episodes during training. Since diabetics vary in their response to insulin, each diabetic athlete, in cooperation with his or her personal physician, must determine the appropriate combination of exercise, diet, and insulin for optimal control of blood glucose concentrations. In general, exercise should take place after a meal and should be part of regular routine. It is often recommended that a reduction in the amount of insulin injected be considered on days in which the athlete is engaged in strenuous training (18, 38, 40). A major concern for the diabetic athlete is the site of the insulin injection prior to exercise. Insulin injected subcutaneously in the leg prior to running (or other forms of leg exercise) results in an increased rate of insulin uptake due to elevated leg blood flow. This could result in exercise-induced hypoglycemia and may be avoided by using an insulin injection site in the abdomen or the arm (40). Conversely, if the training regimen requires arm exercise (e.g., rowing), the site of insulin injection should be away from the working muscle (e.g., abdomen). Having a glucose solution or carbohydrate snack available during training sessions may help avoid hypoglycemic incidents during workouts.

Can diabetics obtain the same benefits from training as nondiabetics? The consensus answer to this question is yes. Although untrained diabetic children tend to be less fit than normal children, young diabetics respond to a conditioning program in a manner similar to healthy children (34). Empirical observations suggest that when the diabetic athlete's blood glucose is carefully regulated, he or she can compete and excel in a variety of competitive sports.

in summary

- Type I diabetics who are free of diabetic complications should not be limited in the type or quantity of exercise.
- The key for safe sports participation for the Type I diabetic is for the athlete to learn to avoid hypoglycemic episodes.

Training for Asthmatics

It is generally agreed that most children, adolescents, and adults with asthma may safely participate in all sports with the exception of SCUBA diving, provided they are able to control exercise-induced bronchospasms via medication or careful monitoring of activity levels (10a, 34). A prerequisite for planning training programs for asthmatics is that the proper therapeutic regimen for managing the athlete's particular type of asthma be worked out prior to commencement of a vigorous training program (chapter 17). Once the asthma is under control, planning the training schedule for asthmatic athletes is identical to that prescribed for athletes without asthma (chapter 21). However, as mentioned in chapter 17, it is often recommended that the asthmatic athlete keep an inhaler (containing a bronchodilator) handy during training sessions, and that workouts be conducted with other athletes in case a major attack occurs.

The issue of the safety of an asthmatic participating in SCUBA diving continues to be debated. The controversy centers around the fact that divers who experience an asthma attack while diving are at high risk for pulmonary barotrauma (damage to the lung due to high pressure) (10a). However, a recent review on the subject suggests that asthmatics with normal airway function at rest, and who do not exhibit exercise-induced asthma, have a risk of barotrauma during diving similar to healthy individuals (10a).

in summary

- Asthmatics can safely participate in all sports with the possible exception of SCUBA diving, provided they are able to control exercise-induced bronchospasms via medication or careful monitoring of activity levels.
- The question of the safety of an asthmatic participating in SCUBA diving continues to be unanswered. Nonetheless, recent evidence suggests that asthmatics who do not exhibit exercise-induced asthma and have normal airways at rest, are at no greater risk during diving than healthy individuals.

Epilepsy and Physical Training

The term **epilepsy** refers to a transient disturbance of brain function, which may be characterized by a loss of consciousness, muscle tremor, and sensory disturbances. Since the occurrence of epileptic seizures are not easily predicted, should epileptics engage in vigorous training programs? Unfortunately, there is little information available to answer this question. Before a clear-cut recommendation for the participation of epileptics in athletics can be made, two fundamental questions must be answered. First, does intense physical activity increase the risk of an epileptic seizure? Secondly, does the occurrence of a seizure during a particular sports activity expose the athlete to unnecessary risk? Let's examine the available evidence concerning each of these questions.

Does Exercise Promote Seizures?

There is one rare type of epileptic seizure that has been shown to be induced by exercise per se (7). These are tonic (continuous motor activity) seizures, which have been reported to occur during a variety of sports activities. Fortunately, this particular type of seizure can be controlled in most instances by anticonvulsant drugs.

As for other types of seizure disorders, physicians remain divided in their opinions as to whether exercise increases the risk of seizure occurrence. A report by Gotze et al. (21) suggests that exercise does not increase the risk of seizures in epileptic children or adolescents. In fact, Gotze (21) argues that exercise appears to reduce the incidence of seizures in epileptics by increasing the threshold for seizures. In support of these claims, a recent review (42) on epilepsy and sports has concluded that there is a reduction in the number of seizures during exercise. In contrast, Kuijer (28) has suggested that the epileptic is at an increased risk of experiencing a seizure during exercise and during recovery from exercise. In this regard, several factors related to exercise have been hypothesized to increase the risk of seizures (42): (1) physical fatigue, (2) hyperventilation, (3) hypoxia, (4) hyperthermia, (5) hypoglycemia, and (6) electrolyte imbalance. In conclusion, division exists in the medical community concerning the risk of exercise and seizures. It seems logical that generalizations about exercise and the epileptic patient cannot be made. Each patient is unique concerning the type, frequency, and severity of epileptic seizures. Therefore, physicians, parents, and coaches must make a case-by-case decision on the wisdom of competitive sports for individual patients.

Another specific concern for the participation of epileptics in contact sports is whether a blow to the head might mediate a seizure. Again, physicians remain divided in their opinions. Some authors believe the risks are high (25), while Livingston (29) argues that no studies exist to prove that repeated head trauma in epileptics causes a recurrence of seizures. Livingston's argument is based on thirty-six years of personal experience with hundreds of seizure patients who have participated in a variety of contact sports such as football, wrestling, and even boxing. While all of these contact sports predispose the athlete to head trauma, Livingston (29) states that he has not observed a single case where recurrent seizures occurred due to head trauma.

Risk of Injury Due to Seizures

Clearly, there are many competitive sports activities (e.g., football, boxing) during which the occurrence of a seizure would expose the athlete to a risk of harm. However, the occurrence of a seizure during many types of daily routine activities (e.g., climbing stairs) or recreational sports (e.g., SCUBA diving, mountain climbing) could also pose a threat to the epileptic. Whether or not the epileptic should participate in physical training or sports must be determined on an individual basis by the use of common sense and advice from a sports physician. The benefit-risk ratio of sports participation may vary greatly from case to case and is dependent on the exact nature of the patient's epilepsy and the sport being considered. A child with only a minor seizure problem may, with the aid of medication, experience only a rare seizure with little visible alteration in behavior or consciousness due to the seizure. This type of epileptic could likely participate in most training activities without harm (4, 21). In contrast, an epileptic who experiences frequent and major seizures would not be a candidate for many types of sports. For a detailed discussion of epilepsy and exercise, see van Linschoten et al. (42).

in summary

- Questions about safe participation for epileptics in training programs must be answered on an individual basis. The benefit-risk ratio of sports participation may vary greatly from case to case, and is dependent on the type of epilepsy involved and the sport being considered.

study questions

1. Outline several possible causes of "athletic" amenorrhea.
2. What is the current recommendation for training and competition during menstruation?
3. Discuss the role of prostaglandins in mediating dysmenorrhea.
4. Based on present information, what are reasonable guidelines for advising the pregnant athlete concerning the intensity and duration of training?
5. Define the female athlete triad.
6. What factors contribute to bone mineral loss in the female athlete?
7. Discuss the notion that intense exercise might result in permanent damage to (a) the cardiovascular system or (b) musculoskeletal system in children.
8. What is the recommendation for Type I diabetics with no physical complications for entering a competitive training program?
9. What factors should be considered when advising the diabetic athlete concerning safe participation in athletic conditioning? Include in your discussion suggestions concerning meal timing, injection sites for insulin, and the availability of glucose drinks during training sessions.
10. What is the current opinion concerning the safe participation of asthmatics in competitive athletics?
11. Define the term *epilepsy*.
12. Discuss the possibility that exercise increases the risk of seizures for epileptics.
13. What factors should be considered in assessing the risk-to-benefit ratio of sports participation for epileptics?

suggested readings

American College of Sports Medicine. 1993. Current comment on the prevention of sport injuries of children and adolescents. *Medicine and Science in Sports and Exercise* 25(Suppl.): 1–7.

Bell, R. et al. 1994. Exercise and pregnancy: A review. *Birth* 21:85–95.

Cypcar, D., and R. Lemanske. 1994. Asthma and exercise. *Clinics in Chest Medicine* 15:351–68.

De Souza, M., and D. Metzger. 1991. Reproductive dysfunction in amenorrheic athletes and anorexic patients: A review. *Medicine and Science in Sports and Exercise* 23:995–1007.

Loucks, A. et al. 1992. The reproductive system and exercise in women. *Medicine and Science in Sports and Exercise* 24:S288–S293.

van Linschoten, R. et al. 1990. Epilepsy and sports. *Sports Medicine* 10:9–19.

references

1. Adams, E. 1938. A comparative anthropometric study of hard labor during youth as a stimulator of physical growth of young colored women. *Research Quarterly* 9:102–8.
1a. American College of Sports Medicine. 1993. Current comment on the prevention of sport injuries of children and adolescents. *Medicine and Science in Sports and Exercise* 25 (Suppl.):1–7.
1b. Andersen, A. Anorexia nervosa and bulimia. *Journal of Adolescent Health Care* 4:15–21, 1983.
2. Åstrand, P. O. et al. 1963. Girl swimmers. *Acta Paediatric Scandanavica* 147(Suppl.):1–75.
3. Baker, E. 1981. Menstrual dysfunction and hormonal status in athletic women: A review. *Fertility and Sterility* 36:691–96.
4. Bennett, D. 1981. Sports and epilepsy: To play or not to play. *Seminars in Neurology* 1:345–57.
4a. Borgen, J., and C. Corbin. 1987. Eating disorders among female athletes. *Physician and Sportsmedicine* 15:89–95.
5. Bullard, J. 1981. Exercise and pregnancy. *Canadian Family Physician* 27:977–82.
6. Bullen, B. et al. 1985. Induction of menstrual disorders by strenuous exercise in untrained women. *New England Journal of Medicine* 312:1349–53.
7. Burger, L., R. Lopez, and F. Elliot. 1972. Tonic seizures induced by movement. *Neurology* 22:656–59.
8. Carpenter, M. et al. 1988. Fetal heart rate response to maternal exertion. *Journal of the American Medical Association* 259:3006.
9. Clapp, J. et al. 1992. Exercise in pregnancy. *Medicine and Science in Sports and Exercise* 24:S294–S300.
10. Curet, L. et al. 1976. Effect of exercise on cardiac output and distribution of uterine blood flow in pregnant ewes. *Journal of Applied Physiology* 40:725–28.
10a. Cypcar, D., and R. Lemanske. 1994. Asthma and exercise. *Clinics in Chest Medicine* 15:351–68.
11. Dale, E., D. Gerlach, and A. Wilhute. 1979. Menstrual dysfunction in distance runners. *Obstetrics and Gynecology* 54:47–53.
12. Dale, E. et al. 1979. Physical fitness profiles and reproductive physiology of the female distance runner. *Physician and Sportsmedicine* 7:83–95.
13. De Souza, M., and D. Metzger. 1991. Reproductive dysfunction in amenorrheic athletes and anorexic patients: A review. *Medicine and Science in Sports and Exercise* 23:995–1007.
14. Dressendorfer, R. 1978. Physical training during pregnancy and lactation. *Physician and Sportsmedicine* 6:74–80.
14a. Drinkwater, B. 1990. Menstrual history as a determinant of current bone density in young athletes. *Journal of the American Medical Association* 263:545–48.

14b. Drinkwater, B. et al. 1984. Bone minerial content of amenorrheic and eumenorrheic athletes. *New England Journal of Medicine* 311:277–81.

15. Ekblom, B. 1969. Effect of physical training on oxygen transport system in man. *Acta Physiologica Scandanavica* 328(Suppl.):1–45.

16. Eriksson, B. 1972. Physical training, oxygen supply and muscle metabolism in 11–13 year-old boys. *Acta Physiologica Scandanavica* 384(Suppl.):1–48.

17. Feicht, C. et al. 1978. Secondary amenorrhea in athletes. *Lancet* 2:1145–46.

18. Felig, P., and V. Koivisto. 1979. The metabolic response to exercise: Implications for diabetes. In *Therapeutics through Exercise*, eds. D. Lowenthal, K. Bharadwaja, and W. Oaks. New York: Grune & Stratton.

19. Galle, P. et al. 1983. Physiologic and psychologic profiles in a survey of women runners. *Fertility and Sterility* 39:633–39.

20. Gilbert, R. et al. 1979. Placental diffusing capacity and fetal development in exercising or hypoxic guinea pigs. *Journal of Applied Physiology* 46:828–34.

21. Gotze, W., S. Kubicki, and M. Munter. 1967. Effect of physical activity on seizure threshold investigated by electroencephalographic telemetry. *Diseases of the Nervous System* 28:664–67.

22. Gray, D., and E. Dale. 1983. Variables associated with secondary amenorrhea in women runners. *Journal of Sports Sciences* 1:55–67.

23. Hale, R. 1984. Factors important to women engaged in vigorous physical activity. In *Sports Medicine*, ed. R. Strauss. Philadelphia: W. B. Saunders.

24. Ingjer, F. 1992. Development of maximal oxygen uptake in young elite cross-country skiers: A longitudinal study. *Journal of Sports Sciences* 10:49–63.

25. Jennett, B. 1974. Early traumatic epilepsy: Incidence and significance after non-muscle injuries. *Archives of Neurology* 30:394–98.

26. Jurkowski, J. et al. 1978. Ovarian hormonal responses to exercise. *Journal of Applied Physiology* 44:109–14.

27. Kolata, G. 1983. Exercise during pregnancy reassessed. *Science* 219:832–33.

28. Kuijer, A. 1980. Epilepsy and exercise, electroencephalographical and biochemical studies. In *Advances in Epileptology: The X Epilepsy International Symposium*, eds. J. Wada and J. Penry. New York: Raven Press.

29. Livingston, S., and W. Berman. 1973. Participation of epileptic patients in sports. *Journal of American Medical Association* 224:236–38.

30. Lokey, E. et al. 1991. Effects of physical exercise on pregnancy outcomes: A meta-analytic review. *Medicine and Science in Sports and Exercise* 23:1234–39.

31. Loucks, A., and S. Horvath. 1985. Athletic amenorrhea: A review. *Medicine and Science in Sports and Exercise* 17:56–72.

32. Loucks, A. et al. 1992. The reproductive system and exercise in women. *Medicine and Science in Sports and Exercise* 24:S288–S293.

33. Lutter, J., and S. Cushman. 1982. Menstrual patterns in female runners. *Physician and Sportsmedicine* 10:60–72.

34. Micheli, L. 1984. *Pediatric and Adolescent Sports Medicine*. Philadelphia: W. B. Saunders.

34a. Micklesfield, L. et al. 1995. Bone mineral density in mature, premenopausal ultramarathon runners. *Medicine and Science in Sports and Exercise* 27:688–96.

35. Mitchell, J. et al. 1992. Acute response and chronic adaptation to exercise in women. *Medicine and Science in Sports and Exercise* 24:S258–S265.

36. Nelson, P., R. Gilbert, and L. Longo. 1983. Fetal growth and placental diffusing capacity in guinea pigs following long-term maternal exercise. *Journal of Developmental Physiology* 5:1–10.

36a. Neuman, T. et al. 1994. Asthma and diving. *Annals of Allergy* 73:344–50.

37. Pivarnik, J. et al. 1992. Menstrual cycle phase affects temperature regulation during endurance exercise. *Journal of Applied Physiology* 72:543–48.

38. Pruett, E. 1985. Insulin and exercise in the non-diabetic man. In *Exercise Physiology*, eds. K. Fotherly and S. Pal. New York: Walter de Gruyter.

38a. Rowland, T. 1992. Trainability of the cardiorespiratory system during childhood. *Canadian Journal of Sports Sciences* 17:259–63.

39. Steinhaus, A. 1933. Chronic effects of exercise. *Physiological Review* 13:103–47.

39a. Sternfeld, B. et al. 1995. Exercise during pregnancy and pregnancy outcome. *Medicine and Science in Sports and Exercise* 27:634–40.

40. Sutton, J. 1984. Metabolic responses to exercise in normal and diabetic individuals. In *Sports Medicine*, ed. R. Strauss. Philadelphia: W. B. Saunders.

41. Terada, J. 1974. Effect of physical activity before pregnancy on fetuses of mice exercised forcibly during pregnancy. *Teratology* 10:141–44.

42. van Linschoten, R. et al. 1990. Epilepsy and sports. *Sports Medicine* 10:9–19.

43. Warren, M. 1980. The effects of exercise on pubertal progression and reproductive function in girls. *Journal of Clinical Endocrinology and Metabolism* 51:1150–57.

44. Williams, M. *Lifetime Fitness and Wellness*. 1996. Dubuque, IA: Wm. C. Brown.

45. Wilmore, J. 1991. Eating and weight disorders in the female athlete. *Internation Journal of Sports Medicine* 1:104–17.

Nutrition, Body Composition, and Performance

objectives

By studying this chapter, you should be able to do the following:

1. Describe the effect of various carbohydrate diets on muscle glycogen and on endurance performance during heavy exercise.
2. Contrast the "classic" method of achieving a supercompensation of the muscle glycogen stores with the "modified" method.
3. Describe some potential problems when glucose is ingested immediately prior to exercise.
4. Describe the importance of blood glucose as a fuel in prolonged exercise, and the role of carbohydrate supplementation during the performance.
5. Contrast the evidence that protein is oxidized at a faster rate during exercise with the evidence that the use of labeled amino acids may be an inappropriate methodology to study this issue.
6. Describe the need for protein *during* the adaptation to a new, more strenuous exercise level with the protein need when the adaptation is complete.
7. Defend the recommendation that a protein intake that is 12%–15% of energy intake is sufficient to meet an athlete's need.
8. Describe the recommended fluid replacement strategies for athletic events of different intensities and durations, citing evidence to support your position.
9. Describe the salt requirement of the athlete, compared to the sedentary individual, and the recommended means of maintaining sodium balance.
10. List the steps leading to iron deficiency anemia and the special problem that athletes have in maintaining iron balance.
11. Provide a brief summary of the effects of vitamin supplementation on performance.
12. Characterize the role of the pregame meal on performance and the rationale for limiting fats and proteins.
13. Describe the various components of the somatotype and what the following ratings signify: 171, 711, and 117.
14. Describe what the endomorphic and mesomorphic components in the Heath-Carter method of somatotyping represent in conventional body composition analysis.
15. Explain why one must be careful in recommending specific body fatness values for individual athletes.

outline

Nutrition and Performance   420
   Carbohydrate   420
   Protein   423
   Water and Electrolytes   426
   Minerals   429

   Vitamins   430
   Pregame Meal   431
Body Composition and
   Performance   432
   Somatotype   432

Body Fatness and
   Performance   434

T his chapter on nutrition, body composition, and performance is an extension of chapter 18, since the primary emphasis must be on achieving health-related goals before performance-related goals are examined. In fact, the information presented here must be examined in light of what the average person needs. Does an athlete need additional protein? What percent body fat is a reasonable goal for an athlete? We will address these questions in that order.

Nutrition and Performance

The nutritional goals of the United States were identified in chapter 18 and are restated here:

Dietary Goals for Health
58% Carbohydrate
30% Fat
12% Protein

The dietary changes required for performance will be discussed relative to these dietary goals needed for health.

Carbohydrate

The dietary goals associated with health recommend that we increase the percent of calories derived from carbohydrate to about 58%. Both Brotherhood (7) and Sherman (73) report that the average percent of carbohydrate in an athlete's diet is only about 50%, which is surprisingly low given the importance of carbohydrate in prolonged moderate to heavy exercise (see chapter 4). This section will consider the use of carbohydrates in the days prior to a performance and, secondly, during the performance itself.

Carbohydrate Diets and Performance

In 1967, three studies were published from the same Swedish laboratory that set the stage for our understanding of the role of muscle glycogen in performance (1, 6, 50). Hermansen et al. (50) showed muscle glycogen to be systematically depleted during heavy (77% $\dot{V}O_2$ max) exercise, and when exhaustion occurred, glycogen content was near zero. Ahlborg et al. (1) found that work time to exhaustion was directly related to the initial glycogen store in the working muscles. Bergstrom et al. (6) confirmed and extended this

by showing that by manipulating the quantity of carbohydrate in the diet the concentration of glycogen in muscle could be altered and, along with it, the time to exhaustion. In their study subjects consumed 2,800 kcal/d using either a low CHO (fat and protein) diet, a mixed diet, or a high-carbohydrate diet in which 2,300 kcal came from carbohydrate. Glycogen contents of the quadriceps femoris muscle were, respectively, 0.63 (low), 1.75 (average), and 3.31 (high) gm/100 g muscle, and performance time for exercise at 75% $\dot{V}O_2$ max averaged 57, 114, and 167 minutes. Figure 23.1 shows these results. In brief, the muscle glycogen content and performance time could be varied with diet. These laboratory findings were confirmed by Karlsson and Saltin (54), who had trained subjects run a 30-km race twice, once following a high-carbohydrate diet and the other time after a mixed diet. The initial muscle glycogen level was 3.5 gm/100 g muscle following the CHO diet and 1.7 gm/100 g muscle following the mixed diet. The best performance of all subjects occurred during the high CHO diet. Interestingly, the pace at the start of the race was not faster; instead, the additional CHO allowed them to maintain the pace for a longer period of time. An important finding in this study was that compared to the high CHO diet, pace did not fall off for those on the mixed diet until about halfway through the race (about one hour or so). This suggests that the normal mixed diet used in their study would be suitable for run or cycle races lasting less than one hour.

Given the importance of muscle glycogen in prolonged endurance performance, it is no surprise that investigators have tried to determine what conditions will yield the highest muscle glycogen content. In 1966 Bergstrom and Hultman (5) had subjects do one-legged exercise to exhaust the glycogen store in the exercised leg while not affecting the resting leg's glycogen store. When this procedure was followed with a high-carbohydrate diet, the glycogen content was more than twice as high in the previously exercised leg, compared to the control leg. Further, they found that in subjects who had the high-carbohydrate diet following the protein/fat diet (plus doing exhausting exercise), the muscle glycogen stores were higher than when the mixed diet preceded the high-carbohydrate treatment (5). This combination of information led to the following *classical method* of achieving a muscle glycogen **supercompensation:**

- prolonged strenuous exercise to exhaust muscle glycogen store,

Figure 23.1

Effect of different diets on the muscle glycogen concentration and work time to exhaustion.

Figure 23.2

Modification of the classic glycogen loading technique to achieve high muscle glycogen levels with minimal changes in a training or diet routine. Glycogen levels are in glucose units (gu) per kilogram (kg).

- a fat/protein diet for three days while continuing to train, and
- a high-carbohydrate diet (90% CHO) for three days, with inactivity.

There were some practical problems with this approach to achieving a high muscle glycogen content given that it required seven days to prepare for a race. Further, some subjects could not tolerate either the extremely low (high fat and protein) or high (90%) carbohydrate diets. Sherman (72) proposed a *modified plan* that causes supercompensation. The plan requires a tapering of the workout from ninety minutes to forty minutes while eating a 50% CHO diet (350 gm/d). This is followed by two days of twenty-minute workouts while eating a 70% CHO diet (500–600 gm/d) and, finally, a day of rest prior to the competition with the 70% CHO diet (or 500–600 gm/d). This regimen was shown to be effective in increasing the glycogen stores to *high values* consistent with good performance (see figure 23.2). However, what should you do if you need to replenish the glycogen stores quickly following heavy exercise?

The limiting factor in muscle glycogen synthesis is glucose transport across the cell membrane. Following a bout of heavy exercise there is an increase in the muscle cell's permeability to glucose, an increase in glycogen synthase activity, and an increase in the muscle's sensitivity to insulin (53). When these factors are combined with the ingestion of at least 0.75 gm/kg of glucose, muscle glycogen is synthesized at a very high rate. The glucose ingestion needs to be initiated immediately after exercise, and should be repeated each two hours for six hours; a delay of only

two hours slows the rate of synthesis. Glucose or **glucose polymers** are better than fructose for synthesizing muscle glycogen, but some fructose should be ingested since it may be better for the replenishing liver glycogen (36, 53, 73). What is needed for the day-to-day replenishment of muscle glycogen?

It takes about twenty-four hours to replenish muscle glycogen following prolonged moderate exercise, provided that about 500–700 gms of carbohydrate are ingested (18, 36, 53). The point that must be emphasized is that a person who is achieving the dietary goal of 58% of calories from carbohydrate is already consuming what is needed to replace muscle glycogen on a day-to-day basis. If an athlete requires 4,000 kcal per day for caloric balance and 58% is derived from carbohydrates, then 2,320 kcal (58% of 4,000 kcal) or 580 gm of carbohydrate will be consumed. This quantity is consistent with what is needed to restore muscle glycogen to normal levels twenty-four hours after strenuous exercise. This is important for training considerations, and this "regular" diet would require little or no change to meet the carbohydrate load (500–600 gm/d) described by Sherman to achieve supercompensation (72).

in summary

- Performance in endurance events is improved by a diet high in carbohydrates due primarily to the increase in muscle glycogen.
- The recommended dietary goal of 58% of caloric intake as carbohydrate provides for a high muscle glycogen content.
- When workouts are tapered over several days while additional CHO (70% of dietary intake) is consumed, a "supercompensation" of the glycogen store can be achieved.

Carbohydrates Prior to or During a Performance

The focus on muscle glycogen as the primary carbohydrate source in heavy exercise has always diminished the role that blood glucose plays in maintaining carbohydrate oxidation in muscle. In Coggan and Coyle's recent review (14) they correct this perception for exercises that last three to four hours, in which blood glucose and muscle glycogen share equally in contributing to carbohydrate oxidation. In fact, as muscle glycogen decreases, the role that blood glucose plays increases until, at the end of three to four hours of exercise, it may be the sole source of carbohydrate. This is what makes blood glucose an important fuel in prolonged work, and why so much attention has been directed at trying to maintain the blood glucose concentration.

Unfortunately, the liver glycogen supply also decreases with time during prolonged exercise, and because gluconeogenesis can supply glucose at a rate of only 0.2 to 0.4 gm/min when the muscles may be consuming it at a rate of 1 to 2 gm/min, hypoglycemia is a real possibility. Hypoglycemia (blood glucose concentration <2.5 mmoles/liter) results when the rate of blood glucose uptake is not matched by release from the liver and/or small intestine. Hypoglycemia has been shown to occur during exercise at 58% $\dot{V}O_2$ max for 3.5 hours (4) and at 74% $\dot{V}O_2$ max for 2.5 hours (21). However, the number of subjects who demonstrate central nervous system dysfunction varied from none (32) to only 25% of the subjects (21). While there is no absolutely clear association between hypoglycemia and fatigue, the availability of blood glucose as an energy source is, without question, linked to the performance of prolonged (three to four hours) exercise (14). How should carbohydrate be taken in before and during exercise to maintain the high rate of carbohydrate oxidation needed for performance?

The timing and the type of carbohydrate taken in to slow down the depletion of the body's carbohydrate stores are important factors. One of the earliest studies showed that when 75 g of glucose were ingested thirty to forty-five minutes before exercise requiring 70%–75% $\dot{V}O_2$ max, plasma glucose and insulin were elevated at the start of exercise, and muscle glycogen was used at

a *faster rate* during the exercise (17). This is counter to the goal of sparing muscle glycogen, and performance has been shown to decrease 19% with such a treatment (34). In contrast to this early study, a recent review of this topic indicated that the blood glucose and plasma insulin responses to pre-exercise glucose feedings are quite variable (some will experience a lowering of blood glucose, most will not), and that, in general, performance in prolonged exercise is either improved or not affected (73). The pre-exercise carbohydrate feeding is viewed as a means of topping off both muscle and liver glycogen stores. Generally, such procedures result in carbohydrates being used at a higher rate, but because of the large amount of carbohydrate ingested, the plasma glucose concentration is maintained for a longer period of time. The following observations and recommendations are offered relative to pre-exercise feedings (73):

- the pre-exercise feeding should contain between one and five gm of carbohydrate per kilogram of body weight, and should be taken one to four hours before exercise;
- the carbohydrate source should be an easily digestible solid high carbohydrate food, but if it is taken one hour before exercise, it should be in liquid form;
- the athlete should test the procedure in training before using it in competition, and
- the athlete should be aware of any sensations (e.g., fatigue) that might indicate a sensitivity to the carbohydrate load, which would not be beneficial to performance.

While ingesting carbohydrates prior to exercise seems to be an appropriate procedure, the most potent effect is when this is combined with carbohydrate feeding during exercise (78a, 87).

In contrast to the pre-exercise feeding studies in which there was some variability in the outcome, there is a great deal of consensus that feeding carbohydrate during exercise delays fatigue and improves performance. Interestingly, the improved performance appears to have nothing to do with sparing the muscle glycogen store. Muscle glycogen is depleted at the same rate during prolonged moderate (70%–75% $\dot{V}O_2$ max) exercise, with or without carbohydrate ingestion; however, liver glycogen is not. The ingestion of carbohydrate appears to spare the liver glycogen store by directly contributing carbohydrate for oxidation. If additional carbohydrate is not ingested during prolonged exercise, the blood glucose concentration decreases as the liver stores are depleted, and fatigue occurs due to an inadequate rate of carbohydrate oxidation by muscle. Figure 23.3 shows Coggan and Coyle's model of how carbohydrate is supplied to muscle during prolonged exercise under fasted and fed conditions. The rate of muscle glycogen depletion is not different; however, when fed carbohydrates, the

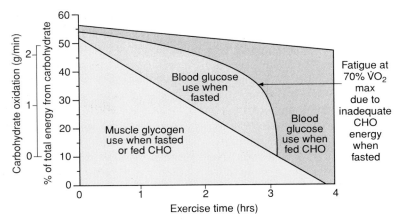

Figure 23.3
Blood glucose and muscle glycogen use when fasted or fed carbohydrates (CHO) during prolonged exercise.

subjects last longer due to the increased availability of blood glucose. When is the best time to consume carbohydrates during exercise?

Coggan and Coyle indicate that carbohydrates can be ingested throughout exercise, or can be taken thirty minutes before the anticipated time of fatigue, with no difference in the outcome (14). This is consistent with their contention that it is the increased availability of glucose late in exercise that delays fatigue. In exercise tests at 75% $\dot{V}O_2$ max, the time to fatigue was extended by about forty-five minutes with carbohydrate ingestion. Since muscles use blood glucose at the rate of about 1 to 1.3 gm/min late in exercise, sufficient carbohydrate should be ingested to provide an additional 45 to 60 gms (45 min × 1 to 1.3 gm/min) of carbohydrate. There is general agreement that this can be achieved when carbohydrates are taken in at the rate of about 30 to 60 gm/hr during exercise (14). The 120 to 240 gm of glucose consumed (4 hrs × 30 to 60 gm/hr) provides for the 45 to 60 gm needed at the end of exercise, but also supports the elevated carbohydrate metabolism throughout exercise. Glucose, sucrose, or glucose polymer solutions are all successful in maintaining the blood glucose concentration during exercise, but the palatability of the solution is improved if glucose polymer solutions are used for concentrations above 10%. Carbohydrate delivery from the stomach to the small intestine increases with the concentration of glucose, but fluid delivery slows down when the carbohydrate concentration exceeds 8%. This trade-off in glucose versus fluid delivery can be balanced by drinking 375 to 750 ml/hr of an 8% solution of carbohydrate, which would deliver 30 to 60 grams of glucose per hour to the blood (20). One final point. Even when the blood glucose concentration is maintained by either glucose infusion or ingestion during exercise, the subject will eventually stop; this indicates that fatigue is related to more than the delivery of fuel to muscles (14).

in summary
- Pre-exercise feedings should contain one to five gm of carbohydrate per kilogram of body weight and should be taken one to four hours before exercise.
- Muscle glycogen is depleted at the same rate, whether or not glucose is ingested during prolonged performance.
- The ingestion of glucose solutions during exercise extends performance by providing carbohydrate to the muscle at a time when muscle glycogen is being depleted.

Protein
The adult RDA for protein is 0.8 gm · kg⁻¹ · d⁻¹ and is easily met by a diet having 12% of its energy (kcal) as protein. For example, the RDA for energy for a nineteen- to twenty-four-year-old male weighing 72 kg is about 2,900 kcal/day. If 12% of that is protein, then 348 kcal are taken in as protein (12% of 2,400 kcal). At 4 kcal/gm, this person would consume approximately 87 gms protein per day, representing 1.2 gm · kg⁻¹ · d⁻¹ (87 g/70 kg), or 50% more than the RDA standard. Does an athlete have to take in more protein than specified in the RDA, or is the normal diet adequate? Confusing as it may seem, the answer to *both* questions appears to be yes.

Protein Requirement During Exercise
Adequacy of protein intake has been based primarily on nitrogen(N)-balance studies. Protein is about 16% N by weight, and when N-intake (dietary protein) equals N-excretion, the person is in N-balance. Excretion of less N than one consumes is called positive N-balance, and the excretion of more N than one consumes is called negative N-balance. This latter condition, if maintained, is inconsistent with good health due to the potential loss of lean body mass.

Based on these N-balance studies it was generally believed that the 0.8 gm · kg^{-1} · d^{-1} RDA standard was adequate for those engaged in prolonged exercise. In these studies, urinary N excretion was usually used as an index of N excretion, since about 85% of N is excreted this way (55). However, some experiments suggest this method of measurement may underestimate amino acid utilization in exercise. Lemon and Mullin (58) found that while there was no difference in urinary N excretion compared to rest, the loss of N in sweat increased 60 to 150-fold during exercise, suggesting that as much as 10% of the energy requirement of the exercise was met by the oxidation of amino acids.

Other studies, using different techniques, supported these observations. Muscle has been shown to release the amino acid alanine in proportion to exercise intensity (33), and the alanine is used in gluconeogenesis in the liver to generate new plasma glucose. A variety of investigators have infused a stable isotope (^{13}C-label) of the amino acid leucine to study the rate at which amino acids are mobilized and oxidized during exercise. In general, the rate of oxidation (measured by the appearance of $^{13}CO_2$) is higher during exercise than at rest in rats and humans (23, 51, 79). Taken as a group, these studies suggest that amino acids are used as a fuel during exercise to a greater extent than previously believed. They also suggest that the protein requirement for those involved in prolonged exercise is higher than the RDA (55). However, there is more to the story.

Oxidation of Amino Acids

Part of the justification for a greater protein requirement in those who exercise is based on work using isotopes of amino acids whose metabolism could be traced during exercise. That is, if an amino acid is metabolized, the "labeled" $^{13}CO_2$ is exhaled and can be used as a marker of its rate of use. The essential amino acid leucine has been used as being representative of the amino acid pool. The previously mentioned work showed that leucine oxidation is increased with exercise (23, 51, 79). This implies that the catabolism of protein is higher during exercise compared to rest. Wolfe et al. (86) confirmed this greater rate of leucine oxidation during exercise but failed to show an increase in urea production, a primary index of protein catabolism. It was concluded that the N contained in leucine does not find its way to plasma urea N as a result of exercise (84, 85); instead the N in leucine is transferred to intermediates (pyruvate) to form alanine, which is later used in the liver in gluconeogenesis.

These results raised additional questions, so another experiment was conducted to see if leucine was, in fact, representative of the amino acid pool. The investigators used the amino acid lysine and found different results for the same experimental procedures. On the basis of their experiments, Wolfe et al. (84) concluded that leucine cannot be used as a model of whole-body protein metabolism during exercise, that changes (or lack of) in urea production during exercise may not reflect an accurate picture of protein breakdown, and finally, that *the data provide no rationale for increasing protein intake when exercising* (84). A recent review supports this proposition, and indicates that even if the leucine requirement is three times the RDA in individuals who exercise, the mixed diet of a typical athlete is sufficient to meet those needs (8). This takes us back to nitrogen-balance studies as a focal point of determining the protein requirements for athletes.

Whole Body Nitrogen Balance Studies

The ability to maintain N-balance during exercise appears to be dependent on

- the training state of the subject,
- the quality and quantity of protein consumed,
- the total calories consumed,
- the body's carbohydrate store, and
- the intensity, duration, and type (resistance vs. endurance) of exercise (8, 10, 55, 56, 57).

If measurements of protein utilization are made during the first few days of an exercise program, formerly sedentary subjects show a negative N-balance (figure 23.4). However, after about twelve to fourteen days of training, this condition disappears and the person can maintain N-balance (41). So, depending on the point into the training program where the measurements are made, one could conclude that either more protein is needed (during the adaptation to exercise) or that protein needs can be met by the RDA (after the adaptation is complete) (10). Butterfield indicates that in N-balance studies the length of time needed to achieve a new steady state depends on the magnitude of the change in the level of N intake, and the absolute amount of N consumed, and that the recommended minimum of a ten-day adaptation period may be inadequate when N intake is very large (8).

Another factor influencing the conclusion one would reach about protein needs during exercise is whether the person is in caloric balance, that is, taking in enough kcal to cover the cost of the added exercise. For example, it has been shown that by increasing the energy intake 15% *more* than that needed to maintain weight, an increase in N retention occurred during exercise when these subjects consumed only 0.57 gm · kg^{-1} · d^{-1} of egg white protein (10). In a parallel study by the same group (77), a 15% *deficit* in energy intake was created while subjects consumed either 0.57 or 0.8 gm · kg^{-1} · d^{-1} egg white protein. When taking in 15% fewer calories than needed, the 0.8 gm · kg^{-1} · d^{-1} protein intake was associated with a negative N balance of 1 g · d^{-1}. However, when the subjects did one or

Table 23.1   Stages of Iron Deficiency

Stages	Description	Test
Iron depletion	Lack of iron stores in the bone and liver due to long-term dietary iron deficiency	Bone marrow biopsy; serum ferritin $<12 \, \mu g \cdot \ell^{-1}$
Iron-deficient erythropoieses	Red blood cell production decreases due to inadequate hemoglobin formation	Unbound protoporphyrin (used in the formation of hemoglobin) increases due to low iron stores
Iron deficiency anemia	Hemoglobin falls to low levels	Men: $<13 \, g \cdot dl^{-1}$ Women: $<12 \, g \cdot dl^{-1}$; *with* evidence that first two stages exist

From Haymes (44).

Allowances must be made for the individual differences in the frequency and volume of ingestion. These authors also provided a drink for recovery that is consistent with the need to replenish electrolytes and muscle glycogen: the drink should contain 30–40 mEq of Na^+, and Cl^-, and deliver 50 gm of carbohydrate per hour. The addition of salt to the drink enhances its palatability, promotes fluid and carbohydrate absorption, and replenishes some of the electrolytes lost during the activity. An additional reason sodium has been added to the drinks is related to concerns that have been raised about the potential for hyponatremia, a dangerously low Na^+ concentration that can occur when a person hydrates only with water during extremely long (4+ hours) ultra-endurance athletic events (64). However, a recent study found that water replacement alone during six hours of exercise at 55% $\dot{V}O_2$ max did not cause the sodium concentration to decrease to the levels associated with hyponatremia. The authors emphasized the importance of fluid replacement to prevent dehydration and hyperthermia, not hyponatremia (3). Sodium can be replaced at meal times.

Salt (NaCl)

One of the Dietary Guidelines for Americans presented in chapter 18 was to decrease the intake of sodium. While the point was made that Americans consume two to three times the amount needed for optimal health, is the dietary intake sufficient for an athlete who participates in regular vigorous physical activity? The mass of sodium in the body determines the water content, given the way water is reabsorbed at the kidney. If a person becomes sodium depleted, body water decreases, and the risk of heat injury increases. An untrained and unacclimatized individual (see chapter 24) loses more Na^+ in sweat than a trained and acclimatized person. If the unacclimatized person has 1.9 gm Na^+ per liter of sweat and loses 5 liters of sweat (11 pounds), the person would lose 9.5 grams of Na^+ per day. As the person becomes acclimatized to heat, the sodium content in sweat decreases to about half that

and Na^+ loss is about 5 gm/day. Given that Na is 40% of NaCl by weight, a person would have to consume 12.5 gm of salt per day to meet that demand. Interestingly, that is about what an average American, eating an average diet, now consumes. It is generally believed that an individual with a high Na^+ loss can stay in sodium/water balance by simply adding salt to food at mealtime, rather than by consuming salt tablets (81). *The best single test of the success of the salt/water replacement procedures is to have an athlete weigh in each day.* The general dietary routine followed by athletes must be successful since early morning body weight remains relatively constant despite large daily sweat losses (7).

in summary

- Fluid replacement during exercise reduces the heart rate, body temperature, and perceived exertion responses to exercise, and the greater the rate of fluid intake, the lower the responses.
- Cold drinks are absorbed faster than warm drinks, and when exercise intensity exceeds 65%–70% $\dot{V}O_2$ max, gastric emptying decreases.
- For exercise lasting less than one hour, the focus is on water replacement only. When exercise duration exceeds one hour, drinks should contain Na^+, Cl^-, and carbohydrate.
- Salt needs are easily met at mealtime and salt tablets are not needed. In fact, most Americans take in more salt than is required.

Minerals

Iron

As mentioned in chapter 18, iron deficiency is the most common nutritional deficiency. The stages of iron deficiency are spelled out in table 23.1, as well as the tests used to detect deficiencies (44). An analysis of the literature suggests that both male and female

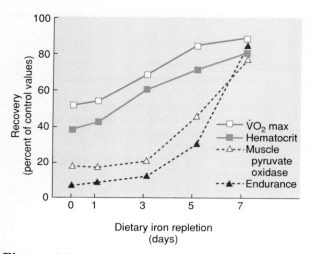

Figure 23.9

Recovery of various physiological capacities with iron repletion. Note that recovery of endurance lagged behind $\dot{V}O_2$ max.

athletes have higher rates of depleted iron stores and/or iron deficiency anemia (7, 13, 44). Given that hemoglobin is a necessary part of the oxygen-transport process, it is not surprising that in individuals with very low hemoglobin values (<11 gm/d), endurance and work performance are decreased (37, 39). Interestingly, when the low hemoglobin condition is corrected in iron-deficient animals by transfusion, $\dot{V}O_2$ max is brought back to normal but not endurance time. This suggests that while hemoglobin levels may be high enough to achieve a normal $\dot{V}O_2$ max, iron deficiency affects the iron-containing cytochromes (electron transport chain) that are involved in oxidative phosphorylation, and endurance performance is adversely affected (25). In a similar study (24), iron supplementation brought the $\dot{V}O_2$ max back to normal values faster than that of mitochondrial activity (measured by pyruvate oxidase activity) and endurance performance (see figure 23.9).

What causes iron deficiency in athletes? Inadequate intake of dietary iron, as in the general population, has been cited as a primary cause of iron deficiency in women athletes (12). In addition, exercise has been associated with increased hemoglobin loss in feces, sweat, and urine (46, 66, 75). When this is combined with evidence showing a greater hemolysis of red blood cells due to simple "pounding" of the feet on the pavement during running, and a reduced level of haptoglobin in the plasma, which is needed to take the hemoglobin to the liver, one can understand why more hemoglobin is lost in the urine and some athletes are at risk of iron deficiency anemia (22, 46). Consistent with this, Diehl et al. (29) have shown decreases in serum ferritin over the course of a field hockey season, and from one hockey season to

the next, in female athletes. The average value at the end of the season on third-year players was 10.5 μg · ℓ^{-1} (below the 12 μg · ℓ^{-1} standard), indicating iron depletion (44).

Generally, when a person has a deficiency in iron stores there is an increased uptake of dietary iron. Unfortunately, athletes do not appear to follow that pattern; studies show that athletes absorb less than half the dietary iron that a comparable group of sedentary anemic individuals absorb (31). This absorption problem increases the difficulty of returning to normal iron status: athletes may have a higher need and yet, when deficient, do not absorb the iron as well as sedentary individuals. Given that the total kcal intake of some athletes (especially women) will be inadequate in terms of iron intake (6 mg iron per 1,000 kcal in the average American diet), supplementation may be needed (12). Women runners lose about 1.7 to 2.3 mg of iron per day while absorbing only about 1.0 mg; this leaves them in negative iron balance. To prevent problems, a daily 18 mg supplement of elemental iron is recommended in order to increase the absorbable iron intake. Further, the female competitive runner should have her serum ferritin checked each year as a part of her general physical to reduce the chance of a major problem (46).

Vitamins

Chapter 18 provided the detail about the RDA for each vitamin. Many of these vitamins are directly involved in energy production, acting as coenzymes in mitochondrial reactions associated with aerobic metabolism. Unfortunately, the old adage that "if a little is good, more will be better," has been applied to the question of whether or not the RDA for athletes is higher than for sedentary people, rather than a factual research base. In general, the major reviews of this issue over the past *thirty years* have systematically concluded that, in general:

- vitamin supplementation is unnecessary for the athlete on a well-balanced diet,
- people who are *clearly deficient* in certain vitamins have improved performance when values return to normal, and
- individuals taking large doses of fat soluble vitamins or vitamin C should be concerned about toxicity (4, 11, 78, 80).

The central concern raised by these reviewers is for the small athlete on a low-energy diet who may not make wise food selections. In fact, some adolescent and adult female athletes have dietary intakes of vitamin E, B-6, B-12, and folate below the RDA standards (45). In these situations a single RDA multivitamin/mineral pill might be appropriate (4). For those who believe the above adage and want to take a high potency multivitamin, a recent study

Table 23.2 Suggested Pregame Meals

Breakfast	Calories	Lunch	Calories
4 ounces orange juice	60	4 ounces tomato juice	25
8 ounces skim milk	80	2 ounces turkey	100
2 slices toast	140	2 slices bread	140
2 tablespoons preserves	110	8 ounces skim milk	80
1 poached egg	80	1 orange	60
		2 plain cookies	120
Total calories	470		525

From M. H. Williams, *Nutritional Aspects of Human Physical and Athletic Performance*, 2d ed. Copyright © 1985. Charles C Thomas, Publisher, Springfield IL. Reprinted by permission.

showed that ninety days on such a pill had no effect on maximal aerobic power, endurance running performance, or strength (74). Additional information on the use of nutritional supplements to improve athletic performance is presented in chapter 25 in which ergogenic aids is discussed.

in summary

- Iron deficiency in American athletes may be related to an inadequate intake of dietary iron as well as a potentially greater loss in sweat and feces. In spite of this deficiency, athletes may absorb less than half of what a sedentary group of anemic individuals absorbs. Iron supplementation (18 mg/day) is recommended for female athletes, as well as an annual clinical assessment of iron status.
- Vitamin supplementation is unnecessary for an athlete on a well-balanced diet. However, for those with a clear deficiency, supplementation is warranted.

Pregame Meal

The two most important nutritional practices associated with optimal performance in endurance exercise are (a) to eat a high (about 70%) carbohydrate diet in the *days preceding* competition when the intensity and duration of workouts are reduced, and (b) to drink liquids at regular intervals *during* the competition. Consistent with our previous discussion, the purposes of the pregame meal are the following (42, 81):

- to provide adequate hydration,
- to provide carbohydrate to "top off" already high carbohydrate stores in the liver,
- to avoid the sensation of hunger on a relatively empty stomach, and
- to minimize G.I. tract problems (gas, diarrhea).

Unfortunately, the type of pregame meal served at various universities throughout this country may rely more on tradition than nutrition. The standard rare steak before a boxing match or football game to bring out the animal instinct, or careful planning to make sure that the color of the Jello® is the same as that when the team won last year's championship, are less than rational, but may be useful in pulling the team together to get ready for competition. Problems arise when the pregame meal is responsible for poor performance because of its own characteristics (high fat and protein) or the inability of the athlete to tolerate the meal without vomiting or experiencing diarrhea due to the emotion associated with competition. These latter conditions would cause a dehydration inconsistent with optimal performance. It is clear that beyond what is recommended in the nutrient make-up of a pregame meal, the ability of the athlete to tolerate it must be considered (81).

Nutrients in Pregame Meal

The number of kcal in a pregame meal should be 500–1,000, and the primary nutrient should be complex carbohydrates because they are easily digested and provide glucose to increase liver glycogen. It is generally recommended that large amounts of simple sugars should not be consumed immediately prior to competition (81). The fat content of the pregame meal should be kept to a minimum since fat is more slowly digested and is not needed as a fuel for exercise since body stores are more than adequate. The protein content of the pregame meal should be small. The digestion and metabolism of protein increases the quantity of acids in the blood that must be buffered and finally excreted by the kidneys (42, 81). Table 23.2 presents two pregame meals that meet these considerations (81). These meals should be eaten about three hours prior to competition.

Jello® is a registered trademark of General Foods, Inc.

Some coaches and athletes prefer one of the commercially available liquid meals as the pregame meal because of convenience. These liquid meals can also be used throughout the day (along with additional water) when events or games are scheduled over long periods of time. Given that some people may not react favorably to any new "food," these liquid meals should be tried on practice days rather than on game day to make sure they are suitable.

in summary

- The pregame meal should provide for hydration and adequate carbohydrate to "top off" stores while minimizing hunger symptoms, gas, and diarrhea. A variety of commercially available liquid meals are consistent with these goals.

Body Composition and Performance

A simple observation of the track and field events at the Olympic Games suggests that the physical characteristics of those successful in the shot put are different from those successful in the marathon. The purpose of this section is to reinforce that observation by providing a brief review of **somatotype** and body fatness related to performance.

Somatotype

In 1940 Sheldon (70) published *The Varieties of Human Physique*, in which he introduced the concept of the somatotype. In his scheme each person could be characterized as possessing a certain amount of the following three components of body form:

Endomorphy   relative predominance of soft roundness and large digestive viscera. He used the prefix *endo* as it relates to the *endo*dermal embryonic layers from which the digestive track is derived.

Mesomorphy   relative predominance of muscle, bone, and connective tissue ultimately derived from the *meso*dermal embryonic layer.

Ectomorphy   relative predominance of linearity and fragility with a great surface area to mass ratio giving great sensory exposure to the environment. The nervous system is derived from the *ecto*dermal embryonic layer.

Sheldon photographed 4,000 college men and ranked each of these three components on a scale of 1 to 7, with 1 representing the least amount of a component and 7 representing the greatest amount. A somatotype is a three-number sequence (e.g., 171 is one-seven-one) characterizing the endomorphic, mesomorphic, and ectomorphic components, respectively. Figure 23.10 shows the extremes of each somatotype. It must be remembered that somatotype considers only body form or shape and does not consider size. Tanner (76) used a two-dimensional plot of the original somatotypes of Sheldon's 4,000 college students on whom the 1 to 7 scale was based. This distribution of somatotypes is shown in figure 23.11 where a contrasting distribution is also presented, showing the somatotypes of 137 Olympic track-and-field athletes. Not surprisingly, the body form or type associated with world-class performance is different from that of the average population and differs by sport and event.

The values used in these figures were based on the Sheldon photographs (71), but according to the somatotyping method of Heath-Carter (47), Sheldon's 1 to 7 scale was too confining in that there are components in certain body types that exceed that given the value of 7. Using their method of somatotyping, Heath-Carter (47) cite the following examples of extremes in somatotypes: (a) extremely obese individuals having endomorphy values as high as 12, (b) members of the Manu tribe of the Admirality Islands with values of 9.5 for mesomorphy, and (c) members of the Nilote tribe in Africa having ectomorphic values of 8 and 9. When Olympic athletes were rated with this Heath-Carter scale, weight lifters and throwers were outside the normal distribution of Sheldon's mesomorphy scale. As one moves from these weight lifters and throwers to the distance runners and basketball players, the somatotype becomes progressively more ectomorphic. The distribution of somatotypes for the women athletes was shifted down and to the left, indicating smaller mesomorphic and larger endomorphic components (28).

Further, the Heath-Carter scale views the somatotype, especially the endomorphic and mesomorphic components, to be dynamic with the potential to change over time. Sheldon had viewed the somatotype as more of a permanent form for a given individual. The Heath-Carter method sees the endomorphic component as being equivalent to relative fatness or leanness and is closely tied to the sum of skinfolds. The mesomorphic component is viewed as being an estimate of the relative musculoskeletal development and similar to lean body mass. This latter translation of somatotype values into body composition values is a good lead into our next section.

Figure 23.10

Extremes of somatotypes: endomorphy, mesomorphy, and ectomorphy.

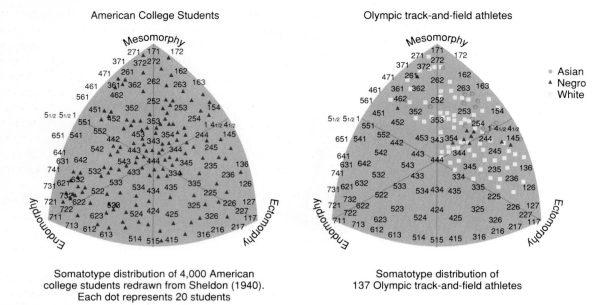

American College Students

Olympic track-and-field athletes

Somatotype distribution of 4,000 American
college students redrawn from Sheldon (1940).
Each dot represents 20 students

Somatotype distribution of
137 Olympic track-and-field athletes

Figure 23.11
Contrast of the somatotypes of American college students with Olympic track-and-field athletes.

Body Fatness and Performance

The somatotypes of the athletes involved in the Olympic Games represent low relative fatness (low endomorphy) and high relative fat-free mass (high mesomorphy). This two-component system of body composition was described in detail in chapter 18, where optimal body fatness goals were presented for health and fitness:

Males: 10%–20% fat
Females: 15%–25% fat

The question is, are these values optimal for athletic performance?

Table 23.3 lists a summary of body fatness values by sport (82). Many are average values and do not represent the range that might be observed in a study. For example, a study might find an average value of 12% body fat for a group of football players, but the range might be 5%–19%. In a sport or activity where body weight must be carried along (e.g., running or jumping), there is a negative correlation between body fatness and performance (82, 83).

There is little question that regular measurements of body composition are useful for athletes in order to monitor changes during the season as well as over the off-season. In this way the athlete will know whether changes in body weight represent gains or losses of body fatness. What is more difficult is providing a fixed absolute recommendation about what body fatness should be for optimal performance for each individual.

One of the main reasons one must be careful in making absolute recommendations, such as "This athlete should reduce her percent body fat from 15.6% to 14.0%," is that the athlete may already be 14% body fat. Each *individual estimate* of body fatness, even done by the underwater weighing technique, has an error in measurement that cannot be ignored. With appropriate methods and careful measurement, percent fat can be estimated with an error of about 3% to 4% fat. So when an athlete is measured as being 15.0% body fat, the true value may be as high as 19% and as low as 11% (52a).

Another reason caution must be used in making an absolute recommendation for each individual athlete is that it ignores the normal variation in body fatness found in elite athletes in any particular sport. An elite group of volleyball players may have an average value of 12%, but the range among the team members might be 6%–16%. No one would think of telling the athlete with 6% body fat to increase body fatness to reach the team average, and the same advice holds true for the one at 16% body fatness who is playing with world-class skill. A recommendation to alter body composition to achieve better performance must be made against the background of present performance

Table 23.3	Percent Body Fat Values for Male and Female Athletes	

Athletic Group or Sport	Male	Female
Baseball	11.8–14.2	—
Basketball	7.1–10.6	20.8–26.9
Canoeing	12.4	—
Football		
Backs	9.4–12.4	—
Linebackers	13.7	—
Linemen	15.5–19.1	—
Quarterbacks, kickers	14.1	—
Gymnastics	4.6	9.6–23.8
Ice hockey	13–15.1	—
Jockeys	14.1	—
Orienteering	16.3	18.7
Pentathalon	—	11.0
Racquetball	8.3	14.0
Skiing		
Alpine	7.4–14.1	20.6
Cross-country	7.9–12.5	15.7–21.8
Nordic combined	8.9–11.2	—
Ski jumping	14.3	—
Soccer	9.6	—
Speed skating	11.4	—
Swimming	5.0–8.5	20.3
Tennis	15.2–16.3	20.3
Track and field		
Distance runners	3.7–18.0	15.2–19.2
Middle distance runners	12.4	—
Sprinters	16.5	19.3
Discus	16.3	25.0
Jumpers/hurdlers	—	20.7
Shot put	16.5–19.6	28.0
Volleyball	—	21.3–25.3
Wrestling	4.0–14.4	

From J. H. Wilmore, "Body Composition in Sport Medicine: Directions for Future Research," in *Medicine and Science in Sports Medicine* 15:21–31, 1983. Copyright © 1983 American College of Sports Medicine, Indianapolis IN. Reprinted by permission.

and general health status as seen in sleeping patterns, adequate diet, mental outlook, and so on. The implementation of longer workouts or a reduction in caloric intake might change the percent body fat in the appropriate direction, but either one could adversely affect the athlete's ability to tolerate a workout or to study for exams. Wilmore's (82) observation of one of the best female distance runners who held most of the American middle distance records should be remembered when making such recommendations: the champion was 17% body fat when most of the elite female runners were <12%.

Monitoring body fatness in athletes by skinfold or underwater weighing is a reasonable procedure to follow because it allows a coach or trainer to observe *changes* in body fatness over the course of a season and from one year to the next. The information is also useful to the athletes who, when they finish their competitive careers, must attend to what is a reasonable body weight in order to be within the optimal body fatness range for health and fitness.

in summary

- A somatotype is a numerical representation on a 1 to 7 scale of the degree to which a person possesses a high level endomorphy, mesomorphy, and ectomorphy. Athletes are clearly different from the ordinary population, indicating a natural predisposition needed for success.
- The body fat percentage consistent with excellence in performance is different for men and women, and varies within gender from sport to sport. Average values for a team should not be applied to any single individual without regard to overall health status as seen in diet, sleep, and mental outlook. Further, it is "natural" for some athletes to have a higher body fatness than others in order to perform optimally.

study questions

1. What procedures would you follow to cause a supercompensation of muscle glycogen?
2. How much of a change in carbohydrate intake would be required for an individual who already achieves the dietary goal for carbohydrate?
3. How could glucose ingestion prior to exercise actually increase the rate of glycogen depletion?
4. Does carbohydrate ingestion during exercise slow down muscle glycogen depletion? Does it improve performance?
5. Is the protein requirement of an athlete higher than that of a sedentary person? Should protein intake be increased?
6. How would you recommend that a person replace water loss due to exercise?
7. How does the fluid replacement strategy differ for short and long races?
8. How would you recommend that a potential iron deficiency anemia condition be dealt with?
9. Does an athlete need additional vitamins for optimal performance? Why?
10. What are the primary considerations in a pregame meal?
11. What is a somatotype and how is it different for athletes compared to the average college population?
12. Given a female distance runner with 17% body fat, what should you consider before making a recommendation for change?

suggested readings

Clarkson, P., and E. Haymes. 1994. Trace mineral requirements for athletes. *International Journal of Sports Nutrition* 4:104–19.

Fogelholm, M. 1995. Indicators of vitamin and mineral status in athletes' blood: A review. *International Journal of Sports Nutrition* 5:267–84.

Lamb, D. R., and M. H. Williams, eds. 1991. *Ergogenics: Enhancement of Performance in Exercise and Sports.* Carmel, IN: Brown & Benchmark.

references

1. Ahlborg, B. et al. 1967. Muscle glycogen and muscle electrolytes during prolonged physical exercise. *Acta Physiologica Scandinavica* 70:129–42.
2. ———. 1982. Lactate and glucose exchange across the forearm, legs, and splanchnic bed during and after prolonged exercise. *Journal of Clinical Investigation* 69:45–54.
3. Barr, S. I., D. L. Costill, and W. J. Fink. 1991. Fluid replacement during prolonged exercise: Effects of water, saline, or no fluid. *Medicine and Science in Sports and Exercise* 23:811–17.
4. Belko, A. Z. 1987. Vitamins and exercise—an update. *Medicine and Science in Sports and Exercise* 19:S191–S196.
5. Bergstrom, J., and E. Hultman. 1966. Muscle glycogen synthesis after exercise: An enhancing factor localized to the muscle cells in man. *Nature* 210:309.
6. Bergstrom, J. et al. 1967. Diet, muscle glycogen and physical performance. *Acta Physiologica Scandinavica* 71:140–50.
7. Brotherhood, J. R. 1984. Nutrition and sports performance. *Sports Medicine* 1:350–89.
8. Butterfield, G. 1991. Amino acids and high protein diets. In *Ergogenics: Enhancement of Performance in Exercise and Sport*, eds. D. R. Lamb and M. H. Williams, 87–117. Carmel, IN: Brown & Benchmark.
9. Butterfield, G. E. 1987. Whole-body protein utilization in humans. *Medicine and Science in Sports and Exercise* 19:S157–S165.
10. Butterfield, G. E., and D. H. Calloway. 1984. Physical activity improves protein utilization in young men. *British Journal of Nutrition* 51:171–84.
11. Clarkson, P. M. 1991. Vitamins and trace minerals. In *Ergogenics: Enhancement of Performance in Exercise and Sport*, eds. D. R. Lamb and M. H. Williams, 123–82. Carmel, IN: Brown & Benchmark.
12. Clement, D. B., and R. C. Asmundson. 1982. Nutritional intake and hematological parameters in endurance runners. *Physician and Sportsmedicine* 10:37–43.
13. Clement, D. B., and L. L. Sawchuk. 1984. Iron status and sports performance. *Sports Medicine* 1:65–74.
14. Coggan, A. R., and E. F. Coyle. 1991. Carbohydrate ingestion during prolonged exercise: Effects on metabolism and performance. In *Exercise and Sport Sciences Reviews*, vol. 19, ed. J. O. Holloszy, 1–40. Philadelphia: Williams & Wilkins.
15. Costill, D. L. 1977. Sweating: Its composition and effects on body fluids. *Annals of the New York Academy of Sciences* 301:160–74.
16. Costill, D. L., and B. Saltin. 1974. Factors limiting gastric emptying during rest and exercise. *Journal of Applied Physiology* 37:679–83.
17. Costill, D. L. et al. 1977. Effects of elevated plasma FFA and insulin on muscle glycogen usage during exercise. *Journal of Applied Physiology* 43:695–99.
18. Costill, D. L. et al. 1981. The role of dietary carbohydrates in muscle glycogen resynthesis after strenuous running. *American Journal of Clinical Nutrition* 34:1831–36.
18a. Coyle, E. F. 1994. Fluid and carbohydrate replacement during exercise: how much and why? *Sports Science Exchange* vol. 7, no. 3. Barrington, IL: Gatorade Sports Science Institute.

24

Exercise and the Environment

objectives

By studying this chapter, you should be able to do the following:

1. Describe the changes in atmospheric pressure, air temperature, and air density with increasing altitude.
2. Describe how altitude affects sprint performances and explain why that is the case.
3. Explain why distance running performance decreases at altitude.
4. Draw a graph to show the effect of altitude on $\dot{V}O_2$ max and list the reasons for this response.
5. Graphically describe the effect of altitude on the heart rate and ventilation responses to submaximal work, and explain why these changes are appropriate.
6. Describe the process of adaptation to altitude, and the degree to which this adaptation can be complete.
7. Explain why such variability exists among athletes in the decrease in $\dot{V}O_2$ max upon exposure to altitude, the degree of improvement in $\dot{V}O_2$ max at altitude, and the gains made upon return to sea level.
8. Describe the potential problems associated with training at high altitude and how one might deal with them.
9. Explain the circumstances that caused physiologists to reevaluate their conclusions that humans could not climb Mount Everest without oxygen.
10. Explain the role that hyperventilation plays in helping to maintain a high oxygen-hemoglobin saturation at extreme altitudes.
11. List and describe the factors influencing the risk of heat injury.
12. Provide suggestions for the fitness participant to follow to minimize the likelihood of heat injury.
13. Describe in general terms the guidelines suggested for running road races in the heat.
14. Describe the three elements in the heat stress index, and explain why one is more important than the other two.
15. List the factors influencing hypothermia.
16. Explain what the Windchill Index is relative to heat loss.
17. Explain why exposure to cold water is more dangerous than exposure to air of the same temperature.
18. Describe what the "clo" unit is and how recommendations for insulation change when one does exercise.
19. Describe the role of subcutaneous fat and energy production in the development of hypothermia.
20. List the steps to follow to deal with hypothermia.
21. Explain how carbon monoxide can influence performance, and list the steps that should be taken to reduce the impact of pollution on performance.

outline

Altitude 440
    Atmospheric Pressure 440
    Short-Term Anaerobic
      Performance 440
    Long-Term Aerobic
      Performance 441
    Maximal Aerobic Power and
      Altitude 442
    Adaptation to High Altitude 443

Training for Competition at
    Altitude 444
    The Quest for Everest 445
Heat 448
    Hyperthermia 448
Cold 451
    Environmental Factors 451
    Insulating Factors 452

Energy Production 453
    Dealing with Hypothermia 454
Air Pollution 454
    Ozone 454
    Sulfur Dioxide 455
    Carbon Monoxide 455

key terms

clo
hypoxia

hyperoxia

normoxia

By now it should be clear that performance is dependent on more than simply having a high $\dot{V}O_2$ max. We have just seen the role of diet and body composition on performance, and in the next chapter we will formally consider "ergogenic" or work-enhancing aids and performance. Sandwiched between these chapters will be a discussion of how the environmental factors of altitude, heat, cold, and pollution can influence performance.

Altitude

In the late 1960s, when the Olympic Games were scheduled to be held in Mexico City, our attention was directed at the question of how altitude (2,300 meters at Mexico City) would affect performance. Previous experience at altitude suggested that many performances would not equal former Olympic standards or, for that matter, the athlete's own personal record (PR) at sea level. On the other hand, some performances were actually expected to be better because they were conducted at altitude. Why? What happens to $\dot{V}O_2$ max with altitude? Can a sea-level resident ever completely adapt to altitude? We will address these and other questions after a brief review of the environmental factors that change with increasing altitude.

Atmospheric Pressure

The atmospheric pressure at any spot on earth is a measure of the weight of a column of air directly over that spot. At sea level the weight (and height) of that column of air is greatest. As one climbs to higher and higher altitudes the height, and of course, the weight of the column is reduced. Consequently, atmospheric pressure decreases with increasing altitude, the air is less dense, and each liter of air contains fewer molecules of gas. Since the *percentages* of O_2, CO_2, and N_2 are the same at altitude as at sea level, any change in the

partial pressure of each gas is due solely to the change in the atmospheric or barometric pressure (see chapter 10). The decrease in the partial pressure of O_2 (PO_2) with increasing altitude has a direct effect on the saturation of hemoglobin and, consequently, oxygen transport. This lower PO_2 is called **hypoxia,** with **normoxia** being the term to describe the PO_2 under sea-level conditions. The term **hyperoxia** describes a condition in which the inspired PO_2 is greater than that at sea level (see chapter 25). In addition to the hypoxic condition at altitude, the air temperature and humidity are lower, adding potential temperature regulation problems to the hypoxic stress of altitude. How do these changes affect performance? In order to answer that question we will divide performances into short-term anaerobic performances and long-term aerobic performances.

Short-Term Anaerobic Performance

In chapters 3 and 19 we described the importance of the anaerobic sources of ATP in maximal performances lasting two minutes or less. If this information is correct, and we think it is, then the short-term anaerobic races shouldn't be affected by the low PO_2 at altitude since O_2 transport to the muscles is not limiting performance. Table 24.1 shows this to be the case when the sprint performances of the 1968 Mexico City Olympic Games were compared to those in the 1964 Tokyo Olympic Games. The performances improved in all but one case, in which the time for the 400-meter run for the women was the same. The reasons for the improvements in performance include the "normal" gains made over time from one Olympic Games to the next and the fact that the density of the air at altitude offers less resistance to movements at high speeds. This latter reason sparked controversy over Bob Beamon's fantastic performance in the long jump in the Mexico City Games (see A Closer Look 24.1).

In the 1968 Olympic Games in Mexico City, Bob Beamon shattered the world record in the long jump with a leap of 29 feet, 2.5 inches. Due to the fact that the record was achieved at altitude where air density is less than at sea level, some questions were raised about the true magnitude of the achievement. Recent progress in biomechanics has made it possible to determine just how much would have been gained by doing the long jump at altitude (77). The calculations had to consider the mass of the jumper, a drag coefficient based on the frontal area exposed to the air while jumping, and the difference in the air density between sea level and Mexico City. The result indicated that approximately 2.4 cm, (less than an inch), would have been gained by doing the jump at altitude where the air density is less. Recently, scientists have tried to predict the effect of altitude on running performances by considering the opposing factors of lower air density and the reduced availability of oxygen (59). The latter factor is discussed below relative to long-distance races.

Table 24.1 Comparison of Performances in Short Races in the 1964 and 1968 Olympic Games

Olympic Games	Short Races: Men				Short Races: Women			
	100 *m*	200 *m*	400 *m*	800 *m*	100 *m*	200 *m*	400 *m*	800 *m*
1964 (Tokyo)	10.0 s	20.3 s	45.1 s	1 m 45.1 s	11.4 s	23.0 s	52.0 s	2 m 1.1 s
1968 (Mexico City)	9.9 s	19.8 s	43.8 s	1 m 44.3 s	11.0 s	22.5 s	52.0 s	2 m 0.9 s
% change*	+1.0	+2.5	+2.9	+0.8	+3.5	+2.2	0	+0.2

*+ sign indicates improvement over 1964 performance.

From E. T. Howley, "Comparison of Performances in Short Races in the 1964 and 1968 Olympic Games," in G. A. Stull and T. K. Cureton, *Encyclopedia of Physical Education, Fitness and Sports: Training, Environment, Nutrition, and Fitness.* Copyright © 1980 American Alliance for Health, Physical Education, Recreation and Dance, Reston VA. Reprinted by permission.

Table 24.2 Comparison of Performances in Long Races in the 1964 and 1968 Olympic Games

Olympic Games	Long Races: Men					
	1,500 *m*	3,000 *m*	5,000 *m*	10,000 *m*	Marathon	50,000 *m* Walk
1964 (Tokyo)	3 m 38.1 s	8 m 30.8 s	13 m 48.8 s	28 m 24.4 s	2 h 12 m 11.2 s	4 h 11 m 11.2 s
1968 (Mexico City)	3 m 34.9 s	8 m 51.0 s	14 m 05.0 s	29 m 27.4 s	2 h 20 m 26.4 s	4 h 20 m 13.6 s
% change*	+1.5	−3.9	−1.9	−3.7	−6.2	−3.6

*+ sign indicates improvement over 1964 performance.

From E. T. Howley, "Comparison of Performances in Short Races in the 1964 and 1968 Olympic Games," in G. A. Stull and T. K. Cureton, *Encyclopedia of Physical Education, Fitness and Sports: Training, Environment, Nutrition, and Fitness.* Copyright © 1980 American Alliance for Health, Physical Education, Recreation and Dance, Reston VA. Reprinted by permission.

Long-Term Aerobic Performance

Maximal performances in excess of two minutes are primarily dependent on oxygen delivery, and, in contrast to the short-term performances, are clearly affected by the lower PO_2 at altitude. Table 24.2 shows the results of the distance running events from 1,500 meters up through the marathon and the 50,000-meter walk, and as you can see, performance was diminished at all distances but the 1,500-meter run. This performance is worthy of special note given that it was expected to be affected as were the others. It is more than just a passing interest that the record setter was Kipchoge Keino, who was born and raised in Kenya at an altitude similar to that of Mexico City. Did he possess a special adaptation due to his birth place? We will come back to this question in a later section. We would like to continue our discussion of the effect of altitude on performance by asking why did the performance fall off by as much as 6.2% in the long distance races?

Maximal Aerobic Power and Altitude

The decrease in distance running performance at altitude is similar to what occurs when a trained runner becomes untrained—it would clearly take longer to run a marathon! The similarity in the effect is related to a decrease in maximal aerobic power that occurs with detraining and with increasing altitude. Figure 24.1 shows that $\dot{V}O_2$ max decreases in a linear fashion, being about 12% lower at 2,400 meters (7,400 feet), 20% lower at 3,100 meters (10,200 feet), and 27% lower at about 4,000 meters (13,100 feet) (8, 14, 16, 20). While it should be no surprise that endurance performance decreases with such changes in $\dot{V}O_2$ max, why does $\dot{V}O_2$ max decrease?

Cardiovascular Function at Altitude

Maximal oxygen uptake is equal to the product of the maximal cardiac output and the maximal arteriovenous oxygen difference, $\dot{V}O_2 = CO \times (CaO_2 - C\bar{v}O_2)$. Given this relationship, the decrease in $\dot{V}O_2$ max with increasing altitude could be due to a decrease in cardiac output and/or a decrease in oxygen extraction.

Maximal cardiac output is equal to the product of maximal heart rate and maximal stroke volume. In several studies the maximal heart rate was unchanged at altitudes of 2,300 meters (18, 62), 3,100 meters (27), and 4,000 meters (8), while changes in maximal stroke volume were somewhat inconsistent (43). If these two variables, maximal stroke volume and maximal heart rate, do not change with increasing altitude, then the decrease in $\dot{V}O_2$ max must be due to a difference in oxygen extraction.

While oxygen extraction ($CaO_2 - C\bar{v}O_2$) could decrease due to a decrease in the arterial oxygen content (CaO_2) or an increase in the mixed venous oxygen content ($C\bar{v}O_2$), the primary cause is the desaturation of the arterial blood due to the low PO_2 at altitude. As you recall from chapter 10, as the arterial PO_2 falls there is a reduction in the volume of oxygen bound to hemoglobin. At sea level, hemoglobin is about 96%–98% saturated with oxygen. However, at 2,300 meters and 4,000 meters, saturation falls to 88% and 71%, respectively. These decreases in the oxygen saturation of hemoglobin are similar to the

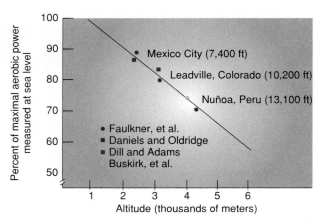

Figure 24.1

Changes in maximal aerobic power with increasing altitude. The sea-level value for maximal aerobic power is set to 100%.

From E. T. Howley, "Comparison of Performances in Short Races in the 1964 and 1968 Olympic Games", in G. A. Stull and T. K. Cureton, *Encyclopedia of Physical Education, Fitness and Sports: Training, Environment, Nutrition, and Fitness.* Copyright © 1980 American Alliance for Health, Physical Education, Recreation and Dance, Reston VA. Reprinted by permission.

reductions in $\dot{V}O_2$ max described earlier at these altitudes. Since maximal oxygen transport is the product of the maximal cardiac output and the arterial oxygen content, the capacity to transport oxygen to the working muscles at altitude is reduced due to desaturation, even though maximal cardiac output may be unchanged up to altitudes of 4,000 meters (43). However, it must be added that a variety of studies have shown a decrease in maximal heart rate at altitude. While some of these decreases have been observed at altitudes of 3,100 meters (16) and 4,300 meters (18), it is more common to find lower maximal heart rates above altitudes of 4,300 meters. For example, compared to sea level, maximal HR was observed to be 24–33 beats/minute lower at 4,650 meters (15,300 feet) and 47 beats/minute lower at about 6,100 meters (20,000 feet) (30, 63). This depression in maximal heart rate is reversed by acute restoration of normoxia, or the use of atropine (30). This altitude-induced bradycardia suggests that myocardial hypoxia may trigger the slower heart rate to decrease the work and, therefore, the oxygen demand of the heart muscle. Given this lower maximal HR, it means that $\dot{V}O_2$ max may decrease at a faster rate at the higher altitudes due to the combined effects of the desaturation of hemoglobin and the decrease in maximal cardiac output.

This desaturation of arterial blood at altitude affects more than $\dot{V}O_2$ max. The cardiovascular responses to submaximal work are also influenced. Due to the fact that each liter of blood is carrying less oxygen, more liters of blood must be pumped per minute in

Figure 24.2
The effect of altitude on the heart-rate response to submaximal exercise.

Figure 24.3
The effect of altitude on the ventilation response to submaximal exercise.

order to compensate. This is accomplished through an increase in the HR response, since the stroke volume response is at its highest point already, or it is actually lower at altitude due to the hypoxia (2). This elevated HR response is shown in figure 24.2 (27). This has implications for more than the performance-based athlete. The average person who participates in an exercise program will have to decrease the intensity of exercise at altitude in order to stay in the target heart rate zone. Remember, the exercise prescription needed for a cardiovascular training effect includes a proper duration of exercise to achieve a total caloric expenditure of about 200–300 kcal, and if the intensity is too high the person will have more difficulty completing the workout.

Respiratory Function at Altitude

In the introduction to this section we mentioned that the air is less dense at altitude. This means that there are fewer O_2 molecules per liter of air, and if a person wished to consume the same number of liters of O_2, pulmonary ventilation would have to increase. At 5,600 meters (18,400 feet) the atmospheric pressure is one-half that at sea level and the number of molecules of O_2 per liter of air is reduced by one-half; therefore, a person would have to breathe twice as much air to take in the same amount of O_2. The consequences of this are shown in figure 24.3, which presents the ventilation responses of a subject who exercised at work rates demanding about a $\dot{V}O_2$ of 1 to 2 $\ell \cdot min^{-1}$ at sea level and at three altitudes exceeding 4,000 meters. The pulmonary ventilation is elevated at all altitudes, reaching values of almost 180 $\ell \cdot min^{-1}$ at 6,400 meters (21,000 feet) (63). This extreme ventilatory response requires the respiratory muscles, primarily the diaphragm, to work so hard that fatigue may occur. We will see more on this in a later section dealing with the assault on Mount Everest.

in summary

- Distance-running performances are adversely affected at altitude due to the reduction in the PO_2, which causes a decrease in hemoglobin saturation and $\dot{V}O_2$ max.
- Up to moderate altitudes (~4000 meters) the decrease in $\dot{V}O_2$ max is due primarily to the decrease in the arterial oxygen content brought about by the decrease in atmospheric PO_2. At higher altitudes, the rate at which $\dot{V}O_2$ max falls may be increased due to a reduction in maximal cardiac output.
- Submaximal performances conducted at altitude require higher heart rate and ventilation responses due to the lower oxygen content of arterial blood and the reduction in the number of oxygen molecules per liter of air, respectively.

Adaptation to High Altitude

The body's response to the low PO_2 at altitude is to produce additional red blood cells to compensate for the desaturation of hemoglobin. In the mining community of Morococha, Peru, where people reside at altitudes above 4,540 meters, hemoglobin levels of 211 $g \cdot \ell^{-1}$ have been measured, in contrast to the normal 156 $g \cdot \ell^{-1}$ of the sea-level residents in Lima. This higher hemoglobin compensates rather completely for the low PO_2 at those altitudes (42):

Sea Level: 156 $g \cdot \ell^{-1}$ times 1.34 ml $O_2 \cdot g^{-1}$ at 98% saturation = 206 ml $\cdot \ell^{-1}$
4,540 m: 211 $g \cdot \ell^{-1}$ times 1.34 ml $O_2 \cdot g^{-1}$ at 81% saturation = 224 ml $\cdot \ell^{-1}$.

Probably the best test of the degree to which these altitude residents have adapted is found in the $\dot{V}O_2$ max values measured at altitude. Average values of

$46-50 \, \text{ml} \cdot \text{kg}^{-1} \cdot \text{min}^{-1}$ were measured on the altitude natives (44, 52, 53, 54), which compares favorably with sea-level natives in that country and in ours. In addition, recreational runners at 3,600 meters have been shown to have $\dot{V}O_2$ max values similar to their sea-level counterparts (26b).

There is no question that any sea-level resident who makes a journey to altitude and stays a while will experience an increase in red blood cell number. However, the adaptation will probably never be complete. This conclusion is drawn from a study that compared $\dot{V}O_2$ max values of several different groups: (a) Peruvian lowlanders and Peace Corps volunteers who came to altitude as adults, (b) lowlanders who came to altitude as children and spent their growing years at altitude, and (c) permanent altitude residents (20). The $\dot{V}O_2$ max values were $46 \, \text{ml} \cdot \text{kg}^{-1} \cdot \text{min}^{-1}$ for the altitude residents and those who arrived there as children. In contrast, the lowlanders who arrived as adults and spent only one to four years at altitude had values of $38 \, \text{ml} \cdot \text{kg}^{-1} \cdot \text{min}^{-1}$. This indicates that in order to have complete adaptation one must spend the developmental years at high altitude. This may help explain the surprisingly good performance of Kipchoge Keino's performance in the 1,500-meter run at the Mexico City Olympic Games mentioned earlier, since he spent his childhood at an altitude similar to that of Mexico City.

in summary

- Persons adapt to altitude by producing more red blood cells to counter the desaturation caused by the lower PO_2. Altitude residents who spent their growing years at altitude show a rather complete adaptation as seen in their arterial oxygen content and $\dot{V}O_2$ max values. Lowlanders who arrive as adults show only a modest adaptation.

Training for Competition at Altitude

It was clear to many of the middle- and long-distance runners who competed in the Olympic Trials or Games in 1968 that the altitude was going to have a detrimental effect on performance. Using $\dot{V}O_2$ max as an indicator of the impact on performance, scientists studied the effect of immediate exposure to altitude, the rate of recovery in $\dot{V}O_2$ max as the individual stayed at altitude, and whether or not $\dot{V}O_2$ max was higher than the pre-altitude value upon return to sea level. The results were interesting, not due to the general trends that were expected, but to the extreme variability in response among the athletes. For example, the decrease in $\dot{V}O_2$ max upon ascent to a 2,300-meter altitude ranged from 8.8% to 22.3% (62), at 3,090 meters it ranged from 13.9% to 24.4% (16), and at 4,000 meters the decrease ranged from 24.8% to 34.3% (8). One of the major conclusions

that could be drawn from these data is that the best runner at sea level might not be the best at altitude if that person had the largest drop in $\dot{V}O_2$ max. Why such variability? Studies of this phenomenon suggests that the variability in the decrease in $\dot{V}O_2$ max across individuals relates to the degree to which athletes experience desaturation of arterial blood during maximal work (45, 46a, 58b). Chapter 10 described the effect that arterial desaturation has on $\dot{V}O_2$ max of superior athletes *at sea level*. If such desaturation can occur under sea-level conditions, then the altitude condition should have an additional impact, with the magnitude of the impact being greater on those who suffer some desaturation at sea level. Consistent with that, exposure to a simulated altitude of 3,000 meters resulted in 20.8% decrease in $\dot{V}O_2$ max for trained subjects and only a 9.8% decrease for untrained subjects (45).

The decrease in $\dot{V}O_2$ max upon exposure to altitude was not the only physiological response that varied among the athletes. There was also a variable response in the size of the increase in $\dot{V}O_2$ max as the subjects stayed at altitude and continued to train. One study, lasting twenty-eight days at 2,300 meters, found the $\dot{V}O_2$ max to increase from 1% to 8% over that time (62). Some found the $\dot{V}O_2$ max to gradually improve over a period of ten to twenty-eight days (4, 15, 16, 62), while others (18, 27) did not. In addition, when the subjects returned to sea level and were retested, some found the $\dot{V}O_2$ max to be higher than before they left (4, 15, 16), while others found no improvements (8, 20, 26). Why was there such variability in response?

There are several possibilities. If an athlete were not in peak condition before ascending to altitude, then the combined stress of the exercise and altitude could increase the $\dot{V}O_2$ max over time while at altitude and show an additional gain upon return to sea level. There is evidence both for (67) and against (1, 17a) the idea that the combination of altitude and exercise stress leads to greater changes in $\dot{V}O_2$ max than exercise stress alone. Another reason for the variability is related to the altitude at which the training was conducted. When runners trained at high (4,000 meters) altitude, the intensity of the runs (relative to sustained sea-level speeds) had to be reduced in order to complete a workout, due to the reduction in $\dot{V}O_2$ max that occurs at altitude. As a result, the runner might actually "detrain" while at altitude, and subsequent performance at sea level might not be as good as it was before going to altitude (8). Daniels and Oldridge (15) provided a way around this problem by having runners alternate training at altitude (seven to fourteen days) and sea level (five to eleven days). Using an altitude of only 2,300 meters, the runners were still able to train at "race pace" and detraining did not occur. In fact, thirteen personal records were achieved by the athletes when they raced at sea level. A recent study using the one-leg training model supports this approach. Subjects trained one leg under hypoxic conditions equivalent to 2,300 meters altitude, while the control leg was exercised under normoxic (sea level) conditions at the same work rate. The subjects exercised three to four times per week for four weeks. The combination of exercise and hypoxia resulted in higher mitochondrial enzyme activity and myoglobin concentration compared to the control leg (75). In contrast, but consistent with our previous discussion, those exposed to extreme altitude (e.g., Mount Everest) experience decreases in muscle fiber area and mitochondria volume (26, 34, 38, 46). See below for additional details.

in summary

- When athletes train at altitude, some experience a greater decline in $\dot{V}O_2$ max than others. This may be due to differences in the degree to which each athlete experiences a desaturation of hemoglobin. Remember, some athletes experience desaturation during maximal work at sea level.
- Some athletes show an increase in $\dot{V}O_2$ max while training at altitude while others do not. This may be due to the degree to which the athlete was trained before going to altitude.
- In addition, some athletes show an improved $\dot{V}O_2$ max upon return to sea level, while others do not. Part of the reason may be the altitude at which they train. Those who train at high altitudes may actually "detrain" due to the fact that the quality of their workouts suffers at the high altitudes. To get around this problem, one can alternate low-altitude and sea-level exposures.

The Quest for Everest

The most obvious tie between exercise and altitude is mountain climbing. The climber faces the stress of altitude, cold, radiation, and, of course, the work of climbing up steep slopes or sheer rock walls. A goal of some mountaineers has been to climb Mount Everest, at 8,848 meters, the highest mountain on Earth. Figure 24.4 shows the various attempts to climb Everest during this century (79). Special note should be made of Hillary and Tensing, who were the first to do it, and Messner and Habeler, who, to the amazement of all, did it without supplementary oxygen in 1978. This achievement brought scientists back to Everest in 1981 asking how this was possible. This section provides some background to this fascinating story.

In 1924, Norton's climbing team attempted to scale Everest without O_2, and almost succeeded—they stopped only 300 meters from the summit (57). This 1924 expedition was noteworthy because data were collected on the climbers and porters by physicians and scientists associated with the attempt. The story of this assault is good reading for those interested in mountain climbing and provides evidence of the keen powers of observation of the scientists. Major Hingston noted the respiratory distress associated with climbing to such heights, stating that at 5,800 meters (19,000 feet) "the very slightest exertion, such as the tying of a bootlace, the opening of a ration box, the getting into a sleeping bag, was associated with marked respiratory distress." At 8,200 meters (27,000 feet) one climber "had to take seven, eight, or ten complete respirations for every single step forward. And even at that slow rate of progress he had to rest for a minute or two every twenty or thirty yards" (57). Pugh, who made observations during a 1960–61 expedition to Everest, believed that fatigue of the respiratory muscles may be the primary factor limiting such endeavors at extreme altitudes (63). Further, Pugh's observations of the decreases in $\dot{V}O_2$ max at the extreme altitudes suggested that $\dot{V}O_2$ max would be just above basal metabolism at the summit, making the task an unlikely one at best. How then did Messner and Habeler climb Everest without O_2?

This was one of the primary questions addressed by the 1981 expedition to Everest. As mentioned earlier, $\dot{V}O_2$ max decreases with altitude due to the lower barometric pressure, which causes a lower PO_2 and a desaturation of hemoglobin. In effect, the $\dot{V}O_2$ max at the summit of Everest was predicated on the observed rate of decrease in $\dot{V}O_2$ max at lower altitudes and then extrapolated to the barometric pressure at the top of the mountain. One of the first major findings of the 1981 expedition was that the barometric pressure at the summit was 17 mm Hg higher than previously believed (81, 82). This higher barometric pressure increased the estimated inspired PO_2 and made a big difference in the predicted $\dot{V}O_2$ max. Figure 24.5 shows that the $\dot{V}O_2$ max predicted from the 1960–61 expedition was near the basal metabolic rate, while the value predicted from the 1981 expedition was closer to 15 ml $\cdot$ kg^{-1} $\cdot$ min^{-1} (81, 82). This $\dot{V}O_2$ max value was confirmed in the Operation Everest II project in which subjects did a simulated ascent of Mount Everest over a 40-day period in a decompression chamber (14, 74). This $\dot{V}O_2$ max value of 15 ml $\cdot$ kg^{-1} $\cdot$ min^{-1} helps to explain how the climbers were able to reach the summit without the aid of supplementary oxygen. However, it was not the only reason.

The arterial saturation of hemoglobin is dependent upon the arterial PO_2, PCO_2, and pH (chapter 10). A low PCO_2 and a high pH causes the oxygen hemoglobin curve to shift to the left, so that hemoglobin is more saturated under these conditions than under normal conditions. A person who can ventilate great volumes in response to hypoxia can exhale more CO_2 and cause the pH to become elevated. It has been shown that those who successfully deal with altitude

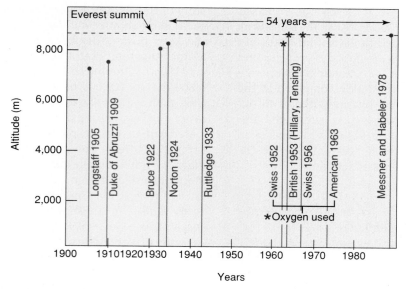

Figure 24.4

The highest altitudes attained by climbers in this century. In 1924 the climbers ascended within 300 meters of the summit without oxygen. It took another fifty-four years to climb those last 300 meters.

Figure 24.5

Plot of maximal oxygen uptake measured at a variety of altitudes, expressed as inspired PO_2 values. The 1964 data of Pugh et al. predicted the $\dot{V}O_2$ max to be equal to basal metabolic rate. The estimation based on the finding that the barometric pressure (and PO_2) was higher than expected as the summit shifts the estimate to about 15 ml · kg⁻¹ · min⁻¹.

have strong hypoxic ventilatory drives, allowing them to have a higher arterial PO_2 and oxygen saturation (71). In fact, when alveolar PCO_2 values were obtained at the top of Mount Everest in the 1981 expedition, the climbers had values much lower than expected (80). This ability to hyperventilate, coupled with the barometric pressure being higher than expected, resulted in higher arterial PO_2, and of course, $\dot{V}O_2$ max values. How high must your $\dot{V}O_2$ max be in order to climb Mount Everest?

Figure 24.5 shows that the climbers in the 1981 expedition had $\dot{V}O_2$ max values at sea level that were higher than those of the 1960–61 expedition. In fact, several of the climbers had been competitive marathon runners (82), and, given the need to transport oxygen at these high altitudes in order to do work, having such a high $\dot{V}O_2$ max would appear to be a prerequisite to success in climbing without oxygen. Subsequent measurements on other mountaineers who had scaled 8,500 meters or more without oxygen confirmed this by showing them to possess primarily Type I muscle fibers and to have an average $\dot{V}O_2$ max of 60 ± 6 ml · kg⁻¹ · min⁻¹ (58). However, there was one notable exception. One of the subjects in this study was Messner, who had climbed Mount Everest without oxygen; his $\dot{V}O_2$ max was 48.8 ml · kg⁻¹ · min⁻¹ (53). West et al. (83) provide food for thought in this regard, "It remains for someone to elucidate the evolutionary processes responsible for man being just able to reach the highest point on Earth while breathing ambient air." However, there is more to consider in climbing Mount Everest than a person's $\dot{V}O_2$ max.

It has been a common experience in mountain climbing, especially with prolonged exposure to high

The Lactate Paradox

When a submaximal test is conducted at altitude the heart rate, ventilation, and lactate responses are higher than what are measured at sea level. This is no surprise for the heart rate and ventilation responses since there is less oxygen per liter of blood and air, respectively. The elevated lactate response is also not unexpected; the assumption being that the hypoxia of altitude provides additional stimulation of glycolysis. What is surprising is that when the same exercise is done after the subject has been acclimatized to altitude for 3 or 4 weeks (chronic hypoxia), the lactate response is substantially reduced. This is the lactate paradox—that the same hypoxic stimulus in chronic hypoxia gives rise to a lower lactate response than observed when the subject is first exposed (acute hypoxia) to altitude (65a).

A wide variety of studies have been done to try and uncover the causes of the reduced lactate response to exercise during chronic exposure to altitude. The results from some of these studies have shown that the lower lactate is not due to a greater oxidative capacity of the muscle, an improved capillary-to-fiber ratio, or an improvement in oxygen delivery (26a, 65a). Instead, the reduction in lactate seems to be associated with a lower plasma epinephrine concentration which, as we know from chapter 5, would provide less stimulation of glycogenolysis via β-adrenergic receptor stimulation (54a, 65a). Evidence supporting this proposition comes from a study in which propranolol (a β-adrenergic receptor blocking drug) was shown to reduce the lactate response to acute hypoxia to a level seen only after chronic hypoxia (65a). However, the changes in epinephrine with acclimatization to altitude cannot entirely explain the lower lactate response (54a). The lower lactate response may also be due to muscular adaptations resulting in tighter metabolic control such that the ADP concentration does not increase as much during exercise; this results in less stimulation of glycolysis (see chapter 13) (26a). Consequently, the lactate paradox may be the result on both hormonal (epinephrine) and intracellular (lower [ADP]) adaptations that occur with chronic exposure to hypoxia.

altitudes, for climbers to lose weight, secondary to a loss of appetite (42a). Clearly, if a large portion of this weight loss were muscle, it would have a potential impact in the climber's ability to scale the mountain. Some recent work from both simulated and real ascents of Mount Everest provide some insight into what changes are taking place in muscle and what may be responsible for those changes. In the Operation Everest II 40-day simulation of an ascent to Mount Everest, the subjects experienced a 25% reduction in the cross-sectional area of Type I and Type II muscle fibers, and a 14% reduction in muscle area (26, 46). These observations were supported by data from a real ascent that combined both heavy exercise and severe hypoxia (34, 38). What could have caused these changes? The Operation Everest II data on nutrition and body composition showed that caloric intake decreased 43% from 3,136 to 1,789 kcal/day over the course of the 40-day exposure to hypoxia. The subjects lost an average of 7.4 kg, with most of the weight from lean body mass, despite the availability of palatable food (66). The hypoxia itself was a sufficient stimulus to suppress the appetite, and alter body composition. Whether or not such changes in muscle mass are linked directly to changes in $\dot{V}O_2$ max, they would clearly affect performance.

in summary

- Mount Everest was climbed without oxygen in 1978. This surprised scientists who thought $\dot{V}O_2$ max would be just above resting $\dot{V}O_2$ at that altitude. They later found that the barometric pressure was higher than they previously had thought and that the estimated $\dot{V}O_2$ max was about 15 ml $\cdot$ kg^{-1} $\cdot$ min^{-1} at this altitude.
- Those who are successful at these high altitudes have a great capacity to hyperventilate. This drives down the PCO_2 and the [H$^+$] in blood, and allows more oxygen to bind with hemoglobin at the same arterial PO_2.
- Finally, those who are successful at climbing to extreme altitudes must contend with the loss of appetite that results in a reduction in body weight and in the cross-sectional area of Type I and Type II muscle fibers.

Table 24.3 Heat-Related Problems

Heat Illness	Signs and Symptoms	Immediate Care
Heat Syncope	Headache Nausea	Normal intake of fluids
Heat Cramps	Muscle cramping (calf is very common) Multiple cramping (very serious)	Isolated cramps: Direct pressure to cramp and release, stretch muscle slowly and gently, gentle massage, ice Multiple cramps: Danger of heat stroke, *treat as heat exhaustion*
Heat Exhaustion	Profuse sweating Cold, clammy skin Normal temperature or slightly elevated Pale Dizzy Weak, rapid pulse Shallow breathing Nausea Headache Loss of consciousness	Move individual out of sun to a well-ventilated area Place in shock position (feet elevated 12–18 in); prevent heat loss or gain Gentle massage of extremities Gentle range of motion of the extremities Force fluids Reassure Monitor body temperature and other vital signs Refer to physician
Heat Stroke	Generally, no perspiration Dry skin Very hot Temperature as high as 106° F Skin color bright red or flushed (blacks—ashen) Rapid and strong pulse Labored breathing—semi-reclining position	This is an *extreme medical emergency* Transport to hospital quickly Remove as much clothing as possible without exposing the individual Cool quickly starting at the head and continuing down the body; use any means possible (fan, hose down, pack in ice) Wrap in cold, wet sheets for transport Treat for shock; if breathing is labored, place in a semi-reclining position

From E. T. Howley and B. D. Franks, *Health/Fitness Instructor's Handbook*. 2d ed. Copyright © 1992 Human Kinetics Publishers, Inc., Champaign IL. Used by permission.

Heat

Chapter 12 described the changes in body temperature with exercise, how heat loss mechanisms are activated, and the benefits of acclimatization. This section will extend that discussion by considering the prevention of thermal injuries during exercise.

Hyperthermia

Our core temperature (37° C) is within a few degrees of a value (45° C) that could lead to death (see chapter 12). Given that, and the fact that distance running races, triathlons, fitness programs, and football games occur during the warmer part of the year, the potential for heat injury is increased (9, 28, 41). Heat injury is not an all-or-none affair, but includes a series of stages that need to be recognized and attended to in order to prevent a progression from the least to the most serious (40). Table 24.3 summarizes each stage, identifying signs, symptoms, and the immediate care that should be provided (12). While it is important to recognize and deal with these problems, it is better to prevent them from happening.

Figure 24.6 shows the major factors related to heat injury. Each one independently influences susceptibility to heat injury:

Fitness   A high level of fitness is related to a lower risk of heat injury (23). Fit subjects can tolerate more work in the heat (17), acclimatize faster (9), and sweat more (6).

Acclimatization   Exercise in the heat, either low intensity (<50% $\dot{V}O_2$ max) and long duration (60–100 min), or moderate intensity (75% $\dot{V}O_2$ max) and short duration (30–35 min), increases the capacity to sweat, and reduces salt loss (37). Acclimatization leads to lower body temperature and HR responses during exercise and a reduced chance of salt depletion (9). Interestingly, although acclimatization increases work tolerance in the heat, exhaustion is experienced at similar core temperatures (56a).

Hydration   Inadequate hydration reduces sweat rate and increases the chance of heat injury

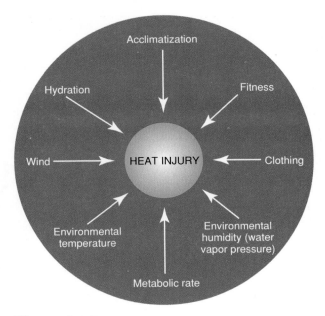

Figure 24.6
Factors affecting heat injury.

Figure 24.7
The effect of different types of uniforms on the body temperature response to treadmill running.

(9, 68, 69, 70). Chapter 23 discussed the procedures for fluid replacement. Generally, there is no difference between water, electrolyte drinks, or carbohydrate-electrolyte drinks in replacing body water during exercise (11, 13, 84).

Environmental Temperature   Convection and radiation heat loss mechanisms are dependent on a temperature gradient from skin to environment. Exercising in temperatures greater than skin temperatures result in a heat *gain*. Evaporation of sweat must then compensate if body temperature is to remain at a safe value.

Clothing   Expose as much skin surface as possible to encourage evaporation. Choose materials, such as cotton, that will "wick" sweat to the surface for evaporation. Materials impermeable to water will increase the risk of heat injury. Figure 24.7 shows the influence of different uniforms on the body temperature response to treadmill running (51).

Humidity (water vapor pressure)   Evaporation of sweat is dependent on the water vapor pressure gradient between skin and environment. In warm/hot environments, the relative humidity is a good index of the water vapor pressure, with a lower relative humidity facilitating evaporation.

Metabolic Rate   Given that core temperature is proportional to work rate, metabolic heat production plays an important role in the overall heat load experienced by the body during exercise. Decreasing the work rate decreases this heat load, as well as the strain on the physiological systems that must deal with it. Carbohydrate and fat metabolism is not affected when moderate exercise is done in a hot environment, compared to a thermoneutral one (84a).

Wind   Wind places more air molecules into contact with the skin and can influence heat loss in two ways. If a temperature gradient for heat loss exists between the skin and the air, wind will increase the rate of heat loss by convection. In a similar manner, wind increases the rate of evaporation, assuming the air can accept moisture.

Implications for Fitness

The person exercising for fitness needs to be educated about all of the previously listed factors. Suggestions might include:

- providing information on heat illness symptoms: cramps, lightheadedness, and so on,
- exercising in the cooler part of the day to avoid heat gain from the sun or structures heated by the sun,
- gradually increasing exposure to high heat/humidity to safely acclimatize,
- drinking water before, during, and after exercise and weighing in each day to monitor hydration,
- wearing only shorts and a tank top to expose as much skin as possible,
- taking heart rate measurements several times during the activity and reducing exercise intensity to stay in the THR zone.

The latter recommendation is most important. The heart rate is a sensitive indicator of dehydration, environmental heat load, and acclimatization. Variation in any of these factors will modify the heart rate response to any fixed submaximal exercise. It is therefore important for fitness participants to monitor heart rate on a regular basis and to slow down to stay within the THR zone.

Implications for Performance

Heat injury has been a concern in athletics for decades. Initially, the vast majority of attention was focused on football because of the large number of heat-related deaths associated with that sport (10). This problem has diminished over the last twenty years due to an emphasis on replacing water *during* practice and games, the use of a preseason conditioning program to increase fitness and initiate acclimatization, weighing in each day to monitor hydration, the development of new materials for jerseys, and the improved recognition of the potential for heat-related injury. While the risk of heat injuries was decreasing for football players, it was increasing in another athletic activity—long-distance road races (28, 41). In response to this problem, and on the basis of sound research, the American College of Sports Medicine developed a Position Stand on The Prevention of Thermal Injuries During Distance Running (3). The elements recommended in this position statement are consistent with what we previously presented:

Medical Director
- Work with race director to prevent heat injury and coordinate first-aid measures.

Race Organization
- Minimize environmental heat load by planning races for the cooler months, and at a time of day (before 8:00 A.M. or after 6:00 P.M.) to reduce solar heat gain.
- Use an environmental heat stress index (see next section) to help make decisions about whether or not to run a race.
- Have a water station every 2–3 km; encourage runners to drink 100–200 milliliters of water per station.
- Clearly identify the race monitors and have them look for those who might be in trouble due to heat injury.
- Have traffic control for safety.
- Use radio communication throughout the race course.

Medical Support
- Medical director coordinates ambulance service with local hospitals and has the authority to evaluate or stop runners who appear to be in trouble.

- Coordinates medical facilities at race site to provide first aid.

Competitor Education
- Provide information about factors related to heat illness that were discussed previously.
- Encourage the "buddy system" (see chapter 17).

The primary focus in these recommendations is on safety.

Environmental Heat Stress

The previous discussion mentioned high temperature and relative humidity as factors increasing the risk of heat injuries. In order to quantify the overall heat stress associated with any environment, a Wet Bulb Globe Temperature (WBGT) guide was developed (3). This overall heat stress index is composed of the following measurements:

Dry Bulb Temperature (T_{db})
- ordinary measure of air temperature taken in the shade

Black Globe Temperature (T_g)
- measure of the radiant heat load measured in direct sunlight

Wet Bulb Temperature (T_{wb})
- measurement of air temperature with a thermometer whose mercury bulb is covered with a wet cotton wick. This measure is sensitive to the relative humidity (water vapor pressure) and provides an index of the ability to evaporate sweat.

The formula used to calculate the WBGT temperature shows the importance of this latter wet bulb temperature in determining heat stress (3):

$$WBGT = 0.7\,T_{wb} + 0.2\,T_g + 0.1\,T_{db}$$

The risk of heat stress is given by the following color-coded flags on the race course:

- Red Flag   WBGT = 23–28° C (73–82° F)   High risk
- Amber Flag   WBGT = 18–23° C (65–73° F)   Moderate risk
- Green Flag   WBGT <18° C (<65° F)   Low risk of heat injury
- White Flag   WBGT <10° C (<50° F)   Low risk of hyperthermia, but possibility of hypothermia

in summary

- Heat injury is influenced by environmental factors such as temperature, water vapor pressure, acclimatization, hydration, clothing, and metabolic rate. The fitness participant should be educated about the signs and symptoms of heat injury, the importance of drinking water before, during, and after the activity, gradually becoming acclimated to the heat, exercising in the cooler part of the day, dressing appropriately, and checking the HR on a regular basis.
- Road races conducted in times of elevated heat and humidity need to reflect the coordinated wisdom of the race director and medical director to minimize heat and other injuries. Concerns include running the race at the correct time of the day and season of the year, frequent water stops, traffic control, race monitors to identify and stop those in trouble, and communication between race monitors, medical director, ambulance services, and hospitals.
- The heat stress index includes dry bulb, wet bulb, and globe temperatures. The wet bulb temperature, which is a good indicator of the water vapor pressure, is more important than the other two in determining overall heat stress.

Cold

Altitude and heat stress are not the only environmental factors having an impact on performance. As mentioned in the "White Flag" category of heat stress, a WBGT of 10° C or less is associated with hypothermia. Hypothermia is the result of a higher rate of heat loss from the body compared to heat production. Cold air facilitates this process in more ways than are readily apparent. First, and most obvious, when air temperature is less than skin temperature a gradient for heat loss exists for convection, and physiological mechanisms involving peripheral vasoconstriction and shivering come into play to counter this gradient. Second, and less obvious, cold air has a low water vapor pressure, which encourages the evaporation of moisture from the skin to further cool the body. The combined effects can be deadly, as witnessed in Pugh's report of three deaths during a "walking" competition over a forty-five-mile distance (60).

Figure 24.8 shows the factors related to hypothermia. These include environmental factors such as temperature, water vapor pressure, wind, and

Figure 24.8
Factors affecting hypothermia.

whether air or water are involved; insulating factors such as clothing and subcutaneous fat; and the capacity for sustained energy production. We will now comment on each of these relative to hypothermia.

Environmental Factors

Heat loss mechanisms introduced in chapter 12 included conduction, convection, radiation, and evaporation. Given that hypothermia is the result of a higher rate of heat loss compared to heat production, understanding how these mechanisms are involved will facilitate a discussion of how to deal with this problem.

Conduction, convection, and radiation are dependent on a temperature gradient between skin and environment; the larger the gradient, the greater the rate of heat loss. What is surprising is that the environmental temperature does not have to be below freezing in order to cause hypothermia. In effect, there are other environmental factors that interact with temperature to create the dangerous condition by facilitating heat loss, namely, wind and water.

Windchill Index

The rate of heat loss at any given temperature is directly influenced by the wind speed. Wind increases the number of cold air molecules coming into contact with the skin so that heat loss is accelerated. The windchill index indicates what the "effective" temperature is for any combination of temperature and wind speed. Siple and Passel (73) developed a formula for predicting how fast heat would be lost at different wind speeds and temperatures:

$$\text{Windchill (kcal} \cdot \text{m}^{-2} \cdot \text{h}^{-1}) = \left[\sqrt{WV \times 100} + 10.45 - WV \right] \times (33 - T_A)$$

Where: WV = wind velocity (m · sec^{-1}); 10.45 is a constant; 33 is 33° C, which is taken as the skin temperature; and T_A = ambient dry bulb temperature in °C.

Table 24.4   Windchill Index

Wind Speed in MPH	Actual Thermometer Reading (°F) 50	40	30	20	10	0	−10	−20	−30	−40	−50	−60
					Equivalent Temperature (°F)							
Calm	50	40	30	20	10	0	−10	−20	−30	−40	−50	−60
5	48	37	27	16	6	−5	−15	−26	−36	−47	−57	−68
10	40	28	16	4	−9	−21	−33	−46	−58	−70	−83	−95
15	36	22	9	−5	−18	−36	−45	−58	−72	−85	−99	−112
20	32	18	4	−10	−25	−39	−53	−67	−82	−96	−110	−124
25	30	16	0	−15	−29	−44	−59	−74	−88	−104	−118	−133
30	28	13	−2	−18	−33	−48	−63	−79	−94	−109	−125	−140
35	27	11	−4	−20	−35	−49	−67	−82	−98	−113	−129	−145
40	26	10	−6	−21	−37	−53	−69	−85	−100	−116	−132	−148

(Wind speeds greater than 40 MPH have little additional effect)

Little Danger (for properly clothed person)

Increasing Danger

Great Danger

Danger from freezing of exposed flesh

Figure 24.9
The effect of different water temperatures on survival of shipwrecked individuals.

If the windchill value equals 800, the conditions are classified as "cold," at 1,200, "bitterly cold," while at 2,000, exposed flesh would freeze in one minute, and at 2,300, exposed flesh would freeze in thirty seconds (22). This information has been translated into a familiar windchill chart shown in table 24.4, which allows you to properly gauge the conditions at a variety of wind velocities and temperatures. The term "danger" refers to the 2,000 windchill value and "great danger" refers to the 2,300 value. Please keep in mind that if you are running, riding, or cross-country skiing into the wind, you must add your speed to the wind speed to evaluate the full impact of the windchill. For example, cycling at 20 mph into calm air at 0° F is equivalent to −35° F! However, wind is not the only factor that can increase the rate of heat loss at any given temperature.

Water

The thermal conductivity of water is about twenty-five times greater than that of air so you can lose heat twenty-five times faster in water compared to air of the same temperature (35). Figure 24.9 shows that it takes only a few hours to cause death when a person is shipwrecked in cold water. Unlike air, water offers little or no insulation at the skin-water interface, so heat is rapidly lost from the body. Given that movement in such cold water would increase heat loss from the arms and legs, the recommendation is to stay as still as possible in long-term immersions (35).

in summary

- Hypothermia is influenced by natural and added insulation, environmental temperature, vapor pressure, wind, water immersion, and energy production.
- The Windchill Index describes how wind lowers the effective temperature at the skin such that convective heat loss is greater than what it would be in calm air at that same temperature.
- Water causes heat to be lost by convection twenty-five times faster than it would be by exposure to air of the same temperature.

Insulating Factors

The rate at which heat is lost from the body is inversely related to the insulation between the body and the environment. The insulating quality is related to the thickness of subcutaneous fat, the ability of clothing to trap air, and whether or not the clothing is wet or dry.

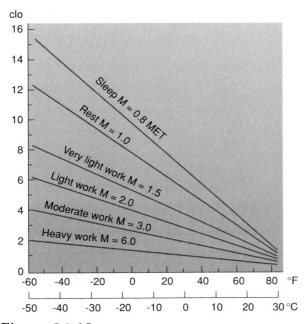

Figure 24.10

Changes in the insulation requirement of clothing (plus air) with increasing rates of energy expenditure over environmental temperatures of −50 to +30° C.

Subcutaneous Fat

An excellent indicator of total body insulation per unit surface area (through which heat is lost) is the average subcutaneous fat thickness (31). Pugh and Edholm's (61) observation that a "fat" man was able to swim for seven hours in 16° C water with no change in body temperature while a "thin" man had to leave the water in thirty minutes with a core temperature of 34.5° C, supports this statement. Long-distance swimmers tend to be fatter than short-course swimmers. The higher body fatness does more than help maintain body temperature; fatter swimmers are more buoyant, requiring less energy to swim at any set speed (33). In addition, body fatness plays a role in the onset and magnitude of the shivering response to cold exposure (see later discussion).

Clothing

Clothing can extend our natural subcutaneous fat insulation to allow us to sustain very cold environments. The insulation quality of clothing is given in **clo** units, where one clo is the insulation needed at rest (1 MET) to maintain core temperature when the environment is 21° C, the RH = 50%, and the air movement is 6 m · min⁻¹ (7). Still air next to the body has a clo rating of 0.8. As the air temperature falls, clothing with a higher clo value must be worn to maintain core temperature, since the gradient between skin and environment increases (58a). Figure 24.10 shows the insulation needed at different energy expenditures

across a broad range of temperatures from −60 to +80° F (7). It is clear that as energy production increases, insulation must decrease to maintain core temperature. By wearing clothing in layers, insulation can be removed piece by piece, since less insulation is needed to maintain core temperature. By following these steps, sweating, which can rob the clothing of its insulating value, will be minimized. A practical example of how clothing helps maintain body temperature (and comfort) can be seen in the following study. Heat loss from the head increases linearly from +32° C to −21° C, with about *half* of the entire heat production being lost through the head when the temperature is −4° C. Wearing a simple "helmet" with a clo rating of 3.5 allows an individual to stay out indefinitely at 0° C (21).

Clothing offers insulation by trapping air, a poor conductor of heat. If the clothing becomes wet, the insulating quality decreases since the water can now conduct heat away from the body at a faster rate (35). A primary goal, then, is to avoid wetness, due either to sweat or to weather. This problem is exacerbated by the cold environment's very low water vapor pressure. Recall from chapter 12 that the water vapor pressure in the environment is the primary factor influencing evaporation and that at low environmental temperatures the water vapor pressure is low even when the relative humidity is high. Think of the time when you have finished playing a game indoors and stepped outside into cold damp weather to cool off. You notice "steam" coming off your body; how is this possible when the RH is near 100%? The water vapor pressure is high at the skin surface since the skin temperature is elevated; so, a gradient for water vapor pressure exists. You will cool off very fast under these circumstances. This is why *cold, wet, windy* environments carry an extra risk of hypothermia. The wind not only provides for greater convective heat loss as described in the windchill chart, but it also accelerates evaporation (29).

Energy Production

Figure 24.10 shows that the amount of insulation needed to maintain core temperature decreases as energy expenditure increases. This is also true for our "natural" insulation, subcutaneous fat. McArdle et al. (56) showed that when fat men (27.6% fat) were immersed for one hour in 20° C, 24° C, and 28° C water, the resting $\dot{V}O_2$ and core temperature did not change compared to values measured in air. In thinner men (<16.8% fat), the $\dot{V}O_2$ increased to counter the rapid loss of heat; however, the core temperature still decreased. When these same subjects did exercise in the cold water, requiring a $\dot{V}O_2$ of 1.7 ℓ · min⁻¹, the fall in body temperature was either prevented or retarded (55), showing the importance of high rates of energy production in preventing hypothermia. More recent studies support these observations, showing an earlier onset and greater magnitude of shivering in lean subjects when exposed to cold air (76). Similar findings have been reported for fit subjects (5). Given the importance of body fatness in the metabolic response to cold exposure, are there differences due to gender?

A review of this topic indicated that women cool faster than men upon exposure to cold water and, despite the greater stimulus to shiver, do not respond with a greater $\dot{V}O_2$. However, when a prescribed amount of exercise is done, men and women respond similarly. In contrast, when the exercise intensity is chosen voluntarily, women exercise at a relatively lower $\dot{V}O_2$ and body temperature falls to a greater extent than in men (24). Interestingly, amenorrheic women exhibit a greater delay (60 min) in activating metabolism when exposed to cold, compared to eumenorrheic women (20 min) and men (10 min). These differences between men and women cannot be explained by differences in body fatness or body surface area (25). In addition, the availability of fuel (muscle glycogen and plasma FFA) seems to have little effect on adaptations to the cold (47, 48, 49, 50, 85).

in summary

- Subcutaneous fat is the primary "natural" insulation and is very effective in preventing rapid heat loss when a person is exposed to cold water.
- Clothing extends this insulation, and the insulation value of clothing is described in clo units, where a value of 1 describes what is needed to maintain core temperature while sitting in a room set at 21° C and 50% RH with an air movement of 6 m · sec^{-1}.
- The amount of insulation needed to maintain core temperature is less when one exercises because the metabolic heat production helps maintain the core temperature. Clothing should be worn in layers when exercising in order to shed one insulating layer at a time as body temperature increases.
- Energy production increases on exposure to cold, with an inverse relationship between the increase in $\dot{V}O_2$ and body fatness. Women cool faster than men when exposed to cold water, exhibiting a longer delay in the onset of shivering and a lower $\dot{V}O_2$, despite a greater stimulus to shiver.

Dealing with Hypothermia

As body temperature falls, the person's ability to carry out coordinated movements is reduced, speech is slurred, and judgment is impaired (72). People can die

from hypothermia, and the condition must be dealt with when it occurs. The following steps on how to do this are taken from Sharkey (72):

- Get person out of the cold, wind, and rain.
- Remove all wet clothing.
- Provide warm drinks, dry clothing, and a warm, dry sleeping bag for a mildly impaired person.
- If semiconscious, keep the person awake, remove clothing, and put into a sleeping bag with another person.
- Find a source of heat (e.g., camp fire).

in summary

- If a person becomes hypothermic, get the person out of the wind, rain, and cold; remove wet clothing and put on dry clothing; use a sleeping bag for warmth; and if it is a severe case, remove clothing from the person and have another person in the sleeping bag to provide warmth; finally, provide some source of heat.

Air Pollution

Air pollution includes a variety of gases and particulates that are products of the combustion of fossil fuels. The "smog" that results when these pollutants are in high concentration can have a detrimental effect on health and performance. The gases can affect performance by decreasing the capacity to transport oxygen, increasing airway resistance, and altering the perception of effort required when the eyes "burn" and the chest "hurts."

The physiological responses to these pollutants are related to the amount or "dose" received. The major factors determining the dose are the concentration of the pollutant, the duration of the exposure to the pollutant, and the volume of air inhaled. This last factor increases during exercise and is one reason why physical activity is curtailed during times of peak pollution levels (19). The following discussion focuses on the major air pollutants: ozone, sulfur dioxide, and carbon monoxide.

Ozone

The ozone we breathe is generated by the reaction of UV light and emissions from internal combustion engines. While a single two-hour exposure to a high ozone concentration, 0.75 parts per million (ppm), decreases $\dot{V}O_2$ max, recent studies show that a six to twelve hour exposure to a concentration of only 0.12 ppm (the U.S. air quality standard) decreases lung function and increases respiratory symptoms. Further, in amateur cyclists who practiced and raced in air containing varying concentrations of ozone, the decrease in pulmonary function following activity was directly related to the ozone concentration (5a). Interestingly, an

Figure 24.11

The effect of the concentration of carbon monoxide in the blood on the change in $\dot{V}O_2$ max.

adaptation to ozone exposure can occur, with subjects showing a diminished response to subsequent exposures during the "ozone season." However, concern about long-term lung health suggests that it would be prudent to avoid heavy exercise during the time of day when ozone and other pollutants are elevated (19).

Sulfur Dioxide

Sulfur dioxide (SO_2) is produced by smelters, refineries, and electrical utilities that use fossil fuel for energy generation. SO_2 does not affect lung function in normal subjects, but it causes bronchoconstriction in asthmatics. These latter responses are influenced by the temperature and humidity of the inspired air, as mentioned in chapter 17. Nose breathing is encouraged to "scrub" the SO_2, and drugs like cromolyn sodium and β_2-agonists can partially block the asthmatic's response to SO_2 (19).

Carbon Monoxide

Carbon monoxide (CO) is derived from the burning of fossil fuel, coal, oil, gasoline, and wood, as well as from cigarette smoke. Carbon monoxide can bind to hemoglobin to form carboxyhemoglobin (HbCO) and decrease the capacity for oxygen transport. This has the potential to affect the physiological responses to submaximal exercise (32) as well as $\dot{V}O_2$ max, as does altitude. The carbon monoxide concentration [HbCO] in blood is generally less than 1% in nonsmokers, but may be as high as 10% in smokers (64). Horvath et al. (36) found that the critical concentration of HbCO needed to decrease $\dot{V}O_2$ max was 4.3%. Figure 24.11 shows the relationship between the blood HbCO concentration and the decrease in $\dot{V}O_2$ max; beyond 4.3% HbCO, $\dot{V}O_2$ max decreases 1% for each 1% increase in HbCO (65).

In contrast, when one performs light work, at about 40% $\dot{V}O_2$ max, the [HbCO] can be as high as 15% before endurance is affected. The cardiovascular system has the capacity to compensate with a larger cardiac output when the HbO_2 concentration is reduced during submaximal work (36, 64, 65). Since it takes two to four hours to remove half the CO from the blood once the exposure has been removed, CO can have a lasting effect on performances (19).

Unfortunately, it is difficult to predict what the actual [HbCO] will be in any given environment. One must consider the previous exposure to the pollutant, as well as the length of time and rate of ventilation associated with the current exposure. As a result, Raven (64) provides the following guidelines for exercising in an area with air pollution:

- Reduce exposure to the pollutant prior to exercise since the physiological effects are time- and dose-dependent.
- Stay away from areas where you might receive a "bolus" dose of CO: smoking areas, high traffic areas, urban environment.
- Do not schedule activities around the times when pollutants are at their highest levels (7–10 A.M. and 4–7 P.M.) due to traffic.

in summary

- Air pollution can affect performance. Exposure to ozone decreases $\dot{V}O_2$ max and respiratory function, while sulfur dioxide causes bronchoconstriction in asthmatics.
- Carbon monoxide binds to hemoglobin and reduces oxygen transport in much the same way that altitude does.
- To prevent problems associated with pollution of any type, reduce exposure time; stay away from "bolus" amounts of the pollutant; and schedule activity at the least polluted part of the day.

study questions

1. Describe the changes in barometric pressure, PO_2, and air density with increasing altitude.
2. Why is sprint performance not affected by altitude?
3. Explain why maximal aerobic power decreases at altitude and what effect this has on performance in long-distance races.
4. Graphically describe the effect of altitude on the HR and ventilation responses to submaximal work and provide recommendations for fitness participants who occasionally exercise at altitude.

5. Describe the process by which an individual adapts to altitude, and contrast the adaptation of the permanent residents of high altitude with that of the lowlander who arrives there as an adult.

6. While training at altitude can be beneficial, how could someone "detrain?" How can you work around this problem?

7. It was formally believed that a person could not climb Mount Everest without oxygen because the estimated $\dot{V}O_2$ max at altitude was close to basal metabolic rate. When two climbers accomplished the feat in 1978, scientists had to determine how this was possible. What were the primary reasons allowing the climb to take place without oxygen?

8. List and describe the factors related to heat injury.

9. What is the heat stress index and why is the wet bulb temperature weighed so heavily in the formula?

10. List the factors related to hypothermia.

11. Explain what the Windchill Index is relative to convective heat loss.

12. What is a clo unit, and why is the insulation requirement less when you exercise?

13. What would you do if a person had hypothermia?

14. Explain how carbon monoxide can influence $\dot{V}O_2$ max and endurance performance.

15. What steps would you follow to minimize the effect of pollution on performance?

suggested readings

Grassi, B. et al. 1995. Maximal rate of blood lactate accumulation during exercise at altitude in humans. *Journal of Applied Physiology* 79:331–39.

Houston, C. 1994. High adventure: The romance between medicine and mountaineering. *Exercise and Sport Science Reviews* 22:1–22.

Reeves, J. T. et al. 1992. Oxygen transport during exercise at altitude and the lactate paradox: Lessons from Operation Everest II and Pikes Peak. In *Exercise and Sport Sciences Reviews*, vol. 20, ed. J. O. Holloszy, 275–96. Baltimore: Williams & Wilkins.

references

1. Adams, W. C. et al. 1975. Effects of equivalent sea-level and altitude training on $\dot{V}O_2$ max and running performance. *Journal of Applied Physiology* 39:262–66.

2. Alexander, J. K. et al. 1967. Reduction of stroke volume during exercise in man following ascent to 3,100 m altitude. *Journal of Applied Physiology* 23:849–58.

3. American College of Sports Medicine. 1985. The prevention of thermal injuries during distance running. *Medicine and Science in Sports and Exercise* 19:529–33.

4. Balke, B., F. J. Nagle, and J. Daniels. 1965. Altitude and maximum performance in work and sports activity. *Journal of the American Medical Association* 194:646–49.

5. Bittel, J. H. M. et al. 1988. Physical fitness and thermoregulatory reactions in a cold environment in men. *Journal of Applied Physiology* 65:1984–89.

5a. Brunekreef, B., G. Hoek, O. Breugelmans, and M. Leentvaar. 1994. Respiratory effects of low-level photochemical air pollution in amateur cyclists. *American Journal of Respiratory, Critical Care Medicine* 150:962–66.

6. Buono, M. J., and N. T. Sjoholm. 1988. Effect of physical training on peripheral sweat production. *Journal of Applied Physiology* 65:811–14.

7. Burton, A. C., and O. G. Edholm. 1955. *Man in a Cold Environment*. London: Edward Arnold.

8. Buskirk, E. R. et al. 1967. Maximal performance at altitude and on return from altitude in conditioned runners. *Journal of Applied Physiology* 23:259–66.

9. Buskirk, E. R., and D. E. Bass. 1974. Climate and exercise. In *Science and Medicine of Exercise and Sport*, eds. W. R. Johnson and E. R. Buskirk, 190–205. New York: Harper & Row.

10. Buskirk, E. R., and W. C. Grasley. 1974. Heat injury and conduct of athletics. In *Science and Medicine of Exercise and Sport*, eds. W. R. Johnson and E. R. Buskirk, 206–10. New York: Harper & Row.

11. Carter, J. E., and C. V. Gisolfi. 1989. Fluid replacement during and after exercise in the heat. *Medicine and Science in Sports and Exercise* 21:532–39.

12. Carver, S. 1986. Injury prevention and treatment. In *Health/Fitness Instructor's Handbook*, eds. E. T. Howley and B. Don Franks, 211–32. Champaign, IL: Human Kinetics.

13. Costill, D. L. et al. 1975. Water and electrolyte replacement during repeated days of work in the heat. *Aviation, Space and Environmental Medicine* 46 (6):795–800.

14. Cymerman, A. et al. 1989. Operation Everest II: Maximal oxygen uptake at extreme altitude. *Journal of Applied Physiology* 66:2446–53.

15. Daniels, J., and N. Oldridge. 1970. The effects of alternate exposure to altitude and sea level on world-class middle-distance runners. *Medicine and Science in Sports* 2:107–12.

16. Dill, D. B., and W. C. Adams. 1971. Maximal oxygen uptake at sea level and at 3,090-m altitude in high school champion runners. *Journal of Applied Physiology* 30:854–59.

17. Drinkwater, B. L. et al. 1976. Aerobic power as a factor in women's response to work within hot environments. *Journal of Applied Physiology* 41:815–21.

17a. Engfred, K. et al. 1994. Hypoxia and training-induced adaptation of hormonal responses to exercise in humans. *European Journal of Applied Physiology* 68:303–9.

18. Faulkner, J. A. et al. 1968. Maximum aerobic capacity and running performance at altitude. *Journal of Applied Physiology* 24:685–91.

19. Folinsbee, L. J. 1990. Discussion: Exercise and the environment. In *Exercise, Fitness, and Health*, eds. C. Bouchard, R. J. Shephard, T. Stevens, J. R. Sutton, and B. D. McPherson, 179–83. Champaign, IL: Human Kinetics.

20. Frisancho, A. R. et al. 1973. Influence of developmental adaptation on aerobic capacity at high altitude. *Journal of Applied Physiology* 34:176–80.

21. Froese, G., and A. C. Burton. 1957. Heat loss from the human head. *Journal of Applied Physiology* 10:235–41.

22. Gates, D. M. 1972. *Man and His Environment: Climate.* New York: Harper & Row.

23. Gisolfi, G. V., and J. Cohen. 1979. Relationships among training, heat acclimation, and heat tolerance in men and women: The controversy revisited. *Medicine and Science in Sports* 11:56–59.

24. Graham, T. E. 1988. Thermal, metabolic, and cardiovascular changes in men and women during cold stress. *Medicine and Science in Sports and Exercise* 20 (Suppl.): S185–S192.

25. Graham, T. E., M. Viswanathan, J. P. van Dijk, and J. C. George. 1989. Thermal and metabolic responses to cold by men and by eumenorrheic and amenorrheic women. *Journal of Applied Physiology* 67:282–90.

26. Green, H. J., J. R. Sutton, A. Cymerman, P. M. Young, and C. S. Houston. 1989. Operation Everest II: Adaptations in human skeletal muscle. *Journal of Applied Physiology* 66:2454–61.

26a. Green, H. J. et al. 1992. Altitude acclimatization and energy metabolic adaptations in skeletal muscle during exercise. *Journal of Applied Physiology* 73:2701–8.

26b. Greksa, L. P., H. Spielvogel, and L. Paredes-Fernandez. 1993. Maximal aerobic power in high-altitude runners. *Annals of Human Biology* 20:395–400.

27. Grover, R. et al. 1967. Muscular exercise in young men native to 3,100 m altitude. *Journal of Applied Physiology* 22:555–64.

28. Hanson, P. G., and S. W. Zimmerman. 1979. Exertional heatstroke in novice runners. *Journal of the American Medical Association* 242:154–57.

29. Hardy, J. D., and P. Bard. 1974. Body temperature regulation. In *Medical Physiology*, 13th ed., vol. 2, ed. V. B. Mountcastle, 1305–42. St. Louis: C. V. Mosby.

30. Hartley, L. H., J. A. Vogel, and J. C. Cruz. 1974. Reduction of maximal exercise heart rate at altitude and its reversal with atropine. *Journal of Applied Physiology* 36:362–65.

31. Hayward, M. G., and W. R. Keatinge. 1981. Roles of subcutaneous fat and thermoregulatory reflexes in determining ability to stabilize body temperature in water. *Journal of Physiology* (London) 320:229–51.

32. Hirsch, G. L. et al. 1985. Immediate effects of cigarette smoking on cardiorespiratory responses to exercise. *Journal of Applied Physiology* 58:1975–81.

33. Holmer, I. 1979. Physiology of swimming man. In *Exercise and Sport Sciences Reviews*, vol. 7, eds. R. S. Hutton and D. I. Miller. Salt Lake City: Franklin Institute.

34. Hoppeler, H., E. Kleinert, C. Schleger, H. Classon, H. Howald, S. R. Kayar, and P. Cerretelli. 1990. II. Morphological adaptations of human skeletal muscle to chronic hypoxia. *International Journal of Sports Medicine* 11:S3–S9.

35. Horvath, S. M. 1981. Exercise in a cold environment. In *Exercise and Sport Sciences Reviews*, vol. 9, ed. D. I. Miller, 221–63. Salt Lake City: Franklin Institute.

36. Horvath, S. M. et al. 1975. Maximal aerobic capacity of different levels of carboxyhemoglobin. *Journal of Applied Physiology* 38:300–303.

37. Houmard, J. A., D. L. Costill, J. A. Davis, J. B. Mitchell, D. D. Pascoe, and R. A. Robergs. 1990. The influence of exercise intensity on heat acclimation in trained subjects. *Medicine and Science in Sports and Exercise* 22:615–20.

38. Howald, H., D. Pette, J. A. Simoneau, A. Uber, H. Hoppeler, and P. Cerretelli. 1990. III. Effects of chronic hypoxia on muscle enzyme activities. *International Journal of Sports Medicine* 11:S10–S14.

39. Howley, E. T. 1980. Effect of altitude on physical performance. In *Encyclopedia of Physical Education, Fitness, and Sports: Training, Environment, Nutrition, and Fitness*, eds. G. A. Stull and T. K. Cureton, 177–87. Salt Lake City: Brighton.

40. Hubbard, R. W., and L. E. Armstrong. 1989. Hyperthermia: New thoughts on an old problem. *The Physician and Sportsmedicine* 17:97–113.

41. Hughson, R. L. et al. 1980. Heat injuries in Canadian mass participation runs. *Canadian Medicine Medical Association Journal* 122:1141–44.

42. Hurtado, A. 1964. Animals in high altitudes: Resident man. In *Handbook of Physiology: Section 4—Adaptation to the Environment*, ed. D. B. Dill. Washington, D.C.: American Physiological Society.

42a. Kayser, B. 1994. Nutrition and energetics of exercise at altitude. *Sports Medicine* 17:309–23.

43. Kollias, J., and E. Buskirk. 1974. Exercise and altitude. In *Science and Medicine of Exercise and Sport*, 2d ed., eds. W. R. Johnson and E. R. Buskirk. New York: Harper & Row.

44. Kollias, J. et al. 1968. Work capacity of long-time residents and newcomers to altitude. *Journal of Applied Physiology* 24:792–99.

45. Lawler, J., S. K. Powers, and D. Thompson. 1988. Linear relationship between $\dot{V}O_2$ max and $\dot{V}O_2$ max decrement during exposure to acute hypoxia. *Journal of Applied Physiology* 64:1486–92.

46. MacDougall, J. D., H. J. Green, J. R. Sutton, G. Coates, A. Cymerman, P. Young, and C. S. Houston. 1991. Operation Everest II: Structural adaptations in skeletal muscle in response to extreme simulated altitude. *Acta Physiologica Scandinavica* 142:421–27.

46a. Martin, D., and J. O'Kroy. 1993. Effects of acute hypoxia on the $\dot{V}O_2$ max of trained and untrained subjects. *Journal of Sports Science* 11:37–42.

47. Martineau, L., and I. Jacobs. 1988. Muscle glycogen utilization during shivering thermogenesis in humans. *Journal of Applied Physiology* 65:2046–50.

48. ———. 1989a. Muscle glycogen availability and temperature regulation in humans. *Journal of Applied Physiology* 66:72–78.

49. ———. 1989b. Free fatty acid availability and temperature regulation in cold water. *Journal of Applied Physiology* 67:2466–72.

50. ———. 1991. Effects of muscle glycogen and plasma FFA availability on human metabolic responses in cold water. *Journal of Applied Physiology* 71:1331–39.

51. Mathews, D. K., E. L. Fox, and D. Tanzi. 1969. Physiological responses during exercise and recovery in a football uniform. *Journal of Applied Physiology* 26:611–15.

52. Mazess, R. B. 1969. Exercise performance at high altitude in Peru. *Federation Proceedings* 28:1301–6.

53. ———. 1969. Exercise performance of Indian and white high-altitude residents. *Human Biology* 41:494–518.

54. ———. 1970. Cardiorespiratory characteristics and adaptations to high altitudes. *American Journal of Physical Anthropology* 32:267–78.

54a. Mazzeo, R. S. et al. 1994. Beta-adrenergic blockade does not prevent the lactate response to exercise after acclimatization to high altitude. *Journal of Applied Physiology* 76:610–15.

55. McArdle, W. D. et al. 1984. Thermal adjustment to cold-water exposure in exercising men and women. *Journal of Applied Physiology: Respiratory, Environmental, and Exercise Physiology* 56:1572–77.

56. McArdle, W. D. et al. 1984. Thermal adjustment to cold-water exposure in resting men and women. *Journal of Physiology: Respiratory, Environmental, and Exercise Physiology* 56:1565–71.

56a. Nielsen, B. et al. 1993. Human circulatory and thermoregulatory adaptations with heat acclimation and exercise in a hot, dry environment. *Journal of Physiology* (London) 460:467–85.

57. Norton, E. F. 1925. *The Fight for Everest: 1924*. New York: Longmans, Green.

58. Oelz, O. et al. 1986. Physiological profile of world-class high-altitude climbers. *Journal of Applied Physiology* 60:1734–42.

58a. Pascoe, D. D., L. A. Shanley, and E. W. Smith. 1994. Clothing and exercise. I. Biophysics of heat transfer between the individual, clothing, and environment. *Sports Medicine* 18:38–54.

58b. Powers, S. K., D. Martin, and S. Dodd. 1993. Exercise-induced hypoxaemia in elite athletes. *Sports Medicine* 16:14–22.

59. Pronnet, F., G. Thibault, and D. L. Cousineau. 1991. A theoretical analysis of the effect of altitude on running performance. *Journal of Applied Physiology* 70:399–404.

60. Pugh, L. G. C. 1964. Deaths from exposure in Four Inns Walking Competition, *Lancet* 1(March 14–15):1210–12.

61. Pugh, L. G. C., and O. G. Edholm. 1955. The physiology of Channel swimmers. *Lancet* 2:761–68.

62. Pugh, L. G. C. E. 1967. Athletes at altitude. *Journal of Physiology* (London) 192:619–46.

63. Pugh, L. G. C. E. et al. 1964. Muscular exercise at great altitudes. *Journal of Applied Physiology* 19:431–40.

64. Raven, P. B. 1980. Effects of air pollution on physical performance. In *Encyclopedia of Physical Education, Fitness, and Sports: Training, Environment, Nutrition, and Fitness*, vol. 2, eds. G. A. Stull and T. K. Cureton, 201–16. Salt Lake City: Brighton.

65. Raven, P. B. et al. 1974. Effect of carbon monoxide and peroxyacetyl nitrate on man's maximal aerobic capacity. *Journal of Applied Physiology* 36:288–93.

65a. Reeves, J. T. et al. 1992. Oxygen transport during exercise at altitude and the lactate paradox: lessons from Operation Everest II and Pikes Peak. In *Exercise and Sport Sciences Reviews*, vol. 20, ed. J. O. Holloszy, 275–96. Baltimore: Williams & Wilkins.

66. Rose, M. S., C. S. Houston, C. S. Fulco, G. Coates, J. R. Sutton, and A. Cymerman. 1988. Operation Everest II: Nutrition and body composition. *Journal of Applied Physiology* 65:2545–51.

67. Roskamm, H. et al. 1969. Effects of a standardized ergometer training program at three different altitudes. *Journal of Applied Physiology* 27:840–47.

68. Saltin, B. 1964. Circulatory response to submaximal and maximal exercise after thermal dehydration. *Journal of Applied Physiology* 19:1125–32.

69. Sawka, M. N. et al. 1984. Influence of hydration level and body fluids on exercise performance in the heat. *Journal of the American Medical Association* 252(9):1165–69.

70. Sawka, M. N. et al. 1985. Thermoregulatory and blood responses during exercise at graded hypohydration levels. *Journal of Applied Physiology* 59:1394–1401.

71. Schoene, R. B. et al. 1984. Relationship of hypoxic ventilatory response to exercise performance on Mount Everest. *Journal of Applied Physiology: Respiratory, Environmental, and Exercise Physiology* 56:1478–83.

72. Sharkey, B. J. 1984. *Physiology of Fitness*. 2d ed. Champaign, IL: Human Kinetics.

73. Siple, P. A., and C. F. Passel. 1945. Measurements of dry atmospheric cooling in subfreezing temperatures. *Proceedings of the American Philosophical Society* 89:177–99.

74. Sutton, J. R. et al. 1988. Operation Everest II: Oxygen transport during exercise at extreme simulated altitude. *Journal of Applied Physiology* 64:1309–21.

75. Terrados, N., E. Jansson, C. Sylven, and L. Kaijser. 1990. Is hypoxia a stimulus for synthesis of oxidative enzymes and myoglobin? *Journal of Applied Physiology* 68:2369–72.

76. Tikuisis, P., D. G. Bell, and I. Jacobs. 1991. Shivering onset, metabolic response, and convective heat transfer during cold air exposure. *Journal of Applied Physiology* 70:1996–2002.

77. Ward-Smith, A. J. 1983. The influence of aerodynamic and biomechanic factors on long jump performance. *Journal of Biomechanics* 16:655–58.

78. West, J. B. Man at extreme altitude. 1982. *Journal of Applied Physiology: Respiratory, Environmental, and Exercise Physiology* 52:1393–99.

79. West, J. B., and P. D. Wagner. 1980. Predicted gas exchange on the summit of Mt. Everest. *Respiration Physiology* 42:1–16.

80. West, J. B. et al. 1983. Pulmonary gas exchange on the summit of Mount Everest. *Journal of Applied Physiology: Respiratory, Environmental, and Exercise Physiology* 55:678–87.

81. West, J. B. et al. 1983. Barometric pressures at extreme altitudes on Mt. Everest: Physiological significance. *Journal of Applied Physiology* 54:1188–94.

82. West, J. B. et al. 1983. Maximal exercise at extreme altitudes on Mt. Everest. *Journal of Applied Physiology* 55:688–98.

83. West, J. B. et al. 1962. Arterial oxygen saturation during exercise at high altitude. *Journal of Applied Physiology* 17:617–21.

84. Yaspelkis, B. B., and J. L. Ivy. 1991. Effect of carbohydrate supplements and water on exercise metabolism in the heat. *Journal of Applied Physiology* 71:680–87.

84a. Yaspelkis, B. B. et al. 1993. Carbohydrate metabolism during exercise in hot and thermoneutral environments. *International Journal of Sports Medicine* 14:13–19.

85. Young, A. J., M. Sawka, P. D. Neufer, S. R. Muza, E. W. Askew, and K. B. Pandolf. 1989. Thermoregulation during cold water immersion is unimpaired by low muscle glycogen levels. *Journal of Applied Physiology* 66:1809–16.

CHAPTER 25

Ergogenic Aids

objectives

By studying this chapter, you should be able to do the following:

1. Define ergogenic aid.
2. Explain why a "placebo" treatment in a "double-blind design" is used in research studies involving ergogenic aids.
3. Describe, in general, the effectiveness of nutritional supplements on performance.
4. Describe the effect of additional oxygen on performance; distinguish between hyperbaric oxygenation and that accomplished by breathing oxygen-enriched gas mixtures.
5. Describe blood doping and its potential for improving endurance performance.
6. Explain the mechanism by which ingested buffers might improve anaerobic performances.
7. Explain how amphetamines might improve exercise performance.
8. Describe the various mechanisms by which caffeine might improve performance.
9. Identify the risks associated with using chewing tobacco to obtain a nicotine "high."
10. Describe the risks of cocaine use and how it can cause death.
11. Describe the physiological and psychological effects of different types of warm-up.

outline

Research Design Concerns   460
Nutritional Supplements   461
Aerobic Performance   462
  Oxygen   463
  Blood Doping   464
Anaerobic Performance   465
  Blood Buffers   465
Drugs   466
  Amphetamines   466
  Caffeine   467
Cocaine   470
Nicotine   470
Physical Warm-Up   471

key terms

autologous transfusion
blood boosting
blood doping
blood packing
dental caries
double-blind research design

ergogenic aid
erythrocythemia
erythropoietin
homologous transfusion
hyperbaric chamber
induced erythrocythemia

normocythemia
placebo
sham reinfusion
sham withdrawal
sympathomimetic

The preceding chapters have described exercise and dietary plans related to performance. However, no presentation of factors affecting performance would be complete without a discussion of **ergogenic aids.** Ergogenic aids are defined as work-producing substances or phenomena believed to increase performance (43).

Ergogenic aids include nutrients, drugs, warm-up exercises, hypnosis, stress management, blood doping, oxygen breathing, music, and extrinsic biomechanical aids. The reader is referred to the texts by Williams (67), Morgan (45), and Lamb and Williams (36) which cover these and more ergogenic aids. Although we discussed nutritional issues related to performance in chapter 23 we will provide additional detail about the role of nutritional supplements as ergogenic aids in this chapter. In addition, we will discuss ergogenic aids related to aerobic performance (oxygen inhalation and blood doping) and anaerobic performance (blood buffers), as well as various drugs (amphetamines, caffeine, cocaine, and nicotine) and physical warm-up. Please note that anabolic steroids and growth hormone were discussed in chapter 5.

While the attention of the reader will be focused on athletic performance, where an improvement of less than 1 percent would alter world records, it must be noted that industrial physiologists have long been concerned about the relationship of lighting, environmental temperature, and background noise (music) to performance in the workplace (45). Research work in this area must be carefully done, with special attention to the research design due to the number of factors that can influence the outcome of the study.

Research Design Concerns

It is sometimes difficult to compare the results of one research study with another. The reason for this is that the effect of an ergogenic aid is dependent on a number of variables (37):

- Amount—too little or too much may show no effect
- Subject—the ergogenic aid may be effective in "untrained" subjects but not "trained" subjects, or vice versa
  —"value" of an ergogenic aid is determined by the subject
- Task—may work in short-term power-related tasks, but not in endurance tasks, or vice versa
  —may work for gross-motor, large-muscle activities and not with fine-motor activities, or vice versa

Figure 25.1
Changes in performance when subjects were told they were taking an anabolic steroid, but were really taking a placebo.

- Use—an ergogenic aid used on an acute (short-term) basis may show a positive effect, but in the long run may compromise performance, or vice versa

Given these variables, scientists must be careful in designing experiments in order not to be "fooled" by the result. For example, an *athlete* may improve performance because he or she believes the substance improves performance, so the "belief" is more important than the substance in determining the outcome. Further, an *investigator* may "believe" in the ergogenic aid and inadvertently offer different levels of encouragement during the testing of athletes under the influence of the ergogenic aid. These problems are controlled for by using a **placebo** as a treatment condition, and using a **double-blind research design,** respectively.

A placebo is a "look-alike" substance relative to the ergogenic aid under consideration, but contains nothing that will influence performance. The need for such a control is seen in figure 25.1, which describes the gain in strength by a group that was taking a placebo but was *told* it was an anabolic steroid. It is contrasted with their performance prior to taking the placebo. The rate of strength gain was higher with the placebo, indicating the need for such a control if one is to isolate the true effect of a substance (2).

A double-blind research design is one in which neither the subject nor the investigator knows who is receiving the placebo or the substance under investigation. The subjects are randomly assigned to receive pill "x" or pill "y." After all data are collected the "code" is broken to find out which pill (x or y) was the placebo and which was the substance under investigation. These designs are very complex and difficult to carry out, but they reduce the chance of subject or investigator bias (45).

The scientist must also be careful in the selection of subjects. If a substance is tested as a potential aid to sprinters, it would be reasonable to select subjects from that population so the results can be generalized to that group. Further, the tests used by the investigator should be as close as, or actually be, the performance task (e.g., 100-meter dash). In short, results obtained on a proper subject population but under controlled laboratory conditions using conventional physiological tests may not be useful when taken to the "field" (45).

in summary

- Ergogenic aids are defined as substances or phenomena that are work-producing and are believed to increase performance.
- Due to the fact that an athlete's *belief* in a substance may influence performance, scientists use a placebo or look-alike substance to control for this effect. In addition, scientists use a double-blind research design in which the investigator and subject are both unaware of the treatment.

Nutritional Supplements

We discussed issues related to basic nutrition in chapter 18, and provided additional detail about the role of nutrition in performance in chapter 23. In this section we go a step further and discuss the role that nutritional supplements play in athletic performance—a point of interest to many athletes. A survey of athletes indicated that 46 percent used nutritional supplements. Elite athletes used supplements more than college or high school athletes, and women used them more than men (57a).

One has to only open a strength-training magazine to become aware of the incredible number of nutritional supplements promoted as improving the effects of a workout, be it size or strength. Williams (68a) provided a summary of a number of these nutritional supplements marketed for strength-trained individuals (STI) (see table 25.1). The middle column contains the purported claim, and the right-most column lists the evidence that supports that claim. A quick reading of that column indicates that little or no support exists for any of the supplements, with the exception of creatine. We all know of the role of phosphocreatine (PC) in high-power events, or at the onset of endurance exercise (see chapters 3 and 4). Recent studies show that the ingestion of four 5-gm doses of creatine for five days will significantly increase intramuscular creatine and PC concentrations prior to exercise. This is associated with high work output during repeated bouts of high-power exercise (30a).

Carnitine, another nutritional supplement listed in table 25.1, is associated with the transport of fatty acids from the cytoplasm into the mitochondria. Table 25.1 indicates that there was no support for its use by STI for the purpose of promoting fat loss. However, endurance athletes are also interested in carnitine because of its putative effect on fat use, which may spare carbohydrates and reduce the lactate concentration during exercise (34a). Although, some studies report a greater use of fat following carnitine supplementation, others found no effect during submaximal exercise, even when plasma FFA were elevated by heparin injection (34a, 63a). Additional research is needed to resolve this issue.

Table 25.1   Nutritional Supplements Marketed for Strength-Trained Individuals

Nutritional Supplement	Promoted Use/Advertised Claim	Valid Research Data with Supplementation to Strength-Trained Individuals (STI)
Protein supplements	Provide adequate protein to support muscle growth, weight gain	No valid data that protein supplements are more effective than natural protein sources; STI may need 1.5–2.0 g protein/kg body weight; easily obtained from healthful diet protein sources, e.g., lean meats, skim milk, complimentary plant proteins
Arginine, lysine, ornithine	Stimulate release of human growth hormone (HGH), insulin; promote muscle growth	May stimulate HGH release; however, HGH itself has not been shown to be ergogenic to STI; research indicates no effect on muscle growth or strength
Creatine	Increase phosphocreatine in muscles; increased energy source and stimulate muscle growth	Preliminary research indicates increased power in short-term, high-intensity exercise; increased weight gain, either contractile protein or water

Continued

From *Sports Science Exchange*, Vol. 6, No. 6, 1993. Copyright © 1993 Gatorade Sports Science Institute, Barrington IL. Reprinted by permission.

Table 25.1   Continued

Nutritional Supplement	Promoted Use/Advertised Claim	Valid Research Data with Supplementation to Strength–Trained Individuals (STI)
Inosine	Increase ATP synthesis; increase strength and facilitate recuperation	No valid studies documenting an ergogenic effect on STI
Choline	Increase acetylcholine or lecithin to increase strength or decrease body fat, respectively	No valid studies documenting an ergogenic effect on STI
Yohimbine	Increase serum testosterone levels; increase muscle growth and strength; alpha-2 adenoreceptor blocker; decrease body fat	No valid studies documenting an ergogenic effect on STI; needs further research to document role as useful agent for weight loss in STI
Glandulars: adrenals, pituitary, testes	Enhance function of analogous gland in humans	No valid studies documenting an ergogenic effect on STI
Vitamin B-12	Enhance DNA synthesis; increase muscle growth	Research indicates no effect on muscle growth or strength in STI
Antioxidant vitamins; C, E, beta-carotene	Prevent muscle damage from unwanted oxidative processes following high-intensity, eccentric muscle contractions	Research data not in agreement; additional research needed to document effect of antioxidants to prevent muscle damage in STI
Carnitine	Increase transport of fatty acids into mitochondria for oxidation; promote fat loss	No valid studies documenting weight loss or an ergogenic effect in STI
Chromium	Potentiate insulin action; promote muscle growth via enhanced amino acid uptake	Research data not in agreement, but more appropriately designed studies show no effect on body composition or strength in STI
Boron	Increase serum testosterone levels; increase muscle growth and strength	Research indicates no effect on serum testosterone levels, lean body mass, or strength in STI
Magnesium	Increase protein synthesis or muscle contractility; increase muscle growth and strength	Research data equivocal, but generally not supportive of an ergogenic effect in STI
Medium chain triglycerides	Increase thermic effect; promote fat loss	No valid studies documenting body fat or weight loss in STI
Omega-3 fatty acids	Stimulate release of HGH	No valid studies documenting an ergogenic effect in STI
Gamma oryzanol	Increase serum testosterone and HGH levels; increase muscle growth	No valid studies documenting an ergogenic effect in STI
Smilax	Increase serum testosterone levels; increase muscle growth and strength	No valid studies documenting an ergogenic effect in STI

in summary

- For the most part there is little evidence that nutritional supplements provide a performance advantage to athletes.

Aerobic Performance

Chapter 20 detailed the various tests used to evaluate the physiological factors related to endurance performance. Clearly, an increased ability to transport O_2 to the muscles and a delay in the onset of lactate production are related to improved performance. Two ergogenic aids have been used to try to influence O_2 delivery: the breathing of O_2-enriched mixtures and blood doping.

Oxygen

Given the importance of aerobic metabolism in the production of ATP for muscular work, it is not surprising that scientists have been interested in the effect of additional oxygen (hyperoxia) on performance. But in order to discuss this issue we must ask the following question: How and when was the O_2 administered to achieve a higher PO_2 in the blood? In his insightful review of this topic, Welch (64) stressed the difficulty of comparing results from studies in which hyperoxia is achieved by increasing the percent of O_2 in the inspired air with those that use a **hyperbaric** (high-pressure) **chamber** with 21% or higher O_2 mixtures. Figure 25.2 shows that performance improves throughout the range of inspired oxygen pressures when O_2-enriched mixtures are used at a normal pressure of 1 atmosphere ("constant pressure"), compared to the use of a hyperbaric chamber ("increasing pressure"). The second part of the question is related to the time of administration of the supplemental O_2. Results vary depending on whether the O_2 is administered prior to, during, or following exercise. For that latter reason, this section on oxygen will be organized by those conditions.

Prior to Exercise

The rationale for the use of supplemental oxygen prior to exercise is to try to "store" additional oxygen in the blood so that more will be available at the onset of exercise. It has been estimated that the hemoglobin in arterial blood is about 97% saturated with O_2 at rest (200 ml O_2/ℓ blood). Breathing 100% O_2 would increase the O_2 bound to hemoglobin by only 3%, or 6 milliliters. However, the amount of oxygen physically dissolved in solution is proportional to the arterial PO_2, and when the PO_2 increases from about 100 mm Hg (breathing 21% O_2 at sea level) to about 700 mm Hg (breathing 100% O_2), the dissolved oxygen increases from 3 ml/ℓ to 21 ml/ℓ. If a person has a total blood volume of 5 liters, approximately 100 milliliters of additional O_2 can be "stored" prior to exercise. However, if the person breathes several times between the time the O_2 breathing stops and the event begins, the O_2 store will return to that associated with air breathing (70).

The focus of attention on the use of oxygen prior to exercise has been on short-term exercise. In general, in runs of 880 yards or less, weight lifting, stair climbing, and swims of 200 yards or less, the O_2 seemed to be beneficial (46, 70). In addition, evidence suggested that the O_2 breathing needed to take place within two minutes prior to the task (70). Some concern has been expressed about these findings due to the fact that in

Figure 25.2

The effect of PO_2 on performance. Constant pressure experiments used oxygen-enriched gas mixtures at sea-level pressure, while the increasing pressure experiments used a hyperbaric chamber to increase the PO_2.

From H. W. Welch, "Effects of Hypoxia and Hyperpoxia on Human Performance" in Kent B. Pandolf, Ed., *Exercise and Sport Sciences Reviews*, Vol. 15. Copyright © 1987 McGraw-Hill, Inc., New York. Reprinted by permission.

some cases the subjects knew they were breathing O_2, a factor that could have affected the results (70). Overall, considering the fact that O_2 cannot be breathed up to the start of a sprint event in swimming or track, any effect would be lost before the starter's gun is fired. Therefore, unless one participates in a breath-holding event, oxygen breathing prior to exercise will have little effect on performance.

During Exercise

The rationale for the use of oxygen during exercise to improve performance is based on the proposition that muscle is hypoxic during exercise and additional O_2 delivery will alleviate the problem (64). If this is the case, then the additional O_2 in the blood during O_2 breathing should increase the delivery of O_2 to the muscle and improve performance. However, Welch et al. (65) showed that when breathing hyperoxic gas mixtures, the increase in the O_2 content of arterial blood (CaO_2) is balanced by a *decrease* in blood flow to the working muscles such that O_2 delivery (CaO_2 × flow) was not different from normoxic (21% O_2) conditions. $\dot{V}O_2$ max is increased by only 2%–5% with hyperoxia, which is about what would be expected since maximal cardiac output doesn't change and the a-$\bar{v}$ O_2 difference does not increase more than 5%–6% (54) [$\dot{V}O_2$ max = $\dot{Q}$ max × (CaO_2 – C $\bar{v}O_2$)].

In spite of similarities in O_2 delivery during hyperoxia and normoxia, *performance* has been shown to increase dramatically as a result of an increase in inspired O_2. Figure 25.2, presented in the introduction to this section, showed a performance increase of 40% while breathing 100% O_2. How could this be if O_2

delivery to muscles is not substantially different? The increased availability of O_2 has been shown to decrease pulmonary ventilation and reduce the work of breathing, a change that should lead to an increase in performance (64, 71, 72). In addition, those athletes who experience "desaturation" of hemoglobin during maximal work (see chapters 9 and 24) while breathing 21% O_2 could benefit by breathing oxygen-enriched gas mixtures (50). Finally, the high PO_2 slows glycolysis during heavy exercise, resulting in a slower accumulation of lactate and H^+ in the plasma and extending the time to exhaustion (32, 64). Given the impracticality of trying to provide O_2 mixtures to athletes *during* performance, this research on hyperoxia is more useful as a tool to answer questions related to the age-old question of what factor, O_2 delivery or the muscle's capacity to consume O_2, limits aerobic performance (64).

After Exercise

The rationale associated with the use of supplemental oxygen after exercise is that the subject might recover more quickly following exercise and be ready to go again. Some of the early work showed just that, but because the subjects knew what gas they were breathing, the results have to be interpreted with caution (46, 70). Wilmore (70) summarized the effects of several studies and concluded that there was no benefit of O_2 breathing during recovery on heart rate, ventilation, and post-exercise oxygen uptake. This conclusion was supported by studies showing no effect of O_2 breathing on subsequent performance in all-out exercise (51).

in summary

- Oxygen breathing before or after exercise seems to have little or no effect on performance, while oxygen breathing during exercise improves endurance performance.

Blood Doping

In chapter 13 we described how $\dot{V}O_2$ max is limited by maximal cardiac output, given the constraint that blood pressure had to be maintained by vasoconstriction of the active muscle mass. Since maximal O_2 transport is equal to the product of maximal cardiac output ($\dot{Q}$ max) and the O_2 content of arterial blood (CaO_2), one way to improve O_2 delivery to tissue when $\dot{Q}$ max cannot change is to increase the quantity of hemoglobin in each liter of blood. **Blood doping** refers to the infusion of red blood cells (RBC) in an attempt to increase the hemoglobin concentration ([Hb]) and, consequently, O_2 transport (CaO_2 is equal to the [Hb] $\times$ 1.34 ml O_2/gm Hb). Other terms to describe this are **blood boosting** and **blood packing,** with **induced erythrocythemia** being the proper medical term.

In blood doping, a subject receives a transfusion of blood, which may be his or her own **(autologous transfusion)** or blood from a matched donor **(homologous transfusion).** The latter procedure is acceptable in times of medical emergencies, but carries the risk of infection and blood-type incompatibility (27); it is therefore not recommended in blood-doping procedures. The constraint to use your own blood in order to achieve the goal of a higher [Hb] creates some interesting problems that led to confusion in the early days of research in this area. The primary problem was related to the mismatch between the maximum time blood could be refrigerated and the time period needed for the subject to produce new RBC and bring the [Hb] back to normal before the reinfusion. Maximum storage time with refrigeration is three weeks, during which time about 1% of the RBC are lost per day. In addition, some RBCs adhere to the storage containers or become so fragile that they will not function upon reinfusion. Due to these problems only about 60% of the removed RBCs could be reinfused (27). The normal time period for replacement of the RBCs following a 400-milliliter donation is three to four weeks, and following a 900-milliliter donation, five to six weeks or more are required. If the blood were reinfused at the end of the three-week maximal storage time, the investigator might not have been able to achieve the condition of an increased [Hb] due to RBC loss (decreased 40%) and the below normal (anemic) values in the subjects. Gledhill (27) makes a strong case for this as a primary reason why studies prior to 1978 showed inconsistent changes in $\dot{V}O_2$ max and performance with blood doping. Another major problem encountered in these early studies was the lack of an adequate research design. There was a need to have a group undergoing a **"sham" withdrawal** (needle placed in the arm but no blood is removed) and a **"sham" reinfusion** (needle placed in the arm but blood is not returned) to act as "placebo" controls.

The central factor allowing a more careful study of blood doping was the introduction of the freezer preservation technique that allows the blood to be stored frozen for years with only a 15% RBC loss. This allows plenty of time for the subject to become **normocythemic** (achieve normal [Hb]), so that any effect of the reinfusion can be correctly evaluated (27).

The general findings were that reinfusions of single units (~450 milliliters) of blood showed small but insignificant increases in [Hb], $\dot{V}O_2$ max, and performance, while the infusion of two units (900 milliliters) significantly increased the [Hb] (8%–9%), $\dot{V}O_2$ max (4%–5%), and performance (3%–34%). The infusion of three units (1,350 milliliters) of blood caused slightly greater increases in [Hb] (10.8%) and $\dot{V}O_2$ max (6.6%). This large reinfusion caused borderline **erythrocythemia** to be approached, so a 1,350-milliliter infusion probably represents the upper limit that can be used. Figure 25.3 shows a gradual reduction in [Hb]

Figure 25.3
Changes in hemoglobin levels in blood following removal (phlebotomy) and reinfusion.

toward the normal value following reinfusion, indicating that increased O_2 transport is maintained for ten to twelve weeks. This is an important point as far as performance gains are concerned (25).

The improvements in performance (3%–34%) were much more variable than the changes in [Hb] or $\dot{V}O_2$ max. Part of the reason for this variation was the type of performance test used. The greatest change was observed in a running test to exhaustion that lasted less than ten minutes, while the smallest change was observed in a 5-mile time trial, with the improvement being fifty-one seconds compared to a preinfusion run time of 30:17 (69). Given that the laboratory results show consistent gains, the question raised by Eichner, "Does it work in the field?," still needs to be answered (17). Until the answer is known, blood doping will continue to be a useful laboratory tool to study the factors limiting $\dot{V}O_2$ max (58).

While the blood doping issue will always raise a question of ethics, Gledhill presents what amounts to a moral dilemma in the use of blood doping in getting athletes ready for performance at altitude. In chapter 24 we have already discussed the changes in $\dot{V}O_2$ max and performance at altitude. Those athletes who stay at altitude experience a natural increase in RBC production to deal with the hypoxia. As Gledhill (27) points out, those athletes who can afford to train at altitude accomplish what blood doping does in a manner that is acceptable to the International Olympic Committee. The recent availability of a recombinant DNA analog of **erythropoietin,** the hormone that stimulates red blood cell production, has complicated the picture.

Erythropoietin is used as a part of therapy for those who have kidney damage and undergo dialysis treatment; the hormone stimulates red blood cell production to reduce the chance of anemia. While normal cross-country training does not seem to increase plasma levels of naturally occurring erythropoietin (4), acute exposure to 3,000 and 4,000 meters simulated altitude has been shown to increase the concentration

1.8- and 3.0-fold, respectively (15). The real concern, of course, is the potential abuse of the DNA-derived analog of this hormone to generate the effects of blood doping, without having to undergo the blood withdrawals and reinfusions. Such abuse is not without its risks, in that RBC production can get out of hand. This could lead to extremely high RBC levels, which would impair blood flow to the heart and brain, resulting in a myocardial infarction or a stroke. However, if an athlete were to use the drug and experience the desired increase in RBC production, the RBC effect would last for some weeks, while the level of erythropoietin would return quickly to resting values, making detection of this blood doping procedure difficult to trace (56).

in summary

- Blood doping refers to the reinfusion of red blood cells in order to increase the hemoglobin concentration and oxygen-carrying capacity of the blood.
- Due to improvements in blood storage techniques, blood doping has been shown to be effective in improving $\dot{V}O_2$ max and endurance performance.

Anaerobic Performance

Improvements in endurance performance focus on the supply of carbohydrate and oxygen to muscle (see previous sections on oxygen and blood doping in this chapter and on carbohydrate in chapter 24). However, in short-term, all-out performances in which anaerobic energy sources provide the vast majority of energy for muscle contraction, the focus of attention shifts to the buffering of the H^+ released from muscle. This section will consider a means by which investigators have tried to buffer the H^+ and improve performance.

Blood Buffers

Elevations in the [H^+] in muscle can decrease the activity of phosphofructokinase (PFK) (62), which may slow glycolysis, interfere with excitation-contraction coupling events by reducing Ca^{++} efflux from the terminal cisternae of the sarcoplasmic reticulum (23), and reduce the binding of Ca^{++} to troponin (47). Decreases in muscle force development have been shown to be linked to increases in muscle [H^+] in both frog muscle (20) and human muscle (61). Finally, when Adams and Welch (1) showed that performance times in heavy exercise (90% $\dot{V}O_2$ max) could be altered by breathing 60% O_2 compared to 21% or 17% O_2, the point of exhaustion was associated with the same arterial [H^+]. The mechanisms involved in the regulation of the plasma [H^+] were described in detail in chapter 11. Briefly, the primary means by which H^+ is buffered *during* exercise is through its reaction with the plasma bicarbonate reserve to form carbonic acid, which subsequently yields CO_2 that is exhaled (respiratory compensation). As the bicarbonate buffer store decreases, the ability to buffer H^+ is reduced and the plasma $[H^+]$ will increase. Knowing this, scientists have explored ways of increasing the plasma buffer store to slow down the rate of H^+ increase during strenuous exercise.

As early as 1932 (13) induced alkalosis (means unknown) was shown to extend run time (min:sec) to exhaustion (5:22 to 6:04). Since that time a wide variety of studies have supported these findings. In recent reviews of this topic, Linderman and Fahey (37), Williams (68), and Horswill (32a) summarized the results in the following way:

- the optimal dose of bicarbonate used to improve performance was 0.3 gm per kilogram of body weight (along with 1 liter of water),
- tasks of a minute or less in duration, even at extremes of intensity, did not seem to benefit from the induced alkalosis, and
- performance gains were shown for tasks of high intensity that lasted about one to ten minutes, or involved repeated bouts of high intensity exercise with short recovery periods.

Sodium citrate has also been shown to be an effective buffer when taken at 0.5 gm/kg and for anaerobic performances of two to four minutes (32a, 44a). The variability in the effectiveness of the sodium bicarbonate treatment suggests that some short-term anaerobic activities are more dependent on the muscle or plasma $[H^+]$ as a primary cause of fatigue than others. Welch (64) indicates that while subjects may stop at the same $[H^+]$ within any exercise protocol, the differences that exist among studies in the "terminal" $[H^+]$ suggest the other factors are more limiting as far as performance is concerned. The use of these agents to cause an alkalosis is not without risks. Large doses of sodium bicarbonate can cause diarrhea and vomiting, both of which are sure to affect performance (26, 37, 68).

in summary

- The ingestion of sodium bicarbonate improves performances of one to ten minutes duration, or in repeated bouts of high-intensity exercise.

Drugs

A variety of drugs have been used to aid performance. Some drugs are as common and "legal" as caffeine and nicotine, while others, like amphetamines and cocaine, are banned from use. We will briefly examine each of these drugs, exploring how they might work to improve performance, as well as the evidence about whether or not they do.

Amphetamines

Amphetamines are stimulants that have been used primarily to recover from fatigue and improve endurance. In 1972 Golding (29) indicated that it was the most abused group of drugs at that time. Amphetamines are readily absorbed in the small intestine, and while the effects reach a peak two to three hours after ingestion, they persist for twelve to twenty-four hours (33, 38). Amphetamines are both a **sympathomimetic** drug (simulates catecholamine effects), and a central nervous system stimulant. The drug produces its effects by altering the metabolism and synthesis of catecholamines, or receptor affinity for catecholamines (33, 38).

The most consistent effect of amphetamines is to increase one's arousal or wakefulness, leading to a perception of increased energy and self-confidence (33). The drug affects the redistribution of blood flow, driving it away from the skin and splanchnic areas and delivering more to muscle or brain. This could lead to problems related to a decrease in lactic acid removal (see chapter 3) and an increase in body temperature (see chapter 12). Animal studies show that amphetamines can increase endurance-type performances. However, the dose of the drug was shown to be important, in that smaller doses (1–2 mg/kg) did not have an effect different from control, and large doses (16 mg/kg) appeared to reduce the ability of the rat to swim. Data collected using run tests on rats indicate the same detrimental effect of high doses (7.5–10 mg/kg) of amphetamines (33).

Ivy (33) concluded from an analysis of studies on human subjects that amphetamines extend endurance and hasten recovery from fatigue. Time to exhaustion was increased in spite of no effect on submaximal or maximal $\dot{V}O_2$ (8, 33). Two explanations have been offered. Ivy (33) feels that the endurance aspect of performance can be improved due to amphetamines' catecholamine-like effect in mobilizing FFA and sparing muscle glycogen, similar to that of caffeine (see the caffeine section, this chapter). Chandler and Blair (8) believe that the amphetamines may simply mask fatigue and interfere with the perception of the normal biological signals that fatigue has occurred. It is this latter conclusion that has raised the most concern about the safety of the athlete, in that during prolonged submaximal work, especially in a hot and/or humid environment, the decreased blood flow to the skin could cause hyperthermia, leading to death (33, 38).

As mentioned at the beginning of this section, amphetamines' major effect is in increasing wakefulness and producing a state of arousal. However, while amphetamines have restored reaction time in fatigued subjects, the drug does not have this effect on alert, motivated, and nonfatigued subjects (11). Given that athletes are usually alert and motivated prior to competition, Golding (29) suggests that

A Closer Look 25.1

Clenbuterol—A New Anabolic Agent

Clenbuterol is a drug that was developed to treat airway diseases (e.g., asthma). Its chemical action in the body is to activate beta-2 receptors in tissue (chapter 5). Although the drug is useful in the treatment of airway diseases, in the early 1980s it was discovered that Clenbuterol is a powerful anabolic agent in skeletal muscles. Indeed, a 14-day treatment of animals with Clenbuterol (2 mg/kg/day) results in a 10%–20% increase in muscle mass [see Yang (73) for a review]. The muscle growth observed in animals following treatment with Clenbuterol is a true hypertrophy and does not involve hyperplasia (41a). Further, the time course of Clenbuterol-induced muscular hypertrophy is rapid with muscle growth beginning within two days after commencement of treatment.

Since the discovery that Clenbuterol is a powerful anabolic agent in skeletal muscle, scientific interest in the clinical use of this drug has grown. For example, this compound is potentially useful in the treatment of conditions that result in muscle wasting (i.e., aging, spinal cord injury, etc.). Unfortunately, many athletes now use Clenbuterol in an effort to increase muscle size and improve performance in power events (e.g., sprinting, football, etc.).

At present, Clenbuterol is not a legal drug in the United States and is a banned substance for use in international athletic competition. Further, use of the drug may also pose serious health risks. Because high doses of Clenbuterol also activate beta-1 receptors, Clenbuterol can increase heart rate and cause potentially serious cardiac arrhythmias. Therefore, use of Clenbuterol as an anabolic agent is unwise (41a, 73).

amphetamines would be counterproductive, making users hyperirritable and interfering with their sleep. Finally, it is risky to extrapolate from data collected under tightly controlled laboratory conditions using discrete measures related to performance ($\dot{V}O_2$ max, endurance time, reaction time) to the actual performance in a skilled sport in front of a hostile audience for a national championship.

in summary

- Amphetamines have a catecholamine-like effect that leads to an increased arousal and a perception of increased energy and self-confidence.
- While amphetamines improve performance of fatigued subjects, the drug does not have this effect on alert, motivated, and nonfatigued subjects.

Caffeine

Caffeine is a stimulant that is found in a wide variety of common foods, drinks, and over-the-counter drugs (see table 25.2). Caffeine has been viewed as an on-again, off-again ergogenic aid. Caffeine was banned by the International Olympic Committee (IOC) in 1962, then removed from the list of banned drugs in 1972. In 1984, the IOC again banned "high levels" in the urine that might have been the result of caffeine injections or suppositories; the standard is now set at 12 μg/ml (63, 66). Caffeine is absorbed rapidly from the GI tract, significantly elevated in the blood at fifteen minutes, and peaking at sixty minutes. Caffeine is diluted by body water and the physiological response is proportional to the concentration in the body water. There is a natural variability in how people respond to caffeine, and chronic users are less responsive than abstainers (63).

While caffeine can affect a wide variety of tissues, figure 25.4 shows that its role as an ergogenic aid is based on its effects on skeletal muscle, the central nervous system, and in the mobilization of fuels for muscular work. The evidence for the enhanced function of skeletal muscle is based primarily on *in vitro* and *in situ* muscle preparations and shows that caffeine can increase tension development (49, 63). This was shown most clearly in fatigued muscle and was believed to be due to enhanced Ca^{++} availability (41). In one human study, caffeine had no effect on maximum voluntary contraction or the maximal tension elicited by electrical stimulation. However, there was greater tension development at lower levels of electrical stimulation in both rested and fatigued muscles. The change in endurance measured by time at 50% of maximal voluntary contraction tension was variable and nonsignificant (40).

Caffeine has long been recognized as a stimulator of the CNS. Caffeine can pass the blood-brain barrier and affect a variety of brain centers, which usually leads to an increased alertness and decreased drowsiness (49, 63). The best evidence supporting caffeine as a CNS stimulant is in the decreased perception of fatigue during prolonged exercise in subjects who took caffeine (12).

Table 25.2   Caffeine Content of Popular Foods, Beverages, Soft Drinks, and Drug Preparations

Caffeine Content of Popular Beverages and Food		Caffeine Content of Various Soft Drinks	
Item	Caffeine (mg)[a]	Soft Drinks	Caffeine (mg per 12-oz Serving)[b]
Coffee (5-oz Cup)		Sugar-Free Mr. PIBB	58
Drip method	110–150	Mountain Dew	54
Percolated	64–124	Mello Yello	52
Instant	40–108	TAB	46
Decaffeinated	2–5	Coca-Cola	46
Instant decaffeinated	2	Diet Coke	46
Tea (Loose or Bags)		Shasta Cola	44
(5-oz Cup)		Shasta Diet Cola	44
One-minute brew	9–33	Mr. PIBB	40
Three-minute brew	20–46	Dr Pepper	40
Five-minute brew	20–50	Sugar-Free Dr Pepper	40
Tea Products		Pepsi Cola	38.4
Instant tea (5-oz cup)	12–28	Diet Pepsi	36
Iced tea (12-oz cup)	22–36	Pepsi Light	36
Cocoa		RC Cola	36
Made from mix	6	Diet Rite	0
Milk chocolate (1 oz)	6	Canada Dry Diet Cola	0
Baking Chocolate (1 oz)	35		

Caffeine in Drug Preparations[c]		Caffeine in Drug Preparations[c]	
Classification	Caffeine (mg per Tablet or Capsule)	Classification	Caffeine (mg per Tablet or Capsule)
Over-the-Counter Stimulants		**Cold Remedies**	
No Doz Tablets	100	Coryban-D	30
Vivarin Tablets	200	Dristan	0
Pain Relievers		Triaminicin	30
Anacin	32	**Weight-Control Aids**	
Excedrin	65	Dexatrim	200
Midol	32	Prolamine	140
Plain aspirin, any brand	0	**Prescription Pain Relievers**	
Vanquish	33	Cafergot	100
Diuretics		Darvon Compound	32.4
Aqua Ban	100	Fiorinal	40
		Migralam	100

[a]Data from Consumers Union, Food and Drug Administration, National Coffee Association, and National Soft Drink Association.
[b]Data from National Soft Drink Association.
[c]Values taken from The Physicians' Desk Reference for Nonprescription Drugs, 1983.
From J. L. Slavin and D. J. Joensen, "Caffeine and Sport Performance" in The Physician and Sportsmedicine, 13:191, 193, May 1985. Copyright © 1985. McGraw-Hill Healthcare Group, Minneapolis, MN. Reprinted by permission. (57)

The role of caffeine in the mobilization of fuel has received considerable attention as the primary means by which it exerts its ergogenic effect. Caffeine has been shown to cause an elevation of glucose and an increase in fatty acid utilization. The elevated glucose could be due to the stimulation of the sympathetic nervous system and the resulting increase in catecholamines, which would increase the mobilization of glucose from the liver. On the other hand, the glucose concentration could be elevated due to a decreased rate of removal related to the suppression of insulin release by catecholamines (see chapter 5) (63).

Lipid mobilization has been shown to be increased as a result of caffeine ingestion. Figure 25.5 shows that the mechanism of action could be related either to the elevated catecholamines increasing the level of cyclic AMP in the adipose cell or to caffeine's blocking of phosphodiesterase activity, which is responsible for breaking down cyclic AMP. Van Handle

METS	Activity	Description
2.5	Sports,	Billiards
3.0	Sports,	Bowling
12.0	Sports,	Boxing, in ring, general
6.0	Sports,	Boxing, punching bag
5.0	Sports,	Children's games (hopscotch, 4-square, dodgeball, playground apparatus, t-ball, tetherball, marbles, jacks, arcade games)
4.0	Sports,	Coaching: football, soccer, basketball, baseball, swimming, etc.
5.0	Sports,	Cricket (batting, bowling)
2.5	Sports,	Croquet
4.0	Sports,	Curling
2.5	Sports,	Darts, wall or lawn
6.0	Sports,	Fencing
9.0	Sports,	Football, competitive
8.0	Sports,	Football, touch, flag, general (T 510)
3.0	Sports,	Frisbee playing, general
3.5	Sports,	Frisbee, ultimate
5.5	Sports,	Golf, carrying clubs
3.0	Sports,	Golf, miniature, driving range
5.0	Sports,	Golf, pulling clubs
3.5	Sports,	Golf, using power cart
4.0	Sports,	Gymnastics, general
4.0	Sports,	Hacky sack
12.0	Sports,	Handball
8.0	Sports,	Handball, team
3.5	Sports,	Hang gliding
8.0	Sports,	Hockey, field
8.0	Sports,	Hockey, ice
4.0	Sports,	Horseback riding
3.0	Sports,	Horseshoe pitching, quoits
12.0	Sports,	Jai alai
10.0	Sports,	Judo, juijtsu, karate, kick boxing, tae kwan do
4.0	Sports,	Juggling
7.0	Sports,	Kickball
8.0	Sports,	Lacrosse
4.0	Sports,	Moto-cross
9.0	Sports,	Orienteering
10.0	Sports,	Paddleball, competitive
6.0	Sports,	Paddleball, casual, general
8.0	Sports,	Polo
10.0	Sports,	Racketball, competitive
7.0	Sports,	Racketball, casual, general
11.0	Sports,	Rock climbing, ascending rock
8.0	Sports,	Rock climbing, rapelling
12.0	Sports,	Rope jumping, fast
10.0	Sports,	Rope jumping, moderate, general
8.0	Sports,	Rope jumping, slow
10.0	Sports,	Rugby
3.0	Sports,	Shuffleboard, lawn bowling
5.0	Sports,	Skateboarding
7.0	Sports,	Skating, roller
10.0	Sports,	Soccer, competitive
5.0	Sports,	Softball or baseball, fast or slow pitch
6.0	Sports,	Softball, pitching
12.0	Sports,	Squash
4.0	Sports,	Table tennis, ping pong
4.0	Sports,	Tai chi
6.0	Sports,	Tennis, doubles
8.0	Sports,	Tennis, singles
4.0	Sports,	Volleyball, competitive
3.0	Sports,	Volleyball, noncompetitive; 6–9 member team
6.0	Sports,	Wrestling (one match = 5 min)
7.0	Sports,	Wallyball
3.0	Walking,	Downstairs
6.0	Walking,	Hiking, cross country
6.5	Walking,	Marching, rapidly, military
2.5	Walking,	Pushing or pulling stroller with child
6.5	Walking,	Race walking
8.0	Walking,	Up stairs, using or climbing up ladder
4.0	Walking,	Using crutches
2.0	Walking,	Walking, less than 2.0 mph, level ground, strolling, household walking, very slow
2.5	Walking,	Walking, 2.0 mph, level, slow pace, firm surface
3.0	Walking,	Walking, 2.5 mph, firm surface
3.0	Walking,	Walking, 2.5 mph, downhill
3.5	Walking,	Walking, 3.0 mph, level, moderate pace, firm surface
4.0	Walking,	Walking, 3.5 mph, level, brisk, firm surface
4.0	Walking,	Walking, 4.0 mph, level, firm surface, very brisk pace
4.5	Walking,	Walking, 4.5 mph, level, firm surface, very, very brisk
4.0	Walking,	Walking, to work or class
4.0	Water activities,	Canoeing, on camping trip
3.0	Water activities,	Canoeing, rowing, 2.0–3.9 mph, light effort
7.0	Water activities,	Canoeing, rowing, 4.0–5.9 mph, moderate effort
12.0	Water activities,	Canoeing, rowing, >6 mph, vigorous effort
3.5	Water activities,	Canoeing, rowing, for pleasure, general
12.0	Water activities,	Canoeing, rowing, in competition, or crew or sculling
5.0	Water activities,	Kayaking
3.0	Water activities,	Sailing, boat and board sailing, wind-surfing, ice sailing, general
5.0	Water activities,	Sailing, in competition
6.0	Water activities,	Skiing, water

METS	Activity	Description
7.0	Water activities,	Skimobiling
5.0	Water activities,	Snorkeling
3.0	Water activities,	Surfing, body or board
10.0	Water activities,	Swimming laps, freestyle, fast, vigorous effort
8.0	Water activities,	Swimming laps, freestyle, slow, moderate or light effort
8.0	Water activities,	Swimming, backstroke, general
10.0	Water activities,	Swimming, breaststroke, general
11.0	Water activities,	Swimming, butterfly, general
6.0	Water activities,	Swimming, leisurely, not lap swimming
10.0	Water activities,	Water polo
3.0	Water activities,	Water volleyball
5.0	Water activities,	Whitewater rafting, kayaking, or canoeing
5.5	Winter activities,	Skating, ice, 9 mph or less
9.0	Winter activities,	Skating, ice, rapidly, more than 9 mph

METS	Activity	Description
15.0	Winter activities,	Skating, speed, competitive
7.0	Winter activities,	Skiing, cross-country, 2.5 mph, slow or light effort, ski walking
8.0	Winter activities,	Skiing, cross-country, 4.0–4.9 mph, moderate speed and effort, general
9.0	Winter activities,	Skiing, cross-country, 5.0–7.9 mph, brisk speed, vigorous effort
14.0	Winter activities,	Skiing, cross-country, >8.0 mph, racing
16.5	Winter activities,	Skiing, cross-country, hard snow, uphill, maximum
5.0	Winter activities,	Skiing, downhill, light effort
6.0	Winter activities,	Skiing, downhill, moderate effort, general
8.0	Winter activities,	Skiing, downhill, vigorous effort, racing
7.0	Winter activities,	Sledding, tobogganing, bobsledding, luge
8.0	Winter activities,	Snow shoeing
3.5	Winter activities,	Snowmobiling

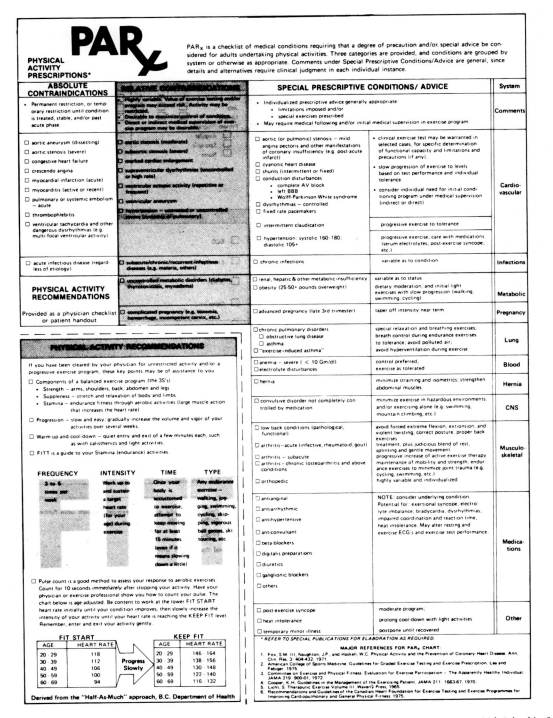

PAR_x

PHYSICAL ACTIVITY PRESCRIPTIONS*

PAR_x is a checklist of medical conditions requiring that a degree of precaution and/or. special advice be considered for adults undertaking physical activities. Three categories are provided, and conditions are grouped by system or otherwise as appropriate. Comments under Special Prescriptive Conditions/Advice are general, since details and alternatives require clinical judgment in each individual instance.

ABSOLUTE CONTRAINDICATIONS	RELATIVE CONTRAINDICATIONS	SPECIAL PRESCRIPTIVE CONDITIONS/ ADVICE	System
• Permanent restriction, or temporary restriction until condition is treated, stable, and/or past acute phase.	(illegible shaded text)	• Individualized prescriptive advice generally appropriate: • limitations imposed and/or • special exercises prescribed • May require medical following and/or initial medical supervision in exercise program.	Comments
☐ aortic aneurysm (dissecting) ☐ aortic stenosis (severe) ☐ congestive heart failure ☐ crescendo angina ☐ myocardial infarction (acute) ☐ myocarditis (active or recent) ☐ pulmonary or systemic embolism – acute ☐ thrombophlebitis ☐ ventricular tachycardia and other dangerous dysrhythmias (e.g. multi-focal ventricular activity)	☐ aortic stenosis (moderate) ☐ subaortic stenosis (severe) ☐ marked cardiac enlargement ☐ supraventricular dysrhythmias (uncontrolled or high rate) ☐ ventricular ectopic activity (repetitive or frequent) ☐ ventricular aneurysm ☐ hypertension – untreated or uncontrolled severe (systemic or pulmonary)	☐ aortic (or pulmonic) stenosis – mild angina pectoris and other manifestations of coronary insufficiency (e.g. post-acute infarct) ☐ cyanotic heart disease ☐ shunts (intermittent or fixed) ☐ conduction disturbances • complete AV block • left BBB • Wolff-Parkinson-White syndrome ☐ dysrhythmias – controlled ☐ fixed rate pacemakers	• clinical exercise test may be warranted in selected cases, for specific determination of functional capacity and limitations and precautions (if any). • slow progression of exercise to levels based on test performance and individual tolerance. • consider individual need for initial conditioning program under medical supervision (indirect or direct)	Cardio-vascular
		☐ intermittent claudication	progressive exercise to tolerance	
		☐ hypertension: systolic 160-180; diastolic 105+	progressive exercise; care with medications (serum electrolytes; post-exercise syncope; etc.)	
☐ acute infectious disease (regardless of etiology)	☐ subacute/chronic/recurrent infectious diseases (e.g. malaria, others)	☐ chronic infections	variable as to condition	Infections
PHYSICAL ACTIVITY RECOMMENDATIONS	☐ uncontrolled metabolic disorders (diabetes, thyrotoxicosis, myxedema)	☐ renal, hepatic & other metabolic insufficiency	variable as to status	Metabolic
Provided as a physician checklist or patient handout		☐ obesity (25-50+ pounds overweight)	dietary moderation, and initial light exercises with slow progression (walking, swimming, cycling)	
	☐ complicated pregnancy (e.g. toxemia, hemorrhage, incompetent cervix, etc.)	☐ advanced pregnancy (late 3rd trimester)	taper off intensity near term	Pregnancy
		☐ chronic pulmonary disorders ☐ obstructive lung disease ☐ asthma ☐ "exercise-induced asthma"	special relaxation and breathing exercises; breath control during endurance exercises to tolerance; avoid polluted air; avoid hyperventilation during exercise	Lung
		☐ anemia – severe (< 10 Gm/dl) ☐ electrolyte disturbances	control preferred; exercise as tolerated	Blood
		☐ hernia	minimize straining and isometrics; strengthen abdominal muscles	Hernia
		☐ convulsive disorder not completely controlled by medication	minimize exercise in hazardous environments and/or exercising alone (e.g. swimming, mountain climbing, etc.)	CNS
		☐ low back conditions (pathological, functional) ☐ arthritis–acute (infective, rheumatoid; gout) ☐ arthritis – subacute ☐ arthritis – chronic (osteoarthritis and above conditions) ☐ orthopedic	avoid forced extreme flexion, extinsion, and violent twisting, correct posture, proper back exercises treatment, plus judicious blend of rest, splinting and gentle movement progressive increase of active exercise therapy maintenance of mobility and strength; endurance exercises to minimize joint trauma (e.g. cycling, swimming, etc.) highly variable and individualized	Musculo-skeletal
		☐ antianginal ☐ antiarrhythmic ☐ antihypertensive ☐ anticonvulsant ☐ beta-blockers ☐ digitalis preparations ☐ diuretics ☐ ganglionic blockers ☐ others	NOTE: consider underlying condition. Potential for: exertional syncope, electrolyte imbalance, bradycardia, dysrhythmias; impaired coordination and reaction time, heat intolerance. May alter resting and exercise ECG's and exercise test performance.	Medications
		☐ post-exercise syncope ☐ heat intolerance ☐ temporary minor illness	moderate program; prolong cool-down with light activities postpone until recovered	Other

* REFER TO SPECIAL PUBLICATIONS FOR ELABORATION AS REQUIRED.

MAJOR REFERENCES FOR PAR_x CHART:

1. Fox, S.M. III, Naughton, J.P., and Haskell, W.C. Physical Activity and the Prevention of Coronary Heart Disease. Ann. Clin. Res. 3: 404-432, 1971.
2. American College of Sports Medicine. Guidelines for Graded Exercise Testing and Exercise Prescription. Lea and Febiger. 1975.
3. Committee on Exercise and Physical Fitness. Evaluation for Exercise Participation – The Apparently Healthy Individual. JAMA 219: 900-01, 1972.
4. Cooper, K.H. Guidelines in the Management of the Exercising Patient. JAMA 211: 1663-67, 1970.
5. Licht, S. Therapeutic Exercise Volume III. Waverly Press, 1965.
6. Recommendations and Guidelines of the Canadian Heart Foundation for Exercise Testing and Exercise Programmes for Improving Cardiopulmonary and General Physical Fitness. 1975.

PHYSICAL ACTIVITY RECOMMENDATIONS

If you have been cleared by your physician for unrestricted activity and/or a progressive exercise program, these key points may be of assistance to you.

☐ Components of a balanced exercise program (the 3S's)
• Strength – arms, shoulders, back, abdomen and legs
• Suppleness – stretch and relaxation of body and limbs
• Stamina – endurance fitness through aerobic activities (large muscle action that increases the heart rate)

☐ Progression – slow and easy; gradually increase the volume and vigor of your activities over several weeks.

☐ Warm-up and cool-down – quiet entry and exit of a few minutes each, such as with calisthenics and light activities.

☐ FITT is a guide to your Stamina (endurance) activities.

FREQUENCY — 2 to 5 times per week

INTENSITY — Work up to and sustain a target heart rate (for your age) during exercise

TIME — Once your body is accustomed to exercise, attempt to keep moving for at least 15 minutes (even if it means slowing down a little)

TYPE — Any endurance exercise – walking, jogging, swimming, cycling, skipping, vigorous ball games, ski touring, etc.

☐ Pulse count is a good method to assess your response to aerobic exercises. Count for 10 seconds *immediately* after stopping your activity. Have your physician or exercise professional show you how to count your pulse. The chart below is age-adjusted. Be content to work at the lower FIT START heart rate initially until your condition improves, then slowly increase the intensity of your activity until your heart rate is reaching the KEEP FIT level. Remember, enter and exit your activity gently.

FIT START			KEEP FIT	
AGE	HEART RATE		AGE	HEART RATE
20 - 29	118		20 - 29	146 - 164
30 - 39	112	Progress	30 - 39	138 - 156
40 - 49	106	Slowly	40 - 49	130 - 148
50 - 59	100		50 - 59	122 - 140
60 - 69	94		60 - 69	116 - 132

Derived from the "Half-As-Much" approach, B.C. Department of Health

Appendix D

1989 Recommended Dietary Allowances

Food and Nutrition Board, National Academy of Sciences—National Research Council Recommended Dietary Allowances,[a] Revised 1989

Designed for the maintenance of good nutrition of practically all healthy people in the United States

Category	Age (years) or Condition	Weight[b] (kg)	Weight[b] (lb)	Height[b] (cm)	Height[b] (in)	Protein (g)	Fat-Soluble Vitamins Vitamin A (μg RE)[c]	Vitamin D (μg)[d]	Vitamin E (mg α-TE)[e]	Vitamin K (μg)	Water-Soluble Vitamins Vitamin C (mg)	Thiamin (mg)
Infants	0.0–0.5	6	13	60	24	13	375	7.5	3	5	30	0.3
	0.5–1.0	9	20	71	28	14	375	10	4	10	35	0.4
Children	1–3	13	29	90	35	16	400	10	6	15	40	0.7
	4–6	20	44	112	44	24	500	10	7	20	45	0.9
	7–10	28	62	132	52	28	700	10	7	30	45	1.0
Males	11–14	45	99	157	62	45	1,000	10	10	45	50	1.3
	15–18	66	145	176	69	59	1,000	10	10	65	60	1.5
	19–24	72	160	177	70	58	1,000	10	10	70	60	1.5
	25–50	79	174	176	70	63	1,000	5	10	80	60	1.5
	51+	77	170	173	68	63	1,000	5	10	80	60	1.2
Females	11–14	46	101	157	62	46	800	10	8	45	50	1.1
	15–18	55	120	163	64	44	800	10	8	55	60	1.1
	19–24	58	128	164	65	46	800	10	8	60	60	1.1
	25–50	63	138	163	64	50	800	5	8	65	60	1.1
	51+	65	143	160	63	50	800	5	8	65	60	1.0
Pregnant						60	800	10	10	65	70	1.5
Lactating	1st 6 months					65	1,300	10	12	65	95	1.6
	2nd 6 months					62	1,200	10	11	65	90	1.6

Reprinted with permission from *Recommended Dietary Allowances: 10th Edition.* Copyright 1989 by the National Academy of Sciences. Published by the National Academy Press, Washington DC.

[a]The allowances, expressed as average daily intakes over time, are intended to provide for individual variations among most normal persons as they live in the United States under usual environmental stresses. Diets should be based on a variety of common foods in order to provide other nutrients for which human requirements have been less well defined. See text for detailed discussion of allowances and of nutrients not tabulated.

[b]Weights and heights of Reference Adults are actual medians for the U.S. population of the designated age, as reported by NHANES II. The median weights and heights of those under 19 years of age were taken from Hamill et al. (1979) (see pages 16–17). The use of these figures does not imply that the height-to-weight ratios are ideal.

[c]Retinol equivalents. 1 retinol equivalent = 1 μg retinol or 6 μg β-carotene. See text for calculation of vitamin A activity of diets as retinol equivalents.

[d]As cholecalciferol. 10 μg cholecalciferol = 400 IU of vitamin D.

[e]α-Tocopherol equivalents. 1 mg d-α tocopherol = 1 α-TE. See text for variation in allowances and calculation of vitamin E activity of the diet as α-tocopherol equivalents.

| Riboflavin (mg) | Niacin (mg NE)[f] | Vitamin B$_6$ (mg) | Folate (µg) | Vitamin B$_{12}$ (µg) | Minerals |||||||||
					Calcium (mg)	Phosphorus (mg)	Magnesium (mg)	Iron (mg)	Zinc (mg)	Iodine (µg)	Selenium (µg)
0.4	5	0.3	25	0.3	400	300	40	6	5	40	10
0.5	6	0.6	35	0.5	600	500	60	10	5	50	15
0.8	9	1.0	50	0.7	800	800	80	10	10	70	20
1.1	12	1.1	75	1.0	800	800	120	10	10	90	20
1.2	13	1.4	100	1.4	800	800	170	10	10	120	30
1.5	17	1.7	150	2.0	1,200	1,200	270	12	15	150	40
1.8	20	2.0	200	2.0	1,200	1,200	400	12	15	150	50
1.7	19	2.0	200	2.0	1,200	1,200	350	10	15	150	70
1.7	19	2.0	200	2.0	800	800	350	10	15	150	70
1.4	15	2.0	200	2.0	800	800	350	10	15	150	70
1.3	15	1.4	150	2.0	1,200	1,200	280	15	12	150	45
1.3	15	1.5	180	2.0	1,200	1,200	300	15	12	150	50
1.3	15	1.6	180	2.0	1,200	1,200	280	15	12	150	55
1.3	15	1.6	180	2.0	800	800	280	15	12	150	55
1.2	13	1.6	180	2.0	800	800	280	10	12	150	55
1.6	17	2.2	400	2.2	1,200	1,200	320	30	15	175	65
1.8	20	2.1	280	2.6	1,200	1,200	355	15	19	200	75
1.7	20	2.1	260	2.6	1,200	1,200	340	15	16	200	75

[f] 1 NE (niacin equivalent) is equal to 1 mg of niacin or 60 mg of dietary tryptophan.

Appendix E

1989 RDAs—Estimated Safe and Adequate Daily Dietary Intakes of Selected Vitamins and Minerals[a]

Category	Age (years)	Vitamins		Trace Elements[b]				
		Biotin (µg)	Pantothenic Acid (mg)	Copper (mg)	Manganese (mg)	Fluoride (mg)	Chromium (µg)	Molybdenum (µg)
Infants	0–0.5	10	2	0.4–0.6	0.3–0.6	0.1–0.5	10–40	15–30
	0.5–1	15	3	0.6–0.7	0.6–1.0	0.2–1.0	20–60	20–40
Children and adolescents	1–3	20	3	0.7–1.0	1.0–1.5	0.5–1.5	20–80	25–50
	4–6	25	3–4	1.0–1.5	1.5–2.0	1.0–2.5	30–120	30–75
	7–10	30	4–5	1.0–2.0	2.0–3.0	1.5–2.5	50–200	50–150
	11+	30–100	4–7	1.5–2.5	2.0–5.0	1.5–2.5	50–200	75–250
Adults		30–100	4–7	1.5–3.0	2.0–5.0	1.5–4.0	50–200	75–250

Reprinted with permission from *Recommended Dietary Allowances: 10th Edition.* Copyright 1989 by the National Academy of Sciences. Published by the National Academy Press, Washington DC.

[a]Because there is less information on which to base allowances, these figures are not given in the main table of RDA and are provided here in the form of ranges of recommended intakes.

[b]Since the toxic levels for many trace elements may be only several times usual intakes, the upper levels for the trace elements given in this table should not be habitually exceeded.

1989 RDAs—Estimated Sodium, Chloride, and Potassium Minimum Requirements of Healthy Persons[a]

Age	Weight (kg)[a]	Sodium (mg)[a,b]	Chloride (mg)[a,b]	Potassium (mg)[c]
Months				
0–5	4.5	120	180	500
6–11	8.9	200	300	700
Years				
1	11.0	225	350	1,000
2–5	16.0	300	500	1,400
6–9	25.0	400	600	1,600
10–18	50.0	500	750	2,000
>18[d]	70.0	500	750	2,000

Reprinted with permission from *Recommended Dietary Allowances: 10th Edition.* Copyright 1989 by the National Academy of Sciences. Published by the National Academy Press, Washington DC.

[a]No allowance has been included for large, prolonged losses from the skin through sweat.

[b]There is no evidence that higher intakes confer any health benefit.

[c]Desirable intakes of potassium may considerably exceed these values (~3,500 mg for adults—see text).

[d]No allowance included for growth. Values for those below 18 years assume a growth rate at the 50th percentile reported by the National Center for Health Statistics (Hamill et al., 1979) and averaged for males and females. See text for information on pregnancy and lactation.

Appendix F

1989 RDAs—Median Heights and Weights and Recommended Energy Intake

Category	Age (years) or Condition	Weight (kg)	Weight (lb)	Height (cm)	Height (in)	REE[a] (kcal/day)	Multiples of REE	Average Energy Allowance (kcal)[b] Per kg	Average Energy Allowance (kcal)[b] Per Day[c]
Infants	0.0–0.5	6	13	60	24	320		108	650
	0.5–1.0	9	20	71	28	500		98	850
Children	1–3	13	29	90	35	740		102	1,300
	4–6	20	44	112	44	950		90	1,800
	7–10	28	62	132	52	1,130		70	2,000
Males	11–14	45	99	157	62	1,440	1.70	55	2,500
	15–18	66	145	176	69	1,760	1.67	45	3,000
	19–24	72	160	177	70	1,780	1.67	40	2,900
	25–50	79	174	176	70	1,800	1.60	37	2,900
	51+	77	170	173	68	1,530	1.50	30	2,300
Females	11–14	46	101	157	62	1,310	1.67	47	2,200
	15–18	55	120	163	64	1,370	1.60	40	2,200
	19–24	58	128	164	65	1,350	1.60	38	2,200
	25–50	63	138	163	64	1,380	1.55	36	2,200
	51+	65	143	160	63	1,280	1.50	30	1,900
Pregnant	1st trimester								+0
	2nd trimester								+300
	3rd trimester								+300
Lactating	1st 6 months								+500
	2nd 6 months								+500

Reprinted with permission from *Recommended Dietary Allowances: 10th Edition.* Copyright 1989 by the National Academy of Sciences. Published by the National Academy Press, Washington DC.

[a]Calculation based on FAO equations, then rounded.

[b]In the range of light to moderate activity, the coefficient of variation is ±20%.

[c]Figure is rounded.

Appendix G

Percent Fat Estimate for Men: Sum of Triceps, Chest, and Subscapula Skinfolds

Sum of Skinfolds (mm)	Age to Last Year								
	Under 22	23–27	28–32	33–37	38–42	43–47	48–52	53–57	Over 57
8–10	1.5	2.0	2.5	3.1	3.6	4.1	4.6	5.1	5.6
11–13	3.0	3.5	4.0	4.5	5.1	5.6	6.1	6.6	7.1
14–16	4.5	5.0	5.5	6.0	6.5	7.0	7.6	8.1	8.6
17–19	5.9	6.4	6.9	7.4	8.0	8.5	9.0	9.5	10.0
20–22	7.3	7.8	8.3	8.8	9.4	9.9	10.4	10.9	11.4
23–25	8.6	9.2	9.7	10.2	10.7	11.2	11.8	12.3	12.8
26–28	10.0	10.5	11.0	11.5	12.1	12.6	13.1	13.6	14.2
29–31	11.2	11.8	12.3	12.8	13.4	13.9	14.4	14.9	15.5
32–34	12.5	13.0	13.5	14.1	14.6	15.1	15.7	16.2	16.7
35–37	13.7	14.2	14.8	15.3	15.8	16.4	16.9	17.4	18.0
38–40	14.9	15.4	15.9	16.5	17.0	17.6	18.1	18.6	19.2
41–43	16.0	16.6	17.1	17.6	18.2	18.7	19.3	19.8	20.3
44–46	17.1	17.7	18.2	18.7	19.3	19.8	20.4	20.9	21.5
47–49	18.2	18.7	19.3	19.8	20.4	20.9	21.4	22.0	22.5
50–52	19.2	19.7	20.3	20.8	21.4	21.9	22.5	23.0	23.6
53–55	20.2	20.7	21.3	21.8	22.4	22.9	23.5	24.0	24.6
56–58	21.1	21.7	22.2	22.8	23.3	23.9	24.4	25.0	25.5
59–61	22.0	22.6	23.1	23.7	24.2	24.8	25.3	25.9	26.5
62–64	22.9	23.4	24.0	24.5	25.1	25.7	26.2	26.8	27.3
65–67	23.7	24.3	24.8	25.4	25.9	26.5	27.1	27.6	28.2
68–70	24.5	25.0	25.6	26.2	26.7	27.3	27.8	28.4	29.0
71–73	25.2	25.8	26.3	26.9	27.5	28.0	28.6	29.1	29.7
74–76	25.9	26.5	27.0	27.6	28.2	28.7	29.3	29.9	30.4
77–79	26.6	27.1	27.7	28.2	28.8	29.4	29.9	30.5	31.1
80–82	27.2	27.7	28.3	28.9	29.4	30.0	30.6	31.1	31.7
83–85	27.7	28.3	28.8	29.4	30.0	30.5	31.1	31.7	32.3
86–88	28.2	28.8	29.4	29.9	30.5	31.1	31.6	32.2	32.8
89–91	28.7	29.3	29.8	30.4	31.0	31.5	32.1	32.7	33.3
92–94	29.1	29.7	30.3	30.8	31.4	32.0	32.6	33.1	33.4
95–97	29.5	30.1	30.6	31.2	31.8	32.4	32.9	33.5	34.1
98–100	29.8	30.4	31.0	31.6	32.1	32.7	33.3	33.9	34.4
101–103	30.1	30.7	31.3	31.8	32.4	33.0	33.6	34.1	34.7
104–106	30.4	30.9	31.5	32.1	32.7	33.2	33.8	34.4	35.0
107–109	30.6	31.1	31.7	32.3	32.9	33.4	34.0	34.6	35.2
110–112	30.7	31.3	31.9	32.4	33.0	33.6	34.2	34.7	35.3
113–115	30.8	31.4	32.0	32.5	33.1	33.7	34.3	34.9	35.4
116–118	30.9	31.5	32.0	32.6	33.2	33.8	34.3	34.9	35.5

From A. S. Jackson and M. L. Pollock, "Practical Assessment of Body Composition" in *The Physician and Sportsmedicine*, 13(5):85, 1985. Copyright © 1985 McGraw-Hill Healthcare Group, Minneapolis MN. Reprinted by permission.

Appendix H

Percent Fat Estimate for Women: Sum of Triceps, Abdomen, and Suprailium Skinfolds

Sum of Skinfolds (mm)	Age to Last Year								
	18–22	23–27	28–32	33–37	38–42	43–47	48–52	53–57	Over 57
8–12	8.8	9.0	9.2	9.4	9.5	9.7	9.9	10.1	10.3
13–17	10.8	10.9	11.1	11.3	11.5	11.7	11.8	12.0	12.2
18–22	12.6	12.8	13.0	13.2	13.4	13.5	13.7	13.9	14.1
23–27	14.5	14.6	14.8	15.0	15.2	15.4	15.6	15.7	15.9
28–32	16.2	16.4	16.6	16.8	17.0	17.1	17.3	17.5	17.7
33–37	17.9	18.1	18.3	18.5	18.7	18.9	19.0	19.2	19.4
38–42	19.6	19.8	20.0	20.2	20.3	20.5	20.7	20.9	21.1
43–47	21.2	21.4	21.6	21.8	21.9	22.1	22.3	22.5	22.7
48–52	22.8	22.9	23.1	23.3	23.5	23.7	23.8	24.0	24.2
53–57	24.2	24.4	24.6	24.8	25.0	25.2	25.3	25.5	25.7
58–62	25.7	25.9	26.0	26.2	26.4	26.6	26.8	27.0	27.1
63–67	27.1	27.2	27.4	27.6	27.8	28.0	28.2	28.3	28.5
68–72	28.4	28.6	28.7	28.9	29.1	29.3	29.5	29.7	29.8
73–77	29.6	29.8	30.0	30.2	30.4	30.6	30.7	30.9	31.1
78–82	30.9	31.0	31.2	31.4	31.6	31.8	31.9	32.1	32.3
83–87	32.0	32.2	32.4	32.6	32.7	32.9	33.1	33.3	33.5
88–92	33.1	33.3	33.5	33.7	33.8	34.0	34.2	34.4	34.6
93–97	34.1	34.3	34.5	34.7	34.9	35.1	35.2	35.4	35.6
98–102	35.1	35.3	35.5	35.7	35.9	36.0	36.2	36.4	36.6
103–107	36.1	36.2	36.4	36.6	36.8	37.0	37.2	37.3	37.5
108–112	36.9	37.1	37.3	37.5	37.7	37.9	38.0	38.2	38.4
113–117	37.8	37.9	38.1	38.3	39.2	39.4	39.6	39.8	39.2
118–122	38.5	38.7	38.9	39.1	39.4	39.6	39.8	40.0	40.0
123–127	39.2	39.4	39.6	39.8	40.0	40.1	40.3	40.5	40.7
128–132	39.9	40.1	40.2	40.4	40.6	40.8	41.0	41.2	41.3
133–137	40.5	40.7	40.8	41.0	41.2	41.4	41.6	41.7	41.9
138–142	41.0	41.2	41.4	41.6	41.7	41.9	42.1	42.3	42.5
143–147	41.5	41.7	41.9	42.0	42.2	42.4	42.6	42.8	43.0
148–152	41.9	42.1	42.3	42.4	42.6	42.8	43.0	43.2	43.4
153–157	42.3	42.5	42.6	42.8	43.0	43.2	43.4	43.6	43.7
158–162	42.6	42.8	43.0	43.1	43.3	43.5	43.7	43.9	44.1
163–167	42.9	43.0	43.2	43.4	43.6	43.8	44.0	44.1	44.3
168–172	43.1	43.2	43.4	43.6	43.8	44.0	44.2	44.3	44.5
173–177	43.2	43.4	43.6	43.8	43.9	44.1	44.3	44.5	44.7
178–182	43.3	43.5	43.7	43.8	44.0	44.2	44.4	44.6	44.8

From A. S. Jackson and M. L. Pollock, "Practical Assessment of Body Composition" in *The Physician and Sportsmedicine*, 13(5):85, 1985. Copyright © 1985 McGraw-Hill Healthcare Group, Minneapolis MN. Reprinted by permission.

Glossary

absolute $\dot{V}O_2$ the amount of oxygen consumed over a given time period; expressed as liters · min^{-1}.

acidosis an abnormal increase in blood hydrogen ion concentration (i.e., arterial pH below 7.35).

acids compounds capable of giving up hydrogen ions into solution.

acromegaly a condition caused by hypersecretion of growth hormone from the pituitary gland; characterized by enlargement of the extremities, such as the jaw, nose, and fingers.

actin a structural protein of muscle that works with myosin in permitting muscular contraction.

action potential the all-or-none electrical event in the neuron or muscle cell in which the polarity of the cell membrane is rapidly reversed and then reestablished.

adenosine diphosphate (ADP) a molecule that combines with inorganic phosphate to form ATP.

adenosine triphosphate (ATP) the high-energy phosphate compound synthesized and used by cells to release energy for cellular work.

adenylate cyclase enzyme found in cell membranes that catalyzes the conversion of ATP to cyclic AMP.

adrenal cortex the outer portion of the adrenal gland. Synthesizes and secretes corticosteroid hormones, such as cortisol, aldosterone, and androgens.

adrenaline *see* epinephrine.

adrenocorticotrophic hormone (ACTH) a hormone secreted by the anterior pituitary gland that stimulates the adrenal cortex.

aerobic in the presence of oxygen.

afferent fibers nerve fibers (sensory fibers) that carry neural information back to the central nervous system.

afferent neuron sensory neuron carrying information toward the central nervous system.

aldosterone a corticosteroid hormone involved in the regulation of electrolyte balance.

alkalosis an abnormal increase in blood concentration of OH^- ions, resulting in a rise in arterial pH above 7.45.

alpha receptors a subtype of adrenergic receptors located on cell membranes of selected tissues.

alveolar ventilation ($\dot{V}_A$) the volume of gas that reaches the alveolar region of the lung.

alveoli microscopic air sacs located in the lung where gas exchange occurs between respiratory gases and the blood.

amenorrhea the absence of menses.

anabolic steroid a prescription drug that has anabolic, or growth-stimulating, characteristics similar to that of the male androgen, testosterone.

anaerobic without oxygen.

anaerobic threshold a commonly used term meant to describe the level of oxygen consumption at which there is a rapid and systematic increase in blood lactate concentration. Also termed the *lactate threshold*.

anatomical dead space the total volume of the lung (i.e., conducting airways) that does not participate in gas exchange.

androgenic steroid a compound that has the qualities of an androgen; associated with masculine characteristics.

androgens male sex hormones. Synthesized in the testes and in limited amounts in the adrenal cortex. Steroids that have masculinizing effects.

angina pectoris chest pain due to a lack of blood flow (ischemia) to the myocardium.

angiotensin I and II these compounds are polypeptides formed from the cleavage of a protein (angiotensinogen) by the action of the enzyme renin produced by the kidneys, and converting enzyme in the lung, respectively.

anorexia nervosa an eating disorder characterized by rapid weight loss due to failure to consume adequate amounts of nutrients.

anterior hypothalamus the anterior portion of the hypothalamus. The hypothalamus is an area of the brain below the thalamus that regulates the autonomic nervous system and the pituitary gland.

anterior pituitary the anterior portion of the pituitary gland that secretes follicle-stimulating hormone, luteinizing hormone, adrenocorticotrophic hormone, thyroid stimulating hormone, growth hormone, and prolactin.

antidiuretic hormone (ADH) hormone secreted by the posterior pituitary gland that promotes water retention by the kidney.

aortic bodies receptors located in the arch of the aorta that are capable of detecting changes in arterial PO_2.

apophyses sites of muscle-tendon insertion in bones.

arrhythmia abnormal electrical activity in the heart (e.g., a premature ventricular contraction).

arteries large vessels that carry arterialized blood away from the heart.

arterioles a small branch of an artery that communicates with a capillary network.

articular cartilage cartilage that covers the ends of bones in a synovial joint.

atherosclerosis a pathological condition in which fatty substances collect inside the lumen of arteries.

ATPase enzyme capable of breaking down ATP to ADP + P_i + energy.

ATP-PC system term used to describe the metabolic pathway involving muscle stores of ATP and the use of phosphocreatine to rephosphorylate ADP. This pathway is used at the onset of exercise and during short-term, high-intensity work.

atrioventricular node (AV node) a specialized mass of muscle tissue located in the interventricular septum of the heart; functions in the transmission of cardiac impulses from the atria to the ventricles.

autologous transfusion blood transfusion where the individual receives his or her own blood.

autonomic nervous system portion of the nervous system that functions to control the actions of visceral organs.

autoregulation mechanism by which an organ regulates blood flow to match the metabolic rate.

axon a nerve fiber that conducts a nerve impulse away from the neuron cell body.

basal metabolic rate (BMR) metabolic rate measured in supine position following a twelve-hour fast, and eight hours of sleep.

bases compounds that ionize in water to release hydroxyl ions (OH$^-$) or other ions that are capable of combining with hydrogen ions.

beta oxidation breakdown of free fatty acids to form acetyl-CoA.

beta receptor agonist (β-agonist) a molecule that is capable of binding to and activating a beta receptor.

beta receptors adrenergic receptors located on cell membranes. Combines mainly with epinephrine and, to some degree, with norepinephrine.

bioenergetics the chemical processes involved with production of cellular ATP.

biological control systems a control system capable of maintaining homeostasis within a cell or organ system in a living creature.

blood boosting a term that applies to the increase of the blood's hemoglobin concentration by infusion of additional red blood cells. Medically termed *induced erythrocythemia*.

blood doping *see* blood boosting.

blood packing *see* blood boosting.

Bohr effect the right shift of oxyhemoglobin dissociation curve due to a decrease of blood pH. Results in a decreased affinity for oxygen.

bradycardia a resting heart rate less than sixty beats per minute.

brain stem portion of the brain that includes midbrain, pons, and medulla.

buffer a compound that resists pH change.

bulimia nervosa an eating disorder characterized by eating and forced regurgitation.

bulk flow mass movement of molecules from an area of high pressure to an area of lower pressure.

calcitonin hormone, released from the thyroid gland, that plays a minor role in calcium metabolism.

calmodulin part of second messenger system involving calcium that results in changes in the activity of intracellular enzymes.

capillaries microscopic blood vessels that connect arterioles and venules. Portion of vascular system where blood/tissue gas exchange occurs.

cardiac accelerator nerves part of the sympathetic nervous system that stimulates the SA node to increase heart rate.

cardiac output the amount of blood pumped by the heart per unit of time; equal to product of heart rate and stroke volume.

cardiovascular control center the area of the medulla that regulates the cardiovascular system.

carotid bodies chemoreceptors located in the internal carotid artery; respond to changes in arterial PO$_2$, PCO$_2$, and pH.

catecholamines organic compounds, including epinephrine, norepinephrine, and dopamine.

cell body the soma, or major portion of the body of a nerve cell. Contains the nucleus.

cell membrane the lipid-bilayer envelope that encloses cells. Called the *sarcolemma* in muscle cells.

cellular respiration process of oxygen consumption and carbon dioxide production in cells (i.e., bioenergetics).

central command the control of the cardiovascular or pulmonary system by cortical impulses.

central nervous system (CNS) portion of the nervous system that consists of the brain and spinal cord.

cerebellum portion of the brain that is concerned with fine coordination of skeletal muscles during movement.

cerebrum superior aspect of the brain that occupies the upper cranial cavity. Contains the motor cortex.

chemiosmotic hypothesis the mechanism to explain the aerobic formation of ATP in mitochondria.

cholesterol a twenty-seven-carbon lipid that can be synthesized in cells or consumed in the diet. Cholesterol serves as a precursor of steroid hormones, and plays a role in the development of atherosclerosis.

clo unit that describes the insulation quality of clothing.

concentric contraction occurs when a muscle is activated and shortens.

conduction transfer of heat from warmer to cooler objects in contact with each other. This term may also be used in association with the conveyance of neural impulses.

conduction disturbances refers to a slowing or blockage of the wave of depolarization in the heart, e.g., first-degree AV block, or bundle branch block.

conductivity capacity for conduction.

convection the transmission of heat from one object to another through the circulation of heated molecules.

Cori cycle the cycle of lactate-to-glucose between the muscle and liver.

coronary artery bypass graft surgery (CABGS) the replacement of a blocked coronary artery with another vessel to permit blood flow to the myocardium.

cortisol a glucocorticoid secreted by the adrenal cortex upon stimulation by ACTH.

coupled reactions the linking of energy-liberating chemical reactions to "drive" energy-requiring reactions.

critical power based on the notion that athletes can maintain a specific submaximal power output without fatigue.

cromolyn sodium a drug used to stabilize the membranes of mast cells and prevent an asthma attack.

cycle ergometer a stationary exercise cycle that allows accurate measurement of work output.

cyclic AMP a substance produced from ATP through the action of adenylate cyclase that alters several chemical processes in the cell.

cytoplasm the contents of the cell surrounding the nucleus. Called *sarcoplasm* in muscle cells.

Daily Value a standard used in nutritional labeling.

deficiency a shortcoming of some essential nutrient.

degenerative diseases diseases not due to infection, which result in a progressive decline in some bodily function.

delayed onset muscle soreness (DOMS) muscle soreness that occurs twelve to twenty-four hours after an exercise bout.

dendrites portion of the nerve fiber that transmits action potentials toward a nerve cell body.

dental caries tooth decay; related to sugar content in foods.

deoxyhemoglobin hemoglobin not in combination with oxygen.

diabetes mellitus a condition characterized by high blood glucose levels due to inadequate insulin. Type I diabetics are insulin dependent, whereas Type II diabetics are resistant to insulin.

diabetic coma unconscious state induced by a lack of insulin.

diacylglycerol a molecule derived from a membrane-bound phospholipid, phosphatidylinositol, that activates protein kinase C, and alters cellular activity.

diaphragm the major respiratory muscle responsible for inspiration. Dome-shaped—separates the thoracic cavity from the abdominal cavity.

diastole period of filling of the heart between contractions (i.e., resting phase of the heart).

diastolic blood pressure arterial blood pressure during diastole.

Dietary Guidelines for Americans general statements related to food selection that are consistent with achieving and maintaining good health.

diffusion random movement of molecules from an area of high concentration to an area of low concentration.

direct calorimetry assessment of the body's metabolic rate by direct measurement of the amount of heat produced.

dose the amount of drug or exercise prescribed to have a certain effect (or response).

double-blind research design an experimental design in which the subjects and the principal investigator are not aware of the experimental treatment order.

double product the product of heart rate and systolic blood pressure; estimate of work of the heart.

dynamic refers to an isotonic muscle contraction.

dynamic stretching stretching that involves controlled movement.

dynamometer device used to measure force production (e.g., used in the measurement of muscular strength).

dysmenorrhea painful menstruation.

dyspnea shortness of breath or labored breathing. May be due to various types of lung or heart diseases.

eccentric contraction occurs when a muscle is activated and force is produced but the muscle lengthens.

ectomorphy category of somatotype that is rated for linearity of body form.

effect change in variable (e.g., $\dot{V}O_2$ max) due to a dose of exercise (e.g., 3 days per week, 40 min/day at 70% $\dot{V}O_2$ max).

effector organ or body part that responds to stimulation by an efferent neuron (e.g., skeletal muscle in a withdrawal reflex).

efferent fibers nerve fibers (motor fibers) that carry neural information from the central nervous system to the periphery.

efferent neuron conducts impulses from the CNS to the effector organ (e.g., motorneuron).

ejection fraction the proportion of end-diastolic volume that is ejected during a ventricular contraction.

electrocardiogram (ECG) A recording of the electrical changes that occur in the myocardium during the cardiac cycle.

electron transport chain a series of cytochromes in the mitochrondia that are responsible for oxidative phosphorylation.

elements a single chemical substance composed of only one type of atom (e.g., calcium or potassium).

endergonic reactions energy-requiring reactions.

endocrine gland a gland that produces and secretes its products directly into the blood or interstitial fluid (ductless glands).

endomorphy the somatotype category that is rated for roundness (fatness).

endomysium the inner layer of connective tissue surrounding a muscle fiber.

endorphin a neuropeptide produced by the pituitary gland having pain-suppressing activity.

end-plate potential (EPP) depolarization of a membrane region by a sodium influx.

energy of activation energy required to initiate a chemical reaction.

energy wasteful systems metabolic pathways in which the energy generated in one reaction is used up

in another that leads back to the first, creating a futile cycle and requiring a higher resting metabolic rate.

enzymes proteins that lower the energy of activation and, therefore, catalyze chemical reactions. Enzymes regulate the rate of most metabolic pathways.

epidemiologic triad a model that shows connections between the environment, agent, and host that cause disease.

epidemiology the study of the distribution and determinants of health-related states or events in specified populations, and the application of this study to control of health problems.

epilepsy a neurological disorder manifested by muscular seizures.

epimysium the outer layer of connective tissue surrounding muscle.

epinephrine a hormone synthesized by the adrenal medulla; also called *adrenaline*.

epiphyseal plate (growth plate) cartilaginous layer between the head and shaft of a long bone where growth takes place.

EPOC an acronym for "excess post-exercise oxygen consumption"; often referred to as the *oxygen debt*.

EPSP excitatory post-synaptic potential. A graded depolarization of a post-synaptic membrane by a neurotransmitter.

ergogenic aid a substance, appliance, or procedure (e.g., blood doping) that improves performance.

ergometer instrument for measuring work.

ergometry measurement of work output.

erythrocythemia an increase in the number of erythrocytes in the blood.

erythropoietin hormone that stimulates red blood cell production.

estrogens female sex hormones, including estradiol and estrone. Produced primarily in the ovary and also produced in the adrenal cortex.

evaporation the change of water from a liquid form to a vapor form. Results in the removal of heat.

exercise a subclass of physical activity.

exergonic reactions chemical reactions that release energy.

extensors muscles that function to extend a limb—that is, increase the angle at a joint.

FAD flavin adenine dinucleotide. Serves as an electron carrier in bioenergetics.

fasciculi a small bundle of muscle fibers.

fast-twitch fibers one of several types of muscle fibers found in skeletal muscle; also called Type II fibers; characterized as having low oxidative capacity but high glycolytic capacity.

ferritin the iron-carrying molecule used as an index of whole-body iron status.

field test a test of physical performance performed in the field (outside the laboratory).

flexors muscle groups that cause flexion of limbs—that is, decrease the angle at a joint.

follicle-stimulating hormone (FSH) a hormone secreted by the anterior pituitary gland that stimulates the development of an ovarian follicle in the female and the production of sperm in the male.

food records the practice of keeping dietary food records for determining nutrient intake.

free fatty acid (FFA) a type of fat that combines with glycerol to form triglycerides. Is used as an energy source.

G protein the link between the hormone-receptor interaction on the surface of the membrane and the subsequent events inside the cell.

gain refers to the amount of correction that a control system is capable of achieving.

General Adaptation Syndrome (GAS) a term defined by Selye in 1936 that describes the organism's response to chronic stress. In response to stress the organism has a three-stage response: (1) alarm reaction; (2) stage of resistance; and (3) readjustment to the stress, or exhaustion.

glucagon a hormone produced by the pancreas that acts to increase blood glucose and free fatty acid levels.

glucocorticoids any one of a group of hormones produced by the adrenal cortex that influences carbohydrate, fat, and protein metabolism.

gluconeogenesis the synthesis of glucose from amino acids, lactate, glycerol, and other short carbon-chain molecules.

glucose a simple sugar that is transported via the blood and metabolized by tissues.

glucose polymer a complex sugar molecule that contains multiple simple sugar molecules linked together.

glycogen a glucose polymer synthesized in cells as a means of storing carbohydrate.

glycogenolysis the breakdown of glycogen into glucose.

glycolysis a metabolic pathway in the cytoplasm of the cell that results in the degradation of glucose into pyruvate or lactate.

Golgi tendon organ (GTOs) a tension receptor located in series with skeletal muscle.

graded exercise test *see* incremental exercise test.

gross efficiency a simple measure of exercise efficiency defined as the ratio of work performed to energy expended, expressed as a percent.

growth hormone hormone synthesized and secreted by the anterior pituitary that stimulates growth of the skeleton and soft tissues during the growing years. It is also involved in the mobilization of the body's energy stores.

HDL cholesterol (high-density lipoprotein cholesterol) cholesterol that is transported in the blood via high-density proteins; related to low risk of heart disease.

hemoglobin a heme containing protein in red blood cells that is responsible for transporting oxygen to tissues. Hemoglobin also serves as a weak buffer within red blood cells.

hemosiderin an insoluble form of iron stored in tissues.

high-density lipoproteins (HDL) proteins used to transport cholesterol in blood; high levels appear to offer some protection from atherosclerosis.

homeostasis the maintenance of a constant internal environment.

homeotherms animals that maintain a fairly constant internal temperature.

homologous transfusion a blood transfusion using blood of the same type but from another donor.

hormone a chemical substance that is synthesized and released by an endocrine gland and transported to a target organ via the blood.

hydrogen ion (H^+) a free hydrogen ion in solution that results in a decrease in pH of the solution.

hyperbaric chamber chamber where the absolute pressure is increased above atmospheric pressure.

hyperoxia oxygen concentration in an inspired gas that exceeds 21%.

hyperplasia an increase in the number of cells in a tissue.

hyperthermia an above-normal increase in body temperature.

hypertrophy an increase in cell size.

hypothalamic somatostatin hypothalamic hormone that inhibits growth hormone secretion; also secreted from the delta cells of the islets of Langerhans.

hypothalamus brain structure that integrates many physiological functions to maintain homeostasis; site of secretion of hormones released by the posterior pituitary; also releases hormones that control anterior pituitary secretions.

hypothermia a condition in which heat is lost from the body faster than it is produced.

hypoxia a relative lack of oxygen (e.g., at altitude).

immunotherapy procedure in which the body is exposed to specific substances to elicit an immune response in order to offer better protection upon subsequent exposure.

incremental exercise test an exercise test involving a progressive increase in work rate over time. Often graded exercise tests are used to determine the subject's $\dot{V}O_2$ max or lactate threshold. (Also called *graded exercise test.*)

indirect calorimetry estimation of heat or energy production on the basis of oxygen consumption, carbon dioxide production, and nitrogen excretion.

induced erythrocythemia causing an elevation of the red blood cell (hemoglobin) concentration by infusing blood; also called *blood doping* or *blood boosting*.

infectious diseases diseases due to the presence of pathogenic microorganisms in the body (e.g., viruses, bacteria, fungi, and protozoa).

inorganic relating to substances that do not contain carbon (C).

inorganic phosphate (P_i) a stimulator of cellular metabolism; split off, along with ADP, from ATP when energy is released; used with ADP to form ATP in the electron transport chain.

inositol triphosphate a molecule derived from a membrane-bound phospholipid, phosphatidylinositol, that causes calcium release from intracellular stores and alters cellular activity.

insulin hormone released from the beta cells of the islets of Langerhans in response to elevated blood glucose and amino acid concentrations; increases tissue uptake of both.

insulin shock condition brought on by too much insulin, which causes an immediate hypoglycemia; symptoms include tremors, dizziness, and possibly convulsions.

integrating center the portion of a biological control system that processes the information from the receptors and issues an appropriate response relative to its set point.

intercalated discs portion of cardiac muscle cell where one cell connects to the next.

intermediate fibers muscle fiber type that generates high force at a moderately fast speed of contraction, but has a relatively large number of mitochondria (Type IIa).

ion a single atom or small molecule containing a net positive or negative charge due to an excess of either protons or electrons, respectively (e.g., Na^+, Cl^-).

IPSP inhibitory post-synaptic potential that moves the post-synaptic membrane further from threshold.

irritability a trait of certain tissues that enables them to respond to stimuli (e.g., nerve and muscle).

isocitrate dehydrogenase rate-limiting enzyme in the Krebs cycle that is inhibited by ATP and stimulated by ADP and P_i.

isokinetic action in which the rate of movement is constantly maintained through a specific range of motion even though maximal force is exerted.

isometric contraction in which the muscle develops tension, but does not shorten; also called a *static contraction*. No movement occurs.

isotonic contraction in which a muscle shortens against a constant load or tension, resulting in movement.

ketosis acidosis of the blood caused by the production of ketone bodies (e.g., acetoacetic acid) when fatty acid mobilization is increased, as in uncontrolled diabetes.

kilocalorie a measure of energy expenditure equal to the heat needed to raise the temperature of 1 kg of water 1 degree Celsius; also equal to 1,000 calories and sometimes written as calorie rather than kilocalorie.

kilogram-meter a unit of work in which 1 kg of force (1 kg mass accelerated at 1 G) is moved through a vertical distance of 1 meter; abbreviated as kg-m, kg · m, or kgm.

kinesthesia a perception of movement obtained from information about the position and rate of movement of the joints.

Krebs cycle metabolic pathway in the mitochondria in which energy is transferred from carbohydrates, fats, and amino acids to NAD for subsequent production of ATP in the electron transport chain.

lactate threshold a point during a graded exercise test when the blood lactate concentration increases abruptly.

lactic acid an end product of glucose metabolism in the glycolytic pathway; formed in conditions of inadequate oxygen and in muscle fibers with few mitochondria.

lateral sac *see* terminal cisternae.

LDL cholesterol form of low-density lipoprotein responsible for the transport of plasma cholesterol; high levels are indicative of a high risk of coronary heart disease.

lipase an enzyme responsible for the breakdown of triglycerides to free fatty acids and glycerol.

lipolysis the breakdown of triglycerides in adipose tissue to free fatty acids and glycerol for subsequent transport to tissues for metabolism.

lipoprotein protein involved in the transport of cholesterol and triglycerides in the plasma.

low-density lipoproteins (LDL) form of lipoprotein that transports a majority of the plasma cholesterol; *see* LDL cholesterol.

luteinizing hormone (LH) also called "interstitial cell stimulating hormone"; a surge of LH stimulates ovulation in middle of menstrual cycle; LH stimulates testosterone production in men.

major minerals dietary minerals including calcium, phosphorus, potassium, sulfur, sodium, chloride, and magnesium.

Margaria power test test of anaerobic power, primarily related to high-energy phosphates, in which a subject runs up stairs with time monitored to the nearest hundredth of a second.

mast cell connective tissue cell that releases histamine and other chemicals in response to certain stimuli (e.g., injury).

maximal oxygen uptake ($\dot{V}O_2$ max) greatest rate of oxygen uptake by the body measured during severe dynamic exercise, usually on a cycle ergometer or a treadmill; dependent on maximal cardiac output and the maximal arteriovenous oxygen difference.

mesomorphy one component of a somatotype that characterizes the muscular form or lean body mass aspect of the human body.

MET an expression of the rate of energy expenditure at rest; equal to approximately $3.5 \ ml \cdot kg^{-1} \cdot min^{-1}$, or $1 \ kcal \cdot kg^{-1} \cdot hr^{-1}$.

mineralocorticoids steroid hormones released from the adrenal cortex that are responsible for Na^+ and K^+ regulation (e.g., aldosterone).

mitochondrion the subcellular organelle responsible for the production of ATP with oxygen; contains the enzymes for the Krebs cycle, electron transport chain, and the fatty acid cycle.

mixed venous blood a mixture of venous blood from both the upper and lower extremities; complete mixing occurs in the right ventricle.

molecular biology branch of biochemistry involved with the study of gene structure and function.

motor cortex portion of the cerebral cortex containing large motor neurons whose axons descend to lower brain centers and spinal cord; associated with the voluntary control of movement.

motor neurons efferent neurons that conduct action potentials from the central nervous system to the muscles.

motor unit a motor neuron and all the muscle fibers innervated by that single motor neuron; responds in an "all-or-none" manner to a stimulus.

muscle spindle a muscle stretch receptor oriented parallel to skeletal muscle fibers; the capsule portion is surrounded by afferent fibers, and intrafusal muscle fibers can alter the length of the capsule during muscle contraction and relaxation.

muscular strength the maximal amount of force that can be generated by a muscle or muscle group.

myocardial infarction   death of a portion of heart tissue that no longer conducts electrical activity nor provides force to move blood.

myocardial ischemia   a condition in which the myocardium experiences an inadequate blood flow; sometimes accompanied by irregularities in the electrocardiogram (arrhythmias and ST-segment depression) and chest pain (angina pectoris).

myocardium   cardiac muscle; provides the force of contraction to eject blood; muscle type with many mitochondria that is dependent on a constant supply of oxygen.

myofibrils   the portion of the muscle containing the thick and thin contractile filaments; a series of sarcomeres where the repeating pattern of the contractile proteins gives the striated appearance to skeletal muscle.

myoglobin   protein in muscle that can bind oxygen and release it at low PO_2 values; aids in diffusion of oxygen from capillary to mitochondria.

myosin   contractile protein in the thick filament of a myofibril that contains the cross-bridge that can bind actin and split ATP to cause tension development.

NAD   coenzyme that transfers hydrogen and the energy associated with those hydrogens; in the Krebs cycle, NAD transfers energy from substrates to the electron transport chain.

negative feedback   describes the response from a control system that reduces the size of the stimulus, e.g., an elevated blood glucose concentration causes the secretion of insulin which, in turn, lowers the blood glucose concentration.

net efficiency   the mathematical ratio of work output divided by the energy expended above rest.

neuroendocrinology   study of the role of the nervous and endocrine systems in the automatic regulation of the internal environment.

neuromuscular junction   synapse between axon terminal of a motor neuron and the motor end plate of a muscle's plasma membrane.

neuron   nerve cell; composed of a cell body with dendrites (projections) that bring information to the cell body, and axons that take information away from the cell body to influence neurons, glands, or muscles.

nitroglycerin   drug used to reduce chest pain (angina pectoris) due to lack of blood flow to the myocardium.

norepinephrine   a hormone and neurotransmitter; released from postganglionic nerve endings and the adrenal medulla.

normocythemia   a normal red blood cell concentration.

normoxia   a normal PO_2.

nucleus   membrane-bound organelle containing most of the cell's DNA.

nutrient density   the degree to which foods contain selected nutrients, e.g., protein.

open-circuit spirometry   indirect calorimetry procedure in which either inspired or expired ventilation is measured and oxygen consumption and carbon dioxide production is calculated.

organic   describes substances that contain carbon.

osteoporosis   a decrease in bone density due to a loss of cortical bone; common in older women and implicated in fractures; estrogen, exercise, and Ca^{++} therapy are used to correct the condition.

overload   a principle of training describing the need to increase the load (intensity) of exercise to cause a further adaptation of a system.

oxidative phosphorylation   mitochondrial process in which inorganic phosphate (P_i) is coupled to ADP as energy is transferred along the electron transport chain in which oxygen is the final electron acceptor.

oxygen debt   the elevated post-exercise oxygen consumption (*see* EPOC); related to replacement of creatine phosphate, lactic acid resynthesis to glucose, and elevated body temperature, catecholamines, heart rate, breathing, etc.

oxygen deficit   refers to the lag in oxygen uptake at the beginning of exercise.

oxyhemoglobin   hemoglobin combined with oxygen; 1.34 ml of oxygen can combine with 1 g Hb.

pancreas   gland containing both exocrine and endocrine portions; exocrine secretions include enzymes and bicarbonate to digest food in the small intestine; endocrine secretions include insulin, glucagon, and somatostatin, which are released into the blood.

parasympathetic nervous system   portion of the autonomic nervous system that primarily releases acetylcholine from its postganglionic nerve endings.

partial pressure   the fractional part of the barometric pressure due to the presence of a single gas, e.g., PO_2, PCO_2, and PN_2.

percent grade   a measure of the elevation of the treadmill; calculated as the sine of the angle.

percutaneous transluminal coronary angioplasty   a balloon-tipped catheter is inserted into a blocked coronary artery and plaque is pushed back to artery wall to open the blood vessel.

perimysium   the connective tissue surrounding the fasciculus of skeletal muscle fibers.

peripheral nervous system (PNS) portion of the nervous system located outside the spinal cord and brain.

pH   a measure of the acidity of a solution; calculated as the negative $\log_{10}$ of the $[H^+]$ in which 7 is neutral, values that are >7 are basic and <7 are acidic.

phosphocreatine   a compound found in skeletal muscle and used to resynthesize ATP from ADP.

phosphodiesterase   an enzyme that catalyzes the breakdown of cyclic AMP, moderating the effect of the hormonal stimulation of adenylate cyclase.

phosphofructokinase   rate-limiting enzyme in glycolysis that is responsive to ADP, P_i, and ATP levels in the cytoplasm of the cell.

phospholipase C   membrane-bound enzyme that hydrolyzes phosphatidylinositol into inositol triphosphate and diacylglycerol that, in turn, bring about changes in intracellular activity.

physical activity   characterizes all types of human movement; associated with living, work, play, and exercise.

physical fitness   a broad term describing healthful levels of cardiovascular function, strength, and flexibility; fitness is specific to the activities performed.

pituitary gland   a gland at the base of the hypothalamus of the brain having an anterior portion that produces and secretes numerous hormones that regulate other endocrine glands and a posterior portion that secretes hormones that are produced in the hypothalamus.

placebo   an inert substance that is used in experimental studies, e.g., drug studies, to control for any subjective reaction to the substance being tested.

pleura a thin lining of cells that is attached to the inside of the chest wall and to the lung; the cells secrete a fluid that facilitates the movements of the lungs in the thoracic cavity.

posterior hypothalamus area of the brain responsible for regulation of the body's response to a decrease in temperature.

posterior pituitary gland portion of the pituitary gland secreting oxytocin and antidiuretic hormone (vasopressin) that are produced in the hypothalamus.

power a rate of work; work per unit time; $P = W/t$.

power test a test measuring the quantity of work accomplished in a time period; anaerobic power tests include the Margaria stair climb test and the Wingate test; aerobic power tests include the 1.5-mile run and cycle ergometer and treadmill tests in which power output and oxygen consumption are measured.

primary risk factor a sign (e.g., high blood pressure) or a behavior (e.g., cigarette smoking) that is directly related to the appearance of certain diseases independent of other risk factors.

progressive resistance exercise (PRE) a training program in which the muscles must work against a gradually increasing resistance; an implementation of the overload principle.

prolactin hormone secreted from the anterior pituitary that increases milk production from the breast.

proprioceptive neuromuscular facilitation technique of preceding a static stretch with an isometric contraction.

proprioceptors receptors that provide information about the position and movement of the body; includes muscle and joint receptors as well as the receptors in the semicircular canals of the inner ear.

protein kinase C part of second messenger system that is activated by diacylglycerol and results in the activation of proteins in the cell.

provitamin a precursor of a vitamin.

pulmonary circuit the portion of the cardiovascular system involved in the circulation of blood from the right ventricle to the lungs and back to the left atrium.

pulmonary respiration term that refers to ventilation (breathing) of the lung.

Quebec 10-second test a maximal effort 10-second cycle test designed to assess ultra short-term anaerobic power during cycling.

radiation process of energy exchange from the surface of one object to the surface of another that is dependent on a temperature gradient but does not require contact between the objects; an example is the transfer of heat from the sun to the earth.

receptor in the nervous system, a receptor is a specialized portion of an afferent neuron (or a special cell attached to an afferent neuron) that is sensitive to a form of energy in the environment; *receptor* is also a term that applies to unique proteins on the surface of cells that can bind specific hormones or neurotransmitters.

reciprocal inhibition when extensor muscles (agonists) are contracted, there is a reflex inhibition of the motor neurons to the flexor muscles (antagonists), and vice versa.

Recommended Dietary Allowances (RDA) standards of nutrition associated with good health for the majority of people. Standards exist for protein, vitamins, and minerals for children and adults.

relative $\dot{V}O_2$ oxygen uptake (consumption) expressed per unit body weight (e.g., $ml \cdot kg^{-1} \cdot min^{-1}$).

releasing hormone hypothalamic hormones released from neurons into the anterior pituitary that control the release of hormones from that gland.

renin enzyme secreted by special cells in the kidney that converts angiotensinogen to angiotensin I.

repetition the number of times an exercise is repeated within a single exercise "set."

residual volume (RV) volume of air in the lungs following a maximal expiration.

respiration external respiration is the exchange of oxygen and carbon dioxide between the lungs and the environment; internal respiration describes the use of oxygen by the cell (mitochondria).

respiratory compensation the buffering of excess H^+ in the blood by plasma bicarbonate (HCO_3^-), and the associated elevation in ventilation to exhale the resulting CO_2.

respiratory exchange ratio (R) the ratio of CO_2 production to O_2 consumption; indicative of substrate utilization during steady state exercise in which a value of 1.0 represents 100% carbohydrate metabolism and 0.7 represents 100% fat metabolism.

resting membrane potential the voltage difference measured across a membrane that is related to the concentration of ions on each side of the membrane and the permeability of the membrane to those ions.

resting metabolic rate (RMR) metabolic rate measured in the supine position following a period of fasting (4–12 hours) and rest (4–8 hours).

rest interval the time period between bouts in an interval training program.

reversibility a principle of training that describes the temporary nature of a training effect; adaptations to training are lost when the training stops.

sarcolemma the cell (plasma) membrane surrounding a muscle fiber.

sarcomeres the repeating contractile unit in a myofibril bounded by Z-lines.

sarcoplasmic reticulum a membranous structure that surrounds the myofibrils of muscle cells; location of the terminal cisternae or lateral sacs that store the Ca^{++} needed for muscle contraction.

Sargent's jump-and-reach test a test of anaerobic power dependent on the high-energy phosphates; a vertical jump test in which the subject jumps as high as possible.

Schwann cell the cell that surrounds peripheral nerve fibers, forming the myelin sheath.

second messenger a molecule (cyclic AMP) or ion (Ca^{++}) that increases in a cell as a result of an interaction between a "first messenger" (e.g., hormone or neurotransmitter) and a receptor that alters cellular activity.

secondary risk factor a characteristic (age, gender, race, body fatness) or behavior that increases the risk of coronary heart disease when primary risk factors are present.

set a basic unit of a workout containing the number of times (repetitions) a specific exercise is done (e.g., do three sets of five repetitions with 100 pounds).

sex steroids a group of hormones, androgens and estrogens, secreted from the adrenal cortex and the gonads.

sham reinfusion an experimental treatment at the end of a blood doping experiment in which a needle is placed in a vein, but the subject does not receive a reinfusion of blood.

sham withdrawal an experimental treatment at the beginning of a blood doping experiment in which a needle is placed in a vein, but blood is not withdrawn.

sinoatrial node (SA node) specialized tissue located in the right atrium of the heart, which generates the electrical impulse to initiate the heart beat. In a normal healthy heart, the SA node is the heart's pacemaker.

SI units system used to provide international standardization of units of measure in science.

sliding filament model a theory of muscle contraction describing the sliding of the thin filaments (actin) past the thick filaments (myosin).

slow-twitch fibers muscle fiber type that contracts slowly and develops relatively low tension but displays great endurance to repeated stimulation; contains many mitochondria, capillaries, and myoglobin.

somatomedins groups of growth-stimulating peptides released primarily from the liver in response to growth hormone.

somatostatin hormone produced in the hypothalamus that inhibits growth hormone release from the anterior pituitary gland; secreted from cells in the islet of Langerhans and causes a decrease in intestinal activity.

somatotype body-type (form) classification method used to characterize the degree to which an individual's frame is linear (ectomorphic), muscular (mesomorphic), and round (endomorphic); Sheldon's scale rates each component on 1–7 scale.

spatial summation the additive effect of numerous simultaneous inputs to different sites on a neuron to produce a change in the membrane potential.

specificity a principle of training indicating that the adaptation of a tissue is dependent on the type of training undertaken; for example, muscles hypertrophy with heavy resistance training but show an increase in mitochondria number with endurance training.

spirometry measurement of various lung volumes.

static stationary; describes a muscle contraction in which tension is developed but the muscle does not shorten (isometric contraction).

static stretching stretching procedure in which a muscle is stretched and held in the stretched position for ten to thirty seconds; in contrast to dynamic stretching, which involves motion.

steady-state describes the tendency of a control system to achieve a balance between an environmental demand and the response of a physiological system to meet that demand to allow the tissue (body) to function over a period of time.

steroids a class of lipids, derived from cholesterol, that includes the hormones testosterone, estrogen, cortisol, and aldosterone.

stroke volume the amount of blood pumped by the ventricles in a single beat.

strong acids an acid that completely ionizes when dissolved in water to generate H^+ and its anion.

strong bases a base (alkaline substance) that completely ionizes when dissolved in water to generate OH^- and its cation.

ST segment depression an electrocardiographic change reflecting an ischemia (inadequate blood flow) in the heart muscle; indicative of coronary heart disease.

summation repeated stimulation of a muscle that leads to an increase in tension compared to a single twitch.

supercompensation an increase in the muscle glycogen content above normal levels following an exercise-induced muscle glycogen depletion and an increase in carbohydrate intake.

sympathetic nervous system portion of the autonomic nervous system that releases norepinephrine from its postganglionic nerve endings; epinephrine is released from the adrenal medulla.

sympathomimetic substance that mimics the effects of epinephrine or norepinephrine, which are secreted from the sympathetic nervous systems.

synapses junctions between nerve cells (neurons) where the electrical activity of one neuron influences the electrical activity of the other neuron.

systole portion of the cardiac cycle in which the ventricles are contracting.

systolic blood pressure the highest arterial pressure measured during a cardiac cycle.

tapering the process athletes use to reduce their training load for several days prior to competition.

target heart rate (THR) range the range of heart rates describing the optimum intensity of exercise consistent with making gains in maximal aerobic power; equal to 70%–85% HR max.

temporal summation a change in the membrane potential produced by the addition of two or more inputs, occurring at different times (i.e., inputs are added together to produce a potential change that is greater than that caused by a single input).

terminal cisternae portion of the sarcoplasmic reticulum near the transverse tubule containing the Ca^{++} that is released upon depolarization of the muscle; also called *lateral sac*.

testosterone the steroid hormone produced in the testes; involved in growth and development of reproductive tissues, sperm, and secondary sex characteristics.

tetanus highest tension developed by a muscle in response to a high frequency of stimulation.

theophylline a drug used as a smooth muscle relaxant in the treatment of asthma.

thermogenesis the generation of heat as a result of metabolic reactions.

thyroid gland endocrine gland located in the neck that secretes triiodothyronine (T_3) and thyroxine (T_4), which increase the metabolic rate.

thyroid-stimulating hormone (TSH) hormone released from the anterior pituitary gland; stimulates the thyroid gland to increase its secretion of thyroxine and triiodothyronine.

thyroxine hormone secreted from the thyroid gland containing four iodine atoms (T_4); stimulates the metabolic rate and facilitates the actions of other hormones.

tidal volume volume of air inhaled or exhaled in a single breath.

tonus low level of muscle activity at rest.

total lung capacity (TLC) the total volume of air the lung can contain; equal to the sum of the vital capacity and the residual volume.

toxicity a condition resulting from a chronic ingestion of vitamins, especially fat-soluble vitamins, in quantities well above that needed for health.

trace elements dietary minerals including iron, zinc, copper, iodine, manganese, selenium, chromium, molybdenum, cobalt, arsenic, nickel, fluoride, and vanadium.

transferrin plasma protein that binds iron and is representative of the whole body iron store.

transverse tubules an extension, invagination, of the muscle membrane that conducts the action potential into the muscle to depolarize the terminal cisternae, which contains the Ca^{++} needed for muscle contraction.

triiodothyronine hormone secreted from the thyroid gland containing three iodine atoms (T_3); stimulates the metabolic rate and facilitates the actions of other hormones.

tropomyosin protein covering the actin binding sites that prevents the myosin cross-bridge from touching actin.

troponin protein, associated with actin and tropomyosin, that binds Ca^{++} and initiates the movement of tropomyosin on actin to allow the myosin cross-bridge to touch actin and initiate contraction.

twenty-four-hour recall a technique of recording the type and amount of food (nutrients) consumed during a twenty-four-hour period.

twitch the tension-generating response following the application of a single stimulus to muscle.

Type I fibers fibers that contain large numbers of oxidative enzymes and are highly fatigue resistant.

Type IIa fibers fibers that contain biochemical and fatigue characteristics that are between Type IIb and Type I fibers.

Type IIb fibers fibers that have a relatively small number of mitochondria, a limited capacity for aerobic metabolism, and are less resistant to fatigue than slow-fibers.

underwater weighing procedure to estimate body volume by the loss of weight in water; result is used to calculate body density and, from that, body fatness.

U.S. Dietary Goals a series of nutritional goals to achieve better health for the American population: 58% carbohydrate; 30% fat (no more than 10% saturated fat); and 12% protein.

vagus nerve a major parasympathetic nerve.

variable resistance exercise strength training equipment in which the resistance varies throughout the range of motion.

veins the blood vessel that accepts blood from the venules and brings it back to the heart.

ventilation the movement of air into or out of the lungs (e.g., pulmonary or alveolar ventilation); external respiration.

ventilatory threshold (Tvent) the "breakpoint" at which pulmonary ventilation and carbon dioxide output begin to increase exponentially during an incremental exercise test.

venules small blood vessels carrying capillary blood to veins.

vestibular apparatus sensory organ, consisting of three semicircular canals, that provides needed information about body position to maintain balance.

vital capacity (VC) the volume of air that can be moved into or out of the lungs in one breath; equal to the sum of the inspiratory and expiratory reserve volumes and the tidal volume.

web of causation an epidemiologic model showing the complex interaction of risk factors associated with the development of chronic degenerative diseases.

whole body density a measure of the weight to volume ratio of the entire body; high values are associated with low body fatness.

Wingate test anaerobic power test to evaluate maximal rate at which glycolysis can deliver ATP.

work the product of a force and the distance through which that force moves (W = F × D).

work interval in interval training, the duration of the work phase of each work-to-rest interval.

Credits

Text and Illustrations

Chapter 3

Figure 3.1: From Ross M. Durham, *Human Physiology*. Copyright © 1989 Times Mirror Higher Education Group, Inc., Dubuque, Iowa. All Rights Reserved. Reprinted by permission of the author.

Figure 3.2, 3.3, 3.4, 3.6, 3.7, 3.10 and **3.15** From Stuart Ira Fox, *Human Physiology*, 5th ed. Copyright © 1996 Times Mirror Higher Education Group, Inc., Dubuque, Iowa. All Rights Reserved. Reprinted by permission.

Figure 3.5: From David Shier, et al., *Hole's Human Anatomy and Physiology*, 7th ed. Copyright © 1996 Times Mirror Higher Education Group, Inc., Dubuque, Iowa. All Rights Reserved. Reprinted by permission.

Figure 3.13 and **3.14:** From Stuart Ira Fox, *Human Physiology*, 4th ed. Copyright © 1993 Times Mirror Higher Education Group, Inc., Dubuque, Iowa. All Rights Reserved. Reprinted by permission.

Chapter 4

Figure 4.4: From S. Dodd, 1984, "Blood Lactate Disappearance at Various Intensities of Recovery Exercise" in *Journal of Applied Physiology*, 57:1462–65. Copyright © 1984 American Physiological Society, Bethesda MD. Used by permission.

Figure 4.11: From G. Brooks and J. Mercier, "Balance of Carbohydrate and Lipid Utilization During Exercise: the 'Crossover Concept'" in *Journal of Applied Physiology*, 76:2253–2261, 1994. Copyright © 1994 American Physiological Society. Reprinted by permission.

Figure 4.13 and **4.14:** From E. Coyle, "Substrate Utilization During Exercise in Active People" in *American Journal of Clinical Nutrition*, 61 (Suppl):9685–9795, 1995. Copyright © 1995 American Society for Clinical Nutrition, Inc., Bethesda MD. Reprinted by permission.

Figure 4.15: From Stuart Ira Fox, *Human Physiology*, 5th ed. Copyright © 1996 Times Mirror Higher Education Group, Inc., Dubuque, Iowa. All Rights Reserved. Reprinted by permission.

Chapter 5

Figure 5.2: From Stuart Ira Fox, *Human Physiology*, 3d ed. Copyright © 1990 Times Mirror Higher Education Group, Inc., Dubuque, Iowa. All Rights Reserved. Reprinted by permission.

Figure 5.5: From Kent M. Van de Graaff and Stuart Ira Fox, *Concepts of Human Anatomy and Physiology*, 4th ed. Copyright © 1995 Times Mirror Higher Education Group, Inc., Dubuque, Iowa. All Rights Reserved. Reprinted by permission.

Figure 5.7: Data from V. A. Convertino, L. C. Keil, and J. E. Greenleaf, 1983, "Plasma Volume, Renin and Vasopressin Responses to Graded Exercises After Training". American Physiological Association, Bethesda MD: *Journal of Applied Physiology: Respiration Environment Exercise Physiology*. 54:508–14.

Figure 5.8: Data from J. T. Maher, et al, 1975, "Aldersterone Dynamics During Graded Exercises at Sea-level and High Altitudes". American Physiological Society, Bethesda MD: *Journal of Applied Physiology* 39:18–22.

Figure 5.12: Data from J. E. Turkowski, et al, 1978, "Ovarian Hormonal Responses to Exercise". American Physiological Society, Bethesda MD: *Journal of Applied Physiology: Respiration Environment Exercise Physiology*. 44:109–14.

Figure 5.13: Reprinted with permission from B. Saltin and J. Karlsson, 1971, "Muscle Metabolism During Exercise", 289-99, edited by B. Pernow and B. Saltin. Copyright © 1971 Plenum Press, New York NY.

Figure 5.14: From M. Kjaer, 1989, "Epinephrine and Some Other Hormonal Responses to Exercise in Man: With Special Reference to Physical Training" in *International Journal of Sports Medicine*, 10:2–15. Copyright © 1989 Georg Thieme Verlag, Stuttgart, Germany. Reprinted by permission.

Figure 5.15: From R. C. Harris, et al., "The Effect of Propranolol on Blycogen Metabolism During Exercise" in *Muscle Metabolism During Exercise*, B. Pernow & B. Saltin, Eds. Copyright © 1971 Plenum Publishing Corporation, New York. Reprinted by permission.

Figure 5.18: Data from C. T. M. Davies and J. D. Few, 1973, "Effects of Exercise on Adrenocortical Function". American Physiological Society, Bethesda MD: *Journal of Applied Physiology*. 35:887–91.

Figure 5.20 A: Data from J. Sutton and L. Lazarus, 1976, "Growth Hormone in Exercise: Comparison of Physiological and Pharmacological Stimuli". American Physiological Society, Bethesda MD: *Journal of Applied Physiology*. 41:523–27.

Figure 5.20 B: Data from J. C. Bunt, et al, 1986, "Sex and Training Differences in Human Growth Hormone Levels During Prolonged Exercise". American Physiological Society, Bethesda MD: *Journal of Applied Physiology*. 61:1796–1801.

Figure 5.22: Data from Scott Powers, et al, 1982, "A Different Cathecolamine Response during Prolonged Exercise and Passive Heating". American College of Sports Medicine, Indianapolis IN: *Medicine and Science in Sports and Exercise*. 14:435-39.

Figure 5.23: From W. W. Winder, et al., 1978, "Time Course of Sympathadrenal Adaptation to Endurance Exercise Training in Man" in *Journal of Applied Physiology: Respiration Environment Exercise Physiology*, 45:370–77. Copyright © 1978 The American Physiological Society, Bethesda MD. Reprinted by permission.

Figure 5.25 A: Data from L. H. Hartley, et al., 1972, "Multiple Hormonal Responses to Graded Exercise in Relation to Physical Training". American Physiological Society, Bethesda MD: *Journal of Applied Physiology*. 33:602–6.

Figure 5.25 B: Data from F. Gyntelberg, et al., 1977, "Effect of Training on the Response of Plasma Glucagon to Exercise". American Physiological Society, Bethesda MD: *Journal of Applied Physiology: Respiration Environment Exercise Physiology*. 43:302–5.

Figure 5.26: Data from F. Gyntelberg, et al., 1977, "Effect of Training on the Response of Plasma Glucagon to Exercise". American Physiological Society, Bethesda MD: *Journal of Applied Physiology: Respiration Environment Exercise Physiology*. 43:302–5.

Figure 5.30 A: From B. Issekutz and H. Miller, "Plasma-free Fatty Acids During Exercise and the Effect of Lactic Acid", 1962, in *Proceedings of the Society for Experimental Biology and Medicine*, 110:237–39. Copyright © 1962 Society For Experimental Biology and Medicine, New York. Reprinted by permission.

Chapter 6

Figure 6.7: From J. Coast and H. G. Welch, 1985, "Linear Increase in Optimal Pedal Rate with Increased Power Output in Cycle Ergometry" in *European Journal of Applied Physiology*, 53:339-42. Copyright © Springer-Verlag, Heidelberg, Germany. Reprinted by permission.

Figure 6.8: From P. Hopkins and S. Powers, 1982, "Oxygen Uptake during Submaximal Running in Highly Trained Men and Women" in *American Corrective Therapy Journal*, 36:130-2 (Now *Clinical Kinesiology: Journal of the American Kinesiotherapy Association*) (formerly the Amrican Corrective Therapy Association). Reprinted by permission.

Chapter 7

Figure 7.1, 7.2, and **7.9:** From Stuart Ira Fox, *Human Physiology*. Copyright © 1984 Times Mirror Higher Education Group, Inc., Dubuque, Iowa. All Rights Reserved. Reprinted by permission.

Figure 7.3, 7.5, 7.6, and **7.13:** From David Shier, et al., *Hole's Human Anatomy and Physiology*, 7th ed. Copyright © 1996 Times Mirror Higher Education Group, Inc., Dubuque, Iowa. All Rights Reserved. Reprinted by permission.

Figure 7.4: From John W. Hole, Jr., *Human Anatomy and Physiology*, 3d ed. Copyright © 1984 Times Mirror Higher Education Group, Inc., Dubuque, Iowa. All Rights Reserved. Reprinted by permission.

Figure 7.7: From Jackson Beatty, *Principles of Behavioral Neuroscience*. Copyright © 1995 Times Mirror Higher Education Group, Inc., Dubuque, Iowa. All Rights Reserved. Reprinted by permission.

Figure 7.8: From John W. Hole, Jr., *Human Anatomy and Physiology*, 5th ed. Copyright © 1990 Times Mirror Higher Education Group, Inc., Dubuque, Iowa. All Rights Reserved. Reprinted by permission.

Figure 7.11: From Kent M. Van de Graaff and Stuart Ira Fox, *Concepts of Human Anatomy and Physiology*, 2d ed. Copyright © 1989 Times Mirror Higher Education Group, Inc., Dubuque, Iowa. All Rights Reserved. Reprinted by permission.

Chapter 8

Figure 8.1, 8.2, 8.4, 8.14 and **8.21:** From David Shier, et al., *Hole's Human Anatomy and Physiology*, 7th ed. Copyright © 1996 Times Mirror Higher Education Group, Inc., Dubuque, Iowa. All Rights Reserved. Reprinted by permission.

Figure 8.3, 8.5 and **8.6:** From Stuart Ira Fox, *Human Physiology*, 5th ed. Copyright © 1996 Times Mirror Higher Education Group, Inc., Dubuque, Iowa. All Rights Reserved. Reprinted by permission.

Figure 8.11: From R. Bottinelli, et al., "Myofibrillar ATPase Activity During Isometric Contractions and Myosin Composition in Rat Single-skinned Muscle Fibers" 1994, in *Journal of Physiology* (London), 481:633-75. Copyright © 1994 Physiological Society, London. Reprinted by permission.

Figure 8.13: Data from G. Adams, et al., 1993, "Skeletal Muscle Myosin Heavy Chain Composition and Resistance Training". American Physiological Society, Bethesda MD: *Journal of Applied Physiology*. 74:911-15.

Figure 8.17: From Stuart Ira Fox, *Human Physiology*, 2d ed. Copyright © 1987 Times Mirror Higher Education Group, Inc., Dubuque, Iowa. All Rights Reserved. Reprinted by permission.

Figure 8.22: From Stuart Ira Fox, *Human Physiology*, 4th ed. Copyright © 1993 Times Mirror Higher Education Group, Inc., Dubuque, Iowa. All Rights Reserved. Reprinted by permission.

Chapter 9

Figure 9.1: From John W. Hole, Jr., *Essentials of Human Anatomy and Physiology*, 5th ed. Copyright © 1995 Times Mirror Higher Education Group, Inc., Dubuque, Iowa. All Rights Reserved. Reprinted by permission.

Figure 9.2: From Kent M. Van de Graaff, *Human Anatomy*, 4th ed. Copyright © 1995 Times Mirror Higher Education Group, Inc., Dubuque, Iowa. All Rights Reserved. Reprinted by permission.

Figure 9.5: From Stuart Ira Fox, *A Laboratory Guide to Human Physiology: Concepts & Clinical Applications*, 4th ed. Copyright © 1987 Times Mirror Higher Education Group, Inc., Dubuque, Iowa. All Rights Reserved. Reprinted by permission.

Figure 9.6 and **9.12:** From David Shier, et al., *Hole's Human Anatomy and Physiology*, 7th ed. Copyright © 1996 Times Mirror Higher Education Group, Inc., Dubuque, Iowa. All Rights Reserved. Reprinted by permission.

Figure 9.7, 9.8, 9.13, 9.15 and **9.16:** From Stuart Ira Fox, *Human Physiology*, 5th ed. Copyright © 1996 Times Mirror Higher Education Group, Inc., Dubuque, Iowa. All Rights Reserved. Reprinted by permission.

Figure 9.9: From Kent M. Van de Graaff and Stuart Ira Fox, *Concepts of Human Anatomy and Physiology*, 4th ed. Copyright © 1995 Times Mirror Higher Education Group, Inc., Dubuque, Iowa. All Rights Reserved. Reprinted by permission.

Figure 9.10: Reprinted by permission of the publisher from Averill: "Critical Decisions in Cardiac Emergencies," *Emergency Medicine*, 2(2):63–79. Copyright 1979 by Excerpta Medica Inc.

Figure 9.11: From Kent M. Van de Graaff and Stuart Ira Fox, *Concepts of Human Anatomy and Physiology*, 4th ed. Copyright © 1995 Times Mirror Higher Education Group, Inc., Dubuque, Iowa. All Rights Reserved. Reprinted by permission.

Figure 9.14: From Stuart Ira Fox, *Human Physiology*, 4th ed. Copyright © 1993 Times Mirror Higher Education Group, Inc., Dubuque, Iowa. All Rights Reserved. Reprinted by permission.

Figure 9.17: Data from L. Rowell, 1993, "Human Cardiovascular Adjustments to Exercise and Thermal Stress". American Physiological Society, Bethesda MD: *Physiological Reviews*. 74:911-15 and L. Rowell, 1986, *Human Circulation Regulation During Physical Stress*. New York NY: Oxford University Press.

Figure 9.21: Data from P. Astrand, et al., 1965, "Intra-arterial Blood Pressure During Exercise with Different Muscle Groups", American Physiological Society, Bethesda MD: *Journal of Applied Physiology*. 20:253–57.

Figure 9.22: Data from G. Brenglemann, 1983, "Circulatory Adjustments to Exercise and Heat Stress", Annual Reviews, Inc., Palo Alto CA: *Annual Review of Physiology*. 45:191–212; E. Fox and D. Costill, 1972, "Estimated Cardiorespiratory Responses during Marathon Running", Heldref Publications, Washington DC: *Archives of Environmental Health*. 24:315–24; and L. Rowell, 1974, "Human Cardiovascular Adjustments to Exercise and Thermal Stress". American Physiological Society, Bethesda MD: *Physiological Reviews*. 54:75–159.

Chapter 10

Figure 10.1, 10.2, 10.5, 10.6 and **10.7:** From Kent M. Van de Graaff, *Human Anatomy*, 4th ed. Copyright © 1995 Times Mirror Higher Education Group, Inc., Dubuque, Iowa. All Rights Reserved. Reprinted by permission.

Figure 10.3: From E. R. Weibel, *Morphmetry of the Human Lung*. Copyright © 1963 Springer-Verlag, Heidelberg, Germany. Reprinted by permission.

Figure 10.4, 10.18 and **10.23:** From David Shier, et al., *Hole's Human Anatomy and Physiology*, 7th ed. Copyright © 1996 Times Mirror Higher Education Group, Inc., Dubuque, Iowa. All Rights Reserved. Reprinted by permission.

Figure 10.9: From John W. Hole, Jr., *Human Anatomy and Physiology*, 6th ed. Copyright © 1993 Times Mirror Higher Education Group, Inc., Dubuque, Iowa. All Rights Reserved. Reprinted by permission.

Figure 10.10, 10.14, 10.15 and **10.17:** From Stuart Ira Fox, *Human Physiology*, 5th ed. Copyright © 1996 Times Mirror Higher Education Group, Inc., Dubuque, Iowa. All Rights Reserved. Reprinted by permission.

Figure 10.16: From Stuart Ira Fox, *Human Physiology*, 3d ed. Copyright © 1990 Times Mirror Higher Education Group, Inc., Dubuque, Iowa. All Rights Reserved. Reprinted by permission.

Figure 10.19: From John W. Hole, Jr., *Essentials of Human Anatomy and Physiology*, 5th ed. Copyright © 1995 Times Mirror Higher Education Group, Inc., Dubuque, Iowa. All Rights Reserved. Reprinted by permission.

Figure 10.20: Data from J. Dempsey and R. Fregosi, 1985, "Adaptability of the Pulmonary System to Changing Metabolic Requirement" Yorke Medical Group, New York NY: *American Journal of Cardiology,* 55:59D–67D; J. Dempsey, et al., 1986, "Is the Lung Built for Exercise?" American College of Sports Medicine, Indianapolis IN: *Medicine and Science in Sports and Exercise,* 18:143–155; and S. Powers, et al., 1985, "Caffeine Alters Ventilatory and Gas Exchange Kinetics during Exercise" American College of Sports Medicine, Indianapolis IN: *Medicine and Science in Sports and Exercise,* 18:101–6.

Figure 10.21: Data from J. Dempsey, et al., 1986, "Is the Lung Built for Exercise?" American College of Sports Medicine, Indianapolis IN: *Medicine and Science in Sports and Exercise,* 18:143–155; and S. Powers, et al., 1982, "Ventilatory and Metabolic Reactions to Heat Stress During Prolonged Exercise" International Federation of Sportive Medicine, Turin, Italy: *Journal of Sports Medicine and Physical Fitness,* 22:32–36.

Figure 10.22: Data from J. Dempsey, et al., 1982, "Limitation to Exercise Capacity and Endurance: Pulmonary System" University of Toronto, Toronto, Ontario, Canada: *Canadian Journal of Applied Sports Sciences,* 7–4–13; and K. Wasserman, et al., 1973, "Anaerobic Threshold and Respiratory Gas Exchange during Exercise" American Physiological Society, Bethesda MD, *Journal of Applied Physiology,* 35:236–43.

Chapter 11

Figure 11.4: Data from E. Hultman and K. Sahlin, 1980, "Acid-base Balance during Exercise", R. Hutton and D. Miller, Eds. Franklin Institute Press, Philadelphia PA: *Exercise and Sport Science Reviews,* 8:41–128; N. Jones, et al., 1977, "Effects of pH on Cardiorespiratory and Metabolic Responses to Exercise". American Physiological Society, Bethesda MD, *Journal of Applied Physiology,* 43:969–64; and A. Katz, et al., 1984, "Maximum Exercise Tolerance after Induced Alkalosis", Stuttgart Germany: *International Journal of Sports Medicine,* 5:107–10.

Figure 11.5: Data from E. Hultman and K. Sahlin, 1986, "Acid-base Balance during Exercise", R. Hutton and D. Miller, Eds. Orlando FL, Academic Press, Inc.: *Exercise and Sport Science Reviews.* 8:41–128.

Chapter 12

Figure 12.10: Data from G. Brengelmann, 1977, "Control of Sweating and Skin Flow During Exercise", E. Nadel, Ed. Academic Press, Inc., Orlando FL: *Problems with Temperature Regulation During Exercise.* and S. Powers, et al., 1982, "Ventilatory and Metabolic Reactions to Heat Stress During Prolonged Exercise" International Federation of Sportive Medicine, Turin, Italy: *Journal of Sports Medicine and Physical Fitness,* 2:32–36.

Chapter 13

Figure 13.5: From T. J. Terjung, "Muscle Adaptations to Aerobic Training" in *Sports Science Exchange,* Vol. 6, No. 6, 1993. Copyright © 1993 Gatorade Sports Science Institute, Barrington IL. Reprinted by permission.

Figure 13.6: Data from S. Powers, et al., 1994, "Influence of Exercise and Fiber Type on Antioxidant Enzyme Activity in Rat Skeletal Muscle" American Physiological Society, Bethesda MD: *American Journal of Physiology,* 266:R375–80.

Figure 13.12: Reprinted with permission from D. Nieman, "Exercise, Infection, and Immunity" in *Int. J. Sports Med.* 75(1994) S131–S141, Georg Thieme Verlag, Stuttgart.

Figure 13.17: From D. G. Sale, 1988, "Neural Adaptations to Resistance Training" in *Medicine and Science in Sports and Exercise,* 20:S135–S143. Copyright © 1988 American College of Sports Medicine, Indianapolis IN. Reprinted by permission.

Chapter 14

Figure 14.1: Data from R. Farmer and D. Miller, 1991, *Lecture Notes on Epidemiology and Public Health Medicine.* Boston MA: Blackwell Scientific Publications, pp. 107–11.

Figure 14.2: Data from R. A. Stallones, 1966, U.S. Government Printing Office, Washington DC: *Public Health Monograph 76;* and I. H. R. Rockett, 1994, "Population and Health: An Introduction to Epidemiology Population Reference Bureau, Washington DC: *Population and Health: An Introduction to Epidemiology,* 49(No. 3):1–48.

Figure 14.4: From C. J. Casperson, "Physical Activity Epidemiology: Concepts, Methods, and Applications to Exercise Science" edited by K. B. Pandolf in *Exercise and Sport Science Reviews,* 17:457, 1989. Copyright © 1989 Williams & Wilkins, Baltimore MD. Reprinted by permission.

Figure 14.5: Data from N. M. Kaplan, 1989, "The Deadly Quartet". American Medical Association, Chicago IL: *Archives of Internal Medicine* 149:1514–20; and A. P. Rocchini, 1991, "Insulin Resistance and Blood Pressure Regulation in Obese and Nonobese Subjects". American Heart Association, Dallas TX: *Hypertension* 17:837–42.

Chapter 16

Figure 16.1: Data from L. S. Goodman and A. Gilman, eds., 1975, *The Pharmacological Basis of Therapeutics.* New York: Macmillan Publshing Company.

Figure 16.2: Data from M. M. Dehn and C. B. Mullins, 1977, "Physiologic Effects and Importance of Exercise in Patients with Coronary Artery Disease" Group Medicine Publications, Inc., New York NY: *Cardiovascular Medicine,* 2:365; and H. K. Hellerstein and B. A. Franklin, 1984. John Wiley & Sons, Inc., New York NY: *Rehabilitation of the Coronary Patient,* 2d ed.

Figure 16.3: Data from R. R. Pate, et al., 1995, "Physical Activity and Public Health" in *Journal of the American Medical Association,* 273:402-407. Chicago, IL: American Medical Association.

Chapter 17

Figure 17.2: From E. R. Richter and H. Galbo, 1986, "Diabetes, Insulin and Exercise" in *Sports Medicine,* 3:275–88. Copyright © 1986 Adis Press, Langhorn PA. Reprinted by permission.

Chapter 18

Figure 18.3: Adapted from M. L. Pollock and J. H. Wilmore, *Exercise in Health and Disease,* 2d ed., 1990. Philadelphia PA: W. B. Saunders.

Figure 18.4: From T. G. Lohman, "The Use of Skinfold to Estimate Body Fatness in Children and Youth" in *Journal of Health, Physical Education, Recreation and Dance,* 98:102, November-December 1987. Copyright © 1987 American Alliance for Health, Physical Recreation and Dance, Reston VA. Reprinted by permission.

Figure 18.7: From E. Jequier, "Calorie Balance vs Nutrient Balance" in *Energy Metabolism: Tissue Determinants and Cellular Corollaries,* John M. Kinney and Hugh N. Tucker, Eds. Copyright © 1992 Raven Press. Reprinted by permission of Lippincott-Raven Publishers, a Wolters Kluwer Company, New York.

Figure 18.8: From A. Keys, et al., *The Biology of Human Starvation,* Vol. I. Copyright © 1950 University of Minnesota Press, Minneapolis MN. Reprinted by permission.

Figure 18.9: From L. O. Schulz and D. A. Scholler, "A Compilation of Total Energy Expenditures and Body Weights in Healty Adults" in *American Journal of Clinical Nutrition,* 60:676–81, 1994. Copyright © 1994 American Society for Clinical Nutrition, Inc., Bethesda MD. Reprinted by permission.

Figure 18.11: From J. Mayer, et al., "Exercise, Food Intake, and Body Weight in Normal Rats and Genetically Obese Mice" in *American Journal of Physiology,* 177:544–48. Copyright © 1954 American Physiological Society, Bethesda MD. Used by permission.

Chapter 19

Figure 19.1: From P. Astrand and K. Rodahl, *Textbook of Work Physiology,* 2d ed. Copyright © 1977 McGraw-Hill, Inc., New York NY. Reprinted by permission.

Figure 19.2: From H. Gibson and R. H. T. Edwards, 1985, "Muscular Exercise and Fatigue" in *Sports Medicine,* 2:120-32. Copyright © 1985 Adis Press, Langhorn PA. Reprinted by permission.

Chapter 20

Figure 20.5: Reprinted with permission from B. Scott and J. Houmard, "Peak Running Velocity is Highly Related to Distance Running Performance" in *Int. J. Sports Med.* 75(1994) 504–507, Georg Thieme Verlag, Stuttgart.

Figure 20.9: From P. Astrand and K. Rodahl, *Textbook of Work Physiology*, 2d ed. Copyright © 1977 McGraw-Hill, Inc., New York NY. Reprinted by permission.

Chapter 21

Figure 21.2: From M. Ikai and T. Fukunaga, 1968, "Calculation of Muscle Strength per Unit of Cross Sectional Area of a Human Muscle by Means of Ultrasonic Measurement" in *Internationale Zeitschrift fuer Angewante Physiologie*,26:26–31. Copyright © 1968 Springer-Verlag, Heidelberg, Germany. Reprinted by permission.

Figure 21.3: From J. Wilmore, et al., 1974, "Alterations in Strength, Body Composition, and Anthrometric Measurements Consequent to a 10-Week Weight Training Program" in *Medicine and Science in Sports*, 6:133–39. Copyright © 1974 American College of Sports Medicine, Indianapolis IN. Reprinted by permission.

Figure 21.4: From R. Armstrong, 1984, "Mechanisms of Exercise-induced Delayed Onset of Muscular Soreness: A Brief Review" in *Medicine and Science in Sports and Exercise*, 16:529–38. Copyright © 1984 American College of Sports Medicine, Indianapolis IN. Reprinted by permission.

Chapter 22

Figure 22.4: From Kent M. Van de Graaff, *Human Anatomy*, 4th ed. Copyright © 1995 Times Mirror Higher Education Group, Inc., Dubuque, Iowa. All Rights Reserved. Reprinted by permission.

Chapter 23

Figure 23.1: From J. Bergstrom, et al., 1967, "Diet, Muscle Glycogen and Physical Performance" in ACTA PHYSIOLOGICA SCANDINAVICA, 71:140-50. Copyright © 1967 Scandinavian Physiological Society, Stockholm Sweden. Reprinted by permission of Blackwell Scientific Publications, Ltd., Oxford, England.

Figure 23.2: From W. M. Sherman, 1983, "Carbohydrates, Muscle Glycogen, and Muscle Glycogen Super Compensation" in *Ergogenic Aids in Sports*, 3–26, edited by M. H. Williams. Copyright © 1983 Human Kinetics Publishers, Inc., Champaign IL. Used with permission.

Figure 23.3: From John O. Halloszy, Ed., in *Exercise and Sport Science Reviews*, 19:982, 1991. Copyright © 1991 Williams & Wilkins, Baltimore MD. Reprinted by permission.

Figure 23.5: Data from P. W. R. Lemon and J. P. Mullin, 1980, "Effect of Initial Muscle Group Glycogen Levels on Protein Catabolism During Exercise" American Physiological Society, Bethesda MD: *American Journal of Applied Physiology* 48:624–29.

Figure 23.6: From C. T. M. Davies, et al., 1982, "Glucose Inhibits CO2 Production from Leucine during Whole Body Exercise in Man" in *Journal of Physiology*, 332:40–1. Copyright © 1982 Cambridge University Press, Cambridge, England. Reprinted by permission.

Figure 23.7: From E. F. Coyle and S. J. Montain, 1995, "Benefits of Fluid Replacement with Carbohydrate During Exercise," in *Medicine and Science in Sports and Exercise*, 24:S324-S330. Copyright © 1995 Williams & Wilkins Company, Baltimore MD. Reprinted by permission.

Figure 23.8: From D. L. Costill and B. Saltin, 1974, "Factors Limiting Gastric Emptying during Rest and Exercise" in *Journal of Applied Physiology*, 37:679–83. Copyright © 1974 American Physiological Association, Bethesda MD. Reprinted by permission.

Figure 23.9: From K. Davies, et al., 1982, "Muscle Mitochondrial Bioenergetics, Oxygen Supply, and Work Capacity during Dietary Iron Deficiency and Repletion in *Journal of Applied Physiology*, 242:E418–E427. Copyright © 1982 American Physiological Society, Bethesda MD. Used by permission.

Figure 23.11: From J. M. Tanner, et al., *The Physique of the Olympic Athlete*. Copyright © 1964 George Allen & Unwin Publishers, Ltd., London, England. Reprinted by permission.

Chapter 24

Figure 24.2: Data from R. Grover, et al., 1967, "Muscular Exercise in Young Men Native to 3,100 m Altitude" American Physiological Society, Bethesda MD: *American Journal of Applied Physiology* 22:555–64.

Figure 24.3: Data from L. G. C. E. Pugh, 1964, "Muscular Exercise at Great Altitudes" American Physiological Society, Bethesda MD: *Journal of Applied Physiology* 19:431-40.

Figure 24.4: From J. B. West and P. D. Wagner, 1980, "Predicted Gas Exchange on the Summit of Mt. Everest" in *Respiration Physiology*, 42:1–16. Copyright © 1980 Elsevier Biomedical Press, Amsterdam, The Netherlands. Reprinted by permission.

Figure 24.5: From J. B. West, et al., 1983, "Barometric Pressures at Extreme Altitudes on Mt. Everest: Physiological Significance" in *Journal of Applied Physiology*, 54:1188–94. Copyright © 1983 American Physiological Society, Bethesda MD. Reprinted by permission.

Figure 24.7: From D. K. Mathews, et al., 1969, "Physiological Responses during Exercise and Recovery in a Football Uniform" in *Journal of Applied Physiology*, 26:611–15. Copyright © 1969 American Physiological Society, Bethesda MD. Reprinted by permission.

Figure 24.9: Data from G. W. Molnar, 1946. American Medical Association, Chicago IL: *The Journal of The American Medical Association* 131:1046-50.

Figure 24.10: From A. C. Burton and O. G. Edholm, *Man in a Cold Environment.* Copyright © 1955 Edward Arnold Publishers. Reprinted by permission of Edward Arnold Publishers, Div. of Hodder & Stoughton Ltd, London, England.

Figure 24.11: From P. B. Raven, et al., 1974,"Effect of Carbon Monoxide and Peroxacetyle Nitrate on Man's Maximal Aerobic Capacity" in *Journal of Applied Physiology*, 36:288–93. Copyright © 1974 American Physiological Society, Bethesda MD. Reprinted by permission.

Chapter 25

Figure 25.1: Data from G. Ariel and W. Saville, 1972. "Anabolic Steroids: The Physiological Effects of Placebos" American College of Sports Medicine, Indianapolis IN: *Medicine and Science in Sports and Exercise* 4:124–26.

Figure 25.3: From N. Gledhill, 1982, "Blood Doping and Related Issues: A Brief Review" in *Medicine and Science in Sports and Exercise*, 14:183–89. Copyright © 1982 American College of Sports Medicine, Indianapolis IN. Reprinted by permission.

Photographs

Chapter 1

Opener: Courtesy of Andrew S. Kozar, University of Tennessee; 1.1A: Courtesy of Carnegie Institute of Washington, D.C.; 1.1B: Courtesy of Quinton Instrument Co.; 1.2& 1.3: Courtesy of W.B. Saunders Company

Chapter 2

Opener: © Bob Daemmrich/Uniphoto Picture Agency

Chapter 3

Opener: © Al Messerschmidt Photos 1995

Chapter 4

Opener: © M. Reibel/Active Images, Inc.

Chapter 5

Opener: © Terry P. Wild/Uniphoto Picture Agency

Chapter 6

Opener: Courtesy of Quinton Instrument Co.; 6.3B: Courtesy of Sensor-Medics, Inc.

Chapter 7
Opener: © Alfred Pasieka/Peter Arnold, Inc.

Chapter 8
Opener: © Manfred Cage/Peter Arnold, Inc.; 8.12A: © Hans Hoppler, "Respiratory Physiology," Vol. 44, p. 94, 1981

Chapter 9
Opener: © Ansel Pitcairn/Peter Arnold, Inc.

Chapter 10
Opener: © Al Messerschmidt Photographs 1992; 10.8: Courtesy of Sensor-Medics, Inc.

Chapter 11
Opener: The Bettmann Archive

Chapter 12
Opener: © Corel Professional Photos

Chapter 13
Opener: © Al Messerschmidt Photos 1995

Chapter 14
Opener: The Bettmann Archive

Chapter 15
Opener: Courtesy of Quinton Instruments Co.

Chapter 16
Opener: © Corel Professional Photos

Chapter 17
Opener: © SuperStock

Chapter 18
Opener: © John Goletti/Uniphoto Picture Agency

Chapter 19
Opener: © Alice Garik/Peter Arnold Inc.

Chapter 20
Opener: © David Frazier Photolibrary; 20.14: Courtesy of CYBEX, Inc.

Chapter 21
Opener: The Bettmann Archive

Chapter 22
Opener: © David Frazier Photolibrary

Chapter 23
Opener: © Marc S. Levine/Active Images, Inc.; 23.10: Courtesy of W.H. Sheldon Trust

Chapter 24
Opener: © Glen Rowell/Peter Arnold, Inc.

Chapter 25
Opener: © 1996 Werner Bortsch/Medical Images Inc.

Art

New illustrations by Bensen Studios, Inc.: 2.1, 2.2, 2.3, 2.4, 2.5, 2.6, 3.1, 3.4, 3.8, 3.9, 3.11, 3.12, 3.13, 3.16, 4.1, 4.2, 4.3, 4.5, 4.6, 4.7, 4.8, 4.9, 4.11, 4.12, 4.13, 4.14, 5.2, 5.6, 5.15, 5.17, 5.28, 5.30A, 5.30B, 6.1, 6.2, 6.3A, 6.5, 6.6, 6.7, 6.8, 7.2, 7.4, 7.8, 8.5, 8.7, 8.8, 8.9, 8.10, 8.11, 8.13, 8.15, 8.16, 8.18, 8.20, 9.3, 9.4, 9.6, 9.13, 9.18, 9.20, 10.13, 10.16, 10.22, 10.24, 10.25, 10.26, 10.27, 11.1, 11.2, 11.3, 11.4, 11.5, 12.1, 12.2, 12.3, 12.4, 12.5, 12.6, 12.7, 12.8, 12.9, 12.10, 13.1, 13.2, 13.3, 13.4, 13.5, 13.6, 13.7, 13.8, 13.9, 13.10, 13.11, 13.12, 13.13, 13.14, 13.15, 13.16, 13.17, 14.1, 14.2, 14.3, 14.4, 14.5, 14.6, 15.1, 15.2, 15.3, 15.4, 15.5, 15.6, 15.7, 15.8, 15.9, 16.1, 16.2, 16.3, 16.4, 16.5, 17.1, 17.2, 17.3, 17.4, 18.1, 18.3, 18.4, 18.5, 18.6, 18.7, 18.8, 18.9, 18.10, 18.11, 19.1, 19.2, 19.3, 19.4, 19.5, 19.6, 19.7, 19.8, 20.1, 20.2, 20.3, 20.4, 20.5, 20.6, 20.7, 20.8, 20.9, 20.10, 20.11, 20.12, 20.13, 20.15, 21.1, 21.2, 21.3, 21.4, 21.5, 21.6, 21.7, 22.1, 22.2, 22.3, 23.4, 23.5, 23.7, 23.8, 23.11, 24.1, 24.2, 24.3, 24.4, 24.5, 24.6, 24.7, 24.9, 24.11, 25.1, 25.4, 25.5, 25.6, 25.7.

Index

Absolute oxygen requirement, 102
Acclimatization
    to cold weather, 226
    to hot weather, 224–26, 448
Acetylcholine, 113–14
    as inhibitory/excitatory, 114–15
    and neuromuscular junction, 129
    release of, 122
Acetylcholinesterase, 113–14, 122
Acetyl-CoA
    formation of, 36
    and glycolysis, 33–34
Acid-base balance
    and endurance training, 240–41
    and exercise performance, 207–8
    extracellular buffers, 208–9
    and hydrogen ion concentration, 206
    intercellular buffers, 208
    and kidneys, 210
    regulation during exercise, 210–11
    and respiratory system, 209–10
    and ventilation, 193
Acidity, increase during exercise, 18
Acidosis, 190
    and lactic acid production, 207
    meaning of, 206
Acids
    definition of, 206
    fixed acids, 207
    organic acids, 207
    strong acids, 206
    volatile acids, 207
Acromegaly, 70–71
Actin, of skeletal muscle, 126, 129–30
Action potential, neurons, 112
Adenosine diphosphate (ADP), and
    adenosine triphosphate (ATP)
    production, 28, 29, 30
Adenosine triphosphate (ATP), 28–41
    and endurance training, 237–38
    and exercise, 29
    and fatigue, 364–65
    and muscular contraction, 131
    structure of, 28
    as universal energy donor, 28–29
Adenosine triphosphate (ATP) production
    and adenosine diphosphate (ADP), 28,
        29, 30
    aerobic production, 33–38, 41
    anaerobic production, 29–32, 41
    ATP-PC system, 29, 40

carrier molecules, 30
computation of ATP production, 39
control systems, 39–40
electron transport chain, 35–38, 40
glycolysis, 29–32, 40
and inorganic phosphate, 28
Krebs cycle, 33–35, 40
methods of, 29
and mitochondria, 35–38
oxidative phosphorylation, 33–34
training to improve ATP-PC system, 397
Adenylate cyclase, 66
Adrenal gland, 72–75
    adrenal cortex, 73–75
    adrenal medulla, 72
    hormones of, 72–75
Adrenaline. See Epinephrine
Adrenocorticotrophic hormone (ACTH), 74
    function of, 69, 79
Aerobic fitness, classifications for
    men/women, 270
Aerobic metabolism
    and adenosine triphosphate (ATP)
        production, 33–38, 41
    and prolonged exercise, 50
    and short-term intense exercise, 49
Aerobic power training, 394–97
    high-intensity, continuous exercise,
        396–97
    interval training, 395–96
    long, slow distance runs, 396
Aerobic respiration, efficiency figure for, 39
Aerobics (Cooper), 8
Afferent fibers, 108
Afterload, and stroke volume, 234–35
Age
    and body temperature and exercise, 224
    and cardiac output, 166
    and loss of strength, 247
    and skeletal muscle, 140–41
    and weight gain, 342
Air, composition of, 185
Air pollution, 454–55
    carbon monoxide, 455
    ozone, 454–55
    sulfur dioxide, 455
Airway resistance, breathing, 182–83
Alanine, 57, 424
Alarm reaction, in stress response, 75
Aldosterone, 73, 80
    functions of, 73, 80

    secretion of, 73
Alkalosis, meaning of, 206
All-or-none law, neurons, 112
Allosteric enzymes, 40
Alpha receptors, 72
Altitude, 440–47
    adaptation to, 443–44
    atmospheric pressure, 440
    and cardiovascular function, 442–43
    and hypoxia/hyperoxia, 440
    and long-term aerobic performance, 441
    and mountain climbing, 445–47
    and respiratory function, 443
    and short-term anaerobic
        performance, 440
    and training for competition, 444–45
    and $\dot{V}O_2$ max, 443–47
Alveolar ventilation, 184
Alveoli
    functions of, 178
    operation of, 180–81
Amenorrhea, and female athletes, 78,
    410–11
American Association for Health, Physical
    Education, and Recreation
    (AAHPER), 5–6, 9
American Association for Health, Physical
    Education, and Recreation (AAHPER)
    Youth Fitness Test, 6
American Association for Health, Physical
    Education, Recreation and Dance
    (AAHPERD)
    Health-Related Fitness Test Manual, 6
    Physical Best, 6
American College of Sports Medicine
    (ACSM), 8, 9, 10
American Journal of Physiology, 9
American Physiological Society (APS), 9
Amino acids
    essential amino acids, 28
    metabolism during exercise, 57-58,
        424–25
    oxidation of, 424
    and proteins, 28, 328
    supplementation by athletes, 424,
        461–62
Amphetamines, 466–67
    effects on performance, 466
Anabolic steroids, 76–77
    abuse by athletes, 77
    adverse effects of, 77
    function of, 76

Anaerobic metabolism, and adenosine diphosphate (ADP), 29–32, 41
Anaerobic power testing, 380–83
    cycling power tests, 382, 382–83
    Margaria power test, 380
    Quebec 10-second test, 382
    running power tests, 380–82, 383
    Sargent's jump-and-reach test, 380
    sports-specific tests, 383
    Wingate test, 382–83
Anaerobic power training, 397–98
    to enhance ATP-PC system, 397
    to enhance glycolytic system, 398
Anaerobic production, adenosine triphosphate (ATP), 29–32
Anaerobic threshold, use of term, 51
Anatomical dead space, 184
Androgenic steroids, function of, 76
Androgens, 73, 80
    functions of, 73, 80
Anemia
    and iron deficiency, 324, 325
    and vitamin deficiencies, 321, 322
Angina pectoris
    meaning of, 268, 309
    and myocardial ischemia, 272
    treatment of, 309
Angioplasty, coronary heart disease, 309
Angiotensin I, 73
Angiotensin II, 73
Anorexia nervosa, 338, 411
    warning signs of, 411
Anterior hypothalamus, 220
Anterior pituitary gland, 68, 69–70
Antidiuretic hormone (ADH), 71, 79
    functions of, 71, 79
    secretion of, 71
Aortic bodies, 196
Apneustic area, brain, 196
Apophyses, 414
Appetite, and exercise, 347
Applied research, nature of, 9
Arbeitsphysiologie (European Journal of Occupational and Applied Physiology), 9
Argine supplementation, 461
Arm exercise, cardiovascular response to, 170
Arrhythmias, nature of, 272, 309
Arterial blood pressure, regulation of, 17
Arteries, function of, 152
Arterioles, function of, 152
Articular cartilage, 414
Asmussen, E., 4
Asthma
    causes of, 304
    and competitive training, 415
    drug therapy, 305
    exercise-induced, 305–6
    preventing attacks, 304, 306
    screening for, 306
Atherosclerosis, 158
    and coronary heart disease, 258
Athletes, training periods for, 402–3
Atmospheric pressure, meaning of, 440

ATPase, and adenosine triphosphate (ATP) production, 28
ATP-PC system
    adenosine triphosphate (ATP) production, 29
    control of, 40
    and short-term intense exercise, 29, 49
Atria
    of heart, 153
    heart, 154
Atrioventricular node (AV node), 158, 160, 161
August Krogh Institute, 4
Autologous transfusion, 464
Autonomic nervous system (ANS), 121–22
    functions of, 121
    parasympathetic division, 121–22
    sympathetic division, 121
Autoregulation, of blood flow, 167
Axon, of neuron, 109, 110

Balance, and vestibular apparatus, 117–18
Balke, Bruno, 8
Balke Standard protocol, 276, 277
Baroreceptor system
    blood pressure regulation, 17
    during exercise, 172
Basal metabolic rate (BMR), 344–46
    and body temperature, 346
    and caloric intake, 345, 346
    and exercise, 345–46
    resting metabolic rate (RMR), 344
Base
    definition of, 206
    strong bases, 206
Basic research, nature of, 9
Behavioral factors, and disease, 258
Bench step, 97–98
    calculation of work performed, 98
Bernard, Claude, 13
Beta-endorphins, and exercise, 74–75
Beta oxidation, 34
    and free fatty acids, 240
    process of, 36
Beta receptor agonists, for asthma, 305
Beta receptors, 72
Bicarbonate, buffering capacity of, 209, 466
Biodynamics Laboratory (University of Wisconsin), 8
Bioenergetics
    control systems, 39–40
    meaning of, 22
Biological control systems, 15
    arterial blood pressure, regulation of, 17
    blood glucose, regulation of, 17–18
    components of, 15–16
    failure of system, effects of, 18
Biotin, 322
Blood
    buffer systems, 208–9
    oxygenation of, 153
    physical characteristics of, 163
Blood buffers. See Buffers

Blood doping, 464–65
    and performance, 464–65
    problems of, 464
Blood flow
    autoregulation, 167
    through heart, 152–53
    to lungs, 187
    pressure/resistance/flow relationship, 163–64
    redistribution during exercise, 167
    regulation during exercise, 167, 169
    vascular resistance, sources of, 164–65
Blood-gas analysis, apparatus for, 4
Blood glucose, 27
    and diabetes, 18, 301–3
    and endurance training, 239–40
    and exercise, 57
    homeostasis during exercise, 82–88
    maintenance of, 82
    regulation of, 17–18
Blood pressure, 155–57
    diastolic blood pressure, 156
    graded exercise test measure, 272
    hypertension, 157
    mean arterial pressure, 156–57
    measurement of, 155–56, 272
    pulse pressure, 156
    regulation of, 17, 157
    systolic blood pressure, 156
Blood sugar. See Blood glucose
Body composition
    and exercise, 348–49
    optimal body weight range, 338
    and performance, 434–35
    somatotype, 432–35
Body composition measures
    Body Mass Index (BMI), 333
    dual energy X-ray absorptiometry (DEXA), 333
    height/weight tables, 331–33
    hydrostatic (underwater) weighing, 333
    isotope dilution, 333
    near infrared interactance (NIR), 333
    nuclear magnetic resonance (NMR), 334
    photon absorptiometry, 333
    potassium-40, 333
    radiography, 333
    skinfold method, 337–38
    skinfold thickness, 334
    total body electrical conductivity (TOBEC), 334
    two/three/four component model for analysis, 334
    ultrasound, 334
    underwater weighing, 335–37
Body Mass Index (BMI), 333
    limitations of, 333
Body temperature
    and basal metabolic rate (BMR), 346
    core temperature measurement, sites of, 216–17
    and enzyme activity, 26
    and fever, 221
    heat loss, 217–19

heat production, 217
homeotherms, 216
hypothalamic regulation of, 220–21
measurement devices, 217
and oxyhemoglobin dissociation
curve, 190
and shivering, 217, 346
use of term, 216
Body temperature and exercise and
age, 224
cold acclimatization, 226
gender differences, 224
heat acclimatization, 225–26
regulation during exercise, 216
thermal events, 221–23
Bohr, Christian, 4
Bohr effect, 189
Bone growth, children, 414
Bone loss, and female athletes, 323, 412
Borg RPE scale, target heart rate (THR)
range, 291–92
Boron supplementation, 462
Boyle's Law, 478
Bradycardia, 234
Brain
brain stem, 118–19
cerebellum, 119
cerebrum, 119
motor centers of, 118–19, 120–21
motor cortex, 119, 120
respiratory control center, 195–96
reticular formation, 118
Brain stem, 118–19
functions of, 118–19
structures of, 118
Breathing, 181–87
airway resistance, 182–83
expiration, 182
inspiration, 182
Bruce protocol, 276
Buffers, 208–9, 465–66
acid-base buffer systems, 208–9
bicarbonate as, 209, 466
carbonic acid as, 209
function of, 208
hemoglobin as, 208
phosphate groups as, 208
proteins as, 208
sodium buffers, 209, 466
Bulimia nervosa, 338–39, 412
warning signs of, 412
Bulk flow, breathing, 181–82
Buskirk, Elsworth R., 9
Bypass surgery, coronary heart disease, 309

Caffeine, 467–70
as ergogenic aid, 467–70
in foods/drinks/drugs, 468
and free-fatty acid mobilization, 468–69
Calcitonin, 72, 79
functions of, 72, 79
Calcium, 323, 325
osteoporosis prevention, 311, 323

Calmodulin, 68, 82
activation and exercise, 54
Caloric intake, and basal metabolic rate
(BMR), 345, 346
Calorie, definition of, 99
Calorimetry
direct, 99
indirect, 100
Canadian Home Fitness Test, 270–71
maximal $\dot{V}O_2$ calculation, 270–71
physical fitness evaluation chart, 271
Capillaries, function of, 152
Carbaminohemoglobin, 191
Carbohydrates, 27, 327, 420–23
carbohydrate metabolism during
exercise, 54–55
classification of, 327
dietary fiber, 327
dietary goals related to, 420
disaccharides, 27
and glycogen synthesis, 27
monosaccharides, 27
oxidation of, 53
and performance, 56, 420–23
polysaccharides, 27
pre-performance intake, 422–23
storage sites of, 56–57
sugars/starches, 327
supercompensation method, 420–21
Carbon dioxide
and blood pH, 209–10
production, calculation of, 477
transport during respiration, 191–92
as volatile acid, 207, 209
Carbonic acid, buffering capacity of, 209
Carbon monoxide, air pollution, 455
Cardiac accelerator nerves, 160
Cardiac contractility, stroke volume, 234
Cardiac cycle
diastole, 154–55
pressure changes during, 155
systole, 154–55
Cardiac output
and age, 166
changes during exercise, 165–66
computation of, 160
definition of, 152
heart rate regulation, 160–61
and maximal oxygen uptake
($\dot{V}O_2$ max), 233
stroke volume regulation, 161–63
Cardiac rehabilitation
exercise effects, 310
exercise prescription, 309–10
initial testing, 309
types of cardiac conditions for, 309
Cardiovascular control center, 160
Cardiovascular disease. See Coronary
heart disease
Cardiovascular drift, 171
Cardiovascular fitness, exercise
prescription for, 290–95
Cardiovascular fitness testing, 50
Canadian Home Fitness Test, 270–71

graded exercise tests, 271–73, 275–81
maximal oxygen uptake ($\dot{V}O_2$)
measurement, 273–75
maximal run tests, 268–69
measurements taken in, 268
readiness questionnaire, 266–68
screening decision tree, 266
walk tests, 270
Cardiovascular system and exercise
and altitude, 442–43
and arm versus leg exercise, 170
central command, 172
emotional influence, 169
and incremental exercise, 170
and intermittent exercise, 171
and prolonged exercise, 171
recovery from exercise, 169–70
rest to exercise transition, 169
Carnitine supplementation, 462
Carotid bodies, 196
Carrier molecules, and ATP production, 30
Catalysts, enzymes and energy
transformation, 24–26
Catecholamines
and body temperature, 217–18
epinephrine, 72, 80
norepinephrine, 72, 80
physiological responses to, 73
Cell
energy transformation in, 24–26
intracellular buffers, 208
Cell body, of neuron, 109, 110
Cell membrane, functions of, 22
Cell structure, 22–23
cell membrane, 22
cytoplasm, 22
nucleus, 22
organelles of cell, 22–23
Cellular control systems, 15
Cellular respiration, definition of, 178
Cellulose, 27
Central chemoreceptors, 196
Central command, meaning of, 172
Central fatigue, 362–63
Central nervous system (CNS), 108
and fatigue, 362–63
sensory information, 115–16
Cerebellum, 119
functions of, 119
Cerebrum, 119
functions of, 119
motor cortex, 119
Certification, of fitness instructors, 10
Charles's Law, 478–79
Chemiosmotic hypothesis, adenosine
triphosphate (ATP) production, 37–38
Chemoreceptors
central chemoreceptors, 196
muscle chemoreceptors, 115–16
peripheral chemoreceptors, 196–97
and respiratory control center, 196–97
and ventilation, 196–97

Children
　　cardiovascular fitness standards, 269
　　cardiovascular system and training,
　　　413–14
　　injuries from sports, 414
　　musculoskeletal system and training, 414
　　overtraining of, 414
　　skinfold method, use of, 338
　　$\dot{V}O_2$ max for, 274
Chloride shift, 192
Cholesterol, 328
　　and coronary heart disease, 28, 258,
　　　260, 328
　　functions of, 28
　　high-density lipoproteins (HDL), 328
　　low-density lipoproteins (LDL), 328
Choline supplementation, 462
Christensen, E.H., 4
Chromium, 326
Chromium supplementation, 462
Chronic obstructive pulmonary disease,
　　307–8
Cigarette smoking, and coronary heart
　　disease, 258, 260
Circulatory system
　　arteries, 152
　　heart, 152–63
　　hemodynamics, 163–65
　　organization of, 152
　　veins, 152
Citric acid cycle. See Krebs cycle
Clenbuterol, as ergogenic aid, 467
Clothing, as cold insulator, 453
Clo units, 453
Cobalt, 326
Cocaine, as ergogenic aid, 470
Cognitive set point model, 341
Cold injuries
　　and cold water, 452
　　factors related to, 451
　　hypothermia, 225, 454
　　treatment of, 454
Cold weather, 451–54
　　cold acclimatization, 225
　　and energy production, 453–54
　　insulating factors, 452–53
　　windchill index, 451–52
Coma, diabetic, 301
Compounds
　　inorganic compounds, 22
　　organic compounds, 22
Concentric contractions, 142
Conducting zone, respiratory system, 179–80
Conduction, heat loss via, 218
Conduction disturbances, nature of, 272
Conductivity, neurons, 111
Control systems of body
　　biological control systems, 15
　　cellular control systems, 15
　　endocrine system, 64
　　gain, 16–17
　　homeostatic control, examples of, 17–19
　　negative feedback, 16
Convection, heat loss via, 218

Cool down, 289
　　objectives of, 394
Cooper Clinic, 9
Cooper's run tests, 268
Copper, 326
Cori cycle, process of, 58
Coronary artery bypass graft surgery, 309
Coronary heart disease, 258–63
　　angioplasty, 309
　　and atherosclerosis, 258
　　bypass surgery, 309
　　cardiac rehabilitation, 309–10
　　and cholesterol, 28
　　epidemiological study, 258–59
　　Framingham study, 258
　　and muscle fiber type, 262
　　myocardial infarction (MI), 309
　　nitroglycerin in, 309
　　and physical inactivity, 259–60, 286
　　research on, 6
　　risk factors, 258–60
　　web of causation for, 258–59
Coronary obstructive pulmonary disease
　　characteristics of, 307
　　exercise prescription for, 308
　　exercise testing in, 307–8
　　grading of disability in, 307
Corticotrophic-releasing hormone (CRH), 74
Cortisol, 73, 74–75, 79
　　exercise effects on, 83–84
　　functions of, 73, 74–75, 79, 83
　　secretion of, 74–75
Coupled reactions, energy transformation, 24
Creatine supplementation, 461
Critical power, measurement of, 377–78
Cromolyn sodium, for asthma, 305, 306
Cross-bridge, and fatigue, 364
Crossed-extensor reflex, 116
Cross-sectional studies, of training, 231
Cureton, Thomas K., Jr., 8
Cycle ergometer, 98, 278
　　calculation of work performed, 98
　　testing protocol, 278–79
　　$\dot{V}O_2$ max calculation, 278, 280
Cyclic AMP
　　and glycogen breakdown, 54
　　and phosphorylase activation, 40
　　second messenger mechanism, 66–68
Cycling power tests, 382
　　anaerobic power testing, 382–83
　　Wingate test, 382–83

Dalton's law, 185
Deadly Quartet, 261–62
Death, leading causes in United States,
　　257, 263
Degenerative disease, nature of, 257
Delayed onset muscle soreness (DOMS)
　　avoidance of, 401
　　causes of, 401
Dendrites, of neuron, 109, 110
Deoxyhemoglobin, 188
Deoxyribonucleic acids (DNA), 22
　　hormones and activation of, 66

Detraining, and $\dot{V}O_2$ max, 236
Dextrose, 327
Diabetes, 300-303
　　causes of, 75
　　and competitive training, 415
　　diabetic coma, 301
　　diseases related to, 300
　　and exercise, 301–3
　　and hypoglycemia, 301, 302
　　ketosis in, 301
　　mechanisms in, 18
　　nutrition therapy, goals of, 303
　　risk factors, 303
　　Type I diabetes, 18, 300, 301–2
　　Type II diabetes, 300, 303
　　warning signs of, 300
Diacylglycerol, 68
Diastole, cardiac cycle, 154–55
Diastolic blood pressure, 156
Diet analysis
　　food records, 329
　　twenty-four hour recall, 329
Dietary fats, 27–28, 328
　　cholesterol, 328
　　dietary goals related to, 420
　　and energy, 27, 328
　　and exercise, 27, 54
　　fat metabolism during exercise, 55, 239
　　fatty acids, 27
　　function of, 328
　　low fat diet, 328
　　oxidation of, 53
　　phospholipids, 27
　　saturated, sources of, 328
　　steroids, 28
　　storage sites of, 56, 57–58
　　triglycerides, 27
　　and weight control, 343–44
Dietary fiber
　　forms of, 327
　　health benefits of, 327
　　recommended daily intake, 327
Dietary Guidelines for Americans, 263, 319,
　　327, 329
　　daily food selections, 329
Diet and athletics. See Nutrition
　　and exercise
Diet and Health, 324
Diffusion, meaning of, 178
Dill, Dr. David Bruce, 4, 5
Direct calorimetry, 99
　　method of, 99
Disaccharides, formation of, 27
Disease
　　chronic obstructive pulmonary disease,
　　　307–8
　　coronary heart disease, 258–63
　　degenerative disease, 257
　　diabetes, 300–303
　　epidemiological study of, 256–57
　　hypertension, 308
　　infectious disease, 257
　　risk factors related to, 258
Dopamine, and Parkinson's disease, 119

Dose-response relationship, exercise prescription, 286–87
Double-blind research design, 460
Double product
    computation of, 170
    of heart, 272
    use for exercise prescription, 170
Douglas, C.G., 4
Dual energy X-ray absorptiometry (DEXA), body composition measure, 333
Duration of exercise, and cardiovascular fitness, 290
Dwarfism, 70
Dynamic contractions, 142
Dynamic stretching, 402
Dynamometer, strength measurement, 385
Dysmenorrhea, and female athletes, 411
Dyspnea, 307
    meaning of, 268

Ear, and vestibular apparatus, 117–18
Eating disorders
    anorexia nervosa, 338, 411
    bulimia nervosa, 338-39, 412
Eccentric contractions, 142
Ectomorph, 432, 433
Education, certification of exercise specialists, 10
Effectors, function of, 15
Efferent nerve fibers, 108–9
Eisenhower, Dwight D., 5
Ejection fraction, 234
Elderly and exercise, 308–12
    benefits of, 310, 312
    and osteoporosis, 310–11
    screening, 311
    training effect, 311
Electrocardiogram (ECG)
    abnormalities detected by, 272
    diagnostic use during exercise, 158
    graded exercise test measure, 272
    waveforms of, 159, 160
Electrolytes
    loss and exercise, 426
    replacement and exercise, 426–29
Electron transport chain
    adenosine triphosphate (ATP) production, 35–38, 40
    control of, 40
Emotions
    and autonomic nervous system (ANS), 121
    cardiovascular changes during exercise, 169
End-diastolic volume (EDV), 161–62, 234
Endergonic reactions, 28
    energy transformation, 24
Endocardium, 153, 154
Endocrine glands
    adrenal gland, 72–75
    ovaries, 77–78
    pancreas, 75–76
    parathyroid gland, 72
    pituitary gland, 68–71

testes, 76–77
thyroid gland, 71–72
Endocrine system
    and homeostasis, 17, 64
    hormone production, 17, 64–80
Endomorph, 432, 433
Endomysium, of skeletal muscle, 126
Endorphins, and exercise, 74–75
End-plate potential (EPP), 129
Endurance performance testing, 375–78
    critical power measure, 377–78
    lactate threshold, 375–77
Endurance training
    and adenosine-triphosphate (ADP), 237–38
    arteriovenous oxygen difference, 235
    and blood glucose, 239–40
    and blood pH, 240–41
    central control of, 244–45
    combined with strength training, 247–48, 399–400
    detraining and $\dot{V}O_2$ max, 236
    and elderly, 311
    and free-fatty acids, 239–40
    and homeostasis, 236
    and injury, 397
    and lactate removal, 241
    and muscular adaptations in, 236–37, 238
    and oxygen deficit, 237–38
    and stroke volume, 234–35
    stroke volume in, 166
    and systemic physiology, 243–45
    and training principles, 231–45
    transfer of training effect to organ systems, 243
    types of activities in, 232
    and ventilatory response, 199
    and $\dot{V}O_2$ max, 231–33
Energy
    biological transformation of, 24–26
    cellular conversion of, 22
    energy of activation, 24
    energy balance equation, 342
    and exercise, 22
    from foods, 27–28
    forms of, 24
    high energy bonds, 24
    and nutrient balance, 342–43
Energy of activation, 24
Energy expenditure
    metabolic equivalent (MET), 101–2
    for selected activities, 481–84
Energy expenditure measures
    direct calorimetry, 99
    indirect calorimetry, 100
Energy production
    and cold weather, 453–54
    energy systems for selected sports, 393
    and incremental exercise, 50–52
    and prolonged exercise, 50
    and short-term intense exercise, 49
    See also Adenosine triphosphate (ATP) production

Energy transformation, 24–26
    and adenosine triphospate (ATP), 28–41
    cellular reactions in, 24–26
    coupled reactions, 24
    endergonic reactions, 24
    and enzymes, 24–26
    exergonic reactions, 24
Energy wasteful systems, 346
Environmental factors, and disease, 258
Environment and exercise, 295
    air pollution, 454–55
    altitude, 440–47
    cold weather, 451–54
    heat/hot weather, 448–51
Enzymes
    allosteric enzymes, 40
    and energy transformation, 24–26
    factors affecting activity of, 26
    molecular structure of, 24
    naming system for, 25–26
    rate-limiting, 39–40
Epicardium, 153, 154
Epidemiology, 255–58
    applications of, 256
    definition of, 256
    diseases studied, 256–57
    epidemiologic triad, 256
    goals of, 256
    and physiological study, 261–62
    synthesis of information, 262–63
    web of causation model, 257
Epilepsy
    exercise and seizures, 416
    injury and seizures, 416
    nature of, 416
Epimysium, of skeletal muscle, 126
Epinephrine, 72, 80
    exercise effects on, 85–86
    and fat metabolism, 55
    functions of, 72, 80
    and glycogen breakdown, 54–55
    and oxygen consumption, 48
    receptors of, 72
Epiphyseal plate, 414
EPOC (excess post-exercise oxygen consumption), 47–49
Equilibrium, and vestibular apparatus, 117–18
Ergogenic aids
    amphetamines, 466–67
    anabolic steroids, 76–77
    blood buffers, 465–66
    blood doping, 464–65
    caffeine, 467–70
    cocaine, 470
    nicotine, 470–71
    nutritional supplements, 461–62
    oxygen supplementation, 463–64
    research on, 460–61
Ergometer
    cycle ergometer, 98
    nature of, 97
Ergometry, nature of, 97

Erythrocythemia, and blood doping, 464–65
Erythropoietin, 465
Essential amino acids, 28
Estrogens, 73, 77–78, 80, 81
    exercise effects, 77–78
    functions of, 73, 77, 80
    types of, 77
Evaporation
    heat loss calculation, 219
    heat loss via, 218–19
    of sweat from skin, 218
Exchange System, foods, 329, 331
Excitation-contraction coupling
    muscle contraction, 130, 131–34
    regulation of, 131–32
    steps in, 134
Excitatory postsynaptic potentials (EPSP), 113–14
    spatial summation, 113
    temporal summation, 113
Excitatory transmitters, 113
Executive fitness programs, 6
Exercise, definition of, 286
Exercise economy testing, 378
    method of, 378
Exercise in Education and Medicine (McKensie), 6
Exercise efficiency
    fiber type, 104
    and movement speed, 103–4
    net efficiency, 102–3
    and work rate, 103
Exercise intensity
    and ATP-PC system, 49
    crossover point, 54
    and fuel selection, 54–55
Exercise Leader, 10
Exercise Lite guidelines, 288, 289
Exercise metabolism
    fat/carbohydrate metabolism during, 55
    fuel selection, factors in, 53–58
    fuel sources, 56–58
    fuel utilization, 53
    during incremental exercise, 50–52
    oxygen debt, 47–48
    oxygen deficit, 46
    during prolonged exercise, 50
    recovery from exercise, 47–48
    rest-to-exercise transition, 46
    during short-term intense exercise, 49
Exercise physiology
    history of. *See* History of exercise physiology
    and physical fitness boom, 10
Exercise prescription
    beginning/end of exercise session, 289
    for cardiac rehabilitation, 309–10
    for cardiovascular fitness, 290–95
    for chronic obstructive pulmonary disease, 307–8
    daily activity recommendations for adults, 288
    for diabetes, 300–303
    dose-response relationship, 286–87

    duration of exercise, 290
    for elderly, 308–12
    example of, 485
    frequency of exercise sessions, 290
    games/sports, 294
    for hypertension, 308
    intensity of exercise, 291–92
    jogging, 293–94
    moderate versus vigorous activity, 289
    pattern of responses in, 288
    physiological variables in, 287–88
    in pregnancy, 312–13
    progression of activities, 289
    screening, 289
    strength training, 294–95
    walking, 292–93
Exercise pressor reflex, 172
Exercise Test Technologist, 10
Exergonic reactions, 28
    energy transformation, 24
Exhaustion stage, in stress response, 75
Expiration, breathing, 182
Extensors, and joint angles, 126
Extracellular buffers, acid-base regulation, 208–9

Fascia, 126
Fasciculi, of skeletal muscle, 126
Fast-acting hormones, 82, 85
Fast-twitch fibers, 51–52, 54, 136–38
Fat cells, and obesity, 339–40
Fatigue, 362–65
    and ATP, 364–65
    central fatigue, 362–63
    and cross-bridge, 364
    and free radical production, 364
    mechanical factors, 364
    muscular, 132
    neural factors, 363
    peripheral fatigue, 363
    sites of, 362, 363
Fats. *See* Dietary fats
Fat-soluble vitamins, 321
Fatty acids
    free fatty acids, 55, 57
    storage of, 27
Feedback, negative feedback, 15
Feedback gain, 16–17
    calculation of, 16–17
Ferritin, 324
Fever
    and body temperature, 220–21
    pyrogens, 221
Fiber. *See* Dietary fiber
Fick's law of diffusion, 186
Field tests
    Canadian Home Fitness Test, 270–71
    maximal run tests, 268–69
    walk tests, 270
Fight or flight, 72
Fitnessgram, 269
Fitness instructors, education/certification of, 10

Fitness testing
    example of, 6
    See also Cardiovascular fitness testing
Fixed acids, 207
Flavin adenine dinucleotide (FAD), and adenosine triphosphate (ATP) production, 30–32
Flexibility training, 402
    dynamic stretching, 402
    static stretching, 402
Flexors, and joint angles, 126
Fluoride, 326
Folic acid, 322
Follicle-stimulating hormone (FSH), 69, 76, 79
    function of, 79
    and menstrual cycle, 77
Follicular phase, menstrual cycle, 77
Food Guide Pyramid, 329, 330
Food label, example of, 320
Food records, diet analysis, 329
Foods
    carbohydrates, 27
    fats, 27–28
    proteins, 28
Framingham Heart Study, 342
    coronary heart disease, 258
Frank-Starling law, 162
Free fatty acids (FFA)
    and caffeine, 468–69
    and endurance training, 239–40
    exercise effects on, 57, 89–90
    in lipolysis, 55
    transport from cytoplasm to mitochondria, 239–40
    transport into muscle, 239
Free nerve endings, 115
Free radicals
    and electron transport chain, 35
    and fatigue, 364
    formation during exercise, 37
Free weights, versus weight machines, 399
Frequency of exercise, and gains, 290
Fructose, 27
Functional syncytium, 154

Gain, 16–17
    of a control system, 16–17
    definition of, 16
    feedback gain, 16–17
Gamma oryzanol supplementation, 462
Gases
    diffusion of, 185–86
    partial pressure of, 185–86
Gas volumes
    correction to reference conditions, 478
    standardization of, 477–78
Gender differences
    body temperature and exercise, 221–22
    and exposure to cold, 454
    response to strength training, 400–401
    response to training principles, 394
    running economy, 104
General Adaptation Syndrome (GAS), 74
    stages of, 75

Genes, composition of, 22
Genetic factors
    and disease, 258
    obesity, 340–41
    response to training, 394
Gigantism, 70
Glandular supplements, 462
Glottis, 179
Glucagon, 76, 80
    exercise effects on, 86–88, 89
    functions of, 76, 80
Glucocorticoids, functions of, 73
Gluconeogenesis
    nature of, 47
    and oxygen debt, 47
Glucose, food sources of, 27
Glucose polymers, 421
Glycogen
    breakdown during exercise, 54
    carbohydrate intake and performance,
        420–23
    conversion from lactic acid, 47, 48
    and exercise, 27
    muscle-glycogen utilization, 81–82
    production of, 27
    storage of, 27
    storage sites of, 56–57
Glycogenolysis
    mechanisms in, 54
    nature of, 27
Glycolysis
    adenosine triphosphate (ATP)
        production, 29–32, 40
    control of, 40
    flowchart of process, 31, 32
    process of, 29–30
    and short-term intense exercise, 49
    training to improve system, 398
Golgi tendon organs (GTOs), 146–47
    functions of, 145, 147
    and strength activities, 147
Golgi-type receptors, 115
G protein, 66
Graded exercise test measures
    blood pressure, 272
    electrocardiogram (ECG), 272
    heart rate, 271–72
    Rating of Perceived Exertion (RPE),
        272–73
Graded exercise tests, 271–73, 275–81
    cycle ergometer, 278–79
    ECG in, 158
    protocols, 275–77
    step test, 279–81
    stopping test, indications for, 273
    treadmill, 277–78
    uses of, 50
Growth hormone (GH), 69, 70–71, 79
    exercise effects on, 84–85
    functions of, 70-71, 79, 84
    imbalances, effects of, 70
    secretion of, 79
    use by athletes, 71

Growth hormone releasing hormone
        (GHRH), 70
Guanosine triphosphate (GTP), and Krebs
        cycle, 33–34
Guidelines for Exercise Testing and Prescription,
        286, 309

Haldane, J.S., 4
Haldane analyzer, 4
Harvard Fatigue Laboratory, 4–5, 8, 9
    distinguished alumni of, 4–5
    journal publishing articles of, 9
    research areas in, 4
Health/Fitness Director, 10
Health/Fitness Instructor, 10
Health history, Physical Activity Readiness
        Questionnaire (PAR-Q), 266–68
Health-Related Fitness Test Manual, 6
Healthy People 2000, 262
    objectives of, 7
Heart, 152–63
    atrioventricular node (AV node), 158, 160
    blood movement within, 153
    cardiac cycle, 154–55
    cardiac output, 160–63
    dual pump system, 153
    electrical activity of, 157–60
    heart rate regulation, 160–61
    layers of heart wall, 153
    measurement of electrical changes, 158
    muscle, characteristics of, 154
    myocardium, 153–54
    pulmonary circuit, 153
    sinoatrial node (SA node), 157, 160
    stroke volume regulation, 161–63
    structure of, 152
Heart rate
    graded exercise test measure, 271–72
    measurement of, 271–72
    regulation of, 160–61
Heart rate abnormalities
    arrhythmias, 272, 309
    conduction disturbances, 272
    myocardial ischemia, 272
    ST segment depression, 272
Heath-Carter method, somatotyping, 432
Heat/hot weather, 448–50
    evaluation for heat stress risk, 450
    heat acclimatization, 225–26, 448
    heat adaptation and training, 225
    sweating effects, 225
Heat injuries
    factors related to, 448–49
    heat cramps, 448
    heat exhaustion, 448
    heat stroke, 448
    heat syncope, 448
    hyperthermia, 223, 448–49
    prevention of, 223, 449–50
    signs of, 448
    treatment of, 448
Height/weight tables, 331–33
    limitations of, 332, 333

Hematocrit, of blood, 163
Hemodynamics, 163–65
    blood, 163
    pressure/resistance/flow relationship,
        163–64
    vascular resistance, 164–65
Hemoglobin
    buffering capacity of, 208
    deoxyhemoglobin, 188
    and iron deficiency, 430
    and oxygen transport, 188–89
    oxyhemoglobin, 188
    oxyhemoglobin dissociation curve,
        189–91
Hemosiderin, 324
Henderson-Hasselbach equation, 209
Henderson, L.J., 4
Henry's law, 186
High-density lipoproteins (HDL)
    and coronary heart disease, 260
    protective effects of, 328
High-intensity, continuous exercise, 396–97
Hill, A.V., 3, 47
History of exercise physiology
    European roots, 3–4
    exercise science, 7–8
    exercise physiology textbook, 7
    graduate study and research, 8–9
    Harvard Fatigue Laboratory, 4–5
    physical fitness promotion, 5–6
    professional societies, 9
    research journals, 9
    university level physical education
        programs, 7–8
Homeostasis
    control systems of body, 15–19
    definition of, 14
    dynamic constancy of, 14
    and endocrine system, 17
    and endurance training, 236
    and exercise, 18–19
    and mechanistic research, 15
    compared to steady state, 14
Homeotherms, nature of, 216
Homologous transfusion, 464
Hooke, Robert, 22
Hormones
    adrenocorticotrophic hormone (ACTH),
        69, 79
    aldosterone, 73, 80
    androgens, 73, 80
    antidiuretic hormone (ADH), 71, 79
    calcitonin, 72, 79
    classification of, 64
    control of secretion, 65
    cortisol, 73, 74–75, 79
    and DNA activation, 66
    and endurance training, 236
    epinephrine, 72, 80
    estrogen, 77–78, 81
    estrogens, 73, 80
    excretion of, 65
    fast-acting hormones, 82, 85
    follicle-stimulating hormone (FSH), 69, 79

functions of, 17, 64
glucagon, 76, 80
growth hormone (GH), 69, 70, 79
insulin, 75–76, 80
interaction with receptors, 66–68
luteinizing hormone (LH), 69, 70, 79
mechanisms of action, 66–68
membrane transport, 66
metabolism of, 65
norepinephrine, 72, 80
oxytocin, 71, 79
parathyroid hormone, 72, 79
permissive hormones, 82, 85
plasma volume, effects of, 65
prolactin, 69, 79
releasing hormones, 68, 70
and second messenger activation, 66, 68
slow-acting hormones, 83
somatostatin, 76
testosterone, 76–77, 80
thyroid-stimulating hormone (TSH), 69, 79
thyroxin (T4), 71–72, 79
and transport protein, 65
triiodothyronine (T3), 71–72, 79
Hormones and exercise
blood glucose homeostasis, 82–88
cortisol, 83–84
epinephrine, 85–86
glucagon, 86–88, 89
growth hormones (GH), 84–85
hormone-substrate interaction, 89
insulin, 86–88
muscle-glycogen utilization, 81–82
norepinephrine, 85–86
thyroxin, 83
Horvath, Steven, 4
Hot weather. See Heat/hot weather; Heat injuries
Human Circulation (Rowell), 9
Humidity, and heat injury, 449
Hydrogen ions
as acids, 206
production during exercise, 207
Hydrostatic (underwater) weighing, body composition measure, 333
Hyperbaric chamber, 463
Hyperglycemia, and diabetes, 18
Hyperoxia, meaning of, 440
Hyperplasia, and strength training, 247, 398
Hyperplastic obesity, 339
Hypertension, 308
classification of, 157
and coronary heart disease, 258, 260
Deadly Quartet, 261
dietary recommendations, 308
exercise prescription, 308
metabolic abnormalities in, 261-62
risk factors, 308
Hyperthermia
development of, 224
factors related to, 448–49
prevention of, 224
Hypertrophic obesity, 339
Hypertrophy, and strength training, 247, 398

Hyperventilation, 53
Hypoglycemia
and diabetes, 301, 302
and exercise, 422
Hypothalamus, 68
anterior and posterior, 220
body temperature regulation, 220–21
fever effects, 221
Hypothermia
development of, 226
factors related to, 451
treatment for, 454
Hypoxemia, exercise-induced, 194
Hypoxia, meaning of, 440
Hypoxic threshold, 197

Illinois Research Laboratory, 8
Immune system
and overtraining, 404
response to exercise, 242
Immunotherapy, for asthma, 304
Incremental exercise
cardiovascular response to, 170
energy production during, 50–52
and pulmonary ventilation, 194
Incremental exercise tests, uses of, 50
Indirect calorimetry, 100
method of, 100
open-circuit spirometry, 100
Infectious disease, nature of, 257
Inhibitory postsynaptic potential (IPSP), 114
Inhibitory transmitters, 114
Injury
and children, 414
and endurance training, 397
and epileptics, 416
Inorganic compounds, nature of, 22
Inorganic phosphate, and adenosine triphosphate (ATP) production, 28
Inosine supplementation, 462
Inositol triphosphate, 68
In-season conditioning, for athletes, 403
Inspiration, breathing, 182
Institute of Environmental Stress, 4
Insulin, 75–76, 80
blood glucose regulation, 17–18
control of release of, 65
and diabetes, 75, 300, 301, 302
and diabetic athlete, 415
exercise effects on, 86–88
factors in secretion of, 75–76
functions of, 75, 86
insulin resistance and hypertension, 261–62
and lipolysis, 55
Insulin resistance
characteristics of, 261
exercise benefits, 262
Integrating center, of control system, 15
Intensity, and target heart rate (THR) range estimation, 291–92
Intercalated discs, 154
Intercellular buffers, acid-base regulation, 208

Intermittent exercise, cardiovascular response to, 171
International Journal of Sports Medicine, 9
Interstitial cell stimulating hormone (ICSH), 76
Interval training, 395–96
advantages of, 395
cardiovascular response to, 171
rest interval, 395
set and repetition in, 396
work interval, 395
Interventricular septum, 153
Iodine, 325
Ion, definition of, 206
Iron, 323–24, 325
Iron deficiency, 429–30
and anemia, 324, 325
causes in athletes, 430
stages of, 429
supplementation for, 430
Irritability, neurons, 111
Islets of Langerhans, 75, 76
Isocitrate dehydrogenase, and control of Krebs cycle, 40
Isokinetic testing, and muscular strength, 386
Isometric contractions, 141–42
Isometric testing, of muscular strength, 384–85
Isotonic contractions, 142
Isotonic testing, of muscular strength, 385
Isotope dilution, body composition measure, 333

Jogging, 293–94
beginning program, 294–95
caloric cost per mile, 350
contraindications to, 294
definition of, 294
program for, 294
Joule, 99
Journal of Applied Physiology, 9
Journal of Aviation Medicine, 9
Journal of Biological Chemistry, 9
Journal of Cardiopulmonary Rehabilitation, 9
Journal of Clinical Investigation, 9
Journal of Nutrition, 9
Journal of Physiology, 9
Journals, of exercise physiology, 9
Jumping power tests, anaerobic power testing, 380

Karvonen method, target heart rate (THR) range, 291
Kennedy, John F., 6
Ketosis, in diabetes, 301
Keys, Dr. Ancel, 8
Kidneys, and acid-base balance, 210
Kilocalorie (kcal), 99
Kinesthesia, and proprioceptors, 115
Kraus, Hans, 5
Krebs, Hans, 33
Krebs cycle
adenosine triphosphate (ATP) production, 33–35, 40

control of, 40
  intermediates in, 55
  stages in process of, 33-35
Krogh, August, 3, 4

Laboratory for Human Performance
    Research, 9
Laboratory for Physiological Hygiene
    (University of Minnesota), 8
Lactate
  and altitude, 447
  Cori cycle, 58
  formation and endurance training, 240-41
  as fuel source in exercise, 58
  resting blood lactate concentration, 241
Lactate threshold
  direct determination of, 376
  in distance running, 379
  in endurance performance testing, 375-77
  factors related to, 51-52
  and high-intensity, continuous exercise,
    396-97
  practical use of, 52
  prediction by ventilatory alterations,
    376-77
Lactic acid
  and acidosis, 207
  cellular formation of, 32
  conversion to glycogen, 47, 48
  and endurance training, 240-41
  enzyme conversion to pyruvic acid, 26
  factors in production during exercise, 210
  lactate threshold, 51
  as organic acid, 207
  and pH of body fluids, 26
  production during exercise, 18, 51-52
  removal during exercise, 48
Lateral sac, 131
Leg exercise, cardiovascular response to, 170
Leucine, 424
Life, Heat, and Altitude (Dill), 4
Lipases, and fat metabolism, 55
Lipolysis, 27
  events in, 55
Loading, hemoglobin, 189
Longitudinal studies, of training, 231
Low-density lipoproteins (LDL), and heart
    disease, 328
Low fat diet, recommendations for, 328
Luft, Dr. Ulrich, 8
Lungs
  air passages, operation of, 179-81
  blood flow to, 187
  function of, 178
  gases, diffusion of, 185-86
  gas exchange organs, 180-81
  and limitations to exercise
    performance, 200
  lung volumes, measurement of, 184-85
  ventilation and diffusion, 178
Luteal phase, of menstrual cycle, 77
Luteinizing hormone (LH), 69, 70, 76, 79
  functions of, 70, 79
  and menstrual cycle, 77
Lysine supplementation, 461

Macrophages, 180
Magnesium, 325
Magnesium supplementation, 462
Maltose, 27
Manganese, 326
Margaria, Rudolpho, 4
Margaria power test, anaerobic power
    testing, 380
Mast cell, 304
Maximal aerobic power testing, 374-75
  protocol for, 374-75
  specificity of, 374
  testing of paraplegics, 375
Maximal oxgyen intake, first use of term, 3
Maximal oxygen uptake ($\dot{V}O_2$ max)
  aerobic power, direct testing of, 374-75
  and altitude, 443-47
  and cardiac output, 233
  for children, 274
  criteria for achievement of, 273
  and detraining, 236
  and endurance training, 231-32
  exercise test protocol, 374-75
  and incremental exercise, 50-52
  longitudinal data on training effects, 233
  physiological factors in, 50-51
  strength/endurance training combined,
    247-48
  and stroke volume, 235
Maximal oxygen uptake ($\dot{V}O_2$ max)
    calculation, 273-75
  for Canadian Home Fitness Test, 270-71
  for cycle ergometer test, 278-79, 280
  from last work rate, 274
  for maximal run test, 268-69
  for paraplegic athletes, 375
  and prediction of athletic
    performance, 374
  reproducibility of, 273-74
  for step test, 281
  from submaximal HR response, 274-75
  for treadmill testing, 277
  usefulness of, 275
  for walk test, 270
Maximal run tests, 268-69
  maximal $\dot{V}O_2$ calculation, 268-69
  types of tests, 268
Measurement
  metric system, 96
  System International (SI), 96
Mechanistic research, nature of, 15
Medicine and Science in Sports, 9
Menstrual cycle
  abnormalities and exercise/training, 78,
    410-11
  hormonal influences, 77-78
  phases of, 77
Mesomorph, 432, 433
Metabolic acidosis, and respiratory
    compensation, 211
Metabolic Cardiovascular Syndrome, 261
Metabolic equivalent (MET), 101-2
  absolute oxygen requirement, 102
  energy expenditure for selected
    activities, 481-84

Metabolism
  and bioenergetics, 22
  definition of, 22
  See also Exercise metabolism
Metric system, 96
  units in, 96
Metropolitan Insurance Company
    height/weight tables, 331-33
Meyerhof, Otto, 3-4
Mineralcorticoids, functions of, 73
Minerals, 323-26
  calcium, 323, 325
  chromium, 326
  cobalt, 326
  copper, 326
  fluoride, 326
  iodine, 325
  iron, 323-24, 325, 429-30
  magnesium, 325
  major minerals, 323
  manganese, 326
  molybdenum, 326
  phosphorus, 325
  potassium, 325
  Recommended Dietary Allowances
    (RDA), 1989 charts, 487-88
  selenium, 326
  sodium, 324
  sulfur, 325
  trace minerals, 323, 325-26
  zinc, 326
Mitochondria
  and adenosine triphosphate (ATP)
    production, 32, 35-38
  and endurance training, 236-37, 238
  free fatty acid transport to, 239-40
  functions of, 22
Mixed venous blood, 152
  oxygen content and exercise, 166
Modulators, of enzymes, 40
Mole, 39
Molecular biology
  and exercise science, 23
  study of, 22
Molybdenum, 326
Monark cycle, 98
Monosaccharides, forms of, 27
Motor cortex, functions of, 119, 120
Motor nerve fibers, efferent nerve fibers, 108-9
Motor neurons
  activation of, 117
  innervation of muscle fiber, 128
Motor unit, 128
Mountain climbing, and altitude, 445-47
Mount Everest, climbing and altitude,
    445-47
Movement speed, and exercise efficiency,
    103-14
Muscle
  heat muscle, 154
  oxygen transport in, 191
  See also Skeletal muscle
Muscle chemoreceptors, 115-16
Muscle soreness, and strength training, 401

Muscle spindle, 146
  composition of, 146
  function of, 145, 146
  innervation of, 146
Muscular endurance, meaning of, 245
Muscular fatigue, causes of, 132
Muscular strength
  definition of, 383–84
  meaning of, 245
  training for. See Strength training
Muscular strength evaluation, 383–86
  isokinetic measurement, 386
  isometric measurement, 384–85
  isotonic measurement, 385
  selection of method, 384
  variable resistance measurement, 386
Myocardial infarction (MI), effects of, 309
Myocardial ischemia, nature of, 272
Myocardium, function of, 153–54
Myofibrils, of skeletal muscle, 126
Myoglobin, oxygen affinity for, 191
Myosin, of skeletal muscle, 126, 129–30

Nagle, Francis J., 8
National Exercise and Heart Disease
    protocol, 276
Nautilus® equipment, 398, 399
Near infrared interactance (NIR), body
    composition measure, 333
Negative feedback, 15
  and control systems, 16
  example of, 16, 17
Negative risk factor, 260
Nervous system
  autonomic nervous system (ANS), 121–22
  central nervous system (CNS), 108
  functions of, 108
  neurons, 108–15
  peripheral nervous system (PNS), 108
Net efficiency, 102–3
Neural adaptations, in strength training, 246
Neural factors, fatigue, 363
Neuroendocrinology
  study of, 64
  See also Endocrine system; Hormones
Neuromuscular junction, 128–29
  and acetylcholine, 129
  and fatigue, 363
Neurons, 108
  action potential, 112
  all-or-none law, 112
  conductivity, 111
  excitatory postsynaptic potentials
      (EPSP), 113–14
  inhibitory postsynaptic potential
      (IPSP), 114
  irritability, 111
  motor neurons, 117
  neurotransmitters, 113–15
  resting membrane potential, 111–12
  sensory neurons, 115–16
  structure of, 109–11
  synapses, 109, 111, 112–13
  synaptic transmission, 112–13

Neurotransmitters, 113–15
  acetylcholine, 113–14
  excitatory transmitters, 113
  function of, 113
  inhibitory transmitters, 114
Nicotinamide adenine dinucleotide (NAD)
  and adenosine triphosphate (ATP)
      production, 30–33
  and NADH, 30–38
Nicotine, 470–71
  and exercise, 470
  smokeless tobacco, 471
Nielsen, M., 4
Nitric oxide, as vasodilator, 168
Nitrogen, partial pressure of, 186
Nitrogen balance, during exercise, 424–25
Nitroglycerin, and coronary heart
    disease, 309
Nixon, Richard, 6
Nodes of Ranvier, 111
Noll Laboratory, 9
Nonshivering thermogenesis, 218
Norepinephrine, 72, 80
  exercise effects on, 85–86
  functions of, 72, 80
  receptors of, 72
  removal of, 121
Normocythemic, 464
Normoxia, meaning of, 440
Nuclear magnetic resonance (NMR), body
    composition measure, 334
Nucleus, functions of, 22
Nutrient balance
  and energy, 342–43
  nutrient balance equations, 342
Nutrients
  carbohydrates, 327
  fats, 328
  minerals, 323–26
  protein, 328
  vitamins, 321–23
  water, 320–21
Nutrition
  diet analysis, 329
  Dietary Guidelines for America, 319
  Exchange System, 329, 331
  Food Guide Pyramid, 329, 330
  nutrient density, 329
  U.S. Dietary Goals, 318–19
Nutritional supplements, 461–62
  effectiveness of, 461
  types of, 461–62
Nutrition and exercise
  carbohydrates, 420–23
  minerals, 429–30
  pregame meals, 431–32
  protein, 423–26
  vitamins, 430–31
  water/electrolytes, 426–29
Nutrition standards
  Daily Value (DV), 319–20
  Recommended Dietary Allowances
      (RDA), 319

Obesity, 339–41
  causes of, 340–41
  definition of, 339
  diseases related to, 339
  and fat cells, 339–40
  hyperplastic obesity, 339
  hypertrophic obesity, 339
  and set point, 341–42
Off-season conditioning, for athletes, 403
Omega-3 fatty acid supplementation, 462
Open-circuit spirometry, method of, 100
Organic acids, 207
Organic compounds, nature of, 22
Ornithine supplementation, 461
Osteoporosis
  and calcium intake, 311, 323
  exercise prescription, 311
  and female athletes, 78, 323, 412
  nature of, 310
  treatment of, 310–11
  Types I and II, 310
Otis, Arthur B., 10
Ovaries, 77–78
  hormones of, 77–78, 81
Overload, training effect, 230–31, 392
Overtraining
  and children, 414
  and immune system, 404
  negative aspects of, 404
  signs of, 404
Oxidation
  of amino acids, 424
  of carbohydrates, 53
  of fats, 53
  nature of, 32
Oxidation-reduction reactions, process of, 32
Oxidative phosphorylation
  and adenosine triphosphate (ATP)
      production, 33–34, 35
  efficiency of, 39
Oxygen
  adenosine triphosphate (ATP)
      production, 38
  blood flow adjustments and exercise, 152
  changes in arterial-mixed blood during
      exercise, 166
  delivery to muscle during exercise, 165–69
  partial pressure of, 185–86
  post exercise elevation of, 47
  requirements in treadmill running, 102
  requirements in treadmill walking, 101
Oxygen consumption, calculation of, 477
Oxygen debt, 47–48
  EPOC (excess post-exercise oxygen
      consumption), 47–49
  and gluconeogenesis, 47
Oxygen deficit
  definition of, 46
  and endurance training, 237–38
Oxygen supplementation, 463–64
  during exercise, 463–64
  post-exercise, 464
  prior to exercise, 463

Oxygen transport, 188–91
  and hemoglobin, 188–89
  in muscle, 191
  oxyhemoglobin dissociation curve, 189–91
Oxygen uptake
  absolute oxygen requirement, 102
  and incremental exercise, 50–52
  oxygen extraction and endurance training, 235
  and prolonged exercise, 50
  relative $\dot{V}O_2$, 104
  See also Maximal oxygen uptake ($\dot{V}O_2$ max)
Oxyhemoglobin, 188
Oxyhemoglobin dissociation curve, 189–91
  Bohr effect, 189
  effect of pH on, 189–90
  and red blood cell concentration, 190–91
  temperature effect on, 190
Oxytocin, 71, 79
  functions of, 71, 79
Ozone, air pollution, 454–55

Pacinian corpuscles, 115
Pancreas, 75–76
  exocrine and endocrine functions of, 75
  hormones of, 75–76
Pantothenic acid, 322
Paraplegic athletes, maximal oxygen uptake ($\dot{V}O_2$ max) estimation, 375
Parasympathetic division, autonomic nervous system (ANS), 121–22
Parasympathetic tone, 160
Parathyroid gland, 72
  hormones of, 72
Parathyroid hormone, 72, 79
  functions of, 72, 79
Parkinson's disease
  and dopamine, 119
  and motor function, 119
Peak running velocity, relationship to finish time, 377
Pennsylvania State University, research laboratory, 8, 9
Peptide bonds, 28
Percentage of maximal HR method, target heart rate (THR) range, 291
Percent grade, treadmill, 98
Percutaneous transluminal coronary angioplasty, 309
Performance
  ethics of study of, 369
  fatigue, 362–65
  intermediate-length performance, 367–68
  long-term performance, 368
  moderate-length performance, 367
  short-term performance, 366
  ultra short-term performance, 366
Performance testing, example of, 6
Perimysium, of skeletal muscle, 126
Peripheral chemoreceptors, 196–97
Peripheral fatigue, 363
Peripheral nervous system (PNS), 108
  somatic motor function, 117
Permissive hormones, 82, 85

pH
  definition of, 206
  and enzyme activity, 26
  and hydrogen ion, 206, 207
  and oxyhemoglobin dissociation curve, 189–90
  pH scale, continuum of, 206
  See also Acid-base balance
Phosphagen system, 29
Phosphocreatine (PC)
  and adenosine triphosphate (ATP) production, 29, 30
  supplementation and exercise, 30
Phosphodiesterase, 66
Phosphofructokinase (PFK), and control of glycolysis, 40
Phospholipase C, 68
Phospholipids, biological function of, 27
Phosphoric acid
  buffering capacity of, 208
  as fixed acid, 207
Phosphorus, 325
Phosphorylase, and control of glycolysis, 40
Photon absorptiometry, body composition measure, 333
Physical activity, definition of, 286
Physical Activity Readiness Questionnaire (PAR-Q), 266–68, 270
Physical Best, 6
Physical education, historical view, 5–6
Physical fitness, historical view, 5–6
Physiological testing
  anaerobic power testing, 380–83
  benefits to athletes, 373
  components of, 373
  endurance performance testing, 375–78
  ethical issues, 372
  exercise economy testing, 378
  maximal aerobic power testing, 374–75
  muscular strength testing, 383–86
  running economy testing, 379
Physiology of Bodily Exercise (Lagrange), 7
Pituitary gland, 68–71
  anterior pituitary, 68, 69–70
  hormones of, 69–71
  posterior pituitary, 68, 71
Placebo, nature of, 460
Plasma, in blood, 163
Plasma volume, and hormone concentration, 65
Platelets, 163
Pleurae, functions of, 178
Pneumotaxic area, brain, 196
Polysaccharides, forms of, 27
Pons, 196
Population attributable risk, 260
Posterior hypothalamus, 220
Posterior pituitary gland, 68, 71
Postganglionic neurons, 121
Potassium, 325
Potassium-40, body composition measure, 333
Power
  definition of, 97
  units of measure related to, 97

Pregame meal, 431–32
Preganglionic neurons, 121
Pregnancy, 312–13
  exercise recommendations, 312–13
  physiological adaptations in, 312
  and training, 412
Preload, 234
Preseason conditioning, for athletes, 403
President's Council on Physical Fitness, 6
President's Council on Physical Fitness and Sports, 6
President's Council on Youth Fitness, 5
Pressure, and blood flow, 163–64
Preventive and Rehabilitation Exercise Specialist, 10
Preventive and Rehabilitation Program Director, 10
Primary risk factors, meaning of, 260
Professional associations, for physiology of exercise, 9
Progressive resistance exercise, nature of, 398
Prolactin, 69, 79
  functions of, 79
Prolonged exercise
  cardiovascular response to, 171
  energy production during, 50
Promoting Health/Preventing Disease, 262
Proprioceptive neuromuscular facilitation (PNF), 402
Proprioceptors, 115
  and kinesthesia, 115
  types of, 115
Proteases, 58
Protein, 28, 328, 423–26
  adult requirement, 328
  and amino acids, 28, 57–58, 328
  dietary goals related to, 420, 425–26
  and energy, 28
  and exercise, 28
  as extracellular buffers, 208
  as intracellular buffers, 208
  nitrogen balance during exercise, 424–25
  requirement and exercise, 423–24
  sources of, 328
  storage sites of, 57–58
Protein kinase C, 68
Protein supplements, 461
Protocols, treadmill testing, 277–78
Provitamin, nature of, 321
Prudential Fitnessgram, 6
Pulmonary circuit, 153
Pulmonary respiration, definition of, 178
Pulmonary ventilation. See Ventilation
Pulmonary volumes
  measurement of, 184–85
  terms related to, 185
Pulse pressure, 156
Pyruvate, and Krebs cycle, 33–35
Pyruvic acid
  enzyme conversion from lactic acid, 26
  and Krebs cycle, 55
  primary function of, 33

Quebec 10-second test, 382

Radiation, heat loss via, 218
Radiography, body composition measure, 333
Rate-limiting enzymes, 39–40
Rating of Perceived Exertion (RPE), graded exercise test measure, 272–73
Receptors
    for epinephrine/norepinephrine, 72
    function of, 15
    hormone-receptor interaction, 66–68
Reciprocal inhibition, 116
Recommended Dietary Allowances (RDA), 319
    for caloric intake, 319
    1989 charts, 486–89
Recovery, from exercise, 169–70
Red blood cells, 163
    and oxyhemoglobin dissociation curve, 190–91
Reflex arc, 116
Reflexes
    crossed-extensor reflex, 116
    pathways for, 116
    spinal reflexes, 119–20
    withdrawal reflex, 116, 119
Relative $\dot{V}O_2$, expression and body weight, 104
Releasing hormones, 68, 70
    functions of, 68
Renin, 73
Repetition, in interval training, 396
Research
    applied research, 9
    basic research, 9
    double-blind research design, 460
    on ergogenic aids, 460–61
    and Harvard Fatigue Laboratory, 4–5
    mechanistic research, 15
    placebo in, 460
    research journals, 9
Research designs
    cross-sectional studies, 231
    longitudinal studies, 231
Residual volume, meaning of, 184
Resistance, and blood flow, 163–64
Resistance stage, in stress response, 75
Respiration
    and altitude, 443
    cellular respiration, 178
    definition of, 178
    pulmonary respiration, 178
Respiratory compensation, and metabolic acidosis, 211
Respiratory control center
    humoral input to, 196–97
    neural input to, 196, 197
    structure of, 195–96
    and ventilation, 195–96
Respiratory exchange ratio (R)
    and fuel utilization during exercise, 53
    nonprotein R, 53
Respiratory gas analyzer, invention of, 4
Respiratory system
    and acid-base balance, 193, 209–10
    air passages, operation of, 179–81
    blood flow to lung, 187

blood-gas response to exercise, 193–94
    breathing, 181–87
    carbon dioxide transport, 191–92
    conducting zone, 179–80
    organs of, 178–79
    oxygen transport, 188–91
    respiratory zone, 180–81
    ventilation during exercise, 197–99
    ventilation-perfusion relationships, 188
    ventilation at rest, 195–97
Respiratory zone, 180–81
Rest to exercise transition
    cardiovascular response, 169
    pulmonary ventilation, 193
Resting membrane potential, neurons, 111–12
Resting metabolic rate (RMR), 344
Rest interval, meaning of, 395
Rest-to-exercise transition, 46
Reticular formation, 118
Reversibility, training principle, 392–93
Risk factors
    negative risk factor, 260
    population attributable risk, 260
    primary and secondary, 260
Robinson, Sid, 4
Runner's high, 75
Running
    caloric cost per mile, 350
    long, slow distance runs, 396
Running economy, 104
    gender differences, 104
    and relative $\dot{V}O_2$, 104
    testing for, 379
Running power tests, 380–82, 383
    anaerobic power tests, 383
    methods of, 380–81
    See also Maximal run test

Sarcolemma
    and fatigue, 363
    of skeletal muscle, 126
Sarcomeres, of skeletal muscle, 126–28
Sarcoplasmic reticulum, of skeletal muscle, 128
Sargent, Dr. Dudley, 5
Sargent's jump-and-reach test, 380
Scholander, Peter F., 4–5
Schwann cells, 109, 111
Screening, exercise prescription, 289
Secondary risk factors, meaning of, 260
Second messengers
    hormone activation of, 66, 68
    types of, 68
Sedentary lifestyle, and coronary heart disease, 259–60, 286
Selenium, 326
Sensory information, 115–16
    muscle chemoreceptors, 115–16
    proprioceptors, 115
    reflexes, 116
Sensory nerve fibers, afferent fibers, 108
Sensory neurons
    muscle chemoreceptors, 115–16
    proprioceptors, 115

Sensory receptors, skeletal muscle, 145
Set, in interval training, 396
Set point, 341–42
    cognitive set point model, 341
    meaning of, 341
Sex steroids, functions of, 73
Sham reinfusion, 464
Sham withdrawal, 464
Shivering, heat production by, 217, 346
Short-term exercise, energy production during, 40
Sinoatrial node (SA node), 157, 160, 161
Skeletal muscle
    and aging, 140–41
    biochemical properties, 135–36
    contractile properties, 136
    and endurance training, 236–37, 238
    extensors, 126
    flexors, 126
    functions of, 126
    Golgi tendon organs (GTOs), 146–47
    muscle spindle, 146
    neuromuscular junction, 128–29
    plasticity of, 140
    sensory receptors, 145
    structure of, 126–28
Skeletal muscle contraction, 129–35
    and ATP, 131
    concentric contractions, 142
    eccentric contractions, 142
    energy for, 131
    excitation-contraction coupling, 130, 131–34
    isometric contractions, 141–42
    isotonic contractions, 142
    sliding filament model, 129–30
    speed of contraction/relaxation, 142
    sustained contractions, 144
    tetanus, 144
    twitch, 142
Skeletal muscle fibers
    alteration and exercise, 139–40
    ATPase activity, 136
    characteristics of fiber types, 138
    contraction speed of, 136
    and coronary heart disease, 262
    efficiency of, 136
    and exercise efficiency, 104
    fast fibers, 136–38
    and force production, 137
    oxidative capacity of, 136
    in rats, new discovery, 137
    slow fibers, 136
    Type I fibers, 136
    Type IIa fibers, 137, 138
    Type IIb fibers, 136–37, 138
    typing, determination of, 138
Skeletal muscle force
    force regulation, factors in, 142, 144
    force-velocity/power-velocity relationships, 144–45
    maximal force production, 136
    and movement speed, 145
    and slow versus fast fibers, 137

Skinfold method
    body composition measure, 334, 337–38
    equations in, 337
    percent fat estimates for men/women, 490–91
    use with children, 338
Sliding filament model, muscle contraction, 129–30
Slow-acting hormones, 83
Slow-twitch fibers, skeletal muscle, 51–52, 136
Smilax, 462
Smokeless tobacco, 471
Sodium, 324
    daily recommended intake, 324
    and hypertension, 308
    intake and athletes, 429
    intake guidelines, 324
Sodium buffers, and exercise performance, 209, 466
Somatic motor function, activities in, 117
Somatostatin, 76
    functions of, 76
    secretion of, 76
Somatotype, 432–35
    ectomorph, 432, 433
    endomorph, 432, 433
    Heath-Carter method, 432
    mesomorph, 432, 433
    and performance, 434–35
Spatial summation, 113
Specificity, training effect, 231, 392
Speed of movement, and exercise efficiency, 103–4
Sperm production, and testosterone, 76
Sphygmomanometer, 155–56
    use of, 156
Spinal cord
    motor functions of, 120
    spinal reflexes, 119–20
Spinal reflexes, 119–20
Spinal tuning, 120
Spirometry, pulmonary volume measurement, 184–85
Sports, in exercise prescription, 294
Sports Medicine, 9
Sports-specific tests, anaerobic power testing, 383
Starches, food sources of, 27, 327
Static contractions, 141–42
Static stretching, 402
Steady state
    definition of, 14
    compared to homeostasis, 14
Step test, 281
    method of, 281
    step ergometers, 281
    $\dot{V}O_2$ max calculation, 279–81
Steroids
    action on target cells, 67
    anabolic steroids, 76, 77
    androgenic steroids, 76
    biological function of, 28
    structure of, 64–65
Strength, and aging, 247

Strength training, 294–95, 398–402
    benefits of, 294–95
    categories of activities, 398
    and central nervous system changes, 398
    combined with endurance training, 247–48, 399–400
    free weights versus machines, 399
    gender differences in response to, 400–401
    guidelines for, 399
    and hyperplasia, 247, 398
    and hypertrophy, 247, 398
    minimum requirements in, 295
    and muscle soreness, 401
    muscular enlargement in, 247
    neural adaptations in, 246
    principles of, 398–99
    progressive resistance exercise, 398
    terms related to, 245–46
    variable resistance exercise, 398
Stress, and coronary heart disease, 260
Stretching
    dynamic stretching, 402
    proprioceptive neuromuscular facilitation (PNF), 402
    static stretching, 402
    in warm-up, 289
Stroke volume, 234–35
    and afterload, 234–35
    and cardiac contractility, 234
    end-diastolic volume (EDV), 161–62, 234
    and endurance athletes, 166, 234–35
    factors increasing stroke volume, 234
    Frank-Starling law, 162
    regulation of, 161–63
    and $\dot{V}O_2$ max increase, 235
Strong acids, nature of, 206
Strong bases, nature of, 206
ST segment depression, 272
Substrate, 24
Substrate-level phosphorylation, 33–34
Sucrose, 27, 327
Sugar
    food label indications for, 327
    sources of, 327
Sulfur, 325
Sulfur dioxide, air pollution, 455
Sulfuric acid, as fixed acid, 207
Summation, muscle contraction, 144
Supercompensation, 420–21
Sweat/sweating
    and electrolyte loss, 426
    evaporation of, 218
    and hot weather, 224
    and water intake, 426
Sympathetic division, autonomic nervous system (ANS), 121
Synapses, 109, 111, 112–13
Synaptic transmission, 112–13
Syndrome X, 261, 262
System International (SI), 96
    units in, 96
Systole, cardiac cycle, 154–55
Systolic blood pressure, 156

Tapering, nature of, 405
Target heart rate (THR) range
    Borg RPE scale, 291–92
    direct estimation, 291–92
    indirect estimation, 291–92
    Karvonen method, 291
    percentage of maximal HR method, 291
Taylor, Henry Longstreet, 8
Tecumseh Community Health Study, 259
Temperature, external
    heat/hot weather, 224–25, 448–50
    heat and pulmonary ventilation, 193–94
Temperature, internal. *See* Body temperature
Temporal summation, 113
Ten percent rule, 397
Terminal cisternae, 132
    of skeletal muscle, 128
Testes, 76–77
    hormones of, 76–77
Testosterone, 76–77, 80
    functions of, 76, 80
    levels and exercise, 76
    secretion of, 76
Tetanus, muscle contraction, 144
Theophylline, for asthma, 305
Thermic effect of feeding, 346
Thermistors, 216, 217
Thermocouples, 216
Thermogenesis, 345, 346
    factors in, 346
Thyroid gland, 71–72
    hormones of, 71–72
Thyroid-stimulating hormone (TSH), 69, 79
    functions of, 69, 79
Thyroxin (T_4), 71–72, 79
    exercise effects on, 83
    functions of, 71–72, 79
Tidal volume, meaning of, 184
Total body electrical conductivity (TOBEC), body composition measure, 334
Total lung capacity (TLC), meaning of, 184
Trace minerals, 323, 325–26
Trachea, 180
Training
    aerobic training methods, 394–97
    anaerobic power training, 397–98
    cool down, 394
    endurance training, 397
    flexibility training, 402
    mistakes related to, 403–6
    and overtraining, 404
    strength training, 398–402
    tapering, 405
    training periods for athletes, 402–3
    warm-up, 394
Training periods for athletes, 402–3
    in-season conditioning, 403
    off-season conditioning, 403
    preseason conditioning, 403
Training principles
    and endurance training, 231–45
    and gender, 393
    genetics and response to, 394
    overload, 230–31, 392

research designs in study of, 231
reversibility, 392
specificity, 231, 392
ten percent rule, 397
Transferrin, 324
Transport protein, and hormones, 65
Transverse tubules
    and fatigue, 363
    of skeletal muscle, 128
Treadmill, 98–99
    calculation of work performed, 98
    oxygen requirement, estimation of,
      101, 102
    percent grade, 98
Treadmill testing, 277–78
    grade/speed settings, 277
    protocols, 276–77
    and $\dot{V}O_2$ max calculation, 277
Triglycerides
    breakdown of, 55, 57
    storage of, 27
Triglyceride supplementation, 462
Triiodothyronine (T_3), 71–72, 79
    functions of, 71–72, 79
Tropomyosin, of skeletal muscle, 126
Troponin, 131
    of skeletal muscle, 126
Twenty-four hour recall, diet analysis, 329
Twitch, skeletal muscle contraction, 142
Type I diabetes, 18, 300, 301–2
Type II diabetes, 300, 303
Type I fibers, 136
Type IIa fibers, 137, 138, 365
Type IIb fibers, 136–37, 138, 365

Ultrasound, body composition measure, 334
Underwater weighing, 335–37
    technique in, 336–37
    whole body density estimate, 335–37
Unloading, hemoglobin, 189
Upper respiratory tract infections (URTI),
    response to exercise, 242
U.S. Dietary Goals, 318–19

Vagus nerve, 160
Valves, of heart, 153
Van Slyke apparatus, 4
Variable resistance exercise, 398
Variable resistance measurement, of
    muscular strength, 386
Vasodilator, nitric oxide as, 168
Vasopressin. See Antidiuretic hormone (ADH)
Veins, function of, 152
Venoconstriction, 162
Venous blood, mixed, 152
Ventilation
    and acid-base balance, 192–93
    alveolar ventilation, 184

and chemoreceptors, 196–97
dead-space ventilation, 184
during exercise, 198–99
meaning of, 178, 184
neural factors, 197
regulation of, 195–97
and respiratory control center, 195–96
at rest, 195–97
Ventilation and exercise
    heat and prolonged exercise, 194
    heavy exercise, 198
    incremental exercise, 194
    rest-to-work transitions, 193
    submaximal exercise, 198, 200
    training, effects of, 199
    ventilatory threshold, 194
Ventilation-perfusion (V/Q) ratio, 188
    exercise effects, 188
    ideal ratio, 188
Ventilatory threshold, meaning of, 194
Venules, function of, 152
Vestibular apparatus, and equilibrium, 117–18
Vital capacity (VC), definition of, 184
Vitamin C, 322
Vitamins, 321–23
    biotin, 322
    deficiency diseases, 321–22
    fat-soluble vitamins, 321
    folic acid, 322
    niacin, 322
    pantothenic acid, 322
    precursor forms, 321
    Recommended Dietary Allowances
      (RDA), 1989 charts, 486–88
    supplementation and athletes,
      430–31, 462
    toxicity of, 321
    Vitamin A, 321
    Vitamin B1, 322
    Vitamin B2, 322
    Vitamin B6, 322
    Vitamin B12, 322
    Vitamin C, 322
    Vitamin D, 321
    Vitamin E, 321
    Vitamin K, 321
    water-soluble vitamins, 322–23
$\dot{V}O_2$ max. See Maximal oxygen uptake
    ($\dot{V}O_2$ max)
Volatile acids, 207

Walking, 292–93
    caloric cost per mile, 350
    program for, 292
    shoes/clothing, 292
Walk tests, 270
    maximal $\dot{V}O_2$ calculation, 270
War, and interest in physical fitness, 5, 7

Warm-up, 289, 471–73
    objectives of, 394
    physiological/psychological aspects
      of, 472
    types of, 472
Water
    daily losses, 320
    drinking and exercise, 320
    as nutrient, 320–21
    pre-exercise intake, 426–27
    replacement during exercise, 427–28
Water-soluble vitamins, 322–23
Web of causation model
    for coronary heart disease, 258–59
    epidemiology, 257
Weight control
    and dietary fat, 343–44
    and energy expenditure, 344–46
    energy and nutrient balance, 342–43
    and exercise, 346–50
    and thermogenesis, 345, 346
    weight loss guidelines, 344
    weight loss versus weight
      maintenance, 349
Weight gain, and age, 342
Weight machines, versus free weights, 399
Weight maintenance, and exercise, 349
Wet Bulb Globe Temperature guide, 450
White blood cells, 163
Whole body density, underwater weighing,
    335–37
Windchill index, 451–52
Wingate test, 382–83
Withdrawal reflex, 116, 119
Women athletes
    bone loss, 323, 412
    eating disorders, 411–12
    female athlete triad, 413
    and iron deficiency, 430
    menstrual cycle, 77–78
    menstrual disorders and
      exercise/training, 410–11
    pregnancy and exercise, 312–13
    pregnancy and training, 412
    See also Gender differences
Work
    definition of, 96–97
    units of measure related to, 97
Work interval, meaning of, 395
Work output measures, 97–98
    bench step, 97–98
    cycle ergometer, 98
    treadmill, 98–99
Work rate, and exercise efficiency, 103

YMCA Way to Physical Fitness protocol, 278–79
Yohimbine, 462

Zinc, 326